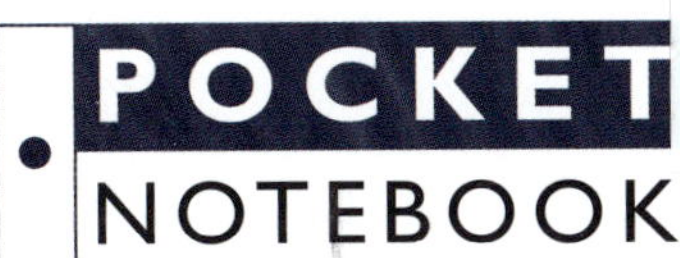

Pocket Emergency MEDICINE

Sixth Edition

Edited by
JOSHUA M. KOSOWSKY, MD, FACEP
Assistant Professor, Department of Emergency Medicine
Harvard Medical School/Mass General Brigham
Boston, Massachusetts

DANIEL RESNICK-AULT, MD, MBA
Assistant Professor of Emergency Medicine
Department of Emergency Medicine
University of Colorado School of Medicine
Aurora, Colorado

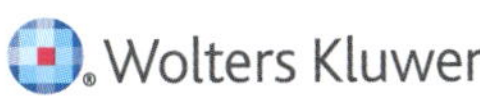

Philadelphia • Baltimore • New York • London
Buenos Aires • Hong Kong • Sydney • Tokyo

Acquisitions Editor: James P. Sherman
Senior Development Editor: Ashley Fischer
Editorial Coordinator: Vinodhini Varadharajalu
Marketing Manager: Janet Feeney
Production Project Manager: Frances Gunning
Manager, Graphic Arts & Design: Stephen Druding
Manufacturing Coordinator: Lisa Bowling
Prepress Vendor: Aptara, Inc.

6th edition

9 8 7 6 5 4 3 2 1

Printed in Mexico

Library of Congress Cataloging-in-Publication Data

Names: Kosowsky, Joshua M. editor | Resnick-Ault, Dan editor
Title: Pocket emergency medicine / edited by Joshua M. Kosowsky, MD, FACEP, Dan Resnick-Ault, MD, MBA.
Description: Sixth edition. | Philadelphia : Wolters Kluwer, [2027] | Series: Pocket notebook | Includes index. | Summary: "Pocket Emergency Medicine is designed as the go-to resource for residents, fellows, practitioners, and physician extenders in the emergency department. Chapters are organized by presenting condition, which allows the reader to use the text the moment a patient presents and encourages development of the thought-processes needed to hone diagnostic decision-making. Chapters are templated to include history, findings, evaluation, treatment, disposition and pearls"– Provided by publisher.
Identifiers: LCCN 2026003052 (print) | LCCN 2026003053 (ebook) | ISBN 9781975258184 spiral bound | ISBN 9781975258191 epub
Subjects: LCSH: Emergency medicine | BISAC: MEDICAL / Emergency Medicine | LCGFT: Handbooks
Classification: LCC RC86.7 .P625 2027 (print) | LCC RC86.7 (ebook)
LC record available at https://lccn.loc.gov/2026003052
LC ebook record available at https://lccn.loc.gov/2026003053

shop.lww.com

CONTRIBUTORS

Diana M. Bongiorno, MD, MPH
Chief Resident
Department of Emergency Medicine
Mass General Brigham
Boston, Massachusetts

Christopher Johns, MD
Resident Physician
Department of Emergency Medicine
Denver Health
Denver, Colorado

Austin Jones, MD, PhD, MPHTM
Resident Physician
Department of Emergency Medicine
Denver Health
Denver, Colorado

Gideon Loevinsohn, MD, PhD
Chief Resident
Department of Emergency Medicine
Mass General Brigham
Boston, Massachusetts

PREFACE

In an era defined by mobile devices, clinical apps, and increasingly powerful AI tools, it is striking—and perhaps telling—that a compact, hardcopy reference continues to resonate with learners and clinicians. Even with instantaneous digital access, many trainees still gravitate toward something they can hold, flip through, annotate, and keep literally in their pocket. Perhaps it is the reliability of a source that never loses its charge or distracts with notifications, or the way a physical reference distills only what matters when cognitive load is high. Or perhaps it reflects something deeper about how we learn at the bedside: that in the intensity of emergency medicine, tactile tools still steady us and help translate knowledge into action.

Pocket Emergency Medicine was created for that purpose. As its name suggests, it is a true pocket reference—designed to live in the white coat or scrubs pocket of anyone practicing acute care. And although the digital landscape has evolved dramatically since the first edition, the core needs of emergency clinicians have not. In the ED, pattern recognition, rapid decision making, and clear organizational frameworks still depend on information that is concise, reliable, and instantly accessible.

As with prior editions, we have maintained a structure that mirrors the way patients present to the emergency department: by symptoms and chief complaints rather than final diagnoses. Each chapter offers an initial approach to the presenting problem, followed by high-yield discussions of key diagnostic considerations. Essential elements of history, examination, testing, and treatment are distilled into practical guidance, supplemented by clinical pearls highlighting pitfalls and must-not-miss findings.

This edition reflects the excellent work of a dedicated team of emergency medicine residents from the Denver Health and Harvard-Affiliated Emergency Medicine Residency programs. Their chapters were refined by experienced senior faculty from the University of Colorado School of Medicine, Brigham and Women's Hospital, and Harvard Medical School, ensuring accuracy, clarity, and relevance.

To our authors, reviewers, and colleagues: thank you for the expertise and care you brought to this project. And to our readers—residents, attendings, PAs, NPs, students, and all who practice acute care—we hope this new edition continues to serve as a reliable companion at the bedside, a steady guide through the unpredictable sea of emergency medicine.

Joshua M. Kosowsky, MD, FACEP
Daniel Resnick-Ault, MD, MBA

ACKNOWLEDGMENTS

I want to acknowledge my late father, Dr Bernard Kosowsky, whose example as a thoughtful clinician and generous teacher continues to shape how I practice. I am grateful as well to the many colleagues, trainees, and mentors who have influenced my thinking through countless conversations and shared clinical moments. And to the patients who have trusted me with their care—thank you; you remain my most important teachers and the reason this work matters.

—Joshua M. Kosowsky

CONTENTS

SECTION I: CARDIOVASCULAR

SECTION II: PULMONARY

SECTION III: GASTROINTESTINAL

SECTION IV: INFECTIOUS DISEASE

SECTION V: NEUROLOGY

SECTION VI: RENAL & GENITOURINARY

SECTION VII: OBGYN

SECTION VIII: DERMATOLOGY

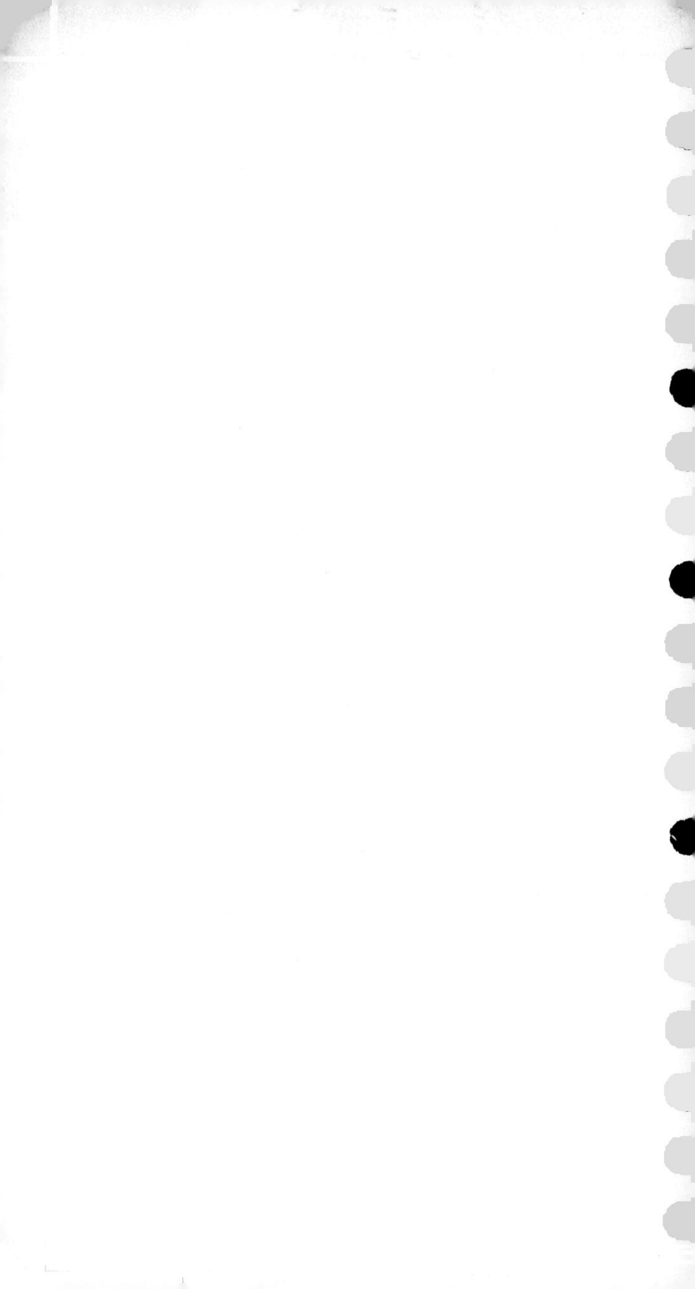

CHEST PAIN

Approach

- Immediate: All nontrivial CP needs IV access, O_2 if hypoxic, cardiac monitoring, ECG, CXR
  - Compare all ECGs to prior, repeat after 15–20 mins if high suspicion for ACS; consider R-sided +/– posterior ECG if high suspicion (see *Electrocardiography* section)
- Hx: Obtain thorough pain HPI (position, quality, radiation, severity, timing, associated sx, alleviating & exacerbating factors), cardiac RFs (eg, for CAD, aortic dz, PE, etc), prior cardiac testing (timing & results of last echo, stress test, catheterization) & prior cardiac events/procedures (eg, MI, CABG, valve repair, PCI, etc)
- Empiric tx: ASA 325 mg (if considering ACS & low suspicion for AoD), NTG for pain if c/f ischemia (unless R-sided ischemia, hypotension, PDE inh use)
- Risk stratify for dxs being considered: ACS (HEART, TIMI, GRACE, or PURSUIT), PE (Wells, PERC), AoD (ADD-RS)

Common or Life-Threatening Causes of Acute Chest Pain	
Pathophysiology	**Etiologies**
Cardiac	ACS (UA/NSTEMI, STEMI), Vasospastic (Prinzmetal)/cocaine-induced angina, myocarditis, pericarditis, cardiac tamponade, constrictive pericarditis, CHF/acute pulm edema, post-MI cx
Vascular	PE, AoD, thoracic aortic aneurysm, pulm HTN
Pulmonary	PNA, PTX, pl effusion/empyema, pleuritis, pulm infarct
GI	GERD, esophageal spasm, Mallory–Weiss tear, Boerhaave synd/esophageal perforation, PUD, biliary dz, pancreatitis
Musculoskeletal	MSK strain/contusion, costochondritis, OA, radiculopathy
Miscellaneous	Herpes zoster, anxiety, sickle cell acute chest synd

ELECTROCARDIOGRAPHY

Approach

- Always check: correct pt, date, lead placement; calibration (mV, paper speed)
- Determine rate, rhythm, axis
- Waves (P, Q, R, S, T, U waves) & segments (PR, QRS, QT intervals, & ST segment)
- Conduction & bundle blocks
- Atrial enlargement, ventricular hypertrophy
- Ischemia/infarction
- Miscellaneous (stigmata of electrolyte abnl, syncope, tox, pacemaker, PE, etc)

Orientation: ECG Calibration & Standardization	
Voltage calibration	Standard ECG voltage is usually set w/ a calibration box encompassing 2 large vertical squares (10 mm tall) & is equal to 1 mV (10 mm/mV): 1 small vertical box = 0.1 mV
Paper recording speed	Standard ECG paper speed if usually set at 25 mm/s: • Large horizontal box (5 mm wide) = 200 ms (0.2 s) • Small horizontal box (1 mm wide) = 40 ms (0.04 s)

Determining Heart Rate *(nl = 60–100 bpm)*	
Quick approach	Count the number of large horizontal squares b/w consecutive QRS complexes and divide 300 by this number: 1 square = 300 bpm, 2 = 150 bpm, 3 = 100 bpm, 4 = 75 bpm, 5 = 60 bpm
Mathematical approach	Multiply the number of QRS complexes on the ECG by 6 (at a standard paper speed of 25 mm/s), each ECG records 10 s of activity

Determining Rhythm (see also section on *Dysrhythmia*)
• Determining the heart's rhythm is a complex process that requires synthesis of other features of ECG interpretation (esp rate, axis, intervals, & waves/segments) • Key questions to help narrow the DDx of dysrhythmias include: 1. Is the rate slow (eg, bradydysrhythmia) or fast (eg, tachydysrhythmia)? 2. Is the QRS narrow (eg, nl sinus rhythm, SVT) or wide (eg, aberrancy, ventricular, electrolyte abnl)? 3. Is the rhythm regular (eg, AFl, SVT, VT) or irregular (eg, AF, AFl w/ variable block, MAT, polymorphic VT)? 4. Are P waves present? (If absent: AF, AFl, nodal/ventricular etiology) 5. Is every P wave f/b a QRS & every QRS preceded by a P wave? 6. For select tachydysrhythmias, is there response to vagal maneuvers or adenosine?

Determining Axis *(nl QRS axis = –30° to +90°, +QRS in lead I & aVF)*		
Type	**Definition**	**Causes**
L axis deviation	QRS b/w –30° & –90° (+QRS lead I, –QRS aVF)	LVH, LBBB, inferior MI, LAFB, ventricular pre-excitation w/ posteroseptal accessory pathway (WPW)
R axis deviation	QRS b/w +90° & +180° (–QRS lead I, +QRS aVF)	RVH, lateral MI, LPFB, ventricular preexcitation w/ free wall accessory pathway (WPW), COPD, dextrocardia
Extreme axis deviation	QRS b/w +180° & –90° (–QRS lead I, –QRS aVF)	VT, hyperkalemia, apical MI, RVH

ECG Waveforms & Segments	
Type	**Definition**
P wave	• Represents atrial depolarization; best seen in leads II & V1 • Nl: Duration <0.12 s, amplitude ≤0.2 mV (frontal) or ≤0.1 mV (transverse), axis upright in I, II, aVF, & V2–V4 & inverted in aVR • Can be absent (AF/AFl, SVT), aberrant shape (AT, MAT, AFL)
PR interval	• Represents time b/w onset of atrial depolarization (start of P) & onset of ventricular depolarization (start of QRS); isoelectric region represents conduction w/i AV node, bundle of His, bundle branches, & Purkinje fibers • Nl: Duration normally 0.12–0.20 s (120–200 ms)
Q wave	• Any initial neg deflection; represents onset of ventricular depolarization (specifically: L to R depolarization of septum) • Nl: Small Qw can be nl in all leads except V1, V2, V3; large Qw can be nl variant in lead III & aVR • Pathologic Q: Any Qw in V1–V3, Qw >0.04 s (1 mm) & ≥0.2 mV (2 mm); or any Qw >25% of QRS complex
R wave	• Any positive deflection w/i QRS; normally, Rw should become greater than Sw by ~V3–V4 (called R-wave progression [RWP]) • Pathology suggested by poor RWP (LVH, LBBB, LAFB, ant-MI, COPD, infiltrative d/o, etc), early RWP/dominant Rw in V1–V2 (RVH, RBBB, post-MI, WPW, HOCM, etc), dominant Rw in aVR (TCA, Na chan o/d)
QRS complex	• Represents ventricular depolarization (1st half: septum & RV; 2nd half: LV) • Nl duration 0.06–0.11 s (60–110 ms) measured in lead w/ widest QRS complex (see *Causes of Abnl Interval Duration Table*) • Pathology suggested by prolongation (see *Causes of Prolonged QRS Table* below) or low voltage (R + S <0.5 mV in limb leads or <0.1 mV precordial; suggests presence of fluid [pericardial/pl effusion], air [COPD], or excess fat/tissue [obesity, infiltrative CMP, myxedema])
ST segment	• Represents plateau from end of ventricular depolarization (end of S) to start of repolarization (beginning of T); jxn of QRS & ST called J-point • Normally isoelectric w/ TP segment • Pathology suggested by ST elevation (≥0.2 mV contiguous precordial leads, ≥0.1 mV limb leads, & ≥0.5 mV in R-sided & posterior leads) or depression (horizontal or downsloping depression ≥0.05 mV in 2 contiguous leads) (see *Causes of ST Elevation*)
T wave	• Represents ventricular repolarization • Normally smooth & round morphology, positive in all leads except aVR; may be biphasic in V1/V2; amplitude generally 2/3 that of the R wave • Pathology suggested by Tw inversions in I, II, aVL, V2–V6 (BBBs, LVH w/ strain pattern, Wellens sign, myocardial ischemia, myopericarditis, cardiac contusion, MVP, SAH, hypokalemia, digoxin effect) or peaked-Tw morphology (hyperkalemia, early myocardial ischemia)
U wave	• Small wave following T wave; represents prolonged repolarization of midmyocardial layer cells "M cells" • Nl amplitude <1.5 mm tall or ~10% on T-wave amplitude • Pathology suggested by prominent Uw (hypokalemia/hypocalcemia, hypothermia, sinus bradycardia, LVH, hyperthyroid, etc)
QT interval	• Measured from start of QRS complex to end of T wave; represents duration of electrical activation & recovery of ventricle • Nl duration 390–450 ms in men; 390–460 ms in women (see *Causes of Abnl Interval Duration Table*)

Normal Intervals & Causes of Abnormal Interval Duration			
Type	**Normal**	**Shortened**	**Prolonged**
PR	120–200 ms	↑ sympathetic tone, ectopic atrial PM, pre-excitation (WPW), junctional rhythm (retrograde P w)	1–3° AVB, meds (digoxin, CCB, BB)
QRS	60–110 ms	↑ sympathetic tone, supra-ventricular tach, lytes (↓ K, ↓ Ca)	BBBs, ventricular conduction (inc pacemakers), cardiomyopathies, lytes (↑ K) & channelopathies, meds (antiarrhythmics, TCAs), hypothermia
QTc	390–450 ms (M)[a] 390–460 ms (F)[a]	↑ sympathetic tone, digoxin tox, lytes (↑ K, ↑ Ca), congenital short QT synds	Myocardial injury: myocarditis, AMI, lytes (↓ K, ↓ Ca, ↓ Mg), hypothyroidism, hypothermia, mitral valve prolapse, increased ICP, meds (antiarrhythmics, psychotics, antihistamines; quinolones, macrolides, methadone, etc), long-QT synds

[a]Several formulas calculate QTc: [1] $QTc = QT/\sqrt{RR}$; [2] $QTc = QT/RR^{1/3}$; [3] $QTc = QT + 0.154 \times (1 - RR)$.

Conduction Delays	
Category	**Definition**
RBBB	1. QRS duration ≥120 ms (≥100–120 ms = "incomplete" RBBB) 2. Late R-wave peak time (AKA intrinsicoid, >0.05 s), M-shaped QRS (rsr′, rSr′, rSR′) in V1–V3 ("rabbit ears") 3. Early R-wave peak time, broad terminal slurred S wave in I, aVL, V5–V6
	Causes: AMI, R-heart strain (PE, pHTN), myopericarditis, endomyocardial fibrosis, Chagas dz, CHD (ASD, VSD, ToF)
LBBB	1. QRS ≥120 ms (≥100–120 ms = "incomplete" LBBB) 2. Wide, notched R wave & absent Q wave in V5–V6, I, aVL 3. Late R-wave peak time (>0.06 s) in V5–V6 4. Wide S wave in V1 w/ rS or QS complex
	Causes: Anterior AMI, LVH, CMP, hyperkalemia, digoxin tox
LAFB	1. QRS duration ≤120 ms 2. LAD (usually ≥–60°) 3. qR pattern in I & aVL 4. rS pattern in II, III, & aVF 5. Late R-wave peak time (>0.045 s) in aVL 6. Increased QRS voltage in limb leads
	Causes: Acute or remote MI, AS, OSA, CMP, endomyocardial fibrosis, Chagas dz, CHD
LPFB	1. QRS duration ≤120 ms 2. RAD (usually ≥+120°) w/o e/o RVH 3. rS pattern in I & aVL 4. qR pattern in II, III, & aVF 5. Late R-wave peak time (>0.045 s) in aVF
	Causes: Acute cor pulmonale, CAD Lenègre dz, CMP, endomyocardial fibrosis, Chagas dz, hyperkalemia
Bifascicular block	RBBB w/ LAFB or LPFB
	Causes similar to LAFB
Trifascicular block	Bifascicular block w/ 3° AVB
Intraventricular conduction delay	1. QRS duration >110 ms 2. Typical waveforms of RBBB & LBBB not present

Atrial Abnormality & Ventricular Hypertrophy	
Type	**Definition**
Right atrial enlargement—RAE (P pulmonale)	1. P amplitude ≥0.15 mV in V1/V2 2. P amplitude ≥0.25 mV in II, III, or aVF 3. P-wave duration (75°–90°)
	Causes: TR, PS; pHTN (eg, ILD, PEs, COPD, CHF); ASD, VSD
Left atrial enlargement—LAE	1. Biphasic P in V1 w/ terminal neg P wave >0.04 s & >0.01 mV 2. Bifid P wave in II, w/ duration b/w peaks in P-wave notches >0.04 s 3. P-wave duration >0.12 s
	Causes: MS/MR, AS; CHF; HTN, HOCM
Right ventricular Hypertrophy—RVH	1. R-axis (>110°) 2. Dominant R in V1 >0.7 mV or R/S ratio >1 3. Dominant S in V5 or V6 >0.7 mV or R/S <1 4. w/ QRS duration (<120 ms)
Left ventricular hypertrophy—LVH	Mx criteria based on QRS voltages (poor sens) (*BMJ* 2007;355(7622):711) Sokolow–Lyon criteria: Sw in V1 + tallest Rw in V5 or V6 ≥3.50 mV (sens 22%, spec 100%) Cornell: Rw in aVL + Sw in V3 >2.8 mV (M) or >2.0 mV (F)

Causes & Morphologies of ST Elevation (*NEJM* 2003;349:2128–2135)	
Differential	**Comments**
STEMI	Upward convex; coronary artery distribution; large T waves
Prinzmetal angina	As above (STEMI), but transient due to coronary spasm etiology
Myo/pericarditis	Upward concave; diffuse (can be regional); +/– PR depression
Massive PE	Inferior & anteroseptal leads
LV aneurysm	Concave or convex; precordium common; ±pathologic Q waves; smaller T waves compared to STEMI. Can occur after MI
LBBB	Concave, usually discordant w/ QRS
LVH	Concave, other features of LVH present
Hyperkalemia	Seen w/ other features of hyperkalemia
Brugada	Usually incomplete RBBB, RAD, rSR′ & downsloping STE V1,V2
Nl	Concave, seen esp in healthy young men, most marked in V2
Early repolarization	Most marked in V4, notching at J-point; tall upright T waves present
Cardioversion	Seen 1–2 mins after DCCV
Transvenous pacing	Presence can be used to ensure correct positioning of pacing wire

ACUTE CORONARY SYNDROME

Overview

- Approach to pt w/ anginal sx: See section on *Chest Pain*
- **Chronic stable angina:** Substernal chest discomfort (pain, tightness, pressure) of less than 10-min duration, provoked by exertion or stress & alleviated by rest or NTG, & nonprogressive (ie, stable) over long periods of time (see *Table*; compare to UA), not considered ACS
  - Chronic angina should be a dx of exclusion in ED, as pts w/ chronic sx often present to ED b/c sxs are somehow different or worsening

Canadian Cardiovascular Society (CCS) Grading of Angina Pectoris	
Grade	**Description** (*Circulation* 1976;54:522)
Grade I	Angina w/ strenuous or rapid or prolonged exertion
Grade II	Slight limitation of ordinary activity. Angina only w/ vigorous physical activity
Grade III	Marked limitation. Angina occurs w/ everyday living activities
Grade IV	Severe limitation. Angina w/ any activity or at rest

- **Acute coronary syndrome:** Clinical spectrum of conditions ranging from UA through MI (NSTEMI & STEMI); due to disrupted vulnerable or high-risk plaque undergoing causing thrombogenesis & causing imbalance b/w myocardial O_2 supply & demand (tissue ischemia)

- **Myocardial infarction** (see *Universal Definition*): death of myocardial cells due to myocardial tissue hypoxia, acutely causing release of intracellular cardiac biomarkers
  - Once diagnosed, important to consider subtype & etiology (see tables below)
    - MI DDx is broad: not always 2/2 acute plaque rupture (see table below)
  - Elevated troponin not always MI: consider nonischemic etiologies (see table below)

Universal Definition of Myocardial Infarction (*Circulation* 2018;138:e618–e651)	
Acute Myocardial Injury	
Detection of a rise &/or fall of cardiac biomarker (typically Troponin I or T) values w/ at least one value above the 99th percentile upper reference limit	
Acute Myocardial Infarction	
Myocardial injury w/ at least one of: • **Symptoms:** sxs of ischemia • **ECG:** new or presumed new significant ST-T chgs, LBBB, Qw • **Imaging:** e/o new loss of viable myocardium or new regional wall motion abnl • **Pathology:** identification of an intracoronary abnlty by angiography or autopsy	
Universal Classification of MI*	
Type 1	Spontaneous MI related to atherosclerotic plaque rupture, ulceration, erosion, or dissection w/ resulting intraluminal thrombosis in 1 or more CAs
Type 2	MI secondary to an ischemic imbalance b/w myocardial O_2 supply & demand (eg, CA spasm, dissection, dysrhythmia, hypotension, anemia)
Type 3	MI resulting in death w/o biomarker values

*Types 4 and 5 refer to procedure-related MIs (CABG, PCI, etc).

Differential for Myocardial Injury & Infarction (*Circulation* 2018;138:e618–e651)		
Causes		**Examples**
Atherosclerotic plaque rupture		Most common cause of 1° ACS
Ischemic injury	Coronary artery dissection	1° (spontaneous, a/w pregnancy), or 2° (a/w type A AoD w/ retrograde RCA dissection, post-PCI)
	Coronary artery spasm	Vasospastic (Prinzmetal/variant, cocaine induced)
	Coronary artery embolism	Thrombus, endocarditis, myxoma
	Fixed atherosclerotic plaque w/ increased O_2 demand	↑ HR, ↑ BP, AS (↑ O_2 demand) ↓ BP, anemia, hypoxia (↓ O_2 supply)
Nonischemic injury		Myocarditis, contusion, infiltrative dz, drug induced, CHF, CMP, procedure, sepsis, CKD, stroke, PE

History

- Classic sxs of angina: Substernal pressure, pain, or tightness; often radiating to neck, jaw, or arms; precipitated by exertion & relieved w/ rest or NTG
  - Associated sxs: dyspnea, diaphoresis, n/v, palpitations, LH
  - Many pts w/ MI present w/o "classic" sx
- Concerning features: new, at rest, or crescendo (frequency, severity, duration, ↓ threshold)

Value of Specific Symptoms in Diagnosis of AMI (*JAMA* 2015;314[18]:1955–1965)		
Pain Descriptor	*+ LR* (95% CI)	*– LR* (95% CI)
Radiation: B/L arms	2.6 (1.8–3.7)	0.93 (0.89–0.96)
Similar to prior ischemia	2.2 (2.0–2.6)	0.67 (0.60–0.74)
Δ in pattern over 24 h	2.0 (1.6–2.5)	0.84 (0.79–0.90)
Worse w/ exertion	1.5–1.8	0.66–0.83
Radiation to neck or jaw	1.5 (1.3–1.8)	0.91 (0.87–0.95)
Radiation: L arm	1.3 (1.2–1.4)	0.88 (0.81–0.96)
Radiation: R arm	1.3 (0.78–2.1)	0.99 (0.96–1.0)
Associated diaphoresis	1.3–1.4	0.91–0.93
Associated dyspnea	1.2 (1.1–1.3)	0.89 (0.82–0.96)
Improvement w/ nitroglycerin	1.1 (0.93–1.3)	0.90 (0.85–0.96)

Physical Examination

- Can be unremarkable unless c/b hypotension, heart block/arrhythmia, signs of R heart failure, pulm edema
- Helpful for assessing for other etiologies: bilateral UE BPs +/– pulse deficits (AoD), lung exam (CHF, PTX, PNA), abdominal exam (biliary & pancreatic etiologies), chest wall TTP (MSK), rash (zoster)

Evaluation

- **ECG:** Always check w/i 10 mins of arrival, if c/f developing ACS, if sxs Δ; compare w/ baseline; if pain persists or chgs present, repeat q15–20min; consider posterior ECG (leads V7–V9) in pts w/ non-dx initial ECG to r/o L circumflex STEMI
  - Acute ischemia chgs: ↑ or ↓ in ST segment or new TWI in anatomic distribution, new LBBB, hyperacute T waves

Anatomic Distribution of ECG Findings Associated with AMI		
Anatomic Area	**ECG Leads**	**Coronary Artery**
Septal	V1–V2	Proximal LAD[1,2]
Anterior	V3–V4	LAD
Apical	V5–V6	Distal LAD, LCx, or RCA
Lateral	I, aVL, V5–V6	LCx
Anterolateral	aVR	L main CA
Inferior[3]	II, III, aVF	RCA (~85%), LCx (~15%)
RV	V1–V2 & V4R (most sens)	Proximal RCA
Posterior	ST depression V1–V2	RCA or LCx (obtain posterior leads)

[1]Wellens syndrome: biphasic or deeply inverted T waves in V2–V3 specific for critical LAD lesion (may be present even after CP has resolved).
[2]De Winter pattern: ST depression & peaked T waves in precordial leads, specific for LAD occlusion.
[3]Obtain R-sided leads in inferior STEMI to evaluate for RV infarct.

  - Old ischemic chgs: Qw or PRWP (indicates presence of CAD even if no known hx)
  - Modified Sgarbossa criteria: used to identify STEMI in the presence of LBBB (see *Table*)

Modified Sgarbossa Criteria for Identifying AMI in Presence of Old LBBB
≥1 lead w/ ≥1 mm STE concordant w/ QRS
≥1 lead w/ ≥1 mm concordant STD in V1–V3
≥1 lead anywhere w/ ≥1 mm STE & ≥25% elevation as compared to depth of preceding S wave

  - **Labs:** Troponin, BMP, CBC, coags, T/S (if intervention planned), tox (if cocaine suspected), D-dimer (if PE suspected)
  - **CXR:** Useful to r/o other causes of CP; check lungs, cardiac silhouette, mediastinum
  - **Transthoracic echo:** If ECG difficult to interpret (prior LBBB, paced) & suspicion for ACS is high, can obtain TTE to assess for regional wall motion abnormalities; +WMA in pt w/ ongoing CP may suggest benefit from earlier PCI (*Circulation* 2021; 144:e368–e454; *BMJ Open* 2024;14(9):e085677)
  - **Risk-stratification testing:** See section on *Risk-Stratification Testing*

Cardiac Biomarkers

- Troponin (I or T): ↑ sens & spec as compared to CK-MB & myoglobin, high-sens assay preferred over standard troponin assay
- Protocols for serial measurement of standard & high-sens troponin vary based on institution (see sample protocols below under dispo)
- Causes of elevated biomarkers other than acute coronary thrombosis: myopericarditis; drug tox; acute neuro dz (eg, ICH); myocardial contusion; myocardial O_2 supply–demand mismatch 2/2 tachyarrhythmia, CHF, HTN, hypotension, PE, sepsis, burns, resp failure
- Δ in serial HS-Tn (1–3 h) may have greater clinical significance than elevation itself for ACS dx, though absolute elevations have prognostic value, esp in high-risk pts (*J Am Heart Assoc* 2014;3(1):e000403)

Treatment

- Give ASA if considering ACS; Only strict CI to ASA is hx of true allergy (anaphylaxis)
- **Chronic stable angina:** ASA (NNT = 50 in pts w/ known or suspected CAD), BP control, mod- to high-intensity statin supported by mx RCTs (*NEJM* 2016;374:1167–1176; *Lancet* 2009;373(9678):1849–1860)
- **ACS:** See UA/NSTEMI & STEMI for details
- **Pain control:** directed at underlying cause, NTG (sublingual, infusion; except in inferior MIs), opiates, NSAIDs, Tylenol PRN

Disposition

- Admit all STEMI, NSTEMI, & UA (see UA/NSTEMI & STEMI for details)
- For pts w/ nondiagnostic hx, ECG, & biomarkers: risk stratify w/ HEART score
  - HEART > TIMI & GRACE in predicting major adverse cardiac events w/i 30 d (score ≥4; sens 95.9%; *Acad Emerg Med* 2019;26(2)140:151)

HEART Score for Chest Pain Patients in the ED (*Neth Heart J* 2008;16(6):191–196)			
History		**Troponin**	
Highly suspicious	2 pts	≥3× Nl limit	2 pts
Moderately suspicious	1 pt	>1 to <3× Nl limit	1 pt
Slightly/nonsuspicious	0 pts	≤ Nl limit	0 pts
ECG		**Risk Factors**[a]	
Significant ST depressions	2 pts	≥3 RFs[b]	2 pts
Nonspecific repolarization	1 pt	1 or 2 RFs	1 pt
Nl	0 pts	No RFs	0 pts
Age		[a]RFs include: current DM, current or recent (<1 mo) smoker, HTN, HLD, FHx CAD, obesity [b]2 pts given for prior PCI, MI, CVA, PAD	
≥65 y	2 pts		
>45–<65 y	1 pt		
≤45 y	0 pts		

Total Score, Prognostic Value, & Disposition		
Score 0–3	2.5% MACE over next 6 wks	D/C home w/ f/u
Score 4–6	20.3% MACE over next 6 wks	Observation & risk-stratification testing
Score 7–10	72.7% MACE over next 6 wks	Admit for early catheterization

- **Sample standard troponin assay protocol:** Perform initial troponin and repeat troponin at 1–3 h after arrival, & at 3 h if intermediate or high suspicion of ACS; if elevated, continue measuring until levels peak & downtrend; risk stratify based on HEART score for dispo

Figure 1.1 Sample high-sensitivity troponin assay protocol (*Crit Pathw Cardiol* 2019;18(1):1)

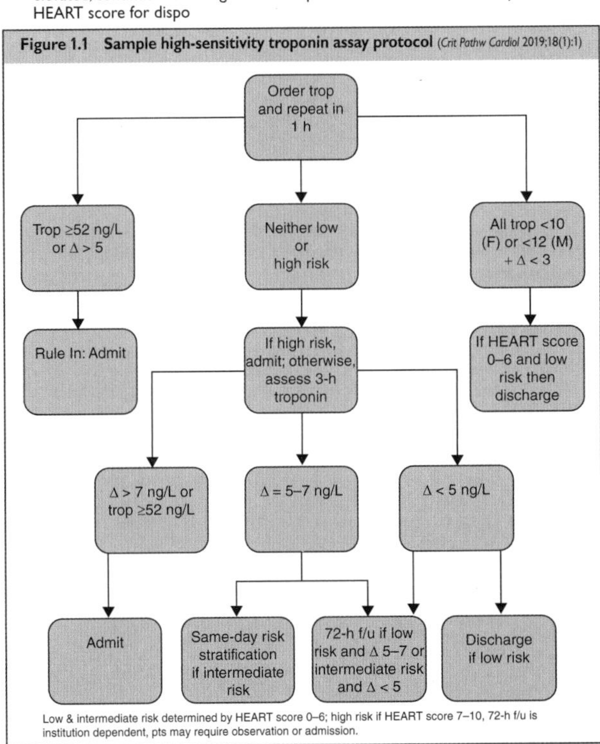

Low & intermediate risk determined by HEART score 0–6; high risk if HEART score 7–10, 72-h f/u is institution dependent, pts may require observation or admission.

- If low risk (HEART score 0–3) & CP for greater than 2 h, single HS-troponin appears to be as safe as serial troponin for pts to be discharged (*JAMA Netw Open* 2021;4(2):e2037930)

STEMI: Overview & Treatment

Definition

- Acute complete occlusion of coronary artery (usually proximal) due to unstable thrombus, causing transmural ischemia & myocardial necrosis; characterized by angina or equivalent, usually at rest, ECG e/o ST elevations & +troponin
- **ECG criteria:** ≥0.1 mV of new ST elevation at the J-point in any lead except V2–V3, & ≥0.5 mV in R-sided & posterior leads in at least 2 contiguous leads
- For leads V2–V3: ≥0.2 mV in men ≥40, ≥0.25 mV in men <40, ≥0.15 mV in women

Treatment Approach (*Circulation* 2025;151(13):e771–2862)

- Initiate early medical therapies (ASA, heparin, nitrates prn, O_2 PRN, analgesia)
  - Antithrombotic/adjunctive therapy should not delay transfer for PCI
- Place defibrillator pads on pt given high risk of VT/VF
- Reperfusion: immediate decision regarding availability of 1° PCI
  - 1° PCI or transfer to PCI-capable hospital preferred for all pts **except** if time b/w first medical contact (FMC) & PCI is expected >120 mins (*Circulation* 2022;145(3):e4–e17)
  - Fibrinolysis may be preferred if delay to PCI expected >120 mins, Goal time from FMC to lysis: <30 mins
    - Pts treated w/ fibrinolysis should undergo delayed angiography (2–24 h)
      - Urgent transfer for expedited angio after fibrinolysis for pts w/ failed reperfusion, sx <12 h or w/ shock or severe acute HF
      - Early PCI after fibrinolysis is associated w/ ↓ mortality and ↓ reinfarction (*Am Heart J* 2008;156(3):564–572)
      - Fibrinolysis is not recommended if sx duration >12 h given lower effectiveness and higher stroke risk (*Lancet* 1994;343(8893):311)
    - If FMC-to-PCI time expected >120 mins, PCI preferred if there are known CIs to lysis, high-risk pt (eg, shock), dx of STEMI in doubt (eg, ? AoD w/ RCA dissection)
    - If planning PCI, call cardiology/PCI lab as early as possible (potentially even before the pt arrives in the ED—if reliable prenotification by EMS)
    - If transferring for PCI, call for transfer early & ensure door-to-balloon time is <90 mins
  - Monitor & treat cxs (eg, CHB, cardiogenic shock, pulm edema, arrhythmias)

Adjunctive Medical Therapies

- **Anti-plt tx:** Always give ASA (162–325 mg PO/PR), ↓ mortality c/w placebo (*Lancet* 1988;2:349); additional benefit from other anti-plt agents (see *Table*); all pts should receive additional anti-plt agents either in the ED or cath lab
- **Antithrombotic tx:** See tables below for recommended regimens
- **Nitrates:** No proven long-term mortality benefit, but may ameliorate sxs; typical dose 0.4 mg SL q5min × 3; contraindicated w/ ↓ BP, RV infarct, Ao stenosis, PD-inh w/i 24–48 h
- **O_2 supplementation:** No e/o benefit & may cause harm, possibly 2/2 free radical formation; use only in hypoxic pts w/ O_2 saturation <90% (*Circulation* 2015;131(24):2143)
- **Beta blockers:** Early BB ↓ VT/VF & reinfarction acutely & ↑ LVEF in long term; However, ↑ risk of acute cardiogenic shock; give oral BB w/i 24 h of STEMI if no CI (shock, bradycardia, HF, bronchospasm)
- **Analgesia:** Morphine formerly routinely used but may be a/w worse outcomes; use opioids only for refractory pain (*Am Heart J* 2005;149(6):1043–1049)

Fibrinolysis

- **Indications:** STEMI *AND* sx onset <12 h prior *AND* time b/w FMC & 1° PCI >120 mins
- **Benefits:** ~20% ↓ mortality in anterior MI or new LBBB; 10% ↓ mortality in IMI
  - Benefits decrease dramatically after 3 h (*Circulation* 2011;124:2512–2521)
- **Risks:** ICH (<1%), major bleeding (1–12%)—likely to be lower w/ TNK rather than TPA (*Circ Cardiovasc Interv* 2020;13(9):e009622)

Contraindications to Fibrinolysis in STEMI (*Circulation* 2025;151(13):e771–2862)

Absolute CIs	Relative CIs
Intracranial neoplasm, aneurysm, AVM H/o any intracranial hemorrhage H/o intracranial/spinal surgery w/i 2 mos H/o i-CVA w/i 3 mos except if w/i 4.5 h H/o closed head/facial trauma w/i 3 mos Active internal bleeding or bleeding d/o Suspected AoD Severe HTN (unresponsive to IV tx)	Any known active intracranial path not listed w/i absolute CIs H/o iCVA >3 mos prior Active PUD, pregnancy, or dementia Current use of oral anticoagulants H/o trauma or major surgery w/i 3 wks H/o recent internal bleeding w/i 2–4 wks H/o severe poorly controlled HTN, or SBP >180 or DBP >110 on presentation Traumatic or prolonged CPR (>10 mins) Noncompressible vascular punctures Pregnancy Active peptic ulcer

Fibrinolytic Agents for STEMI (*Circulation* 2025;151(13):e771–2862)

Agent	Dosing	Patency, 90 mins
Tenecteplase (TNK-tPA)	Single IV bolus: <60 kg (30 mg), 60–69 kg (35 mg), 70–79 kg (40 mg), 80–89 kg (45 mg), ≥90 kg (50 mg)	85%
Reteplase (rPA)	10 U + 10 U IV bolus given 30 mins apart	84%
tPA	Bolus 15 mg, infusion 0.75 mg/kg for 30 mins (max 50 mg), then 0.5 mg/kg (max 35 mg) over 60 mins; total dose not to exceed 100 mg	73–84%

Adjunctive Therapies for Fibrinolysis in STEMI (*Circulation* 2025;151(13):e771–2862)

P2Yi2 receptor inh (loading dose)	**Clopidogrel:** 300 mg for pts ≤75 y/o, 75 mg for pts >75 y/o; ↑ artery patency, ↓ MACE if given w/ ASA (*NEJM* 2005;352:1179; *Lancet* 2005;366:1607)
Antithrombotic tx	**UFH:** IV bolus 60 U/kg (max 4,000 U) then gtt at 12 U/kg/h (max 1,000 U), maintain aPTT ~50–70 s × 48 h or until revasc (Note: preferred in pts undergoing delayed PCI)
	Enoxaparin: If <75 y/o, 30 mg IV bolus, then 15 mins later, 1 mg/kg SC q12h; if >75 y/o, no bolus, 0.75 mg/kg SC q12h; if CrCl <30 mL/min, 1 mg/kg q24h
	Fondaparinux: Initial 2.5 mg IV, then 2.5 mg SC the following day; continue × 8 d or until revasc; esp useful if hx of HIT; CI if CrCl <30; may ↓ mortality w/o ↑ bleeding c/w UFH (*JAMA* 2006;295(13):1519–1530)

Primary PCI

- **Indications:** Preferred modality if expected <120 mins from FMC; STEMI sx onset <12 h prior; STEMI sx onset <12 h if CI to fibrinolytics regardless of time delay from FMC; presence of severe acute HF or cardiogenic shock; ongoing ischemia 12–24 h
- **Goal:** door-to-balloon <90 mins by skilled operator at high-volume center
- **Benefits:** 27% ↓ death, 65% ↓ re-MI, 54% ↓ stroke, 95% ↓ ICH c/w lysis (*Lancet* 2003;361:13)
- PCI w/i 3 h of lytics in stable pts (w/o e/o failed reperfusion) may cause harm (*PLoS One* 2015;10(11):e0141855)

Adjunctive Therapies for PCI in STEMI (*Circulation* 2025;151(13):e771–2862)

$P2Y_{12}$ receptor inh (loading dose) *Note: There is a lack of strong evidence supporting early (ED-based) administration of $P2Y_{12}$ receptor inh*	**Clopidogrel:** 600 mg load; ↓ infarct size, cardiac fxn, stent thrombosis, & ↓ 30-d MACE c/w 300 mg load (*J Am Coll Cardiol* 2011;58(15):1592–1599; *Lancet* 2010;376(9748):1233–1243) but ↑ bleeding & ICU LOS if need for urgent CABG (*Am Heart J* 2011;161(2):404–410); discuss w/ cardiology if potential CABG w/i 5 d
	Prasugrel: 60 mg load; mild ↓ ischemic cx but ↑ bleeding c/w clopidogrel; best if young & no need for surgery w/i 1 y; avoid if hx of CVA/TIA (*NEJM* 2007;357:2001; TRITON-TIMI, *Lancet* 2009;373:732)
	Ticagrelor: 180 mg load; mild ↓ mortality, MI, stroke c/w clopidogrel, but ↑ nonprocedural bleeding (eg, ICH) (*NEJM* 2009;361:1045–1057)

Antithrombotic tx	**UFH:** IV bolus 50–70 U/kg IV, then 12 U/kg/h (max 1,000 U), maintain aPTT ~50–70 s
	Bivalirudin: 0.75 mg/kg IV bolus, then 1.75 mg/kg/h infusion w/ or w/o UFH; preferred over UFH w/ GP IIb/IIIa inh in pts at high risk of bleeding; useful if hx of HIT

Note: 2025 ACCF/AHA Guideline for Mgmt of STEMI recommends GIIb/IIIa inh (abciximab, tirofiban, or eptifibatide) in select pts, though often performed in cath lab.

Disposition

- If no PCI available: Transfer to PCI-capable center regardless of decision to use lytics
- If PCI available: Admit to cath lab → CCU/cardiology

Unstable Angina/NSTEMI: Overview & Treatment

Definition

- Pathogenesis: Nonocclusive coronary thrombus on pre-existing plaque, causing dynamic & progressive obstruction, inflammation, & ischemia
- **Unstable angina:** Any angina that is new onset (if CCS III–IV severity), occurring at rest, or crescendo in nature (frequency, severity, duration, or more easily triggered), but *lacking* both ST elevations & positive troponin. Note: Dx of UA is rare if measuring high-sens troponins
- **NSTEMI:** Similar to UA, but characterized by elevated troponin
- **ECG criteria:** None; can have nl ECG, territorial STD, TWI, or NSSTW chgs

Treatment Approach

- Initiate early medical therapies (ASA, heparin, nitrates prn, O_2 PRN, analgesia)
- Determine risk using TIMI or GRACE risk scores to guide early vs delayed timing of angiography (see section below)
- Monitor & treat cxs (eg, heart blocks, arrythmias shock, pulm edema)

Early Invasive vs Selective Invasive Approach

- Ultimately, approach decided by interventional cardiology based on mx factors: risk score, procedural risks, recent angiography results, clinical stability & sx, pt goals, etc
- Selective invasive approach includes noninvasive risk stratification to determine need for angiography (ie, stress test or CT angiography)

Angiography Selection & Timing in UA/NSTEMI (*Circulation* 2025;151(13):e771–2862)

Immediate (<2 h) invasive	**Unstable or very high risk** Cardiogenic shock Signs or sx of HF (pulm edema, mitral regurg) Hemodynamic instability electrical instability (sustained VT or VF) Refractory angina
Early (<24 h) angiography	**Unstable or very high risk** Steep rise in troponin despite optimized medical therapy Ongoing dynamic ST-segment chgs GRACE Risk Score >140
Routine (<72 h) angiography	**Intermediate-risk** GRACE Risk Score 109–140 No ongoing ischemic sx Stable or downtrending troponin values
Either routine angiography or selective invasive strategy	**Lower-risk (Any of the following:)** GRACE Risk Score <109 TIME Risk Score <2 No ongoing ischemic sx Stable or downtrending troponin values Troponin <99th percentiles

- **Selective invasive approach:** Best for initially stabilized pts w/o high-risk scores, ongoing sxs, arrhythmias, heart failure; 2/2 marginal benefit but ↑ risks of early invasive approach (*Cochrane Database Syst Rev* 2016;26(5):CD004815)
  - Medical therapies (see above) for 48 h minimum, pre-D/C stress test or CT angio
  - Invasive angiography only if recurrent ischemia, arrhythmias, heart failure, positive stress test

- **Early invasive approach:** In meta-analysis, no ↓ all-cause mortality/nonfatal MI, may ↓ risk of MI, refractory angina, & rehosp at 6–12 mos c/w selective approach; however, also ↑ bleeding risk & procedure-related MI (*Cochrane Database Syst Rev* 2016;26(5):CD004815)
- Higher-risk pts benefit most from earlier angiography

GRACE Risk Score for UA/NSTEMI (*BMJ* 2006;333(7578):1091)

Age (y)							
≤30	30–39	40–49	50–59	60–69	70–79	80–89	≥90
0 pts	*8 pts*	*25 pts*	*41 pts*	*58 pts*	*75 pts*	*91 pts*	*100 pts*

Heart Rate (bpm)						
≤50	50–69	70–89	90–109	110–149	150–199	≥200
0 pts	*3 pts*	*9 pts*	*15 pts*	*24 pts*	*38 pts*	*46 pts*
Systolic Blood Pressure (mmHg)						
≤80	80–99	100–119	120–139	140–159	160–199	≥200
58 pts	*53 pts*	*43 pts*	*34 pts*	*24 pts*	*10 pts*	*0 pts*

Killip Class			
I (No heart failure)	II (Crackles in lower lung fields)	III (Crackles in whole lung field)	IV (Cardiogenic shock)
0 pts	*20 pts*	*39 pts*	*59 pts*

Serum Creatinine Level (mg/dL)						
0–0.38	0.39–0.79	0.80–1.19	1.20–1.58	1.59–1.90	2.0–3.99	≥4
1 pt	*4 pts*	*7 pts*	*10 pts*	*13 pts*	*21 pts*	*28 pts*

Cardiac Arrest at admx		**ST-Segment Deviation**		**Troponin Elevation**	
Yes	No	YES	No	Yes	No
39 pts	*0 pts*	*28 pts*	*0 pts*	*14 pts*	*0 pts*

Risk Classification & Prognosis		
Total score ≤100	Low risk	In-hospital death <1%
Total score 101–170	Medium risk	In-hospital death 1–3%
Total score ≥171	High risk	In-hospital death >3%

TIMI Risk Score for UA/NSTEMI (*JAMA* 2000;284:825)

Age ≥65 y	1 pt	Severe angina (≥2 episodes w/i 24 h)	1 pt
≥3 RFs for CAD	1 pt	ST deviation ≥0.5 mm	1 pt
Known CAD (stenosis ≥50%)	1 pt	+cardiac biomarker (Tn, CK-MB)	1 pt
ASA use in past 7 d	1 pt		

Risk Classification & Risk of Death/MI/Urgent Revascularization w/i 14 d

Total score	14-d Risk: D/MI/Urg Revasc (%)	Total score	14-d Risk: D/MI/Urg Revasc (%)
0–1 pt	5	4 pts	20
2 pts	8	5 pts	26
3 pts	13	6–7 pts	41

Adjunctive Medical Therapies (*Circulation* 2025;151(13):e771–2862)
- **Analgesia, O_2 supplementation, nitrates, statins, beta blockers:** See previous section, *same as adjunctive medical therapies for STEMI*
- **Anti-plt tx:** Always give ASA (162–325 mg PO/PR)
  - **Regardless of PCI approach:** $P2Y_{12}$ inh (clopidogrel or prasugrel) or ticagrelor. Ticagrelor may be preferred due to reduction in mortality (*NEJM* 2009;361:1045)
  - Inconclusive benefit from ED administration (vs cath lab/inpt unit) of DAPT in either early invasive or selective approach, though generally earlier tx is better if UA/NSTEMI dx certain & low bleeding risk, consider in discussion w/ cardiology
- **Antithrombotic tx:** See table for recommended regimens; continue until angiography (early invasive approach) or 48 h vs hospital LOS (selective approach, if stress results indicate no need for angiography); hold anticoagulation if on warfarin until INR <2.0; anticoagulants have short-term benefit (UFH ↓ mortality 33–56% at 2–12 wks), but long-term benefit unclear, as dz process resumes once anticoagulation discontinued

Antithrombotic Therapy in UA/NSTEMI (*Circulation* 2025;151(13):e771–2862)
UFH: IV bolus 60 U/kg (max 4,000 U) then gtt at 12 U/kg/h (max 1,000 U), maintain aPTT ~50–70. Preferred in early invasive approach
Enoxaparin: 1 mg/kg SC q12h; if CrCl <30 mL/min, 1 mg/kg q24h. Not preferred w/ early invasive approach
Bivalirudin: 0.1 mg/kg IV bolus, then 0.25 mg/kg/h infusion. Rarely preferred over heparin/ enoxaparin
Fondaparinux: Initial 2.5 mg IV, then 2.5 mg SC daily, preferred if hx of HIT. Not recommended if undergoing PCI given risk of catheter thrombosis

Disposition

- Admx to CCU/cardiology based on risk, clinical stability, arrhythmia risk
- If UA, low-risk score, –Tn, nondiagnostic ECG: Consider admitting to a CP/observation unit for serial troponin testing & cardiac risk stratification; admx if recurrent sx, Δ ECG, +Tn

RISK-STRATIFICATION TESTING

Approach

- **Definition:** noninvasive eval for obstructive CAD in low-risk pts w/ acute CP or other sx c/f ACS
- **Indications:** dx obstructive CAD, assess Δ clinical status in pt w/ known obstructive CAD, localize ischemia in pts w/ known symptomatic obstructive CAD
- **Contraindications:** severe acute illness, AMI w/i 48 h, high-risk UA, alternative critical dx (PE, AoD, myopericarditis, acute decompensated CHF, arrhythmias, severe AS)
- Low-risk (HEART 0–3, TIMI 0–1, GRACE <109) pts may be safely discharged w/o stress testing if close o/p FU can be arranged
  - ED stress testing in low-risk pts is low yield & high cost (*Am J Cardiol* 2015;116(2):204–207)
  - 6-mo risk of MACE is low & may be unchanged regardless of whether pt receives stress in ED (*Crit Pathw Cardiol* 2016;15(4):145–151)
- Based on clinical judgment, can D/C pts w/ nl stress test w/i 12 mos, recent (<5 y) nonobstructive angiography test, and those w/ coronary CTA (CCTA) w/o stenosis w/i 2 y (*Acad Emerg Med* 2021;28(7):718)

Exercise Treadmill Testing

- Pt runs on treadmill; monitoring includes ECG, sxs, Δ hemodynamics (HR, BP)
  - "Diagnostic" test requires pt to achieve min of 85% of predicted HR (pHR = 220 – age)
- **Test characteristics:** 68% sens, 77% spec among pts w/ intermediate risk (*Prog Cardiovasc Dis* 1989;32(3):173–206)
- **Benefits:** lowest cost of risk-stratification tests
- **Downsides:** requires nl resting ECG; ↓ sens if low-risk pt; ↓ sens & spec in women; ↓ sens if anti-ischemic drugs not D/C-ed

Pharmacologic/Exercise Stress w/ Nuclear SPECT Imaging

- Ischemia induced by pharmacologic agents (eg, dobutamine, adenosine, dipyridamole, regadenoson) or exercise; radio-labeled tracers (eg, sestamibi) enter myocardial cells & reflect regional perfusion; ↓ tracer uptake during stress that resolves w/ time suggests viable area of tissue ischemia; fixed defect suggest existing infarct
- **Test characteristics:** adenosine SPECT sens 90%, spec 75%; dipyridamole SPECT sens 89%, spec 65%; dobutamine SPECT sens 82%, spec 75% (*Am Heart J* 2001;142(6):934–944)
- **Benefits:** Can use if abnl baseline ECG or unable to exercise; can localize ischemia
- **Downsides:** More expensive than exercise stress; ↓ sens & spec in women; ↓ sens if anti-ischemic drugs not D/C-ed, requires radioisotopes & personnel to administer them

Pharmacologic/Exercise Stress w/ Echo Imaging

- Ischemia induced by pharmacologic agents (eg, dobutamine, adenosine, dipyridamole, regadenoson) or exercise; echocardiography performed to assess for regional WMAs compared to rest
- **Test characteristics:** adenosine echo sens 72%, spec 91%; dipyridamole echo sens 70%, spec 93%; dobutamine echo sens 80%, spec 84% (*Am Heart J* 2001;142(6):934–944)
- **Benefits:** Can use if abnl baseline ECG or unable to exercise; can localize ischemia; can provide information re LVEF & valvular fxn

- **Downsides:** More expensive than exercise stress; ↓ sens if anti-ischemic drugs not D/C-ed, user variability, injury involving >20% of wall required to be able to be detected

Coronary Computed Tomographic Angiography

- CT angiography of coronary arteries; images timed in conjunction w/ HR; assesses CAD burden & severity, presence of CA calcification; does not assess myocardial perfusion
- **Test characteristics:** sens 97%, spec 78 (*Eur Heart J* 2018;39(35):3322)
- **Benefits:** ↓ LOS & ↓ costs c/w conventional stress testing; esp useful for low-risk pts or intermediate-risk & nl serial ECGs/biomarkers
- **Downsides:** Increased risk of downstream testing (2/2 ↓ spec & detection of incidental findings), radiation exposure, requires relative bradycardia (often requires beta blockers)
  - Less effective for excluding obstructive CAD in pts w/ high pretest probability & high calcium score
- Combination of single neg conventional troponin & neg coronary CTA has equivalent risk of MACE c/w conventional stress (*Heart* 2018;103(3):215)

Disposition

- Inadequate quality study: discuss case w/ cardiology
- Adequate quality + Neg result + Low risk: D/C w/ f/u
- Adequate quality + Neg result + Int risk: discuss case w/ cardiology, likely D/C w/ f/u
- Adequate quality + Pos result: discuss w/ cardiology, admit
- For adequate study w/ high-risk test results, consider coronary angiography, ± admx depending on clinical presentation

Pearls

- False-positives: Positive risk-stratification testing in a pt who presented to ED w/ CP does not necessarily mean CP was 2/2 by CAD; esp if low pre-TP & other causes possible
  - Causes: valve dz, HCM, HTN, AV fistula, anemia, low CO, COPD, BBB
- False-negs: neg risk-stratification testing in a pt who presented to ED w/ CP does not necessarily mean CP was not 2/2 by CAD; esp if high pre-TP

CARDIAC CATHETERIZATION

Overview

- **Indications:** ACS (see STEMI & UA/NSTEMI above for timing of PCI); high-risk stress test result *OR* indeterminate-risk stress test result & high pre-TP for obstructive CAD; ongoing angina despite tx; r/o CAD in pts w/ CP suspected from nonatherosclerotic etiology (ie, spasm) or systolic dysfxn suspected of nonischemic etiology (ie, ni-CMP); after ROSC in pts w/ cardiac arrest (see below for criteria)
  - Post-arrest PCI recommended if STEMI &/or absence of mx unfavorable features (unwitnessed arrest, no bystander CPR, initial non-VF rhythm, >30 mins to ROSC, ongoing CPR, noncardiac/traumatic arrest, pH <7.2, lactate >7, age >85, ESRD); decision individualized for each case (*J Am Coll Cardiol* 2015;66(1):62–73)
  - COACT Trial: strategy of immediate angiography not superior to delayed angiography for resuscitated pts w/ OHCA w/o STEMI (*JAMA Cardiol* 2020;5:1358)
- Types of percutaneous coronary interventions:
  - Balloon angioplasty: effective but ↑ risk of CA dissection & restenosis 2/2 remodeling
  - Bare metal stent: Rarely used today given higher restenosis rates and MI
  - Drug-eluting stent: Preferred. ↓ restenosis & ↓ MI (*Lancet* 2019;393(10190):2503–2510)

Post-PCI Complications

- **Bleeding (arterial access site):** Apply pressure, reverse/stop anticoagulation
- **Bleeding (retroperitoneum—from femoral access site):** May c/o back pain, ±Hct drop, ↓ BP, ↑ HR; obtain abd/pelvic CT; reverse/stop anticoagulation, c/s IR/surgery
- **Pseudoaneurysm:** P/w pain, expanding mass, systolic bruit; obtain US; tx w/ manual compression, ±thrombin injection/surgery
- **AV fistula:** May p/w sx 2/2 ↓ perfusion to LE (2/2 emboli, dissection, thrombus), continuous bruit, ↓ distal pulses; obtain US ± angiogram; c/s cards &/or surgery for repair (percutaneous or operative)
- **Renal injury:** 2/2 atheroemboli, contrast, or low BPI; supportive care
- **Stent thrombosis:** P/w acute CP & ST elevations; c/s cards/cath lab, for urgent catheterization; more common in BMS than DES; commonly 2/2 underexpanded stent, dissection, or D/C anti-plt Rx
- **Stent restenosis:** P/w subacute or chronic return of anginal sx months after PCI (but 10% p/w ACS); occurs 2° postprocedure tissue remodeling, not atherosclerosis; incidence ~2% of pts/year (BMS > DES) (*J Am Coll Cardiol* 2020;75(6):590)

POST-MI COMPLICATIONS

Immediate Complications

- **LV systolic dysfunction/cardiogenic shock:** Common w/ large anterior AMI; Dx w/ JVD, CXR or BSUS (B/L B-lines, ↓ EF); Tx w/ O_2 for hypoxia, ↓ preload (NTG SL → gtt), ↓ afterload (avoid hydral 2/2 reflex ↑ HR), inotropy PRN (norepi ± dobutamine esp if SVR high; avoid epinephrine), diuretics, careful titration of PEEP (if intubated), emergent reperfusion (lytics/PCI), may need mechanical circulatory support (eg, IABP).
- **RV systolic dysfunction/cardiogenic shock:** Common in RV AMI; BSUS (few B-lines, ↑ RV:LV ratio, dilated IVC); Tx w/ O_2 for hypoxia, ↑ preload (IVF until e/o nonfluid responsive; ongoing IVF may aggravate), ↓ PVR (bronchodilators, inh NO or prostacyclins), inotropy PRN (milrinone > norepi), minimize PEEP/TV (if intubated), emergent reperfusion (lytics/pPCI); avoid nitrates as they reduce RV preload
- **Tachyarrhythmias (eg, VT/VF, AF):** Ischemia causes re-entry circuits in myocardium; place defibrillation pads on pt immediately on arrival; If unstable, tx per ACLS; If stable VT, tx w/ IV BB/membrane stabilization (amiodarone, metoprolol), check & replete lytes; emergent reperfusion (lytics/pPCI)
- **Bradyarrhythmias:** Heart block can be 2/2 strong vagal tone (1° HB) &/or ischemia to AV node (1°–3° HB); place pacer pads on pt immediately on arrival; Tx w/ IVF (for BP), atropine, TC/TV pacing if unstable; emergent reperfusion (lytics/pPCI)

Early Complications

- **Infarct expansion, reinfarction, postinfarction ischemia:** Usually w/i 4 d of MI; can present similarly to initial MI or w/ new sx; dx can be challenging: Δ ECG (2/2 nl evolution from prior MI vs new ischemia), +Tn (may be elevated from prior MI; new ↑ is concerning), +CK-MB (suggests new ischemia); tx as w/ ACS; discuss w/ cardiology; depending on prior mgmt (PCI vs lytics; BA vs DES), may need PCI
- **Ventricular wall rupture:** Usually w/i 2–7 d after untreated MI; RFs include ↑ age, female, anterior infarct, ↑ wall strain (↑ HR, ↑ afterload), unsuccessful reperfusion; Presents w/ sudden death, PEA, deterioration. Dx w/ echo
  - **Free wall rupture:** Rapid bleeding into pericardium causing s/sx of tamponade; Tx w/ IVF/blood; emergent pericardiocentesis & cardiac surgery; mortality >90%
  - **Pseudoaneurysm:** Bleeding contained w/i myocardial wall; may p/w arrhythmias, heart failure, systemic embolization, or be asx & dx'ed only on imaging; once identified, c/s cardiology & cardiac surgery
  - **Septal rupture:** Often occurs early (<24 h after untreated MI). Maybe asx or p/w sx of L → R shunt & ↓ L-sided CO (angina, shock, pulm edema); new holosystolic murmur; dx by echo; tx w/ urgent surgical closure
- **Papillary muscle rupture:** Usually w/i 7 d of untreated MI; frequency i-MI & p-MI > a-MI; p/w sx of acute pulm edema, systolic murmur; BSUS differentiate from post-MI VSD; tx w/ ↓ preload & afterload (NTG), diuretics, O_2, IABP, emergent surgical repair
- **Pericarditis:** Usually w/i 7 d of MI; most common w/ a-MI; p/w low-grade fever, CP, friction rub; ECG w/ diffuse STE w/o reciprocal chgs; BSUS ± pericardial effusion; tx w/ ASA, avoid other NSAIDs for initial 7–10 d post-MI. Note: Early post-MI pericarditis is distinct from Dressler synd (below)

Delayed Complications

- **Left ventricular aneurysm:** Suspect if ECG w/ persistent STE post-MI; can p/w HF, embolic sx, arrhythmias; dx w/ echo; c/s cardiology (reperfusion), cardiac surgery
- **Left ventricular thrombus:** Most common in a-MI; RFs include ↓ EF, severe MVR, LV aneurysm (eg, slow, nonlaminar flow); P/w cardioembolic dz; tx w/ anticoagulation
- **Dressler syndrome:** Usually weeks-months after MI; presumed autoimmune mediated; p/w fever, CP, pleurisy; BSUS w/ pericardial & pl effusions; tx w/ NSAIDs (ASA preferred)

VASOSPASTIC (VARIANT/PRINZMETAL) ANGINA

Overview

- **Definition:** Distinct synd of ischemic CP classically occurring at rest 2/2 focal coronary artery spasm, & a/w transient STE
- Commonly occurs in areas of pre-existing atherosclerotic plaque
- Can be a/w infarction, arrhythmia, & sudden cardiac death; consider in all pts w/ healthy SCD

History
- Often young (35–50 y/o), F > M, tobacco, EtOH, stimulant use; PMH/FHx migraine, Raynaud's, pericarditis, MV prolapse; may have no known cardiac hx but CAD not uncommon
- Sxs include substernal pressure radiating to jaw & arm; can respond to NTG; often occur midnight to early AM (↑ vagal tone), or after hyperventilation or cold
- May be a/w marked diurnal variation in exercise tolerance (↓ tolerance in AM, ↑ in PM)

Evaluation
- ECG reveals transient territorial STE & reciprocal ST Δs; may induce a variety of conduction disturbances or arrhythmias
- Stress testing to evaluate for fixed obstructive lesion may induce no ST Δs, STDs, or STEs, or STEs may be seen during recovery phase of stress testing if exercise induced
- Dx definitively w/ angiography & provocative intracoronary ACh &/or ergot derivative

Treatment
- High-dose CCB (nifedipine, verapamil, diltiazem), nitrates PRN; D/C smoking & triggers
- Avoid beta blockers (can aggravate sxs), consider long-term nitrates in those w/ persistent sxs despite CCB

Disposition
- Admit, given risk of MI & arrhythmia during acute episodes

COCAINE-INDUCED ANGINA

Overview
- Definition: Anginal sx occurring after cocaine use, 2/2 ↑ myocardial O_2 demand (↑ HR, ↑ afterload, ↑ contractility & end-systolic wall stress) & ↓ O_2 supply (coronary artery vasoconstriction); generally not 2/2 acute thrombosis, though cocaine a/w premature CAD/ACS
- Cocaine is associated w/ ~25% of MIs in those <45 years old (*Circulation* 2001;103(4):502)
  - Most cocaine-associated MIs occur w/o significant underlying CAD
- Can be c/b arrhythmia & heart failure (~90% occur w/i 12 h of presentation)

History
- CP may be a/w dyspnea, anxiety, palpitations, diaphoresis, dizziness, or nausea
- Sxs typically occur w/i 3 h of ingestion, but cocaine metabolites may persist up to 24 h to cause delayed or recurrent vasoconstriction
- RF for cocaine-induced MI: current smoker, EtOH use, pregnancy

Evaluation
- Similar to ACS (see above)
- Maintain high index of suspicion for AoD
- Urine toxicology: Usually detects cocaine metabolite benzoylecgonine (urine $t_{1/2}$ of 6–8 h) up to 24–48 h (range 16–66 h); however, chronic cocaine users may have detectable levels for weeks after last use

Treatment
- Given risk of MI, tx similarly to ACS (see ACS, "Adjunctive Medical Therapies")
  - ASA, analgesia PRN, O_2 PRN, NTG PRN, antithrombotic tx all as per ACS guidelines
  - Avoid BB given (largely theoretical) risk of unopposed α-adrenergic effect (↑ CA vasospasm, ↑ BP)
- IV Benzodiazepines (↓ central stimulatory effects of cocaine)
- IV Anti-HTN (NTG, sodium nitroprusside, phentolamine; avoid BB)
- If STEMI: 1° PCI preferred over lytics 2/2 ↑ ICH risk after cocaine
- VT/VF immediately after cocaine is 2/2 Na channel blockade & may respond to sodium bicarbonate tx in addition to standard therapies

Disposition
- Admit: If +Tn, ongoing CP, persistent unstable VS
- EDOU: If sx & VS controlled, –Tn, nonischemic ECG; no difference in 30-d outcomes if pts w/ & w/o stress testing, consider if CAD RFs & f/u plan (*Circulation* 2008;117:1897–1907)
- Provide drug-abuse counseling to all pts prior to D/C

SPONTANEOUS CORONARY ARTERY DISSECTION (SCAD)

(*Circulation* 2018;137(19):e523–e557)

Overview
- Nontraumatic separation of coronary artery wall
- Rare cause of ACS but may account of 25% of cases among women <50 y old (*Circulation* 2012;126(5):579)

History
- Anginal CP ± dyspnea, diaphoresis, n/v
- RF for SCAD: female sex (>85%), fibromuscular dysplasia, connective tissue/autoimmune dz, migraines, multiparity, hormone tx
- Consider in young pt presenting w/ MI or card arrest

Evaluation
- Similar to STEMI/NSTEMI (see above)
- EKG chgs common inc STE
- Cardiac CT angiography may not be sens
- Dx is made in the cath lab w/ invasive coronary angiography

Treatment
- Tx similarly to ACS (see ACS, "Adjunctive Medical Therapies"). Consider DAPT
- Revascularization may be deferred in stable pts. Unstable pts require PCI vs CABG
  - Fibrinolysis should be avoided
- BB tx associated w/ ↓ recurrence

Disposition
- Admx to CCU/cardiology based on risk, clinical stability

DVT AND PULMONARY EMBOLISM

Deep Vein Thrombosis

Overview
- Definition: In situ thrombosis of LE/UE deep veins, often provoked by stasis/turbulence, hypercoagulability, endothelial injury (Virchow triad)
- RFs: hypercoagulable state (eg, cancer, pregnancy, OCPs, APS, systemic inflammation, inherited thrombophilia); recent surgery or trauma; prolonged immobilization; venous outlet obstruction; excess extremity use (eg, sports, occupation; for UE DVT); ↑ age; obesity; PMH or FHx of DVT/PE; smoking; recent hospitalization
- Lower-extremity DVT: ~90% of DVTs, but as many as 50% may be isolated distal DVT of the calf (only require tx if severe sx or propagating; see below)
- Upper-extremity DVT: ~10% of DVTs; c/w LE DVT, ↓ risk of PE (6% vs 15–32%), ↓ risk of recurrence (2–5% vs 10%); can be 1° (20%) or 2° (80%) (*NEJM* 2011;364(9):861–869; *Circulation* 2012;126:768–773)
  - Primary: thoracic outlet compression of subclavian (SC) vein (eg, ribs, clavicle), microtrauma to SC vein from repeated UE movements (often young, athletes or occupation), idiopathic
  - Secondary: catheter-associated, cancer-associated (hypercoag, compression), surgery (immobilization, endothelial trauma), systemic hypercoag state (preg, etc)
  - Mgmt based on location (proximal vs distal), depth (deep vs superficial)

History & Physical Examination
- Hx & Ex: May have unilateral discomfort, swelling, paresthesia, weakness, erythema, warmth, palpable cord, tenderness along deep venous system, dilation of collaterals
  - Always ask about RFs; perform ROS to assess for s/sx of concurrent PE
  - Physical exam notoriously insensitive for DVT. Difference in calf diameter is most useful PE finding (*Ann Intern Med* 2005;143(2):129)

Evaluation
- Use Wells score to determine pre-TP of DVT (see *Table*), dx confirmed by + US

Modified Wells Criteria for DVT (From *NEJM*. 2003;349(13):1227–1235. Table 1.)				
Active cancer (tx ongoing or w/i 6 mos or palliative)				1 Pt
Paralysis, paresis, or recent immobilization of LE				1 Pt
Recently bedridden >3 d or major surgery w/i 4 wks				1 Pt
Localized tenderness along deep venous system				1 Pt
Entire leg swelling				1 Pt
Calf swelling by >3 cm c/w asx (10 cm below tibial tuberosity)				1 Pt
Pitting edema (greater in symptomatic leg)				1 Pt
Collateral superficial veins (nonvaricose)				1 Pt
Previously documented DVT				1 Pt
Alternative dx as likely or greater than that of DVT				–2 Pts
Points	**Pre-Test Prob**	**D-dimer Sens (%)**	**Prevalence of DVT (%)**	**NPV of D-dimer (%)**
–2–0 pts	Low	86	3%	99
1–2 pts	Mod	85	17	95
≥3 pts	High	90	53	81

- Low and mod pre-TP pts can be ruled out for DVT w/ neg D-dimer, high-risk pts should undergo compression US
  - Standard D-dimer cutoff = 500 ng/mL; high-sens D-dimer, sens 96% spec 34% (*Blood Adv* 2020;4(7):1250–1264)
  - Age-adjusted and pre–TP-adjusted cutoffs can increase spec

Figure 1.2 Diagnosis of DVT.

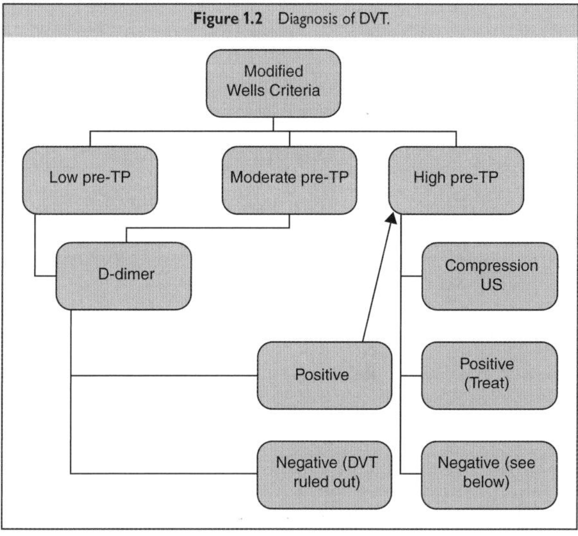

- UE DVT: Compression US (sens 97%, spec 96%) (*NEJM* 2011;364(9):861–869; *Ann Intern Med* 2014;160(7):451–457)
- LE DVT (initial eval): Imaging test results based on pre-TP and extent of US: whole leg (WL; superior) or proximal vein (PV) US
  - Low pre-TP: neg US (PV or WL) rules out DVT
  - Mod pre-TP:
    - Neg WL: DVT ruled out
    - Neg PV: obtain WL or repeat PV at 7 d
  - High pre-TP:
    - Neg WL: Consider iliac vein thrombosis if proximal s/sx
    - Neg PV: obtain WL or repeat PV at 3 and 7 d

- CT venography: High sens but ↑ radiation & contrast; consider if mod or high pre-TP, pos D-dimer & neg PC-US but unable to obtain WL-US or repeat PC-US
- LE DVT (recurrent on the same side): high risk of false-positives (2/2 scarring, post-thrombotic synd); compare US findings to prior

Figure 1.3 Diagnosis and treatment of DVT, mod or high pretest probability. (**A**) Starting with D-dimer assessment, and (**B**) Starting with ultrasonography (preferred for high PTP). (*Chest* 2012;141(2 suppl):e351S)

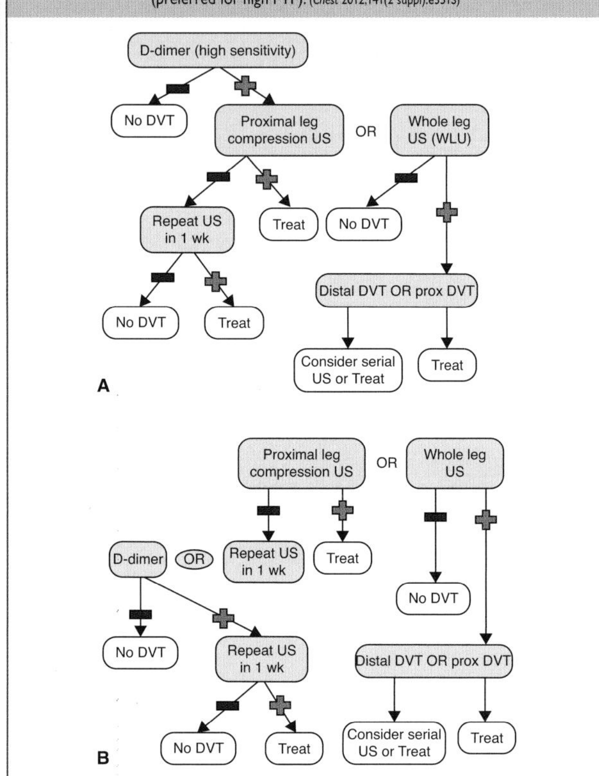

Treatment (*Blood Adv* 2020;4(19):4693–4738)

- UE DVT: Anticoagulation × 3–6 mos minimum, though comparative data lacking on specific regimens
  - Cather-associated DVT: Catheter removal only indicated if catheter malfxn or infxn, no further need for catheter, or strong CIs to systemic A/C
  - Isolated basilic/cephalic vein thrombosis: Very low risk of PE, A/C rarely required
- LE DVT: Anticoagulation × 3–6 mos minimum unless strong CIs. DOACs are usually preferred
  - If strong CIs to A/C: IVC filter until bleeding risk resolves
- Isolated distal DVT: Tx as above if severe sx or high-risk (extension on repeat US, previous VTE, age >50, cancer, unprovoked, persistent immobilization, >1 calf vein, known thrombophilia), can consider prophylactic AC dosing (*Eur Heart J* 2018;39(47):4208)
- Duration of tx generally depends if provoked (3 mos) or unprovoked (no identifiable RFs) or active malignancy (extended if no bleeding risk, 3 mos if bleeding risk)

Anticoagulation Regimens

- Anticoagulation regimen should be selected based on comorbidities, ability to take PO medications, pt preference (monitoring, etc), risks of bleeding:
  - DOACs are most commonly started for o/p mgmt
- PO Rivaroxaban (15 mg BID × 3 wks, 20 mg QD thereafter)
- PO Apixaban (10 mg BID × 7 d, 5 mg BID thereafter)
- SC LMWH (1 mg/kg BID; renally dose): slight ↓ risk of death, recurrence, major bleeding c/w UFH; preferred w/ malignancy & pregnancy; relative CIs include CKD & obesity
- IV UFH (80 U/kg bolus, 18 U/kg/h gtt): As above, may be preferred over LMWH if CKD/ESRD; risk of HIT higher than LMWH
- SC Fondaparinux (5 mg QD [<50 kg], 7.5 mg QD [50–100 kg], 10 mg QD [>100 kg]; renally dose): similar risk of death, recurrence, major bleeding c/w LMWH; preferred w/ hx of HIT
- PO Warfarin (INR 2.0–3.0): Bridge w/ LMWH/Fondaparinux until INR therapeutic

Complications

- **Phlegmasia alba dolens (Painful white leg):** emergent cx; P/w swollen white leg 2/2 extensive DVT obstructing collaterals (but not involving them), largely impeding arterial inflow, a/w arterial spasm; Tx w/ IV heparin (in case need for surgery), +/– catheter-directed thrombolytic tx
- **Phlegmasia cerulea dolens (Painful blue leg):** emergent cx; P/w severely swollen cyanotic leg 2/2 extensive iliofemoral DVT inc thrombosis of collaterals & capillary beds, fully impeding arterial flow, causing massive fluid sequestration in affected limb (2/2 hydrostatic pressure), circulatory shock, death (20–40% cases); Tx w/ IV heparin (in case need for surgery), catheter-directed thrombolytic tx, aspiration thrombectomy, or open surgical thrombectomy, transfer to IR capable facility

Disposition

- Most pts can be managed in o/p setting w/ anticoagulation
- Pts w/ severe pain, severe swelling, signs of cxs, or high risk for AC-related bleeding or AC failure (eg, inherited thrombophilia, malignancy) should be admitted
  - Pts who fail AC or w/ cxs or massive iliofemoral DVT may require thrombolysis or thrombectomy

---

PULMONARY EMBOLISM

Overview

- Definition: embolization of venous thrombus into pulmonary arterial system
  - Diff from amniotic fluid embolism (RF: peripartum) & fat embolism (RF: long-bone fx)
- RFs: See section on DVT above; major identifiable RFs include recent surgery (OR 21.0), trauma (OR 12.7), immobility (hosp or nursing home; OR 8.0), cancer (OR 4.1–6.5), paraplegia (OR 3.0), estrogen tx (OR 3.0) (*JAMA* 2003;290(21):2849–2858)
- Most PEs arise from lower extremity DVTs.
  - Over 50% of pts w/ diagnosed proximal DVTs have co-occurring PEs (*Am J Med* 2007; 120(1):871)

Approach

- IV access, ECG, O_2 prn, Monitor, CXR to r/o alternative dx
- If HD stable: diagnostic testing based on pre-TP
- If unstable, consider empiric antithrombotic tx ± lysis if potential benefit > bleeding risk

History & Physical Examination

- Hx: SOB, CP (+/– pleuritic), cough, syncope, hemoptysis
  - Sx may be mild or absent, even in pts w/ large PE
- Assess pre-TP: In low-risk pts, may use PERC criteria to decide whether any testing is necessary or Wells criteria for risk stratification (to decide whether D-dimer is sufficient initial w/u)
- Ex: unexplained ↑ HR, ↑ RR, ↓ SpO_2, fever, JVD, ↓ BP, signs of DVT, SOB w/ clear lungs

Pulmonary Embolism Rule Out Criteria (PERC) for Pts w/ Low Risk of PE	
Age <50	No recent trauma or surgery or hosp w/i 4 wks
HR <100	No hemoptysis
O_2 Sat on room air ≥95%	No exogenous estrogen use
No prior hx of DVT/PE	No unilateral leg swelling

If all of above criteria present in low-risk pt, PE can be r/o (false negative rate ~1%). If not ruled out, obtain PE w/u w/ additional dx tests (*Thromb Haemost* 2008;6:772).

Evaluation

- ECG: sinus tach is most common, S1Q3T3 pattern not sens/spec, diffuse TWI (V1–V4), RBBB
- Labs: CBC, PT/PTT, BMP, cardiac enzymes, BNP, D-dimer if low or mod risk
- CXR: r/o other dx; "classic" PE findings (Hampton's hump: pl wedge-shaped infarct, Westermark sign: unilateral lung oligemia) not sens/spec
- Determine pre-TP using Wells score or revised Geneva score
- If low risk and PERC criteria neg, no need for further testing
- If low or mod risk, but cannot r/o using PERC, obtain D-dimer
  - Standard cutoff of <500 ng/mL is highly sens (98%) but nonspec (55%) (*Thromb Res* 2018;166:63)
  - Age-adjusted D-dimer cutoff = Age (years) × 10 FEU for pts >50, increases spec while maintaining high sens (PLOS Med 2022;19(1):e1003905)
  - YEARS algorithm incorporates differential D-dimer cutoff values based on clinical pre-TP (see *Table* below). Validated in all trimesters of pregnancy (*NEJM* 2019;380(12):1139)
  - False-positive D-dimer: pregnancy, trauma, infxn, malignancy, inflammatory conditions, surgery, ↑ age, SCD, AF, ACS, CVA, acute UGIB, DIC

Wells Criteria for PE (*Thromb Haemost* 2000;83(3):416–420; *JAMA* 2006;295(2):172–179)	
Criteria	**Original**
Clinical signs & sx of DVT	3 pts
Tachycardia >100 bpm	1.5 pts
Immobilization or surgery w/i 4 wks	1.5 pts
Previous DVT/PE	1.5 pts
Hemoptysis	1 pt
Malignancy	1 pt
PE more likely than alternative dx	3 pts
Original Wells Criteria Probability Scoring	
Low[a]	<2.0 pts
Mod[a]	2.0–6.0 pts
High[b]	>6.0 pts
Modified Wells Criteria Probability Scoring	
PE unlikely[a]	<4.0 pts
PE likely[b]	>4.0 pts
Revised Geneva Score for PE (*Ann Intern Med* 2006;144(3):165–171)	
Criteria	**Original**
Age >65	1 pt
Previous DVT/PE	3 pts
Surgery (under GA) or fx (LE) w/i 1 mo	2 pts
Active malignancy or cure <1 y	2 pts
Unilateral LE pain	3 pts
Hemoptysis	2 pts
HR 75–94	3 pts
HR ≥95	5 pts
Pain w/ LE deep vein palpation & unilateral edema	4 pts
Scoring	
Low[a]	<3 pts
Mod[a]	4–10 pts
High[b]	>11

[a]Order D-dimer to r/o out PE.
[b]Order imaging (CTA, V/Q) to r/o PE.

YEARS Algorithm (*Lancet* 2017;390(10091):289)	
Criteria (+1 pt each)	**D-dimer Cutoffs**[a]
S/s of DVT	0 pts = if D-dimer <1,000 then PE excluded
Hemoptysis	1+ pts if D-dimer = <500 then PE excluded
PE most likely Dx	[a]Decreased CT by 14% as compared to Wells

- If high risk by Wells/Geneva score, + D-dimer, or + YEARS criteria, obtain additional testing:
  - Bedside US: Echo for RV dilatation (RV:LV > 1) or dysfxn (HK, paradoxical septal wall motion, McConnell sign [akinesis of RV free wall w/ preserved apical movement]) can suggest dx but not r/o (sens 50%, spec 98%, PPV 88%, NPV 88%) *(Ann Emerg Med 2014;63(1):16–24)*
  - CT pulm angiography (sens 94%, spec 98%) *(Blood Adv 2020;4(18):4296)* is first line
    - May miss small/subsegmental PEs (of uncertain clinical significance), requires contrast load (consider risk/benefits in pts w/ contrast allergy or low GFR)
    - Can identify alternate diagnoses
  - V/Q scan (sens 58–98%, spec 36–95%): Obtain if CI to CT-PA, requires nl baseline CXR; tx if results are high probability; 2/3 of all cases may result in low/intermediate probability or be nondiagnostic *(Blood Adv 2020;4(18):4296)*
  - MR angiography (MRA sens 78%, spec 99%; MRA/MRV sens 92%, spec 96%): Use in pts w/ CI to CTA; high proportion of studies w/ limited qual *(Ann Intern Med 2010;152(7):434–443)*
  - Catheter-based pulm angiogram: Gold standard, though rarely used

Risk Stratification

- HR, ↓ BP, ↓ SpO_2, CTA RV/LV dimension >0.9, ↑ Tn or BNP, US e/o RV dysfxn or w/ R-sided thrombus, older age all predict bad outcomes
- PESI (pulmonary embolism severity index): Can be used to predict 30-d outcome

PESI Score *(Am J Respir Crit Care Med 2005;172(8):1041)*	
Criteria	**Points**[a]
Age	Age in years
Sex	Female = 0, Male = 10
Hx of cancer	Yes = +30
Hx of heart failure	Yes = +10
Hx of chronic lung Dz	Yes = +10
HR >/110 bpm	Yes = +20
SBP <100 mmHg	Yes = +30
RR >/30/min	Yes = +20
T <36°	Yes = +20
AMS (lethargy, disorientation, coma, stupor)	Yes = +60
O_2 saturation <90%	Yes = +20

Risk Based on Score *(Thromb Haemost 2008;100(5):943)*					
Risk	Very low	Low	Intermediate	High	Very high
Score	<66	66–85	86–105	106–125	>125
30-d mort	0–1.6%	1.7–3.5%	3.2–7.1%	4–11.4%	10–24.5%

[a]If risk low or very low, consider o/p mgmt if no other criteria for admx, for higher scores consider ICU given high risk of morbidity & mortality.

Simplified PESI Score *(Arch Intern Med 2010;170(15):1383)*	
All criteria = +1 point	
Age >80	
Hx of cancer	
Hx of chronic cardiopulmonary dz	0 pt = low risk (consider o/p) ≥1 pt = high risk
HR ≥110 bpm	
SBP <100 mmHg	
O_2 saturation <90%	

Treatment

- Supportive: O_2, IV fluids & pressors for ↓ BP (avoid excessive IVF as can worsen RV dsfxn)
- Anticoagulation *(see A/C regimens under DVT)*
- IV thrombolysis (tPA: 10 mg IV bolus f/b 90 mg over 2 h): Indicated if HD instability (SBP <90 mmHg) w/ confirmed PE or HD unstable & high suspicion of PE, or submassive PE (not hypotensive but w/ ↑ Tn or BNP or RV dysfxn) w/ high risk of hypotension (e/o significant pHTN or RV dysfxn, low bleeding risk)
  - Consider lytics in unexplained PEA arrest if possibly 2/2 massive PE
- Catheter-directed or surgical thrombectomy: For pts w/ HD instability & massive PE if (1) CI to lysis, (2) failed lysis, or (3) experienced center & +RV dysfxn. C/s cardiac surgery *(Circulation 2023;147(9):e628–e647)*
- IVC filter: When a/c fails or CI; no long-term mortality benefit *(NEJM 1998;338:409)*

Disposition

- Low risk, HD stable, few comorbidities, no e/o RV strain: initiate AC, echo, D/C w/ close FU vs observation based on local guidelines
- HD stable, comorbidities, e/o RV strain: Admit, tele floor
- HD unstable, mx comorbidities, e/o RV strain, AMS, resp distress: Admit, ICU

DECOMPENSATED HEART FAILURE

Overview

- Heart failure: When the heart's ability to pump blood at rate needed to meet the body's metabolic demands is impaired; either 2/2 ↓ systolic fxn (reduced EF: HFrEF) or ↓ diastolic relaxation (preserved EF: HFpEF); can be primarily L-sided, R-sided, or biventricular; although a chronic illness, characterized by intermittent decompensations 2/2 volume disequilibrium
- Manifestations of decompensated L-sided HF: pulm edema and pl effusions (2/2 ↑ hydrostatic pressure), atrial arrhythmias (2/2 ↑ atrial size), systemic hypoperfusion (HFrEF: ↑ LV end-diastolic volume → ↓ contractility [once over Frank–Starling curve] → ↓ EF & CO; HFpEF: ↓ LV end-diastolic volume 2/2 impaired relaxation → ↓ CO)
- Manifestations of decompensated R-sided HF: SOB, peripheral edema (↑ systemic venous pressure), liver dysfxn (congestion), JVD
- Acute decompensations can occur 2/2 many causes (see *Table*)

Common Precipitants of ADHF	
Medication Δ or nonadherence[a]	Hypertensive crisis (↑ afterload)
Dietary indiscretion (↑ Na, ↑ fluid)	O/ds (BB, CCB), Illicit drugs or EtOH
Bradyarrhythmia	Anemia
Myocardial infarct/ischemia	Myopericarditis, endocarditis
Tachyarrhythmia (eg, AF)	Sepsis, infxn
COPD/PE (↑ RH pressures, hypoxia)	*Valvular heart dz (see Table at end of section)*
Renal failure (↑ volume)	*Structural heart dz (see Table at end of section)*

[a]Esp diuretics, anti-HTN, or rate-controlling agents; however, review any med chgs, as may have pharmacokinetic properties that affect cardiac meds.

Approach

- Initiate immediately: IV access, O_2 PRN, ECG, monitor, CXR
- If e/o severe resp distress, early CPAP/BiPAP, NTG gtt (unless ↓ BP)
- Early use of bedside US (thoracic & echo) can reduce time to dx

History & Physical Examination

- Hx: SOB/DOE, CP, cough (clear → pink sputum), orthopnea/PND, LE/abd swelling, weight gain
  - Always ask: timing (acuity), severity (fxnal capacity), behavioral chgs (sleeping upright), chgs in home O_2, frequency of weight monitoring & any Δ from dry weight
  - Always assess for possible precipitants & concurrent illness (see Table above)
- Ex: ↑ HR, ↑ RR, ↑ BP (usually), cardiac dysrhythmia; +S3 (HFrEF), +S4 (HFpEF); rales or ↓ BS, wheeze (L-sided); leg edema, JVD, ↑ liver size, +hepatojugular reflex, cold vs warm

Acute Decompensated HF: Hx & PEx Findings (*JAMA 2005;294:1944*)			
Increase Likelihood of ADHF		**Decrease Likelihood of ADHF**	
Historical Factor	**Likelihood Ratio (95% CI)**	**Historical Factor**	**Likelihood Ratio (95% CI)**
H/o heart failure	5.8 (4.1–8)	No h/o HF	0.45 (0.38–0.53)
H/o MI	3.1 (2–4.9)	No DOE	0.48 (0.35–0.67)
PND	2.6 (1.5–4.5)		
Orthopnea	2.2 (1.2–3.9)		
Historical Features w/ Minimal Diagnostic Utility			
H/o CAD, HLD, DM, HTN, COPD, smoking. Sxs of edema, cough, fatigue, & weight gain			

Increase Likelihood of ADHF		Decrease Likelihood of ADHF	
Exam Factor	Likelihood Ratio (95% CI)	Exam Factor	Likelihood Ratio (95% CI)
S3 on auscultation	11 (4.9–25)	No rales	0.51 (0.37–0.7)
JVD	5.1 (3.2–7.9)		
Rales	2.8 (1.9–4.1)		
Any murmur	2.6 (1.7–4.1)		
LE edema	2.3 (1.5–3.7)		
Exam Features w/ Minimal Diagnostic Utility			
Abdominojugular reflex, SBP <100 mmHg or >150 mmHg, wheezing, ascites			

Evaluation

- Acute decompensated HF is primarily a clinical dx, aided by lab & imaging evals
- ECG: L-atrial enlargement, LVH, tachyarrhythmia, ischemia, e/o old infarction(s)
- Labs: CBC, lytes, Cr, troponin, LFTs, VBG, BNP/NT-proBNP (see below)
- Bedside thoracic US: >3 B-lines/field in 2+ lung fields bilaterally; operator dependent, but w/ skilled operator may be superior to CXR in dx of L-sided HF (*JAMA Netw Open* 2019;2(3):e190703); can evaluate for:
  - Pl effusions (2/2 CHF or other dx)
  - Focal B-lines (eg, 2/2 PNA, infarct > asymmetric pulm edema)
  - Reduced EF & pericardial effusion
  - IVC inspiratory collapsibility: <30–50% collapsibility w/ inspiration & diameter >2 cm suggests volume overload; cannot be used if pt on PPV (*J Ultrasound Med* 2020;39(7):1367–1378)
- CXR (sens 73%, spec 90%): pulm edema, pl effusion, ↑ heart size HF (*JAMA Netw Open* 2019;2(3):e190703)
- BNP (>100 ng/L), NT-proBNP (>300 ng/L): Compare w/ dry weight BNP if hx of CHF; levels correlate w/ dz severity of underlying CHF (*NEJM* 2002;347:161–167)
  - False-negs: obesity, very acute heart failure
  - False-positives: Renal failure/ESRD, ↑ age, valvular dz, cor pulmonale, AMI, sepsis

Pooled Sensitivity & Specificity of BNP/NT-proBNP for AD-CHF (*BMJ* 2015;350:h910)					
BNP Level	**Sens (%)**	**Spec (%)**	**NT-proBNP Level**	**Sens (%)**	**Spec (%)**
≤100 ng/L	95	63	≤300 ng/L	99	43
100–500 ng/L	85	86	300–1,800 pg/mL	90	76
≥500 ng/L	35	78	≥1,800 ng/L	67	72

Treatment

- **Diuresis (↓ volume):** Pts w/ refractory edema have impaired PO absorption & may need IV diuresis; give 2× home loop diuretic dose in IV form; give home nonloop diuretics (eg, metolazone) for sequential nephron blockade
  - Conversions: furosemide:torsemide:bumetanide 40:20:1 IV; furosemide (PO:IV) 2:1; torsemide (PO:IV) 1:1; bumetanide (PO:IV) 1:1
  - If allergy to furosemide/torsemide/bumetanide, can use ethacrynic acid
- **Nitrates (↓ preload):** nitrates (0.4 mg SL q5min or 10–300 mcg/min IV): Caution in pts w/ AS → ↓ BP 2° preload depnitroprusside if NTG ineffective
- **Positive pressure ventilation:** CPAP/BiPAP for ↓ SpO_2 or increase WOB (if no CIs); ↓ mortality, ↓ need for intubation (*Cochrane Syst Rev* 2019;4(4):CD005351); intubate profound AMS, resp failure
- **Inotropes:** for cardiogenic shock (see section on *Shock*)
- **Other:** Positioning (sit up > supine), O_2 to maintain sat >/90%, Foley may be necessary to assess I/Os, PCI if ACS, IABP/LVAD (severe cardiogenic shock), VA-ECMO for severe unresponsive shock

Disposition

- Low risk: mild exacerbation, known dx, benign etiology (ie, dietary indiscretion), & close f/u: D/C after discussion w/ cardiologist; may ↑ diuretic for a few days
- Select HF pts can be managed by a rapid tx protocol in short stay/observation unit w/ similar outcomes to admitted pts (*JAMA Netw Open* 2024;7(1):e2350511)
- Most pts require admx/Δs to tx regimen before D/C home: cardiology/tele
- All pts on PPV, severe resp distress, signs of poor perfusion: ICU

Structural Causes of Heart Failure	
Dilated CMP	**Pathophys:** Ventricular dilatation → ↓ contractility → ↑ EDV → ↓ EF **Causes:** Idiopathic, familial, ischemia, valvular, infxn (Chagas), EtOH, cocaine, autoimmune **Presentation:** L or R HF sx; embolic events; arrhythmia **Evaluation:** ECG (PRWP, Qw, BBB, AF), CXR (↑ heart size), echo (LV dilatation, ↓ EF, LV ± RV HK) **Treatment:** See standard HF tx **Pearl:** Always consider in chronic EtOH users w/ SOB
Hypertrophic CMP	**Pathophys:** LV outflow tract obstruction, worse if ↓ EDV → ↓ EF **Causes:** 50% are familial; asymmetric septal hypertrophy (eg, 2/2 HTN) may result in HOCM physiology (not true HOCM) **Presentation:** SOB/angina; arrhythmias; sudden death **Evaluation:** Systolic crescendo/decrescendo murmur; ECG (LVH, septal Qw), CXR (↑ heart size), echo (↑ septal thickness) **Treatment:** BB, CCB **Pearl:** Avoid diuretics/preload reduction (inc PPV), digoxin, exercise
Restrictive CMP	**Pathophys:** ↓ compliance → ↓ EDV → ↓ EF **Causes:** Amyloidosis, sarcoidosis, hemochromatosis, XRT, cancer **Presentation:** R > L HF; embolic events; poor response to diuretics **Evaluation:** ↑ JVP, S3, S4, ECG (low voltage), CXR (pulm edema w/o ↑ heart size), echo (symmetric wall thickening, LAE/RAE) **Treatment:** Treat underlying cause, gentle diuresis
Constrictive pericarditis	**Pathophys:** ↓ compliance → ↓ EDV → ↓ EF **Causes:** Postviral, XRT, TB, postcardiac surgery, idiopathic **Presentation:** R > L HF **Evaluation:** ↑ JVP, pericardial knock; echo (septal bounce) **Treatment:** Diuresis, pericardiotomy

Valvular Heart Disease (*Circulation* 2021;143:e72)	
Aortic stenosis	**Causes:** Calcification (age >70 y), bicuspid valve, rheumatic heart dz **Presentation:** Angina, exertional syncope, CHF **Exam:** Midsystolic, crescendo–decrescendo @ RUSB that radiates to carotids, S4 gallop, soft S2, delayed & diminished carotid pulses (pulsus tardus & parvus) **Eval:** Echo (transvalvular velocity, EF, aortic valve area [AVA]) **Acute tx:** ↓ Afterload; minimize ↓ preload & neg inotropy (avoid vasodilators, diuretics); if severe acute HF decompensation 2/2 critical AS, c/s cardiac surg for consideration of urgent AVR, balloon valvuloplasty as bridge **Pearl:** Indications for AVR (if sx) include: V_{max} ≥4 m/s or ΔP_{mean} ≥40 mmHg; V_{max} <4 m/s + AVA ≤1.0 cm^2 + EF <50%; or V_{max} <4 m/s + AVA ≤1.0 cm^2 + SVI <35 mL/m^3
Aortic regurg	**Causes:** Rheumatic heart dz, bicuspid valve, endocarditis, aortic root abnormalities (aneurysm, dissection) **Presentation:** Acute or chronic CHF **Exam:** Diastolic decrescendo murmur, wide pulse pressure, water hammer pulse, spontaneous nailbed pulsations, to-and-fro murmur over femoral artery **Eval:** Echo: Severity of AI → width of regurgitant jet **Acute tx:** ↓ Afterload (nifedipine, ACEi); vasodilators ± dobutamine; if severe & unstable, c/s cardiac surg for consideration of urgent AVR **Pearl:** Indications for AVR (if sx): VC >0.6 cm, holodiastolic aortic flow reversal, Regurg Vol ≥60 mL, Regurg F ≥50%, ERO ≥0.3 cm^3
Mitral stenosis	**Causes:** Rheumatic heart dz, congenital, annular calcification **Presentation:** CHF, AF, emboli, hemoptysis, hoarseness **Exam:** Diastolic murmur, opening snap in early diastole, loud S1 **Eval:** ECG (LAE, AF, RVH), echo (valve area, pressure gradients), CXR (LAE->straightening of L heart border) **Acute tx:** Careful diuresis, BBs; however, percutaneous balloon valvuloplasty (PBV) & MVR have best outcomes **Pearl:** Most pts have sx if MVA <1.5 cm^2; MVR vs PBV based on sx; PBV favorable c/w MVR, but 10–40% may have delayed restenosis & require repeat tx (*Lancet* 2009;374:1271–1283)

Mitral regurg	**Causes:** Chronic (MVP, endocarditis, dilated CMP, connective tissue dz, rheumatic heart dz), acute (AMI, ruptured chordae, papillary muscle dysfxn) **Presentation:** Pulm edema **Exam:** Blowing holosystolic murmur **Eval:** ECG (LAE, ischemia, AF), echo (width of regurgitant jet), CXR (LAE, pulm edema) **Acute tx:** Vasodilators (ACEi, nitrates), BB, diuretics; MV repair is preferred tx for pts w/ sx and severe MR (generally preferred over replacement for pts w/ degenerative MR)

AORTIC DISSECTION

Overview

- **Definition: AoD:** Tearing of the aortic *tunica intima* that allows blood to enter into & traverse the aortic wall b/w *tunica intima* & *tunica media* layers
  - Intramural "false lumen" can obstruct nl flow in true aortic lumen, inc critical vascular branches (esp carotid, celiac, sup/inf mesenteric, renal, & spinal arteries), can rupture through adventitia into pl or pericardial space
  - Can also manifest w/ intramural hemorrhage, penetrating ulcer, pseudoaneurysm, & traumatic rupture
- Classification of dissection impacts mgmt & prognosis (see *Table*)

Prognosis for Aortic Dissection (*Circulation* 2018;137(17):1846–1860)					
Stanford Type	**% of Cases**	**Anatomical Distribution**	**Organs at Risk**	**In hospital Mortality w/ Medical Tx**	**In hospital Mortality w/ Surgical Tx**
Type A	67%	Ascending aorta +/– descending	Brain Coronary artSpinal cord Abd/kidneys Legs	57%	18%
Type B	33%	Descending aorta w/o ascending	Spinal cord Abd/kidneys Legs	10%	30%

Approach

- Immediate IV, ECG, pCXR, analgesia, BP control (if hypertensive)
- c/s cardiothoracic surgery early, esp for type A dissection if clinically suspected
- Key factors: extent of dissection, size of T/F lumens, involvement of branches, presence of periaortic/mediastinal hematoma or pl effusion

Risk Factors for Aortic Dissection (*Circulation* 2010;121:e266)	
Mechanism	**Associated Disorders**
↑ Aortic wall stress	HTN, cocaine/stimulant use, extreme valsalva (eg, power lifting), blunt trauma/deceleration injury, exertion, aortic coarctation, pheochromocytoma
Vulnerability of Ao wall	Genetic disorders (Ehlers–Danlos, Marfan, Turner, Loeys–Dietz, Noonan synds, congenital bicuspid valve, familial dissection), inflammatory vasculitides (SLE, GCA, Behcet, Takayasu), infectious vasculitides (syphilis, TB)
Iatrogenic wall injury	Cardiac/valve surgery, IABP use, aortic cannulation, cath
Other	Male, >50 y, pregnancy, PCKD, chron steroids, immunosupp, FHx

History & Physical Examination

- Individual elements of hx in isolation notoriously insensitive &/or nonspecific (see *Table*)
- Hx: Abrupt onset & often severe CP (ascending), interscapular back pain (descending), or neck pain; often maximal at onset, ripping/tearing in quality, & can migrate; can be a/w syncope, neuro deficits
  - Up to 10% of pts may not p/w pain (more common in chronic dissection)
  - Ask about RFs & consider in all blunt trauma pts w/ CP or back pain

- Ex: Check for murmur (AR), B/L UE BP asymmetry >20 mmHg (↓ sens), pulse deficit, neuro deficits inc Horner synd, abd pain, flank pain, signs of tamponade (JVD, muffled heart sounds, tachycardia, hypotension)

Aortic Dissection: Frequency of History, Exam, & CXR Findings				
	Component	**Overall (%)**	**Type A (%)**	**Type B (%)**
History	Severe/worst-ever pain	90	90	90
	Abrupt onset of pain	90	91	89
	Chest or back pain	85	85	86
	Pain presenting w/i 6 h of sx		79	
	Abdominal pain	30	22	43
Exam	HTN at presentation	49	36	69
	Hypotension, shock, or tamponade	18	27	3
	Any focal neuro deficit	12	17	5
	Any pulse deficit	27	31	21
	Aortic regurgitation	32	44	12
CXR	CXR w/ widened mediastinum	60	63	56
	CXR w/ abnl aortic contour	48	47	49
	CXR nl	16	11	21

IRAD, *Circulation* 2004;110(11 Suppl 1):237; *Lancet* 2008;372:55–66.

Evaluation

- ECG: Assess for inf-STEMI (type A dissection can involve RCA; ~4–8% of thoracic dissections will present w/ signs of STEMI), LVH (e/o chronic HTN), ST-segment chgs
  - In pts w/ inferior STEMI, always consider type A dissection
- Labs: Type & Cross, coags, CBC, lytes, CMP (Cr ↑ w/ renal ischemia), troponin, lactate (↑ w/ any ischemia, ↑↑ may suggest abd viscera ischemia), PT/PTT
- CXR: May be nl; characteristic findings include wide mediastinum, abnl aortic knob, L apical cap, trachea shift → R, depressed L bronchus, L pl effusion, double density appearance of aorta (suggesting true & false lumen)
- Growing data support combined use of D-dimer & ADD-RS to risk stratify for AoD
  - ADD-RS 0–1 & neg D-dimer: sens 98.8% in r/o AoD; ADD 0 & neg D-dimer: sens 99.6%
  - D-dimer not appropriate in pts w/ ADD 2–3, given high false-neg rates
- Bedside cardiac US: positive study includes: intimal flap, intramural hematoma, ascending Ao dilatation, AV insuff, pericardial effusion; operator dependent
- Definitive diagnostic modalities: CTA (sens 100%, spec 98%—first line based on current guidelines), TEE (sens 98%, spec 95%—may be preferred in unstable pts), MRI (sens 98%, spec 98%) (*Circulation* 2022;146(24):e334–e482; *Arch Intern Med* 2006;166:1350–1356)

Aortic Dissection Detection Risk Score (ADD-RS)		
High-Risk Conditions (+1 pt)	**High-Risk Pain Features (+1 pt)**	**High-Risk Exam Features (+1 pt)**

• Marfan synd
• FHx aortic dz
• Known AoV dz
• Recent aortic manipulation
• Known thoracic AA
	• Chest, back, or abd pain described as:
	  • Abrupt in onset
	  • Severe in intensity
	  • Ripping or tearing
		• E/o perfusion deficit (pulse deficit, SBP differential)
		• Focal neuro deficit in conjunction w/ pain
		• Hypotension/shock

Test Characteristics of ADD & Combined Approach Using ADD + D-Dimer[a]				
	ADD-RS Alone		**ADD-RS + Negative D-Dimer**	
ADD-RS	**Sens (%)**	**Spec (%)**	**Sens (%)**	**Spec (%)**
0 (Low risk)	94.6	34.7	99.8	21.8
0–1	43.4	89.3	98.3	51.4

[a]*PLoS One* 2024;19(6):e0304401.

Treatment (*Circulation* 2022;146(24):e334–e482)

- In general, surgical tx preferred for type A, medical tx for type B
- Tx revolves around tight impulse control (BP & HR); Goal HR <60–80, SBP <120 mmHg
  - IV BB gtt preferred to bolus (esmolol, labetalol)
  - If need for further impulse control, particularly BP control: IV CCB gtt (eg, nicardipine). Ensure concomitant BB to avoid reflex tachycardia

- If refractory HTN/tachy: vasodilator (nitroprusside > NTG: w/ concomitant BB)
- A-line for close monitoring (pref RUE or farthest from false lumen)
- Analgesia: Short-acting narcotics preferred in case of hemodynamic chgs
- Urgent surgical consultation should be obtained (cardiothoracic surgery for type A, vascular surgery for type B) for all pts diagnosed w/ thoracic AoD regardless of the location as soon as the dx is made or suspected
  - Type A: Evaluate for emergent surgical repair (1–2% mortality/h in 1st 24 h)
  - Type B: Manage medically w/ consideration for endovascular repair (esp if e/o organ malperfusion, enlarging aneurysm, leaking/rupture, inability to control BP/sx)

Disposition

- All pts w/ acute AoD should be admitted to ICU (+/– via OR)

THORACIC AORTIC ANEURYSM

Overview

- Nl aortic diameter ↑ w/ age, sex (M > F), body surface area, imaging modality
- **Thoracic aortic aneurysm:** Permanent localized dilatation of aortic wall involving tunica intima, tunica media, AND tunica externa, >1.5 × nl aortic diameter; dilatation 1–1.5 × nl is ectatic. (nl size is <3 cm), can occur at root, ascending, arch, or descending
  - Usually 2/2 degenerative dz (see RF for AoD above), ~25% of pts also have an AAA
- **Thoracic aortic pseudoaneurysm:** See TAA, but involves <3 aortic wall layers
- Cxs vary based on diameter; average rate of expansion 0.10–0.42 cm/y

Yearly Complication Rates as a Function of Aortic Size (*Ann Thorac Surg* 2002;74:S1877)

Aortic Size	>3.5 cm (%)	>4 cm (%)	>5 cm (%)	>6 cm (%)
Rupture	0	0.3	1.7	3.6
Dissection	2.2	1.5	2.5	3.7
Death	5.9	4.6	4.8	10.8
Any of above	7.2	5.3	6.5	14.1

History, Physical Examination, & Evaluation

- Hx/Ex: Often discovered incidentally on imaging; sx can vary widely:
  - Compressive sx: hoarseness (compression of recurrent laryngeal nerve), dyspnea (lung compression), dysphagia (esophageal compression), SVC synd
  - Heart failure (2/2 aortic regurgitation), embolization, AoD, rupture
- Imaging: CTA (first line; good sens, quick, noninvasive); MRI (best for aortic root); TTE (limited for eval of aortic root or descending TA); TEE (better than TTE for aortic root & descending TA)

Treatment

- RF modification: lipid profile optimization, smoking cessation, BP control (BB, ACEi), avoid heavy lifting or valsalva
- Urgent open vs endovascular repair as indicated; surveillance w/ repeat imaging if asx and do not yet meet criteria for elective repair

Indications for Urgent Cardiac Surgical Consultation (*Circulation* 2010;121:e266)
• Asx pts w/ degenerative TAAs, chronic AoD, intramural hematoma, penetrating atherosclerotic ulcer, mycotic aneurysm, or pseudoaneurysm for whom the ascending aorta or aortic sinus diameter is ≥5.5 cm
• Pts w/ Marfan synd or other genetically mediated disorders (see above) for whom the ascending aorta or aortic sinus diameter is 4–5 cm
• Pts who have a growth rate of more than 0.5 cm/y in an aorta that is <5.5 cm
• Pts w/ sxs suggestive of expansion of TAA

Disposition

- Admit all pts meeting indications for emergency repair, symptomatic pts
- For asx pts w/o need for urgent intervention, D/C w/ vascular/cardiac surgery f/u & PCP f/u for RF modification

ACUTE PERICARDITIS

(*NEJM* 2014;371(25):2410–2416)

Definition

- Acute inflammatory dz of the pericardium due to a variety of causes:
  - Idiopathic (80% in developed nations)—Presumed postviral
  - Infectious (TB, fungal, less likely staph/strep, viral, parasitic)
  - Post-MI (Early post-MI vs Dressler synd)
  - Systemic dz (cancer, connective tissue disorder, myxedema, uremia)
  - Trauma or tx (postsurgical, XRT, posttraumatic, medication related)
- Dx requires at least 2 of the following:
  1. Characteristic CP (see table below)
  2. Pericardial friction rub (high-pitched, scratch sound heard best at L sternal border)
  3. Suggestive ECG findings (see below)
  4. Pericardial effusion (more than trivial size)

History & Physical Examination

- Hx: characteristic CP—Sudden onset, retrosternal, pleuritic, positional (better w/ leaning forward or upright); pain can radiate to neck, arms, shoulders, similar to ACS
  - Ask about recent viral illness, other associated conditions above
  - May have low-grade fever, SOB, dyspnea, myalgias
- Exam: friction rub (high-pitched, scratch sound heard best at LLSB apex w/ pt leaning forward in full expiration); ↑ HR, ↑ RR, nl BP

Evaluation

- ECG: Findings occur in 4 stages (see table), generally characterized by diffuse STE & PR depressions, though subtle PR depressions may be only sign
  - Classic CP & ECG findings present in only ~2/3 of pts (*Emerg Med J* 2013;30:1003)
  - Assess for electrical alternans (suggests pericardial tamponade, see next section)

Stages of ECG Changes in Pericarditis		
Stage 1	Acute (hours to days)	Diffuse ST ↑ (I, V5, V6); reciprocal STD aVR & V1; PR ↓ II, aVF, V4–V6; PR ↑ aVR
Stage 2	Early resolution	Normalization of ST & PR segments
Stage 3	Late resolution	TWI I, V5, V6 which can be widespread
Stage 4	Complete resolution	Normalization of ECG

- Labs: CBC, BMP (r/o uremia), LFTs, ESR/CRP (↑ CRP in 75%), cardiac enzymes (DDx includes ACS, as much as 1/3 cases a/w myocarditis) (*NEJM* 2014;371(25):2410–2416)
  - If dx pericarditis clinically additional testing unnecessary unless comorbidities/hx suggests important underlying etiology
- CXR: r/o other dx; can see cardiomegaly if >250 cc pericardial effusion
- Bedside echo: Assess for (1) pericardial effusion, (2) tamponade physiology (late diastolic collapse of RA, persistence of RA collapse >1/3 cardiac cycle, early diastolic collapse of RV, collapse of LA, distended IVC)
  - Nl echo does not r/o pericarditis
- Although not routinely indicated, CT & MRI can help make dx (pericardial thickening)

Treatment

- Pharmacologic tx is mainstay:
  - NSAIDs + colchicine initial recommended tx, provided no CIs
  - NSAIDs: ibuprofen (600–800 mg q6h–q8h), indomethacin (25–50 mg q8h), or aspirin (2–4 g QD in divided doses) for 1–2-wk course; give w/ PPI for gastric protection
    - ASA preferred among NSAIDs in early post-MI period
    - NSAIDs should also be restarted if develop recurrence
  - Colchicine (0.5 mg QD if ≤70 kg; 0.5 mg BID if >70 kg for 3 mos): used in conjunction w/ NSAIDs; c/w placebo, ↓ risk of recurrence & persistent sx at 72 h by 50% (*NEJM* 2013;369:1522–1528), tx of choice in recurrent pericarditis; risk of tox
    - Use cautiously w/ CKD, hepatobiliary dz, bleeding dyscrasias, GI motility d/o
    - In conjunction w/ NSAIDs, usually improves sx w/i 1–3 d
  - Steroids (prednisone 0.2–0.5 mg/kg/d w/ slow taper after 2–4 wks): only 1st line for autoimmune or uremic etiologies; o/w should not be routinely used 1st line, can consider use in those who fail NSAID or colchicine therapy; use in initial tx ↑ risk of recurrence
  - Optimal duration of tx unclear: 3-mo course recommended (*NEJM* 2013;369:1522–1528)

- Tx underlying condition as needed (abx, dialysis for uremia, chemo, etc)
- Pericardiocentesis indicated for purulent (postsurgical, TB, etc) or neoplastic pericarditis or cardiac tamponade
- CT surgery c/s: Recent cardiac surgery or if pericardial window needed

Disposition
- Most pts can be discharged home
- Admit if HD abnlty, fever, myocarditis, uremia, large effusion, tx failure

Pearls
- Acute idiopathic pericarditis is self-limited, responsive to tx in majority of cases
- Can be recurrent in 10–30%: smaller proportion incessant (relapse in <6 wks) or intermittent (sxs-free intervals >6 wks, but recurs)
- Can be a/w pericardial effusion w/ or w/o tamponade
- Late cxs such as constrictive pericarditis are very rare

CARDIAC TAMPONADE

Overview (*NEJM* 2003;349:684)
- Definition: A life-threatening state in which intrapericardial pressure (2/2 fluid, blood, pus) > RVEDP → ↓ RV preload → ↓ LV preload → ↓ LVEDP → equilibration of L & R heart pressures → ↓ CO → obstructive shock
- Tamponade more related to rate of fluid accumulation than volume of fluid (fluid accumulates faster than the rate of pericardium's ability to stretch)
- Can be caused by blood (type A AoD, post-MI free wall rupture, postsurgical, trauma), pus (TB, postsurgical), air, or other fluid (myxedema, uremia, malignancy, SLE)

History & Physical Examination
- Hx: If atraumatic, can p/w progressive SOB/DOE, orthopnea, PND, CP, lightheadedness, AMS, weakness; traumatic usually w/ gross penetrating wound or blunt aortic injury
- Ex: ↑ HR, ↑ RR, **Beck triad** (↓ BP, distended neck veins, muffled heart sounds), narrow pulse pressure, pulsus paradoxus (see below)

Performing Pulsus Paradoxus Test: Assessing the Reversed Bernheim Effect
• Inflate BP cuff to 20 mmHg above SBP, deflate until the 1st Korotkoff sound is heard during expiration only. Record number. Next, deflate the cuff until Korotkoff sounds are heard equally during both inspiration & expiration. Subtract this number from the 1st
• Abnl if the difference b/w these 2 numbers is >10 mmHg
• DDx: Cardiac tamponade, severe asthma/COPD, PE, constrictive pericarditis

Evaluation
- ECG: Low voltage, electrical alternans, ±signs of pericarditis
- CXR: Globular heart, but may be nl if rapid accumulation, minimum of ~200 cc of fluid required to produce visible cardiomegaly on CXR
- Echo (Test of choice): Can confirm dx; effusion (can be variable size) w/ septal shift, systolic collapse of RA (earliest sign), persistence of RA collapse >1/3 cardiac cycle, diastolic collapse of RV (most specific, collapse of LA, exaggerated resp cycle chgs in mitral & tricuspid in-flow velocities (pulsus surrogate), plethoric IVC w/ minimal respiratory variation (high sens) (*Am J Emerg Med* 2019;37(3):321–326)
- Pericardial fluid: if atraumatic, consider sending fluid culture & Gram stain, BUN, Cr, ANA, RF, malignancy screen/cytology

Treatment
- IVF bolus: preload dependent state; ↑ preload to RV causes ↑ RVEDP > intrapericardial pressure → ↑ LV preload → ↑ CO
  - Preload is purely temporizing to pericardiocentesis; w/ excess IVF pts will develop pulm edema & hypoxia
  - PPV (eg, intubation and mechanical ventilation) should avoided if at all possible until tamponade is addressed, given profound effect on ↓ preload
- Definitive tx is pericardiocentesis or pericardial window: Cardiac tamponade w/ HD compromise requires urgent drainage (bedside if unstable; vs in cath lab or OR if time)

Disposition
- Admit all pts w/ cardiac tamponade. If drained effectively & stable, can admit to tele floor (ie, cardiology); If admitted while awaiting drainage, admit to ICU

MYOCARDITIS

Overview (*NEJM* 2022;387(16):1488–1500)

- Definition: Acute lymphocytic inflammatory dz of the myocardium of varying severity ranging from subclinical dz to fulminant systolic failure & death
- Frequently a/w viral infxns (coxsackie, adenovirus, influenza, parvovirus B19, COVID-19), bacterial infxns (eg, strep, mycoplasma), Chagas dz, postvaccine, toxins/meds (cocaine, doxorubicin), autoimmune dz (sarcoidosis, giant cell myocarditis)

History & Physical Examination

- Hx: dyspnea, CP, arrhythmias; may have systemic sxs inc fever, fatigue, arthralgia, malaise, vomiting, diarrhea; Can present similar to HFrEF; viral prodrome (10–80%)
- Exam: Ranges from asx to subtle signs of systolic dysfxn (unexplained sinus tachycardia, LE edema) to fulminant heart failure (JVD, rales), arrhythmia, or cardiac arrest
  - VS abnormalities: fever, ↑ HR, ↑ RR, less commonly ↓ BP
  - May be toxic appearing or present w/ tachycardia out of proportion to fever

Evaluation

- ECG: sinus tachycardia, STE/STD, nonspecific ST Δs (can mimic ACS), VT/VF, widened QRS, prolonged QTc, heart block, Δs of pericarditis (see above)
- CXR: ↑ cardiac size, may have pulmonary edema
- Labs: cardiac enzymes (Troponin > CKMB; ↑ sens w/ ↑ extent of dz), BNP, CBC w/ diff (can see eosinophilia), ↑ ESR/CRP (*NEJM* 2009;360:1526–1538)
- Cardiac MRI: useful for establishing definitive dx and/or planning bx, initial test of choice
- Endocardial biopsy is historical gold standard, but now generally recommended for select pts

Treatment

- Largely supportive; treat HF, cardiogenic shock (may require inotropes, mechanical circulatory support), and arrhythmias

Pearls

- Should restrict competitive sports for 3–6 mos following acute myocarditis

HYPERTENSION AND HYPERTENSIVE EMERGENCIES

Approach

- Must differentiate chronic elevations in BP from an acute elevation, esp if symptomatic
- Must differentiate transient elevations (ie, from anxiety or pain) from other causes
- Search for life-threatening causes of elevations in BP and e/o end-organ damage (see HTN emergency)

Differential for Hypertension	
Pathophysiology	**Differential**
Other	Anxiety, pain, medication or substance induced (stimulants, steroids, TCAs, decongestants, NSAIDs), rebound HTN (clonidine, BBs), EtOH withdrawal, preeclampsia/eclampsia, ICH, CVA, OSA, tyramine crisis
Cardiovascular	Essential (primary) HTN, ADHF, AoD, coarctation of aorta
Renal	CKD, renal artery stenosis, glomerulonephritis, fibromuscular dysplasia
Endocrine	Cushing, pheochromocytoma, hyperaldosteronism, hyperthyroidism

Definition

- Categories of HTN: nl is SBP <120 & DBP <80 mmHg, elevated is SBP 120–129 & DBP <80, Stage 1 HTN is SBP 130–139 or DBP 80–89, Stage 2 is SBP ≥140 or DBP ≥90 (on 2+ occasions or via 24-h ambulatory monitoring)
- Asx HTN (previously hypertensive urgency): SBP ≥180 or DBP ≥120 w/ no acute organ damage; this term is also referred to as "hypertensive crisis" & has largely fallen out of favor
- HTN emergency: elevated BP w/ s/s acute organ damage (eg, cardiac, vascular, CNS, renal)

History & Physical Examination

- H/o CAD, HF, TIA/stroke, PAD, CKD, meds/noncompliance, EtOH/substance use
- Look for precipitants: progression of primary HTN, medication noncompliance, rebound HTN (clonidine), worsening renal dz, pheochromocytoma, Cushing dz, drug use (cocaine, amphetamines, MAOIs + tyramine), cerebral injury

- Assess for organ damage: CP, SOB, severe headache, neuro sx, visual chgs, AMS, oliguria, hematuria
- Exam: MS, neuro exam (e/o papilledema, visual acuity), signs of AHF

Evaluation (*Hypertension* 2024;81(8):e94–e106)
- Check BP in both arms, check cuff/cuff size
- In ED pts w/ asx markedly elevated BP, routine screening for acute target organ injury (ie, serum Cr, US) is not required
- In select pt populations (eg, those w/ poor f/u), screening for an elevated Cr level may identify kidney injury that affects mgmt

Treatment: Chronic HTN
- In general goal BP <130/80 mmHg (*Hypertension* 2018;71:e13)
- Tx cHTN results in 50% ↓ CHF, 40% ↓ stroke, 20–25% ↓ MI (*Lancet* 2000;356:1955)
- Even for pts w/ markedly elevated BP (ie, ≥180/≥110), initiation of BP mgmt in the ED is not required if asx
- In select pt populations (eg, those w/ poor f/u), EPs can consider treating markedly elevated BP in the ED and/or initiate therapy for long-term control w/ plan for o/p f/u

Treatment: Hypertensive Emergency
- ↓ MAP by 25% w/i 1–2 h using IV meds, then f/u w/ PO version w/ goal 160/100 in next 2–6 h, & BP nl in 24–48 h, treat based on underlying cause (see below)
- Avoid tx HTN during acute stroke (permissive HTN) unless pt is getting lysed, has extreme HTN (>220/120), AoD (*Stroke* 2013;44:870)

Antihypertensive Medications for Specific Causes		
Dz	**Drug Choice**	**Dose**
Cardiac ischemia	Metoprolol NTG	2.5–10 mg IV 10–200 mcg/min IV
CHF	NTG	10–200 mcg/min IV
ICH, CVA, HTN encephalopathy	Nicardipine Labetalol	0–15 mg/h IV 10 mg IV
AoD	Esmolol + nicardipine, or labetalol alone	Esmolol: Bolus 0.25–0.5 mg/kg over 1–2 mins, then 10–200 mcg/kg/min gtt; see above for nicardipine & labetalol
Preeclampsia–eclampsia	Magnesium Hydralazine	If sz: 2–6 g IV load, then infusion 10 mg IV

Disposition & Pearls
- Asx pts may be D/C home w/ PCP f/u
- True hypertensive emergencies require ICU admx for BP tx/monitoring
- HTN in the ED is often a/w anxiety/pain. Always repeat BP once pt is calm, pain improved
- In neonates, suspect renovascular dz, coarctation of the aorta, or kidney malformation

Hypertensive Encephalopathy
- Results from diffuse vasogenic cerebral edema 2/2 failure of autoregulation
- Presents w/ severe HA, vomiting, AMS, may progress to szs or coma
- May have retinal involvement, papilledema, focal neuro deficits in >1 pattern
- CT: obtain if neuro s/s or signs elevated ICP to eval for alternative etiologies; can be unremarkable or show diffuse edema & small hemorrhage
- Generally reversible w/ prompt BP reduction (30–40%)

Posterior Reversible Encephalopathy Syndrome
- Pathophys & presentation similar to hypertensive encephalopathy, localized to posterior circulation
- Sxs related to post-cerebral impairment (visual sxs HA, AMS, sz)
- Brain MRI w/ white matter edema in posterior parietal–temporal–occipital regions
- A/w HTN, CKD, malignancy, cytotoxic therapy, autoimmune dz
- Tx directed at BP control, underlying cause

HYPOTENSION AND SHOCK

Approach
- ABCs (airway, breathing, circulation) are first priority
- Differentiate hypotension from shock (end-organ damage 2/2 inadequate perfusion)

Definition
- Hypotension: BP below pt's baseline, often defined as SBP <90 or MAP <65 mmHg
- Shock: insufficient perfusion pressures for organs' metabolic needs

Pathophysiology of Shock[a]		
Mechanism	**Differential**	
↓ Intravascular volume	Hypovolemic shock—hemorrhagic (traumatic or non-traumatic) vs nonhemorrhagic (eg, dehydration)	
↓ CO	Cardiogenic shock (CHF, arrhythmia)	
	Obstructive shock	PE
		Cardiac tamponade
		Tension PTX
Peripheral vasodilation (ie, distributive)	Septic shock, anaphylactic shock, neurogenic shock, adrenal crisis	

[a]Also consider hypotension could be 2/2 medication effect, measurement error.

History & Physical Examination

- Hx: sxs a/w specific cause (CP, SOB, bleeding, infectious sxs, trauma)
- Exam: Ill appearing, ↓ BP, ↑ HR, +/– hypoxia, ↑ RR, UOP ↓, AMS, +/– fever or hypothermia, warm vs cool extremities

Evaluation

- CBC, Chem 7, PT/PTT, cardiac markers, LFTs, blood gas, lactate, type and screen, stool guaiac, ECG to assess for e/o ischemia or arrhythmia
- POCUS: RUSH exam (*Crit Care Res Pract* 2012:503254) incorporates a 3-part bedside physiologic assessment simplified as:
  - ***the pump***—cardiac POCUS to assess for pericardial effusion/tamponade, LV contractility, RV size
  - ***the tank***—IVC POCUS to assess volume status, as well as thoracic and abdominal POCUS to assess for pathology that could alter vascular volume; ie, PTX, pl effusion, B-lines/pulmonary edema, free intra-abdominal fluid
  - ***the pipes***—aorta POCUS to assess for AoD/AAA & DVT POCUS to evaluate for clot

Treatment

- Priority should be to obtain adequate IV access. If peripheral large-bore IVs cannot be placed in timely manner, consider IO (humeral/tibial) or stat central venous access w/ large internal diameter catheters (eg, cordis)
- Priority should be to restore hemodynamics before time-consuming diagnostic w/u:
  - If likely to be volume responsive, 1–2 L of isotonic crystalloid infusion as rapid as possible (ie, pressure bag if indicated)
  - Consider stat uncrossmatched blood if c/f life-threatening hemorrhage; consider using rapid infuser device; consider permissive hypotension (goal SBP 70 or MAP 60) in hemorrhagic shock (*J Trauma* 2002;52(6):1141–1146)
  - Consider peripheral vasoactive agents if persistently hypotensive after IVF bolus as bridge to obtaining central venous access (*Emerg Med Australas* 2020;32(2):220–227); norepinephrine often initial pressor of choice, though consider etiology of shock and other pt factors (eg, ability to tolerate adverse effects of that pressor)
- Use mental status, UOP, & MAP as early e/o adequate end-organ perfusion, trend lactate

Vasoactive Agents & Dosing (*Emerg Med Clin N Am* 2008;26:759)				
Vasoactive Agent	**Primary Receptor Activity**	**Relative Effects**	**Typical IV Dosing**	**Adverse Effects**
Phenylephrine	α1 +++	↑ SVR ↓ HR	20–200 mcg/min	Reflex bradycardia
Norepinephrine	α1 ++++ α2 +++ β1 +++ β2 0(+)	↑ HR ↑ SV ↑ SVR	1–40 mcg/min	Tachydysrhythmia
Epinephrine	α1 ++++ α2 +++(+) β1 +++ β2 0(+)	↑↑↑ HR ↑↑↑ SV ↑↑↑ SVR bronchodilate	1–20 mcg/min	Tachydysrhythmia Splanchnic ischemia
Dopamine	*Dose dependent:* α2+, β1+, β2+, D++ α1/2+, β1++, β2+, D++ α1+(++), α2+, β1++, β2+, D++	Natriuresis ↑↑ HR ↑↑ SV ↑ SVR	*Dose dependent:* 1–5 mcg/kg/min 5–10 mcg/kg/min 10–20 mcg/kg/min	Tachydysrhythmia (higher risk than norepinephrine)

Vasopressin	V1 receptor	↑ SVR ↓ HR	0.01–0.08 U/min	Limb ischemia Acute MI Bradycardia
Dobutamine	α1 0(+) α2 0(+) β1 ++++ β2 +++	↑↑ HR ↑↑↑ SV ↓ SVR	2–20 mcg/kg/min	Tachydysrhythmia HypoTN Acute MI
Milrinone	PDE inhibition	↑ HR ↑↑↑ SV ↓ SVR	0.25–0.75 mcg/kg/min	Tachydysrhythmia HypoTN

Pearls

- Not all hypotension is clinically significant. Use clinical context, pt's baseline BP & check the BP cuff (too large of cuff underestimates BP)
- Palpating pulse can provide a marker of SBP, but may overestimate the absolute value

Cited Correlations of Pulse & SBP (BMJ 2000;321:673) (Note: poorly evidence based)	
Pulse Present	**Minimum SBP (mmHg)**
Radial artery	80
Femoral artery	70
Carotid	60

HYPOVOLEMIC SHOCK

Approach

- Dehydration is a dx of exclusion; consider other etiologies; see below

Definition

- Intravascular volume depletion → ↓ perfusion

Differential for Hypovolemic Shock	
Hemorrhage	Trauma (internal, external), GI bleed, ruptured AAA, ruptured ectopic, vaginal bleeding, other vascular injury
Dehydration	Decreased PO intake, GI losses (eg, diarrhea, vomiting), burns (insensible losses), increased UOP (eg, medication or osmotic diuresis)

History

- Trauma, melena, hematochezia, hematemesis, ↓ PO intake, vomiting, diarrhea, meds

Physical Examination

- E/o trauma, guaiac + stool, pelvic exam, may have cool extremities, pallor

Evaluation

- As above +UA/hCG, FAST (blood in abdomen or chest)/RUSH exam; consider CT chest/abd/pelvis, pelvic US, type/screen based on differential

Treatment

- **Identify/treat cause**, IV fluid bolus; consider early PRBCs; **consult** immediately for life-threatening disorders requiring definitive tx (surgery, GI, Ob/Gyn)

Disposition

- Admit vs OR/endoscopy

CARDIOGENIC SHOCK

Approach

- Consider intubation early, look for & **treat underlying cause**

Definition

- ↓ CO + nl intravascular volume → ↓ systolic contractility + ↑ diastolic filling

Differential
STEMI, fulminant myocarditis, dysrhythmia, valvular failure, advanced HF/ cardiomyopathy, cardiac contusion

History & Physical Examination

- May have SOB, CP, AMS, edema depending on etiology
- HR, ↓ BP, ↑ RR, hypoxia, pulm rales, S3, S4, murmur, cool & diaphoretic

Evaluation
- CBC, Chem 7, Ca, Mg, PO_4, ECG, CXR, POCUS/stat echo (systolic/diastolic dysfxn, papillary muscle rupture, valvular failure, VSD, pericardial effusion, R heart strain)

Treatment
- Treat underlying dz, caution w/ IV fluids, require frequent reassessment of perfusion & breathing (if ↓ intravascular volume can consider small aliquots, eg, 250 cc)
- Reasonable 1st-line vasopressor is norepinephrine (*Curr Opin Crit Care* 2020;26(4):411)
- Dopamine: ↑ myocardial contractility & BP, but ↑ O_2 demand, increased risk of arrhythmia as compared to norepinephrine or epinephrine
- Dobutamine: ↑ HR & inotropy, less O_2 demand, but causes vasodilation (best if not tachycardic or severely hypotensive)
  - Often 1st list inotrope but no sufficient data to support any specific inotrope to reduce mortality (*Cochrane Database Syst Rev* 2020;11(CD009669))
- Central venous catheter: Consider for CVP monitoring, administration of pressors
- Cardiology c/s, particularly given may progress to require mechanical support
- Revascularization if ACS: early revasc → ↓ mortality (*NEJM* 1999;341:625; *JAMA* 2001;285:190)
- Other: thrombolytics, IABP, ventricular assist device, ECMO, valve repair

Disposition
- Admit to ICU (likely CCU)

SEPTIC SHOCK

Approach (*Crit Care Med* 2021;49(11):e1063)
- Identify & treat early → best outcomes when treated w/i 6 h
- Evaluate for source of infxn & achieve source control

Definition
- Sepsis = life threatening organ dysfxn 2/2 dysregulated host response to infxn
- Septic shock: sepsis & vasopressor requirement for MAP >/65 & lactate >2 despite adequate fluid resuscitation
- There is no ideal screening tool for sepsis; source of infxn plus SIRS criteria (SIRS: ≥2 of the following: Temp ≥38 °C or ≤36 °C, HR >90, RR >20 or $PaCO_2$ <32 mmHg, WBC >12,000, <4,000, or >10% bands) has been used. qSOFA score (GCS <15, RR ≥22, SBP ≤100) no longer recommended as single screening tool

Common Causes of Sepsis	
Pathophysiology	**Differential**
Respiratory	PNA, empyema
Abdominal	Peritonitis/perforation, abscess, cholangitis, typhilitis
Skin	Cellulitis, necrotizing skin and soft tissue infxn
GU/Gyn	UTI, pyelonephritis, PID/TOA
CNS	Meningitis, brain abscess
Other	Bacteremia/endocarditis, septic arthritis, osteomyelitis, epidural abscess, influenza, and other viral infxns

Evaluation
- CBC w/ diff, Chem 10, LFTs, serial lactate, BCx (×2)/urine/sputum culture, PT/PTT, cardiac markers, VBG, CXR; imaging based on differential

Supporting Criteria for Sepsis
Inflammatory variables: Leukocytosis (WBC >12,000 μL^{-1}) Leukopenia (WBC <4,000 μL^{-1}) Nl WBC w/ >10% immature cells (band forms) Plasma CRP >2 SD above nl Plasma procalcitonin >2 SD above nl
Organ dysfxn variables: Arterial hypoxemia (diffuse alveolar damage, ARDS, PaO_2/FiO_2 <300) Acute oliguria (UOP <0.5 mL/kg/h for at least 2 h despite fluid resuscitation) Cr increase >0.5 mg/dL Coagulation abnormalities (INR >1.5 or aPTT >60 s, DIC) Ileus Cardiovascular dysfxn (myocardial depression, distributive shock) TCP (plt count <100,000 μL^{-1}) Hyperbilirubinemia (plasma Tbili >4 mg/dL, elevated transaminases)

Tissue perfusion variables:
Hyperlactemia (>2–4 mmol/L)
Decreased cap refill/mottling

Treatment (*Crit Care Med* 2021;49(11):e1063)

- **IV fluid resuscitation:** at least 30 mL/kg of IV crystalloid (NS or LR) w/i the 1st 3 h (unless CI to 30 mL/kg, lower volume may be reasonable), additional fluids guided by frequent reassessment of hemodynamic status/perfusion inc serial lactate measurement; note recent downgrade in 2021 guidelines from strong to weak recommendation based on low quality of evidence
- **Target MAP of 65 mmHg** w/ early vasopressors as needed (norepinephrine 1st choice, vasopressin 0.04 U/min can be added)
- Consideration of central access, arterial line, & further hemodynamic assessment
- POCUS to evaluate volume status & cardiac dysfxn
- **Abx:** broad spectrum, draw cultures prior (cover gram+, gram–, anaerobes; consider double coverage for pseudomonas)
  - Start abx w/i 1 h of sepsis recognition, regardless of whether source is known
  - Example regimen: cefepime (gram+/–, psa), vanc (MRSA), flagyl (anaerobes)
  - Source control (surgery, indwelling device/line removal, etc)
- **Hydrocortisone:** Consider (50 mg q6h) in pts w/ severe sepsis refractory to IV fluids & pressors & for pts on chronic steroids/hx of adrenal insufficiency; corticotropin test + routine steroid use → no benefit & possibly harm (*NEJM* 2008;358:111)
- **Blood products:** PRBCs to target Hgb >7 g/dL; PLT tfx if <10,000 μL^{-1} w/o bleed, <20,000 μL^{-1} w/ risk of bleeding, <50,000 μL^{-1} for active bleeding, surgery, procedure; assess for DIC & coagulopathy
- **Oxygenation/ventilation:** supplemental O_2; consider need for intubation early; if intubated use lung protective ventilation (low TV of 6 cc/kg IBW, plateau <30 cm H_2O, high PEEP) (*NEJM* 2000;342:1301) use of sedation/paralytics → ↓ O_2 consumption
- **Glucose control:** q1–2h measurements; initiate protocolized blood glucose mgmt when 2 consecutive measurements **>180** mg/dL to a target **>180** mg/dL
- **Renal replacement therapy:** Monitor I/Os strictly; Use continuous therapies (ie, CVVH) to facilitate managing fluid balance in HD unstable pts

Disposition

- Admit, ICU if unstable from resp or hemodynamic standpoint vs OR if need source control

NEUROGENIC SHOCK

Approach

- Evaluate according to ATLS, always consider w/ e/o injury to cervical/thoracic spine
- Cervical spine injury → risk of apnea, may require intubation; evaluate according to ATLS

Definition & Pathophysiology

- Spinal cord injury at the level of T6 or above → disruption of sympathetic pathways → loss of vascular sympathetic tone → vasodilation & bradycardia

History

- Trauma w/ severe injury to the spinal cord, neuro deficits
- Less common causes: GBS, transverse myelitis, spinal anesthesia

Findings

- ↓ HR, ↓ BP, flushed & warm skin, anesthesia, paralysis below a spec dermatome; saddle anesthesia, ↓ rectal tone, areflexia, Horner synd, absent bulbocavernosus reflex, priapism (unopposed PNS stimulation)

Evaluation

- CT spine (esp cervical, thoracic); consider CT head, chest, abd/pelvis if h/o trauma

Treatment

- C-spine immobilization, strict log-roll precautions
- Should maintain goal MAP >85–90 after SCI (*Neurosurgery* 2013;60(CN_suppl_1):82)
- IV fluids: prior to starting pressors
- Pressors: norepinephrine preferred, phenylephrine (avoid if bradycardic, may worsen HR)
- c/s neurosurgery immediately, may require surgical decompression

Disposition

- Admit ICU

Pearls

- Differentiate from spinal shock, which describes acute loss of motor, sensory & reflex function due to spinal cord injury
- Any trauma pt w/ hypotension should be suspected of having hemorrhagic shock until proven o/w. Thus, neurogenic shock should be treated if suspected, but should not be the 1° DDx in the hypotensive trauma pt

SYNCOPE

Definition

- Syncope: sudden loss of consciousness & postural tone arising from an abrupt drop in cerebral perfusion w/ spontaneous recovery, quick return to baseline mental status
- Pre-syncope, near syncope: As above, but sxs resolve before complete LOC or loss of tone; may experience AMS & weakness before return to nl
- Objective in ED is to distinguish from other causes of sudden LOC (syncope mimics), & differentiate benign syncope etiologies from those requiring further eval or tx (see table)

Common or Concerning Causes of Syncope	
Primary Cardiac Etiologies	
Tachydysrhythmia	**Mechanism:** ↑ HR (eg, VT, VF, AF, AT, SVT, WPW, TdP, long QT, Brugada), ↓ LVEDV, ↓ CO; **Hx:** May be unheralded or prodrome of LH, palpitations, SOB
Bradydysrhythmia	**Mechanism:** ↓ HR (eg, Sick sinus synd, BB, CCB, Heart block Mobitz type II second-degree or 3rd-degree CHB, PPM malfxn), ↓ CO; **Hx:** May be unheralded or associated w/ position/exertion; prodrome of LH, weakness, DOE
Valvular heart dz (usually AS)	**Mechanism:** ↓ Preload w/ fixed severe AS, ↓ CO; **Hx:** often a/w position (standing), dehydration, exertion, dysrhythmia (↓ CO), can have chronic DOE/known AS
HFrEF (eg, acute MI, post-MI, CMP)	**Mechanism:** ↓ EF, ↓ CO; **Hx:** Weakness, DOE, PND/orthopnea, recent MI or hx HF, med or dietary chgs
Hypertrophic cardiomyopathy (HCOM)	**Mechanism:** ↑ HR, ↓ EDV, ↓↓ SV 2/2 outflow obstruction (can also ↑ risk of VT/VF); **Hx:** Often a/w exercise (↑ HR), missed meds (↑ HR), or dehydration (↓ preload)
Tamponade	**Mechanism:** ↑ intrapericardial pressures > RV filling pressure, ↓ L-sided filling pressures, ↓ CO; **Hx:** Progressive weakness, SOB, DOE, CP, orthopnea
Primary Vascular Etiologies	
Pulmonary embolism	**Mechanism:** ↑ PA obstruction, ↓ L-sided preload, ↓ CO; **Hx:** may be unheralded, or sudden SOB, CP, sense of doom, may have s/s of DVT
Pulmonary HTN	**Mechanism:** ↓ LV preload 2/2 any ↑ PVR; **Hx:** Often a/w exertion, PMH of idiopathic pulmonary HTN, CTD, MS/MR, COPD
AoD (Type A>B)	**Mechanism:** False lumen ↓ carotid inflow, OR tamponade present; **Hx:** Sudden severe CP, back pain, flank pain or abdominal pain, diaphoresis
TAA/AAA	**Mechanism:** Sudden expansion, contained leak, or rupture of aortic aneurysm; **Hx:** Sudden but not always severe CP, back pain, flank pain, abdominal pain
Subclavian (SCA) steal synd	**Mechanism:** Retrograde vert artery flow → ↓ posterior circulation perfusion 2/2 sudden ↓ SBP or ↑ SCA flow a/w proximal ipsilateral SCA stenosis/occlusion; **Hx:** Can be a/w movements of affected UE, dehydration, med Δs, arm ischemia, sometimes also w/ vertigo/posterior circulation neuro sxs
Vertebrobasilar insufficiency	**Mechanism:** ↓ SBP (any cause) w/ chronic VB stenosis (eg, atherosclerosis) can ↓ cerebrovascular perfusion (if impaired autoreg), ↓ CPP → syncope; **Hx:** May be unheralded, often a/w position (standing), dehydration, dysrhythmia (↓ CO), a/w dizziness/vertigo, dysarthria, ataxia, vision chgs

Noncardiovascular Etiologies	
Vasovagal	**Mechanism:** ↑ vagal tone a/w emotional or physiologic stressor; **Hx:** Common emotional precipitants include sight of blood, instrumentation, sudden emotional shock; physiologic stressors inc fatigue, prolonged standing, warmth, pain, n/v, coughing, swallowing, micturition, defecation (Valsalva); **DX:** Clinical dx, ↓ HR (sinus brady) & BP during event; **TX:** None needed; **DISPO:** Home
Carotid sinus hypersensitivity	**Mechanism:** ↑ vagal tone after mechanical pressure on carotid sinus; **Hx:** Often after shaving, head turning; **TX:** None indicated; **DX:** Clinical; **DISPO:** Home
Orthostatic hypotension	**Mechanism:** ↓ vascular compliance → ↓ SBP w/ position chgs; **Hx:** Often elderly (stiff vessels), can be associated w/ bleeding/ symptomatic anemia; **DX:** CBC, consider imaging if c/f anemia, orthostatic VS ↓ sens (sxs w/ standing may be more helpful & sens than VS) warranting admx, generally DC home if none identified
Autonomic dysfxn	**Mechanism:** Impaired function of autonomic nervous system; **Hx:** May be a/w other autonomic dysfxn (GI, bladder, sweating), may have hx of DM, EtOH, SLE, Neuro dz (Parkinson's); check med Δs; often hx of similar episodes in the past
Medications/Toxic	Common medications (new or ↑ dose) a/w syncope: Vasodilators (α-blockers, nitrates, ACEI/ARB, CCB, hydralazine, phenothiazines, antidepressants), diuretics, neg chronotropes (BB, CCB), antiarrhythmics (class IA, IC, III), psychoactive meds (antipsych, TCAs, barbs, benzos), substances (EtOH), hypoglycemics, anticonvulsants, CO, etc
Syncope mimics[a]	sz, TIA/stroke, ICH, migraine, cataplexy, hypoglycemia, hypoxia

[a]Can mimic syncope, but not considered true syncopal events.
Modified from *NEJM* 2002;347:878; *JACC* 2006;47:473.

History & Physical Examination (*Circulation* 2017;136:e60)

- HPI: Always ask about preceding activity (exertion, posture), other potential precipitants, prodromal sxs (palpitations, dyspnea, CP, LH), rate of onset & recovery to baseline mental status, tongue biting and/or urinary incontinence, duration, associated sxs (CP, SOB, palpitations, focal neuro deficits, HA, abdominal pain, nausea), hx prior syncope, any concern for injuries
  - Abrupt onset w/o prodrome, occurrence while sitting/supine are more c/f serious pathology
  - Differentiate from sz: syncope typically more abrupt, shorter duration, quicker return to nl (seconds–minutes vs more prolonged postictal period w/ generalized sz), no tongue biting or incontinence, lack of rigidity or aura; note syncope commonly can occur w/ slow & irregular myoclonic jerking (convulsive syncope) mistaken as sz/convulsive activity
- PMH (cardiac dz, prior episodes), meds, & FHx (sudden cardiac death) are very important, collateral information from witnesses, associated trauma from fall
  - High-risk hx: older age, structural heart dz, CAD or h/o arrythmia
- Lower-risk hx: young, healthy, nonexertional, no hx or e/o cardiac dz, no FHx sudden cardiac death
- Exam: guided by hx; evaluate neuro exam (inc stability w/ standing/gait), evidence tongue bite (suggesting sz), murmurs, carotid bruits, consider orthostatic vitals

Evaluation

- ECG in all pts: in addition to direct e/o dysrhythmia (bradycardia, tachycardia, heart block, extrasystoles), look for findings associated w/ ventricular dysrhythmias (HOCM, ARVD, Brugada synd, prolonged QTc, pre-excitation, acute ischemia or e/o prior MI

Characteristic ECG Findings in Patients with Selected Cardiac Causes of Syncope	
Cardiac Dz	**ECG Findings**
Brugada synd (*Circulation* 2012;5:606)	• *Type I:* Coved ST-segment elevation ≥2 mm in V1–V3 f/b a neg T wave in >1 R precordial lead • *Type II:* STE w/ saddle-back appearance w/ a high takeoff STE ≥2 mm, a trough displaying STE ≥1 mm, & then either a + or biphasic T wave • *Type III:* Either saddleback or coved appearance w/ STE <1 mm • Other: Prolonged QT, hx of VT/VF, family hx sudden cardiac death or Brugada

HOCM (*Am J Emerg Med* 2007;25:72)	• Characteristic findings of LVH (see *ECG* section) • Deep narrow Q waves in inferior (II, III, aVF) & lateral (I aVL, V5,V6) leads in pts w/ septal hypertrophy • Deep inverted T waves in mid & lateral precordial leads in pts w/ isolated apical hypertrophy
Arrhythmogenic R ventricular dysplasia (ARVD) (*Am J Med* 2004;117:685)	• Epsilon waves (small amplitude deflections at transition of QRS & ST segment) in R precordial leads • Prolonged QRS complex to >110 ms in V1–V3 w/o RBBB • Inverted T waves V1–V3 in absence of RBBB • Reduced R-wave amplitude
Long QT synd (*Circulation* 1995;92:2929; *Circulation* 2000;102:2849)	• Prolongation of QT interval, usually >500 ms • LQT1 has a broad T wave, LQT2 has small &/or notched T wave, LQT3 has unusually long onset T wave
Pre-excitation synd (WPW) (*Am Heart J* 1930;6:685)	• Short PR interval <120 ms • Slurred upstroke of QRS complex (delta wave) • Increased QRS duration >110 ms

- Labs & imaging: All guided by hx/exam & specific dx's being considered; consider CBC, electrolytes (+/– hCG), POC glucose in most pts; however, obvious vasovagal syncope in a young o/w young, healthy male w/o ongoing sxs may not require any labs
  - Consider based on clinical presentation: cardiac markers, pro-BNP, D-dimer, CXR, TTE, UA, stool guaiac, head CT in elderly, orthostatic vitals, continuous tele monitoring
- Any pt w/ PPM and/or ICD who has syncope or presyncope should have their device interrogated in the ED given higher likelihood of dysrhythmia in such pts

Disposition (*Ann Emerg Med* 1997;29:4; *Circulation* 2017;136:e60)
- Home if no high-risk cardiac features: (1) age <45, (2) nl ECG, (3) nl exam (4) o/w reassuring eval. Consider o/p f/u, consider Holter monitor to assess for paroxysmal arrhythmia
- O/w, perform risk assessment

Risk Assessment
- Note: at present no single clinical decision rule should outweigh clinical judgment, no single clinical decision rule is specifically recommended

Short- & Long-Term Risk Factors (*Circulation* 2017;136:e60)	
Short Term </30 d	**Long Term >30 d**
Male sex	Male sex
Older age >60 y	Older Age
No prodrome	Ventricular arrhythmias
Preceding palpitations	Cancer
Exertional syncope	Structural heart dz
Structural heart dz	Cerebrovascular dz
CHF	CHF
Cerebrovascular dz	Diabetes
FHx of sudden cardiac death	High CHADS-2 score[a]
Trauma	Abnl ECG
E/o bleeding	Lower GFR
Persistently abnl vitals	
Abnl ECG	
Positive Troponin	

[a]CHADS-2: CHF (+1), HTN (+1), Age >/75 (+1), DM (+1), previous CVA/TIA (+2) (*Clin Cardiol* 2013;36(5):262).

San Francisco Syncope Rule	
Clinical Features ("CHESS")	
CHF (past or present)	SBP <90 mmHg initially
Hct <30%	SOB
ECG abnl (new Δ or not sinus rhythm)	

Using San Francisco Syncope Rule to Guide Disposition Decisions
• If any of above features present, consider admx, further w/u
• Predicts risk of serious outcome (mortality, MI, arrhythmia, PE, CVA, SAH, significant hemorrhage, return to ED) w/i 7 d; sens 86% (CI 83–89%), spec 49% (CI 48–41%) (*Ann Emerg Med* 2010;56(4):362)
• If none of above features present, consider D/C

Ann Emerg Med 2004;4:224; 2006;47:448; 2007;49:420; 2008;427:e1; *CMAJ* 2011;183(15):E1116.

Canadian Syncope Rule (*JAMA Intern Med* 2020;180(5):737)	
Predisposition to vasovagal sx (−1)	Elevated troponin (+2)
Hx of heart dz (+1)	Abnl QRS axis <−30 or >100 (+1)
Any SBP <90 or >180 mmHg (+2) ED Dx of vasovagal (−2) ED Dx of cardiac syncope (+2)	QRS duration >130 ms (+1) Qtc >480 (+2)
Using Rule to Guide Disposition Decisions	
• Score −3 to −2: very low risk (sens 99.3%, spec 28.5%)[a], likely safe for D/C • Score −1 to 0: low risk (sens 95.7%, spec 58.2%)[a], likely safe for D/C • Score 1–3: medium risk (sens 91.4–66.2%, spec 78.1–91.6%)[a], shared decision making • Score 4–5: high risk (sens 38.9–51.8%, spec 97.3–95.3)[a], admit to hospital • Score >5: very high risk (sens 28.8%, spec 99%)[a], admit to hospital	

[a]For 30-d serious outcomes.

- Other clinical decision rules: FAINT score (not externally validated) (*Ann Emerg Med* 2020; 75(2):147–158); Rose Rule (*J Am Coll Cardiol* 2010;55:713–721); OESIL (*Eur Heart J* 2003;24(9):811–819); Boston (*J Emerg Med* 2007;33:233)

DYSRHYTHMIA

Approach
- Always obtain an ECG & rhythm strip
- Follow ACLS protocols for anyone unstable or significantly symptomatic

Differential			
Type			**Differential**
Bradycardia			Sinus bradycardia, sick sinus synd, AV blocks (2° & 3° AV block), PPM malfxn,
Tachycardia	Regular	Narrow complex	Sinus tach, SVT (AVNRT, AVRT), AT, AFL
		Wide complex	VT, SVT w/ aberrancy, SVT w/ pre-excitation (eg, WPW), tachycardia w/ PM
	Irregular	Narrow complex	AF, AFL w/ variable AV block, multifocal atrial tachycardia, sinus tachycardia w/ ectopy
		Wide complex	AF or AFL w/ aberrancy, polymorphic VT

BRADYCARDIA

Approach (*Circulation* 2019;140:e382–e482)
- Anticipate need for external/transvenous pacing & cardiology c/s early
- Medication hx is crucial (BB, CCB, antidysrhythmics, recent chgs)
- In children, highly consider toxic ingestion; in neonates, consider congenital cardiac dz

Definition
- HR <60 in an adult, <80 in a child <15 y/o, <100 in an infant <1 y/o. Caused by depressed function of the SA node or conduction system block/delay

Sinus Bradycardia, SA Node Block, & Escape Rhythms (*NEJM* 2000;342:703)

History
- Fatigue, syncope/presyncope, DOE, medication hx (esp beta blockers, CCB), often no sxs

Differential
- Physiologic (athletic young adults), medications (nodal agents), hypothyroidism, ↑ vagal tone (inc inferior MI, hemoperitoneum), hypothermia, ↑ ICP, hypoxia, intrinsic SA node dz, hyperkalemia

- Escape rhythm occurs when rate of supraventricular impulses is less than the intrinsic rate of ectopic pacemaker cells
  - Intrinsic rates: SA node (60–100 bpm), atria (<60 bpm), AV node (40–60 bpm), ventricles (20–40 bpm)

Intrinsic Pacemaker Rates	
SA Node: 60–100 bpm	AV Node: 40–60 bpm
Atria: <60 bpm	Ventricles: 20–40 bpm

Evaluation
- Sinus bradycardia ECG: HR <60 in adults, nl PR intervals, P wave preceding each QRS
- SA node block: absent atrial depolarization & missing P waves
- Junctional escape rhythm: HR 40–60 bpm, narrow QRS (<120), no relation b/w QRS complexes & P waves
- Ventricular escape rhythm: HR 20–40 bpm, wide QRS (>/120 ms), may have LBBB or RBBB morphology
- Assess rhythm strip, consider CMP, TSH, cardiac markers

Treatment
- Asx sinus bradycardia does not require tx. Tx if symptomatic or life-threatening cause is suspected w/ atropine (1st line), epinephrine (2nd line) and/or pacing

Disposition
- Admit anyone who is symptomatic

Sinus Node Dysfunction (Sick Sinus Syndrome/Tachy–Brady Syndrome)

Definition
- Sinus node dysfxn includes a series of ECG abnormalities characterized by failure to generate appropriate cardiac potentials from the sinus node
- In sick sinus synd, there are frequent long sinus pauses that may degenerate to absent atrial depolarization for a period of time before the resumption of regular cardiac conduction (sinus arrest)
- In tachy–brady synd, episodes of sinus bradycardia or sinus arrest are interspersed w/ episodes of supraventricular tachycardia (often AF)

History
- Syncope, presyncope, fatigue, weakness, DOE, palpitations
- Typically observed in 70–80 y/o, suggesting age-related degeneration of the SA node
- May be due to fibrosis, infiltrative dz (eg, amyloidosis, sarcoidosis)
- Consider medication effects (BB, CCB, digoxin)

Evaluation
- ECG (frequent sinus pauses, bradycardia/tachycardia rhythms); consider electrolytes, cardiac markers, CBC, TSH; Holter monitoring; TTE to assess for structural cause

Treatment
- Acute tx only for symptomatic or life-threatening arrhythmia; ultimately may require combination of PPM for bradycardia & rate control for tachycardia

Disposition
- Admit anyone who is symptomatic for permanent PM placement
- If minimal or no sxs are present, consider D/C home w/ close f/u

AV NODE BLOCK

Definition
- Results when conduction from the atria to the AV node & into the His bundle is disrupted
- Blocks can anatomically be located in the atria, AV node, or His–Purkinje system
- Classified as 1°, 2° Mobitz I (Wenckebach), 2° Mobitz II, & 3° blocks based on characteristic ECG patterns:

Differential		
Classification	**ECG Findings**	**Differential**
1° AV block	Prolonged PR interval >0.2 s, nl QRS	↑ vagal tone, MI, age-related degeneration, drugs (BB, CCB, digoxin), infxn, cardiomyopathy

2° AV block Mobitz type I	• Progressive ↑ PR interval w/ RR interval shortening until QRS dropped • Appears as grouped beats • Block at level of AV node	↑ vagal tone, *inferior* MI, age-related degeneration, drugs (BB, CCB, digoxin), infxn, endocarditis, cardiomyopathy
2° AV block Mobitz type II	• Stable PR & RR interval w/ occasional dropped QRS • Can be regular (2:1) or irregular • Block at level of His–Purkinje	Age-related degeneration, *anteroseptal* MI, CMP, Lenegre dz, drug tox, myocarditis (eg, Lyme), endocarditis, cardiomyopathy (eg, infiltrative)
3° AV block (CHB)	• Complete AV dissociation • P waves are not conducted & never produce a QRS • Escape rhythm is a regular narrow junctional or wide ventricular response	MI (inferior MI w/ AV node ischemia or anteroseptal MI w/ H-P ischemia), age-related degeneration, drugs (BB, CCB, digoxin), infxn, endocarditis, myocarditis (eg, Lyme), congenital, cardiomyopathy (eg, infiltrative)

Approach
- Differentiate 1°, 2° Mobitz I (Wenckebach), 2° Mobitz II, & 3° blocks
- 2° Mobitz II & 3° blocks are never nl → look for underlying cardiac dz
- In children, be highly suspicious of toxic ingestion
- In neonates, consider congenital cardiac dz
- Determine (1) rate, (2) wide or narrow QRS, (3) rhythm regular or irregular, (4) P waves present or absent, (5) is every P wave f/b QRS & every QRS preceded by P

History
- 1°: Asx, incidental finding on ECG, can be nl finding in 2% of adults
- 2°: Mobitz I (Wenckebach): Often asx; irregular HR, fatigue, ↑ vagal tone
- 2°: Mobitz II: May be asx; presyncope/syncope, fatigue, DOE
- 3°: Usually symptomatic; presyncope/syncope, fatigue, weakness, DOE

Evaluation
- ECG & rhythm strip, tele
- 2° Mobitz II & 3°: labs in anticipation of PPM placement & search for cause

Treatment
- 1° & 2° Mobitz I: No tx generally necessary
- 2° Mobitz II & 3°:
  - Symptomatic pts require transcutaneous &/or transvenous pacing; if HD unstable, consider a beta-adrenergic agent (dopamine, epinephrine) as bridge to pacing
  - Dopamine has been demonstrated to have equivalent survival outcomes & adverse events to transcutaneous pacing (*Resuscitation* 2008;76(3):341)
  - Assess for & treat reversible causes (drugs, hypothermia, hypoxia, electrolytes, hypothyrodism, infx, ischemia)
  - Atropine often ineffective in high-degree AV blocks, avoid atropine in heart transplant pts (heart is denervated, risk of 3° AVB or sinus arrest)
  - Have transcutaneous pacer attached (remember to treat associated pain of shocks) & ready for use in high-risk pts; consider transvenous pacing
  - C/s cardiology

Disposition & Pearls
- Pts w/ 1° & 2° Mobitz I: D/C home w/ f/u
- Pts w/ 2° Mobitz II & 3°: Admit all to Tele ward for cardiology c/s & PPM
- Mobitz II is concerning b/c risk of progression to CHB

TACHYCARDIA/PALPITATIONS

Approach
- Determine stable vs unstable as well as (1) rate, (2) wide or narrow QRS, (3) rhythm regular or irregular

Differential Diagnosis of Tachycardia			
Narrow		Wide	
Regular	**Irregular**	**Regular**	**Irregular**
Sinus tach	AF	VT	Polymorphic VT
SVT	MAT	AFL/SVT w/ aberrancy	Atrial fibrillation/SVT w/ aberrancy
AFL	AFL w/ variable block	Antidromic AVRT	Atrial fibrillation/SVT w/ pre-excitation

Supraventricular Tachycardia (*Circulation* 2016;133:e506–e574)

Approach

- Differentiate type based on ECG, rhythm strip, & response to adenosine/vagal maneuvers (see below)

Definition

- Rhythm arises above the ventricles (either atrium or AV junction) w/ narrow QRS unless pre-excitation or aberrant conduction

History

- H/o pulm or cardiac dz → AT, MAT, AFL, AF, NPJT
- In an o/w healthy adult → AVNRT, AVRT
- Gradual onset → ST, AT; abrupt onset → AVNRT, AVRT

Evaluation

- Consider CBC, BMP, TSH, tox screen; in some cases, ECG/rhythm strip is sufficient

SVT Pathophysiologies			
	Type of SVT	**Pathophysiology**	**Features**
Atrial	ST	Pain, fever, infxn, anxiety, hypovolemia, PE, medication, anemia, hyperthyroidism, CHF/heart dz, exertion	Typically <150 bpm, regular, P waves are UPRIGHT before QRS, slowed by vagal maneuver & adenosine (↑ AV block)
	AT	Originates in atria but not SA node; a/w COPD, CAD, EtOH, digoxin	
	MAT	Originates in atria at ≥3 separate sites (therefore ≥3 p-wave morphologies), a/w lung dz	
	AFL	Atrial macroreentry, typically R atrium	Often ~150 bpm (if 2:1 AV block), sawtooth P waves, regular, ↑ AV block unmasks
	AF	Mx irregular atrial impulses, typically from pulm veins	Irregular, fibrillation or no P waves, slowed by ↑ AV block
AV jxn	AVNRT	Reentrant pathway w/i AVN	Typically >150 bpm, retrograde P waves after QRS or w/I, terminated by vagal maneuver & adenosine (↑ AV block)
	AVRT	Reentrant pathway using AVN + accessory pathway b/w atria & ventricles	
	NPJT (Accelerated AV junctional)	Originates at AV jxn, a/w myo/endocarditis, cardiac surgery, IMI, digoxin	Typically 70–130 bpm, AV dissociation, retrograde P waves

From *NEJM* 1995;332:162; 2006;354:1039; 2012;367:1438–1448.

Treatment

- Synchronized cardioversion for any unstable rhythm
- ST: Treat underlying condition
- AT/MAT: Treat underlying condition; consider AV nodal blocker
- AF/AFL: rhythm vs rate control; txt also different if pre-excitation (see section on *AF/AFL*)
- AVNRT/AVRT: Vagal maneuvers, adenosine, CCB preferable to beta blockers → avoid adenosine/nodal agents if e/o pre-excitation (see WPW below)
- NPJT: CCB, beta blockers, amiodarone

Disposition

- Most pts w/ ST, AVNRT, AVRT can be D/C home once rhythm is controlled if → asx & no acute underlying condition. Admx for other rhythms is variable, but often necessary due to underlying condition
- c/s cardiology for any pt w/ unstable SVT & those difficult to control w/ standard tx

Pearl

- MAT is often misdiagnosed as AF. Look closely at P-wave morphology

Atrial Fibrillation & Atrial Flutter

Definition (*JACC* 2006;48:e149; *Circulation* 2014;64(21):e1–e76)

- AF is a supraventricular tachyarrhythmia characterized by uncoordinated atrial activity w/ consequent deterioration of mechanical function
- Can be 1st episode, paroxysmal (terminates w/i 7 d of onset, recur w/ variable frequency), persistent (>7 d), long-standing persistent (>1 y) &/or permanent (joint decision b/w pt & clinician to stop further attempts to maintain NSR)

- Valvular → rheumatic heart dz, or postvalve surgery (bioprosthetic, mech, &/or MVR)
- AFL is characterized by atrial depolarizations in a regular rate at ~300 bpm caused by a reentrant mechanism, ventricular conduction limited by AV node refractory period in a fixed or variable ratio to atrial conduction (2:1 AV block is most common)

Differential of Triggers of Atrial Fibrillation	
Pathophysiology	**Differential**
Other	Idiopathic (50%)
Cardiac	CHF, peri/myo/endocarditis, MI/ischemia, s/p cardiac surgery, HTN
Pulm	COPD, PNA, PE
Endo	Hyperthyroid, stress, infxn, postop
Drugs	EtOH "holiday heart syndrome," cocaine, amphetamines, sympathomimetics, caffeine

History & Physical Examination
- Timing, abrupt vs gradual onset (palpitations, SOB, DOE, fatigue presyncope/syncope, CP); recent illness or procedure, drug & alcohol use, prior similar sxs, on AC
- Irregularly irregular pulse; may be regular w/ AFL

Evaluation
- ECG, CBC, lytes, Ca, Mg, PO_4; CXR
- Consider cardiac markers (if active CAD is suspected); TSH, D-dimer, dig level if appropriate; echo (LA size, thrombus, valves, LV/RV fxn)
- Consider o/p Holter in pts w/ suggestive hx who arrive in NSR
- ECG in AF: Replacement of consistent P waves by rapid oscillating or fibrillatory waves that vary in amplitude, shape, & timing, a/w irregularly irregular, frequently RVR
- ECG in AFL: Atrial rate 250–350 bmp w/ ventricular response rate typically 150 bpm (2:1 conduction), presence of "sawtooth" flutter ("F") waves. Can be ***typical*** (spiky V1, neg in II, III, aVF, opposite pattern known as reverse typical) or ***atypical*** (appearance other *than* typical). F waves revealed via adenosine or vagal maneuvers

Treatment (*J Am Coll Cardiol* 2019;74(1):104; *Circulation* 2014;64(21):e1–e76)
- Main objectives: Rate or rhythm control, prevention of thromboembolism, relief of sxs
- When deciding on mgmt strategies in the ED, several things to consider include:
  a. Is the pt stable or unstable?
  b. Is this 1st episode or recurrent episode, & is this part of a paroxysmal, persistent, or permanent duration paradigm?
  c. If 1st episode or paroxysmal, how long have sxs been present (ie, <48 h)?
  d. What is the pt's stroke risk? (Calculate $CHADS_2VASC$ score)
  e. Is there an underlying precipitant of AF that should be treated?
  f. Does the pt have a cardiologist/PCP w/ whom you can make joint decision or poor f/u?
- **Rate control vs rhythm control:** There appears to be no difference in symptomatic improvement, CHF, thromboembolic cx, severe bleeding, or mortality when comparing the 2 strategies (*Lancet* 2000;356:1789; *NEJM* 2002;347:1825; *J Am Coll Cardiol* 2003;41:1690; *Chest* 2004;126:476); however, rhythm control seems to be a/w increased rates of hospitalization & adverse medication effects (*Lancet* 2000;356:1789; *NEJM* 2002;347:1825); more recent data suggest that early rhythm control a/w lower risk of poor cardiovascular outcomes in pts w/ CV conditions (*NEJM* 2020;383:1305–1316)
  - May not be generalizable to ED pt presenting w/ 1st episode or paroxysmal AF
- **Treatment algorithms** (*Can J Cardiol* 2020;36(12):1847; *Circulation* 2014;64(21):e1; 2019;140:e125)

Figure 1.4 Unstable patient with atrial fibrillation. ([a]Note: see Direct current cardioversion and anticoagulation below.)

Unstable patient (SBP <90 mmHg, AMS, acute pulmonary edema, AMI, wide complexes suggesting pre-excitation syndrome)

↓

Emergent direct current cardioversion (DCCV) using 150–200 J biphasic defib
[a]Give heparin bolus and gtt to goal aPTT 1.5–2 times reference range to prevent embolism

Figure 1.5 Stable patient, first episode or paroxysmal atrial fibrillation. ([a]Note: Can consider cardioversion in these patients; however, consider delaying DCCV and anticoagulate for 3 wks if high risk of stroke.)

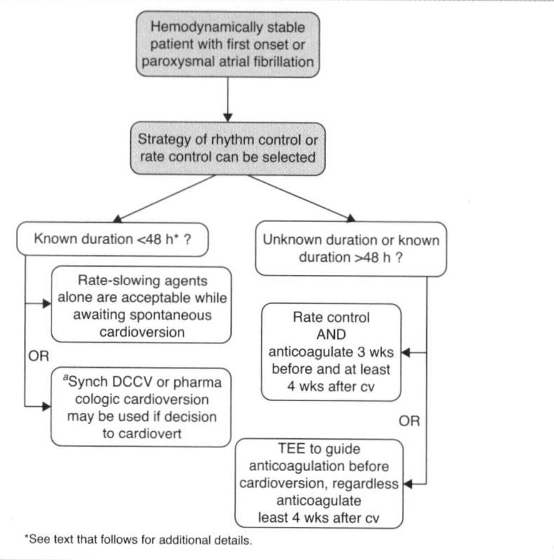

- Note there is limited data supporting safety of cardioversion w/o AC for AF up to 48 h duration, since some data suggests higher risk of thromboembolic Cx vs threshold of <12 h (*J Am Coll Cardiol* 2019;74(1):104). Consider pt RFs particularly if stable pt w/ onset <48 h but >12 h

Figure 1.6 Stable patient, persistent or permanent atrial fibrillation.

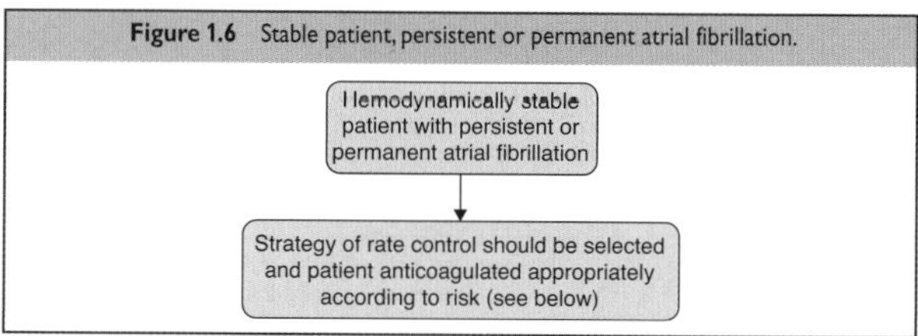

- **Rate control:** IV Beta blockers or nondihydropyridine CCBs recommended as 1st-line therapy for rate control in acute setting as long as no hx pre-excitation synd. CCB, however, should be used w/ caution in pts w/ reduced EF, and should avoid IV nondihydropyridine CCBs and IV BBs in pts w/ decompensated HF
- IV administration of digoxin or amiodarone is recommended to control HR w/ AF & HF
- Can consider IV calcium pre-tx to reduce risk of diltiazem-associated hypotension in AF/AFL w/ RVR (*Am J Emerg Med* 2025:88:23–28)
- Digoxin or amiodarone can be added to therapy w/ beta blockers or CCB if HR is not controlled
- Consider IV amiodarone for rate control in critically ill pts w/ no hx pre-excitation
- Lenient rate strategy (HR <110 bpm) reasonable if pt asx & nl LV function (*NEJM* 2010;362:1362–1373)
- IV procainamide or ibutilide recommended for HD stable pts w/ AF involving conduction over an accessory pathway. For pts w/ WPW and AF, IV CCB, amiodarone, adenosine, or digoxin should be avoided as they may paradoxically accelerate the ventricular response, and BB have similar potential risk (*Circulation* 1982;65:348–354; *Circulation* 2014;64(21):e1–e76)

Rate Control Agents for Atrial Fibrillation/Atrial Flutter (*Circulation* 2014;64(21):e1–e76)			
Medication		**Initial Dose**	**Maint Dose**
BB	Metoprolol	2.5–5 mg IV bolus q5min × 3	Start 25–100 mg PO BID
	Esmolol	500 mcg/kg IV	50–300 mcg/kg/min IV gtt
	Propranolol	1 mg IV q2min × 3	Start 10–40 mg PO TID or QID
CCB	Diltiazem	0.25 mg/kg IV × 1; may repeat 0.25–0.35 mg/kg IV after 15 mins	5–15 mg/h IV gtt or start 30–90 mg PO QID or
	Verapamil	0.075–0.15 mg/kg IV; may give additional 10 mg after 30 mins	Start 40–80 mg PO TID
Digoxin (onset in hours)		0.25 mg IV q2h, up to 1.5 mg maximum over 24 h	
Amiodarone		300 mg IV over 60 mins (alternative dosing strategies exist)	10–50 mg/h over 24 h

- **Direct current cardioversion:** Recommended dose 150–200 J biphasic waveform
  - There may be higher 1st-shock success for DCCV if initial energy used 200 J vs 100 J (BEST-AF, *Heart* 2008;94:884)
  - Pre-tx w/ amiodarone, flecainide, ibutilide, propafenone, or sotalol can be used to enhance the success of DCCV & prevent recurrent AF
- **Pharmacologic cardioversion:** Administration of flecainide, dofetilide, propafenone, or ibutilide is recommended for pharmacologic cardioversion if no CIs
  - Procainamide has been shown to be effective in ED population w/ 52% cardioversion w/ drug alone, w/ 96% success rate if f/b DCCV in nonresponders as compared to 92% w/ shock alone (*Lancet* 2020;395(10221):339)
  - Amiodarone is a reasonable option & safe in pts w/ CHF, but digoxin & sotalol may be harmful & are not recommended
  - Beta blockers or nondihydropyridine CCBs should be given ≥30 minutes before administering class Ic antiarrhythmic agents (eg, propafenone, flecainide as below)

Rhythm Control Agents for Atrial Fibrillation/Atrial Flutter			
Medication		**Initial Dose**	**Special Considerations**
Class Ia	Procainamide	20–50 mg/min to maximum of 15–17 mg/kg IV	• Preferred w/ WPW • May cause hypotension, QRS prolongation (stop if QRS increases >50%, hypotension)
Class Ic	Propafenone	450 mg PO (<70 kg) 600 mg PO (>70 kg)	• May cause hypotension, bradycardia, ventricular proarrhythmia • Contraindicated in pts w/ ischemic HD, LV dysfxn, structurally abnl heart
	Flecainide	200 mg PO (<70 kg) 300 mg PO (>70 kg)	• May cause hypotension, bradycardia, ventricular proarrhythmia • ↓ dose in renal insuff • Contraindicated in pts w/ ischemic HD, LV dysfxn, structurally abnl heart
Class III	Dofetilide	0.5 mg PO (eGFR >60) 0.25 mg PO (eGFR 40–60) 0.125 mg PO (GFR 20–40) Contraindicated if eGFR <20	• 2–3% risk torsades de pointes; contraindicated if long QT, bradycardia • Require hospitalization for initiation given risk of QTc prolongation
	Ibutilide	1 mg over 10 mins (>60 kg) 0.01 mg/kg, 10 mins (<60 kg) *May repeat once at same dose if doesn't terminate*	• Contraindicated in pts w/ hypokalemia, prolonged QTc, torsades de pointes
	Amiodarone	150 mg IV over 10 mins, 1 mg/min for 6 h, then 0.5 mg/min for 18 h	• QT prolongation, hypotension • SE: Hepatotoxicity, hypothyroid, thyrotoxicosis, pneumonitis, pulm fibrosis, corneal microdeposits

- **Anticoagulation:** All pts w/ AF or AFL should be stratified using a predictive index for stroke (ie, CHA_2DS_2-VASc), risk of bleeding (ie, HAS-BLED); most should receive AC (*Circulation* 2014;64(21):e1–e76; *J Am Coll Cardiol* 2019;74(1):104)
- Pts w/ very low risk of CVA (CHA_2DS_2-VASc = 0 for men and 1 for women), reasonable to omit AC unless MS or mechanical heart valve

- Pts w/ mod risk of CVA (CHA_2DS_2-VASc ≥2 for men or ≥3 for women) should receive oral anticoagulation w/ either warfarin or DOAC
- Most pts should receive DOAC, pts w/ valvular AF (a/w mod–severe MS or MVR) should receive warfarin
- DOAC include rivaroxaban 20 mg QD (ROCKET-AF, *NEJM* 2011;365:883) & apixaban 5 mg PO BID (ARISTOTLE, *NEJM* 2011;365:981), doses require renal adjustment
- For pts w/ sxs <48 h undergoing cardioversion (electric or pharm) anticoagulate for at least 4 wks regardless of CHA_2DS_2-VASc score. If sxs >48 h, anticoagulated for 3 wks prior to cardioversion or obtain TEE to assess for LA thrombus
- In unstable pts undergoing cardioversion, start AC as soon as possible & continue for at least 4 wks post cardioversion

CHA2DS2-VASC Score for Estimating Stroke Risk in Patients with AF (*Chest* 2010;137(2):263; *Eur Heart J* 2012;33(12):1500–1510)	
Risk Criteria	**Score**
CHF	1
HTN	1
Age	<65 = 0, 65–74 = 1, ≥75 = 2
DM	1
Female gender	1
Prior stroke, TIA, Thromboembolism	2
Vascular dz (prior MI, PAD, aortic plaque)	1
Score	**Risk of Stroke/TIA/Thromboembolism %/y**
0	0.3
1	0.9
2	2.9
3	4.6
4	6.7
5	10.0
6	13.6
7	15.7
8	15.2
9	17.4

HAS-BLED Score for Estimating Major Bleeding Risk in Patients with AF (*Chest* 2010;138:1093)	
Clinical Characteristic	**Score**
HTN (SBP >160 mmHg)	1
Abnl renal or liver fxn (1 pt each)[b]	1 or 2
Stroke	1
Major bleeding or predisposition to bleeding	1
Labile INRs	1
Elderly (age >65 y/o)	1
Medications w/ predisposition to bleeding or EtOH use (1 pt each)[c]	1 or 2
HAS-BLED Score	**Major Bleeds/100 Patient-Years[a]**
0	1.13%
1	1.02%
2	1.88%
3	3.74%
4	8.70%
5	12.50%
6–9	Not reported

[a]Major bleeding defined as any bleeding requiring hospitalization &/or causing a decrease in Hgb of >2 g/L &/or requiring blood tfx that was not a hemorrhagic stroke.
[b]Abnl renal fxn defined as chronic dialysis, renal transplant, or Cr >200 µmol/L (2.3 mg/dL). Abnl liver fxn defined as chronic hepatic dz (ie, cirrhosis), Tbili >2× ULN, in association w/ AST/ALT. ALP >3× ULN.
[c]Medications included anti-plt agents & NSAIDs.

Disposition
- Home: Pts who convert to sinus, or are rate controlled, & anticoagulated if necessary
- All discharged pts should get close PCP or cardiology f/u
- EDOU: depending on local clinical protocols
- Admit: pts w/ acute underlying illness, ongoing sxs, or poor rate control

Pearls
- Risk of stroke is similar in all forms of AF/AFL (recurrent paroxysmal, persistent, & permanent AF, & AFL)
- Spontaneous cardioversion occurs w/i 48 h in 50–67% acute AF
- 5–8% elderly have recurrent AF
- Atrial fibrillation w/ RVR may be compensatory tachycardia, search for underlying cause (sepsis, PE, etc)

Pre-excitation (*Circulation* 2016;133:e506–e574)

Definition
- **Accessory pathway:** A bypass tract that conducts impulses b/w atria and ventricles
- **Wolff–Parkinson–White:** Accessory conduction pathway evident on resting ECG and hx of sxs typical of SVT
- **Orthodromic AVRT:** Impulse travels down AV node (fast), then conducts retrograde, up the accessory pathway (slowly) → thus generally narrow-complex QRS w/ retrograde p waves in early part of ST segment (therefore short RP interval)
- **Antidromic AVRT:** Impulse travels down the accessory pathway (slowly), then conducts retrograde, up the AV node (fast) → thus wide-complex QRS

Evaluation
- ECG & rhythm strip
- WPW: short PR <120 ms, prolonged QRS >110 ms, delta wave (slurring uprise of initial portion of QRS)
- Orthodromic AVRT: narrow-complex tachycardia (unless BBB)
- Antidromic AVRT: wide complex tachycardia
- AF/AFL in WPW: irregular rhythm, wide QRS complexes that Δ in shape & morphology, may degenerate into VT/VF

Treatment
- As above, synchronized cardioversion if unstable
- Orthodromic AVRT: vagal maneuvers, adenosine; consider IV beta blockers, CCB (must be ready to perform cardioversion when giving any of these medications); avoid digoxin
- AF/AFL w/ pre-excitation → cardiology c/s, DC cardiovert, or use procainamide; meds inc beta blockers & CCB are ineffective or can precipitate VF (see section on *AF/AFL*)

Ventricular Tachycardia

Approach
- Determine if pt is stable or unstable → use ACLS protocol for any pt w/ unstable VT
- Differentiate VT from nonsustained VT (NSVT), & other causes of wide complex tachycardia (see above)
- Differentiate monomorphic from polymorphic VT

Definition
- NSVT: VT lasting <30 s
- SVT w/ aberrancy: VT look-alike b/c abnl conduction → wide complex tachycardia. Caused by fixed BBB, rate-related BBB, or accessory pathway
- Torsades de pointes: polymorphic VT + prolonged QT

Causes
- **Monomorphic, structurally abnl heart:** prior MI, cardiomyopathy, arrhythmogenic RV dysplasia (ARVD)
- **Monomorphic, structurally nl heart:** idiopathic VT
- **Polymorphic:** ischemia, cardiomyopathy, torsades de pointes, Brugada synd (see below)

History
- Palpitations, lightheadedness, CP, SOB, nausea, syncope, unresponsiveness; PMH: CAD, cardiomyopathy, mx CAD RFs, & FHx sudden cardiac death all ↑ risk VT

Evaluation
- ECG, rhythm strip, lytes, Ca, Mg, PO_4, cardiac markers; CXR; digoxin level if appropriate
- Brugada algorithm: 4-step approach to differentiate VT from SVT w/ aberrancy

Brugada Algorithm (*Circulation* 1991;83:1649)	
Criterion	**Sens & Spec for VT if Criteria Present**[a]
Absence of an RS complex in all precordial leads	21%, 100%
R to S interval >100 ms in one precordial lead	66%, 98%
AV dissociation	82%, 98%
Morphology criteria for VT present in both precordial leads V1–V2 & V6	99%, 97%

[a]Stepwise. If "no" to all questions then consistent w/ SVT w/ aberrant conduction (Sens 97%, Spec 99%)

Criteria for WCT Suggesting VT (From *Arrhythm Electrophysiol Rev.* 2013;2(1):23–29. Table 2.)	
Criterion	**ECG Appearance**
AV dissociation	Independent P waves; capture beats, fusion beats
Wide QRS	RBBB type: QRS >140 ms suggests VT LBBB type: QRS >160 ms suggests VT R to S interval >100 ms in any precordial lead
Extreme axis deviation	QRS axis b/w +180° & –90° (+QRS in aVR, –QRS in I, aVF)
Atypical QRS morphology for BBB	–QRS b/w +180° & –90° (–QRS lead I, & –QRS aVF) RBBB type: Absence of tall R′ in V1, r/S ratio <1 in V6 LBBB type: Onset to nadir >60–100 ms in V1, Q wave in V6
Concordance	Of QRS in precordial leads w/ same pattern & direction

Treatment

- **Unstable VT:** ACLS protocol, cardioversion (if + pulse) vs defibrillation (if no pulse)
- **Stable VT:** Consider synchronized cardioversion or can also use either:
  - Lidocaine: 1–1.5 mg/kg IV load, then 1–4 mg/min
  - Amiodarone: 150 mg IV load, then 1 mg/min for 6 h, then 0.5 mg/min for 18 h
  - Procainamide 20–50 mg/min until maximum of 15–17 mg/kg IV, or until arrythmia suppressed, develops hypotension or QRS duration increases >50%
- **Polymorphic VT:** Magnesium 2–4 g IV bolus
- **Other:** Replete electrolytes (Ca, Mg, PO_4); treat coincident ischemia if present

Treatment of Wide-Complex Tachycardias	
	Tx
VT	Amiodarone, lidocaine, procainamide, DCCV
Polymorphic VT	Magnesium
SVT w/ [a]aberrancy (ie, BBB)	Adenosine (avoid if irregular), vagal maneuvers, DCCV
SVT w/ pre-excitation	Procainamide, DCCV
Tachycardia + PM	Treat cause of tachycardia, apply magnet if PM-mediated

[a]Causes of aberrancy: bundle branch blocks (fixed, rate-related, Ashman phenomenon), accessory pathways (ie, WPW), meds (ie, class Ia/Ic antiarrhythmics, TCAs), pseudo-STEMI, PM, hyperkalemia, hypothermia, cardiomyopathies, channelopathies.

Disposition

- Admit to cardiac step-down unit or cardiac ICU

Pearls

- Assume all wide complex tachycardias to be ventricular unless proven o/w
- Best clinical predictors that WCT is VT → prior MI, CHF, LV dysfxn (*Am J Med* 1998;84:53)

Brugada Syndrome (*Circulation* 2012;5:606)

Definition

- Characteristic EKG findings (see *Syncope* section above) plus qualifying clinical characteristics; incomplete RBBB w/ STE V1–V3 caused by alteration of the myocyte Na channel, associated w/ VT & sudden cardiac death

History

- Classically young, o/w healthy male, FHx sudden cardiac death; sxs: presyncope, syncope, palpitations, cardiac arrest; may have hx VT/VF; ECG findings may be unmasked in the setting of stressor (eg, fever)

Evaluation

- ECG, electrolytes, Ca, Mg, PO_4

Treatment

- Tele; electrophysiology c/s

Disposition

- If incidental finding, refer to cardiology for f/u. O/w, admit to Tele bed for EP study, possible ICD placement.

PACEMAKER AND AICD MALFUNCTION

Definition

- PM: Intracardiac device used for significant AV block &/or sinus node dysfxn
- AICD: Intracardiac device for the termination of VF/VT, & prevention of sudden cardiac death → for pts s/p VF/unstable VT arrest, persistent EF ≤30–35%, Brugada, or long QT synd (*Circulation* 2007;115:1170; *NEJM* 1997;337:1576)
- Biventricular pacing (cardiac resynchronization therapy): RA, RV, & coronary sinus leads → synchronize RV & LV function → ↓ CHF sxs & hospitalization, ↑ survival (*NEJM* 2004;350:2140; 2005;352:1539)

Approach

- Obtain an ECG & rhythm strip immediately
- Obtain the make & model of the device (most pts have a card, o/w obtain AP CXR → magnify device to obtain model number → internet search for type)
- Common PM codes: DDD (dual chamber paced, sensed, & response to sensed beat) & VVI (ventricle paced, sensed, & inhibitory response to sensed beat)

Evaluation

- Magnet placed over device
  - PM: Inhibits sensing, paces at fixed rate regardless of intrinsic cardiac activity (asynchronous pacing)
  - AICD: Inhibits further firing (while magnet applied), though not bradycardic pacing

Pacemaker Malfunction	
Pathophysiology	**Differential**
Failure of output → no pacer spike despite indication to pace	Battery depletion
Failure to capture → pacing spikes *not* followed w/ depolarization	Lead fracture or dislodgement, ↑ pacer threshold, electrolyte abnormalities, local ischemia, or scar
Oversensing → pacer spike despite *no* indication to pace	Lead fracture or dislodgement, sensing threshold too low
Undersensing → *no* pacer spike despite indication to pace	Lead fracture or dislodgement, sensing threshold too high
PM-mediated tachycardia	Reentrant tachycardia in pts w/ D-paced PM, b/w the PM leads (act as an accessory pathway → anterograde conduction) & the AV node (retrograde conduction)

History & Physical Examination

- Lightheadedness, palpitations, syncope
- ↑, ↓, and/or irregular HR, ↓ BP

Evaluation

- ECG, CXR (to visualize device & leads)
- Device interrogation
- Biventricular pacing seen as 2 simultaneous pacing spikes preceding paced QRS, predominantly QRS in lead I & + in V1 (opposite in R ventricular pacing)
- Biventricular pacing has unique cxs: coronary sinus dissection or perforation
- Pacemaker cxs not related to malfxn: infxn, thrombophlebitis, pacemaker synd (due to loss of AV synchrony), perforation, tamponade

Treatment

- Transcutaneous pacing: for unstable pts
- **MAGNET: FOR PM-mediated tachycardia or oversensing:** Magnet over the PM → paces @ 80 bpm

Disposition

- Pending eval and interrogation results, may need to c/s EP for device reprogramming; to cath lab if need lead/battery replacement

AICD Firing (*JAMA* 2006;296:2839; *NEJM* 2003;349:1836; *JACC* 2006;48:1064)	
Pt Sxs	**AICD Interrogation**
Pt-sensed AICD[a] firing	No firing
	Inappropriate firing
	Appropriate firing

[a]AICDs can also malfxn like PMs (see *PM* section above).

History & Physical Examination
- **AICD firing:** sudden jolt of pain
- **Premonitory sxs:** palpitations, LH, dyspnea, CP
- **Precipitants:** exercise, illness, noncompliance w/ antiarrhythmics, new meds
- ECG (ischemia, ↑ QT), CBC, Chem 7, cardiac markers, CXR

Evaluation
- C/s EP or device rep. for interrogation & reprogramming
- No firing (nl interrogation despite sxs): Look for other cause of sxs → D/C home
- Inappropriate firing (based on interrogation): Treat underlying condition; reprogram if necessary
- Look for precipitants: VT, abnl electrolytes, ↑ QT, ischemia, medication noncompliance or substance related

Treatment
- Treat primary-illness; follow ACLS protocol for arrhythmia

Disposition
- If appropriate firing (based on interrogation): Admit to Tele unit or CCU

Pearl
- If make/model # of device unknown, magnification of PA CXR will reveal device-sp code in small print

MECHANICAL SUPPORT DEVICES

Overview (*Emerg Med Australas* 2014;26(2):104)
- LVAD: Often bridge to transplant, or destination therapy in pts who do not qualify for transplant
  - Supports cardiac output by mechanical pump that draws blood from the LV & pumps it into the ascending aorta
  - Pump is connected via a driveline that exits the pt's epigastrium to an external controller box w/ batteries that are worn on a harness
- Other mechanical support devices include BiVAD, TAH, and ECMO

Findings
- Most devices do not have pulsatile flow, so pts will not have pulse or BP that can be measured w/ automatic cuff
- Perform perfusion assessment w/ skin, mental status, etc
- To measure BP manually, inflate cuff & place Doppler over brachial or radial artery, deflate until a continuous sound is heard, which is the MAP
- Auscultate chest to assess for continuous noise of machine if pump is working

Evaluation
- ECG, CXR, Tele, echo, labs (CBC, coags, lytes, cardiac biomarkers, cultures) per clinical suspicion
- Assess batteries & pump function
- Immediately attempt to contact VAD center or VAD team

LVAD Complications	
Problem & Presentation	**Treatment**
RV failure (pump does not support RV unless BiVAD, e/o RV dysfxn) presents w/ poor perfusion (AMS, cool, pale, clammy, low flow)	Small fluid boluses, inotropes, assess for RV MI or failure, consider afterload reduction w/ nitrates
Infxn (driveline or others)	Drivelines can become infected, also at risk for other infxns inc bacteremia, pneumonia, UTI, etc. Treat w/ abx
Bleeding (GIB, etc)	All pts on AC, also w/ acquired PLT dysfxn, transfuse PRN
Pump thrombosis (check alarms, AC compliance)	Heparin or thrombolysis, consider heparin in the setting of prolonged hemostasis
Dysrhythmia (many pts also have AICD)	Device continues to function so pt may remain awake in VF, treat w/ cardioversion/defib, antidysrhythmics
Machine malfxn	Check batteries, flow, check alarms, c/s w/ VAD team

Cardiac arrest	Chest compressions risk dislodging device leading to massive hemorrhage, mx methods should be used to confirm absence of circulation prior to initiation of compressions & attempt to correct pump or use device's external hand pump if available first: • Evaluate for any e/o device malfxn (eg: replace battery, etc) • Consider early transition to cardiopulmonary bypass • In a case series of pts who received compressions none had dislodgement & 50% survived *(Resuscitation* 2014;85:702–704)

Disposition
- C/s VAD center or VAD team, admit to cardiology or CCU

ECHOCARDIOGRAPHY

Overview
- Uses: assess for pericardial effusion & signs of tamponade, assess LV function, assess for RV dilation, assess volume status
- Views: parasternal long, parasternal short, subxiphoid, apical 4 chamber
- Echo views and positioning below based on EM convention w/ indicator on L of screen

Echo Views & Findings		
View	**Probe Positioning**	**Normal Findings**
Parasternal long	Place transducer in 3rd–4th L intercostal space adjacent to sternum w/ probe marker facing L hip	Allows visualization of the RV, aortic outflow tract, LA, & LV, & assessment of chamber size and LV function
Parasternal short	Place transducer in 3rd–4th L intercostal space adjacent to sternum w/ probe marker facing R hip (rotate ~90° clockwise from PSL)	Allows visualization of RV & LV (inc papillary muscles) & LV function and wall motion abnormalities
Apical 4 chamber	Place transducer at the apex w/ the probe marker facing the R hip (view can be improved w/ pt in L lateral position)	Allows visualization of all 4 chambers & for assessment of chamber size & function, eval for RV dilation
Subxiphoid	Place the transducer just inferior to the xiphoid w/ the probe marker facing the pt's R side & flatten the probe	Allows assessment for effusion
IVC	Place the transducer just inferior to the xiphoid w/ the probe marker facing the pt's head (rotate ~90° clockwise from subxiphoid view)	Allows for assessment of IVC size & resp variation

Echo Findings		
Finding & View	**Technique**	**Significance**
Parasternal long: End-point septal separation (EPSS) *(Am Heart J* 1983;106(1):21–28)	Use M-mode w/ marker placed over most distal tip of anterior mitral leaflet, the M-mode image appears as 2 peaks, the E-point (larger peak; corresponding to early diastolic filling) & the A-point (corresponding to the atrial kick), measure distance in mm b/w peak of E-point & septum, EPSS >7 mm corresponds to LVEF <50% (sens 87%, spec 75%), EPSS ≥13 corresponds to EF ≤35%; limitations: mitral stenosis, aortic regurgitation can give false-positive	LV function can be estimated visually; mitral valve EPSS can be measured & aid in estimation. EPSS is a measurement of the distance b/w the interventricular septum & anterior mitral valve leaflet in early diastole

Apical 4 chamber: Tricuspid annular plane systolic excursion (TAPSE)	Assess RV size (LV should be larger) & movement in the apical 4-chamber view. Place M-mode cursor over lateral tricuspid annulus, measure in mm the distance annulus moves over 1 cardiac cycle, can use average over mx cycles to improve accuracy	TAPSE measurement can be used to evaluate for RV dysfxn, no consensus for cutoff for TAPSE, American Society of Echocardiography guidelines indicate TAPSE <17 mm is abnl (*J Am Soc Echocardiogr* 2015;28(1):1–39.e14). Limitations: not specific for acute vs chronic RV dysfxn or cause of RV dysfxn
Apical 4 chamber: McConnell's sign	Assess RV movement in apical 4-chamber view McConnell's sign = akinesia of mid free wall but nl motion at apex	77% sens & 94% spec for acute PE (*Am J Cardiol* 1996;78:469)
Parasternal short: D-sign	Obtain parasternal short view & assess shape of LV	Abnl D-shaped LV w/ septum pushing into LV indicates increased RV pressure
IVC	Use M-mode to assess IVC size & variability w/ resp cycles	If IVC diameter <0.9 cm & IVC collapse >50% w/ each breath (in nonventilated pts), likely fluid responsive; if IVC diameter >2 cm & IVC collapse <15% w/ each breath, likely not fluid responsive. However limited high-quality evidence, and must be interpreted in clinical context
Apical 4 Chamber: Transvalvular flow in Tamponade	Use pulsed wave Doppler over the mitral valve to measure peak E-wave velocity and respiratory variation	Peak E-wave velocity variation of 25% or more over the respiratory cycle is suggestive of tamponade physiology (*J Am Coll Cardiol* 1988;11(3):572); should have plethoric IVC in tamponade

COUGH

Pneumonia

Definitions (*Am J Respir Crit Care Med* 2019;200(7):e45–e67)
- CAP: Out of hospital or </48 h since admit
- HAP: >/48 h after hospital admit
- VAP: >/48 h after intubation
- HCAP: Eliminated in most recent ATS/IDSA guidelines due to data showing over-treatment for MRSA PNA w/o improvement in outcomes

History
- Typical CAP (eg, Strep, Klebsiella, Haemophilus): fever/chills, SOB, CP, cough, sputum
- Atypical CAP (eg, Mycoplasma, legionella): mild fever, mild/mod SOB, CP, cough, GI sx
- Aspiration PNA: a/w neurologic dz, esophageal dz, vomiting, AMS or intoxication, & poor dental hygiene
- MRSA/PsA: prior resp isolation of MRSA &/or PsA, IV abx w/i 90 d, other local RFs (ie, chronic HD, immunosupp, recent influenza [MRSA], CF/bronchiectasis [PsA], asplenia)
- Legionella: severe PNA in elderly, a/w hyponatremia & GI sx
- Viral PNA (influenza, SARS-CoV-2) fevers/chills, myalgias, HA, sore throat, dry cough
- TB: Undomiciled, HIV+/immunosuppressed, IVDU, incarcerated, travel to endemic region; presents w/ blood-tinged sputum, night sweats, fevers, wt loss
- PJP: poorly controlled HIV (CD4 <200, lymph <1 k); presents w/ subacute tachypnea

Physical Examination
- Fever, tachycardia, tachypnea, hypoxia, rales, decreased breath sounds
- PNA less likely w/ nl VS & clear lungs, except in elderly, infants, immunosuppressed

Evaluation
- Who needs labs? Reserve for pts needing hospitalization, eg, w/ abnl VS, extremes of age, w/ concerning comorbidities, &/or poor f/u
  - Labs: CBC, BMP, resp viral panel, consider lactate (if c/f sepsis)
  - Labs to consider: blood/sputum cx (if MRSA/PsA RFs, cavitary lesion, effusion, ICU admit), Pneumococcal urine antigen (if ICU admit), Legionella urine antigen (if recent exposure to area w/ outbreak, ICU admit), ABG & LDH (if c/f PJP)
- CXR: focal consolidation (typical PNA); diffuse interstitial pattern (atypical PNA); bat-wing pattern (PJP); hilar adenopathy, calcified or cavitary apical lesions (TB)

Treatment

Scenario/ Etiology	Empiric Treatment Guidelines
Outpt	Healthy & no MRSA/PsA risks: amoxicillin (1 g PO TID) OR doxycycline (100 mg PO BID) OR azithromycin (500 mg PO on d 1, then 250 mg daily) Comorbidities: 1) Amoxicillin/clavulanate (500 mg PO TID or 875 mg PO BID) OR cephalosporin (such as cefpodoxime 200 mg PO BID) +2) Azithromycin (500 mg PO on d 1, then 250 mg daily) OR doxycycline (100 mg PO BID) OR Levofloxacin (750 mg PO QD)
Inpt, no MRSA/ PsA risks	1) 3rd-gen cephalosporin (such as CTX 1 g IV QD) OR ampicillin/sulbactam 2 g IV q6h +2) azithromycin OR doxycycline OR Levofloxacin
Inpt, MRSA/ PsA risks	MRSA RF: Add Vancomycin (15–20 mg/kg loading dose) OR linezolid (600 mg IV q12) PsA RF: antipseudomonal PCN/cephalosporin (such as cefepime 2 g IV Q8) OR carbapenem (500 mg IV Q6) OR aztreonam (2 g IV Q8). Refer to local antibiogram
Severe PNA (ICU)	Emerging evidence supporting use of steroids (eg, 200 mg hydrocortisone IV daily) to reduce mortality (*NEJM* 2023;(388):1931–1941)
Aspiration PNA	Same as inpt CAP. If abscess/empyema, add metronidazole (500 mg IV q8), b-lactam/b-lactamase inhibitor
Influenza A & B	Oseltamivir (75 mg PO BID × 7 d) Oseltamivir should be considered in pts w/ sx <48 h or w/ high-risk comorbidities. Oseltamivir tx reduces duration of sx (*Cochrane Dat. Sys. Rev* 2014;(4):CD008965)

COVID-19	Consider nirmatrelvir/ritonavir for elderly, immunocompromised, or pts w/ multiple comorbidities; consider remdesivir for pts at risk for severe dz requiring hospitalization, consider dexamethasone for pts requiring supplemental O_2 (*NIH COVID-19 Treatment Guidelines*; https://www.covid19treatmentguidelines.nih.gov/)
PJP	Room Air SaO_2 ≥92%/PaO_2 ≥70 mmHg: TMP/SMX 14–20 mg/kg/d of trimethoprim divided TID RA SaO_2 ≤92%/PaO_2 ≤70 mmHg: Add glucocorticoids (prednisone 40 mg PO BID or methylprednisolone 30 mg IV BID)
TB	**RIPE: R**ifampin (10 mg/kg, max 600 mg, PO QD) + **I**NH (5 mg/kg PO QD) + Vit B_6 (25–50 mg PO QD, prevents neuropathy) + **P**yrazinamide (15–30 mg/kg, max 2 g, PO QD) + **E**thambutol (15–25 mg/kg, max 2.5 g, PO QD)

Disposition

- CAP: Consider using PSI (preferred by IDSA) or CURB-65 score (see *Table* below) together w/ comorbidities & ambulatory sat to determine need for admission
- PJP: Admit unless SpO_2 >95% w/o desaturation on exertion
- TB/Legionella: Admit & report to Department of Public Health

Pneumonia Severity Index (PSI) (*NEJM* 1997;336(4):243–250)			
Variable	**Points Assigned**		
Demographics	If male: (+Age); if female, (+Age – 10); nursing home resident (+10)		
Comorbidities	Neoplastic dz (+30); liver dz (+20); CHF (+10); cerebrovascular dz (+10); renal dz (+10)		
Physical exam	AMS (+20); HR ≥125 (+20); RR >30 (+20); SBP <90 (+15); temp <35 °C or ≥40 °C (+10)		
Labs & CXR	pH <7.35 (+30); BUN ≥30 mg/dL (+20); Na <130 (+20); glucose ≥250 mg/dL (+10); Hct <30 (+10); PaO_2 <60 (+10); pleural eff (+10)		
PORT Score (Recommended Triage & Prognosis) Calculated from PSI			
Class	**Score**	**Mortality (%)**	**Disposition**
I	<50	<1	Outpt
II	≤70	<1	Outpt
III	71–90	2.8	Observation
IV	91–130	8.2	Floor
V	>130	29.2	ICU
CURB-65 Score (*Thorax* 2003;58(5):377)			
1 point each	**C**onfusion, **U**rea >20 mg/dL, **R**R >30, S**B**P <90, DBP <60, age **>65**		
Score <2	Outpt; mortality 0.7% (if 0), 3.2% (if 1)		
Score = 2	Inpt vs observation; mortality 3%		
Score >2	Flor vs IC; mortality 17% (if 3), 41.5% (if 4), 57% (if 5)		

Pearls

- Special considerations: IVDU/endocarditis (multifocal PNA, esp b/l), malignancy (postobstructive PNA), post-influenza (MRSA PNA), recent elective surgery (aspiration PNA risk increases w/ age, duration of anesthesia, periop NG tube)
- In severe PNA, high-flow NC (vs NIPPV) reduces 30-d mortality & may reduce need for intubation (esp if PaO_2:FiO_2 <200) (*NEJM* 2015;372(23):2185–2196)

Acute Bronchitis

Etiology

- Most commonly viral (parainfluenza, adenovirus, rhinovirus, coronavirus, RSV, influenza) but atypical bacteria ~5% of cases (*chlamydia p., mycoplasma, B. pertussis*)

History

- Cough >5 d (dry or wet), low-grade fever, myalgias, wheezing, often after URI sxs
- Consider pertussis: posttussive emesis, whoop, duration >1 wk

Physical Examination

- Fever uncommon (if present consider influenza or PNA); may have chest wall tenderness from muscle strain; lungs often clear, but up to 40% have bronchospasm/wheeze

Evaluation

- Labs/CXR not routinely needed; reserve for abnl VS, pts w/ comorbidities, & at extremes of age

Treatment
- Supportive care: lack of strong evidence supporting, decongestants, or antihistamines (*Chest* 2017;152(5):1021–1037)
- If wheezy or asthma hx: bronchodilator (albuterol MDI 2 puffs QID) & consider inhaled corticosteroids × 7 d. Also consider COPD exacerbation as cause
- Abx not routinely indicated (*Cochrane Syst Rev* 2017;6(6):CD000245)
- Abx reserved for elderly, significant comorbidities

Disposition
- Discharge home w/ PCP f/u; will likely recover in 2–3 wk

DYSPNEA (SHORTNESS OF BREATH)

Definition
- Difficult or labored breathing (acute or progressive) often due to primary pulm or cardiovascular etiologies, but w/ broad DDx (eg, endo, heme, tox, neuromuscular)
- Always assess for resp distress: RR >24 or <8, tripoding, accessory muscle use, inability to speak in full sentences, AMS, abnl chest movement

Approach to the Patient		
Etiology	**H&P**	**Evaluation**
	Upper Airway Causes	
Airway obstruction • Angioedema • FB aspiration • Epiglottitis • Croup • Abscess/Hematoma • Neoplasm	Hx: Often sudden onset, ask about vaccinations (epiglottitis) PEx: Stridor, resp distress, pooled secretions (severe); check airway patency, neck ROM/swelling	XR chest &/or neck CT neck if considering abscess or hematoma Laryngoscopy/ Bronchoscopy
	Cardiac Causes	
Myocardial ischemia	Hx: Exertional, but UA can present at rest. Often w/ pain, n/v, diaphoresis, LH	ECG, troponins, +/– stress tests vs coronary CTA
Arrhythmia (SVT, NSVT)	Hx: Can be paroxysmal or constant (AF). Sometimes w/ palpitations, CP, LH	ECG, tele, electrolytes
Valve dz • L heart (AV, MV) • R heart (PV, TV)	Hx: Exertional, often indolent PEx: Murmur, periph edema, lung crackles	ECG, echo
Cardiogenic pulmonary edema • CHF • AV/MV dz • Myocarditis • Constrictive pericarditis • Tamponade	Hx: Exertional, orthopnea, PND, can have CP PEx: Basilar crackles, LE edema/JVD (if RHF present), murmur	CXR: Edema, Kerley B lines, cephalization, effusion Lung U/S: B lines BNP (less sens in obese pts)
	Pulmonary Causes	
Noncardiogenic pulm edema • ARDS • Opioid OD • Salicylates • HAPE	Hx: Often exertional, increasing O_2 req PEx: Crackles, tachypnea	CXR: Edema, opacities, Kerley B lines Lung U/S: B lines
PTX • Spontaneous (tall/thin pts, emphysema) • Traumatic • Barotrauma (scuba, inhalation)	Hx: Acute onset, +/– w/ CP usually unilateral PEx: Unequal breath sounds & chest rise; tracheal deviation + JVD & hypotension if tension	CXR: Can be subtle. Visceral pleural line seen + no lung markings beyond Lung U/S: Absent lung sliding, lung point
PE	Hx: Often acute, can have pleuritic CP, s/sx of DVT; consider RFs PEx: If massive –> hypoxemia, hypotension, JVD	D-dimer if low/mod pretest prob CXR: Wedge infarct ECG: R heart strain Bedside echo: RV dilation CTA chest or V/Q scan

Obstructive lung dz • Asthma • COPD • Bronchospasm (bronchitis, anaphylaxis)	Hx: Chronic or acute irritants (allergens, URI, tobacco), hx atopy; assess freq & severity of exacerbations PEx: Wheezing, prolonged expiration, accessory muscles, air movement	Decreased peak expiratory flow rate (PEFR) suggests obstructive etiology CXR (if needed to r/o PNA): Nl or hyperinflated (emphysema)
Pleural eff (PNA, HF, cancer, cirrhosis)	Hx: Slow onset, orthopnea (often due to atelectasis) PEx: Diminished breath sounds at base & tactile fremitus	CXR: Blunted costophrenic angle, layering Lung U/S: Hypoechoic fluid Diagnostic thoracentesis (use Light criteria)
PNA	Hx: Fever, cough, +/– CP PEx: Rales or rhonchi, tachypnea, tachycardia	CXR: +/– Infiltrate
Interstitial lung dz • Occupational & environmental • Medications (MTX, Ritux, Amio) • XRT • Autoimmune (RA, sarcoid, scleroderma) • IPF	Hx: Chronic nonproductive cough PEx: Rales, Look for evidence of associated extrapulm dz	CXR: (can be hard to interpret) +/– reticular or nodular opacities CT chest for better characterization of parenchyma
Malignancy	Hx: Chronic cough, wt loss, hemoptysis, smoker PEx: Cachexia, clubbing	CXR: +/– Mass CT chest for better characterization

Other Etiologies	
Pathophysiology	**Differential**
Metabolic/endocrine	Hypermetabolic state (fever, thyrotoxicosis), metabolic acidosis from any cause w/ resp compensation (look for Kussmaul respirations), electrolyte derangements (Ca, Mg)
Hematologic	Anemia (heme malignancy, hemolysis, occult bleeding), TRALI
Toxins	Opioid (resp acidosis), salicylate (resp alkalosis), organophosphate (bronchorrhea), CO (binds Hgb >O_2, inhibiting O_2 delivery), cyanide (disrupts mitochondrial oxidative phosphorylation)
Mechanical	Abd distension (eg, pregnancy, massive ascites), morbid obesity
Neuromuscular	Myasthenia gravis, Guillain–Barré, ALS, stroke, botulism, West Nile virus, phrenic nerve dz (eg, tumor infiltration, surgery)
Psychogenic	Anxiety/panic attack, somatization disorder

Asthma

Definition

- Chronic recurrent inflammatory disorder w/ airway hyperresponsiveness, bronchospasm, & reversible airway obstruction

Clinical Features

- Progressive wheezing, dyspnea, chest tightness, cough (especially nocturnal)
- Always assess sx frequency, severity, duration, home tx
  - Evaluate for triggers: smoke, dust, air pollution, pests (roaches, mice), pet dander, mold, disinfectants, cold air, exercise, URI, stress, meds (NSAIDs, BBs)
- Assess asthma hx: past txs, baseline PEFR, ED visits/y, admissions, ICU admissions, prior intubations

Physical Examination

- Tachypnea, tachycardia, inspiratory/expiratory wheezes, prolonged expiration, decreased or no air movement, use of accessory muscles, tripoding, cyanosis. Wheezing may be absent w/ minimal air movement

Evaluation

- CXR: Avoid in routine exacerbations; order to r/o PNA/PTX, in elderly, w/ comorbidities
- PEFR: Compare to pt's baseline. Varies by age, gender, & height. Average adult female: 300–470; adult male: 400–660. Values below 200 suggest severe obstruction (except in elderly)
  - Mixed evidence regarding impact of PEFR monitoring on outcomes

- Blood gases are not routinely indicated to assess for severity, but normocarbia in severe asthma may be a sign of "tiring out," impending respiratory failure

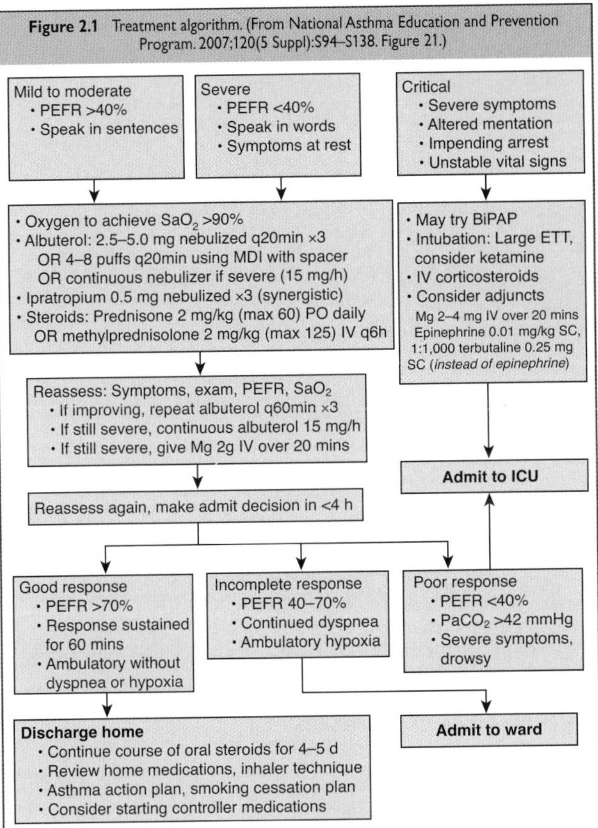

Figure 2.1 Treatment algorithm. (From National Asthma Education and Prevention Program. 2007;120(5 Suppl):S94–S138. Figure 21.)

Pearls

- MDI w/ spacer as effective as nebulizers (but harder for ill pts)
- Consider prescribing ICS at discharge if pt is not already taking. All pts >6 y should be prescribed ICS (*Lancet Respir Med* 2023;11(7):589)

Chronic Obstructive Pulmonary Disease (COPD)

Definition

- Progressive incompletely reversible airflow obstruction, w/ impaired gas exchange, usually w/ smoking hx. Formal diagnosis needs PFTs (postbronchodilator FEV_1/FVC <70% predicted)
  - Mild (FEV_1 ≥80%), mod (FEV_1 50–80%), severe (FEV_1 30–50%), very severe (FEV_1 <30%)

History

- Exacerbation: cough (worse than baseline), increased sputum (purulence & volume), dyspnea, wheeze
- Precipitants: infxn (viral > bacterial), cold weather, poor air quality, cardiopulmonary dz, PE (17% of acute exacerbations; *Int J Chron Obstruct Pulmon Dis* 2023;18:907), medication changes

Physical Examination

- Chronic bronchitis ("Blue Bloater"): cough w/ ↑ sputum production, cyanotic, plethoric, not in overt respiratory distress, scattered rhonchi & rales
- Emphysema ("Pink Puffer"): thin, dyspneic, tachypneic, noncyanotic, tripoding, pursed-lip exhalation (for auto-PEEP), diminished breath sounds

Evaluation

- ECG for dysrhythmia (AF or MAT), cor pulmonale (P pulmonale: big P wave in II)
- CXR to r/o PNA, PTX, effusion, edema, malignancy
- Consider D-dimer/CTA chest given high prevalence of PE in COPD exacerbations
- Blood gas to evaluate pH & $PaCO_2$, BMP & CBC (especially if admitted)
  - If chronic respiratory acidosis present, compare $PaCO_2$ w/ expected (calculated from HCO_3)
- Viral PCR testing (if epidemic), sputum cx (if severe COPD & PNA)
- Exacerbation severity: Mild (subjective dyspnea <5, RR <24, HR <95, SpO_2 ≥93% on baseline O_2 & change ≤3% from baseline, CRP <10 mg/L [if obtained]), mod ([3+ of the following] subjective dysnpea ≥ 5, RR≥24, HR≥95, SpO_2 <93% on baseline O_2 &/OR change >3% from baseline CRP ≥ 10 mg/L) , Severe (mod criteria + blood gas w/ new/worsening hypercapnia/acidosis) (GOLD 2025 Report. https://goldcopd.org/2025-gold-report/)

Treatment

- Titrate supplemental O_2 (goal SpO_2 88–92%): Chronic hypoxemia w/ inc risk of O_2-induced hypercapnia; increased mortality w/ SpO_2 >92% (*Emerg Med J* 2021;38(3):170)
- Albuterol (short-acting beta-agonist): 2.5–5 mg neb q30min × 3, then q2–4h OR MDI w/ spacer
- Ipratropium bromide (anticholinergic): 0.5 mg nebulized q30min × 3 doses, then q2–4h (synergistic effect w/ albuterol, so give together)
- Steroids: Prednisone 40 mg PO QD (5 d) OR methylprednisolone (for severely ill pts)
- Abx recommended if requiring hospitalization or ≥2 of increased SOB, increased sputum purulence, increased sputum volume
  - There is emerging evidence for use of CRP & procalcitonin in guiding abx administration (*BMC Pulm Med* 2022;22(1):194)
  - Outpt w/o risks: macrolide, doxycycline, or 2nd/3rd-gen cephalosporin (eg, cefdinir, cefpodoxime)
  - Outpt w/ risks: amoxicillin/clavulanate or fluoroquinolone
  - Inpt: 3rd-gen cephalosporin OR resp fluoroquinolone. Cefepime/Pip-taz If PsA RFs
- Noninvasive PPV (BiPAP): resp acidosis, severe SOB or fatigue, refractory hypoxemia; watch for PTX w/ PPV
  - Decreases mortality by 46% (NNT 12), intubation by 65% (NNT 5), tx failure by 50 (*Cochrane Database Syst rev* 2004;(3):CD004104)
- Invasive (intubation): Not tolerating BiPAP, impending respiratory failure, CV instability, AMS
- Mg 2 g for severe/refractory exacerbation

Disposition

- Home: mild sxs, ambulatory SpO_2 >90%, <q4h bronchodilators, outpt f/u, home support
  - Early f/u associated w/↓ mortality; 20% pts not back at prior baseline by 2 mo (GOLD 2017 Report. *Am J Respir Crit Care Med* 2017;195(5):557–582)
- Admit: Incomplete tx response, sig below baseline, multiple comorbidities, severe COPD/freq exacerbations, elderly, poor home support (*Am J Respir Crit Care Med* 2017;7(7))

Acute Respiratory Distress Syndrome

Berlin Definition (*JAMA* 2012;307(23):2526–2533)

- Acute (sx <1 wk) diffuse inflammatory lung injury, characterized by vascular leak, diffuse alveolar damage, imaging w/ b/l opacities, not secondary to cardiac failure or fluid overload, w/↓ PaO_2: FiO_2 200–300 (mild), 100–200 (mod), <300 (severe) when PEEP ≥5 cm H_2O

Pathophysiology

- Impaired gas exchange, poor compliance (stiff lungs), intrapulmonary shunt

Etiology

- Direct lung injury: PNA (inc COVID-19), aspiration, near drowning, hydrocarbons, inhalational injury, embolism (thrombotic, fat, air, amniotic)
- Systemic: sepsis, shock, DIC, trauma, burns, transfusion, pancreatitis, meds

Clinical Features

- Rapidly progressive dyspnea (<1 wk), cyanosis, crackles, & eventual respiratory failure

Evaluation

- Definitive dx requires ABG (PaO_2:FiO_2 <300) & CXR w/ b/l pulm edema
- May need TTE to r/o cardiac etiology, bronchoscopy to r/o diffuse alveolar hemorrhage

Treatment

- Supportive w/ focus on treating the underlying condition
- Lung-protective ventilation: decreased 28 d mortality by 10% (NNT 10) (*Cochrane Database Syst Rev* 2013;(2):CD003844)
- Minimize barotrauma: Low TV (<6 mg/kg), keep P_{Plat} <30
- Maintain high PEEP to keep alveoli open
- Avoid excess IVF. Excess volume in ED may negate subsequent benefit from conservative fluid management in ICU (*Crit Care Med* 2016;44(4):782–789)
- Refractory hypoxia: best PEEP trial, paralysis, inhaled prostacyclins, prone positioning, ECMO

Upper Airway Obstruction/Foreign Body (FB)

History

- RFs: extremes of age, neurocognitive disorders, seizure, substance abuse
- DDx: angioedema, infectious etiology (eg, epiglottitis), soft tissue abscess/hematoma
- Subacute (eg, malignancy, expanding goiter): often a delayed diagnose (eg, wheezing unresponsive to bronchodilators)

Physical Examination

- General appearance: May arrive cyanotic & in respiratory arrest if high-grade obstruction
- In breathing pt, respiratory exam depends on degree & location of obstruction: Decreased air movement, stridor, wheezing, secretion intolerance.

Evaluation

- CXR, XR neck rarely shows FB. CT may be helpful for radio-opaque or neoplastic causes
- Diagnostic & therapeutic flex bronchoscopy is standard

Treatment

- If still breathing: Airway equipment, inc cricothyrotomy kit, at bedside. Prepare for transfer to OR to remove FB in a controlled environment (bronchoscopy or DL)
- If not breathing: Attempt direct laryngoscopic visualization & removal of FB w/ forceps. If unsuccessful, perform cricothyrotomy
- If FB moves inferior to vocal cords but still occluding, push object into one lung by pressure from Ambu bag/ETT; once intubated, position ETT to ventilate contralateral lung

Disposition

- Flex bronchoscopy successful in 90% cases (*Respir Care* 2015;60(10):1438–1448)
- If object is safely removed & pt stable, can discharge home

HEMOPTYSIS

Definition

- Expectoration of blood or blood-stained sputum from below the vocal cords
- "Massive" hemoptysis: No defined volume (generally >500 cc/d or >100 cc/h), but any volume inhibiting breathing should be treated similarly; high-mortality via asphyxiation

Differential	
Pathophysiology	**Differential**
Pulm	COPD, CF, bronchiectasis, pulm HTN, PE, AVM, lung trauma
Cardiac	Pulm edema (eg, 2/2 CHF, mitral valve pathology)
Infectious	Acute bronchitis (#1 cause), PNA, TB, abscess, fungal infxn
Neoplastic	Malignancy (primary or met), carcinoid
Autoimmune	Goodpasture (anti-BM), granulomatosis polyangiitis (ANCA+)
Other	Recent instrumentation, tracheoarterial fistula (recent thoracic/vasc surgery), FB aspiration, inh cocaine, Osler–Weber–Rendu (telangiectasias), spontaneous (coagulopathy)

Approach to Patient

History

- Onset (sudden vs progressive); quantity of blood; differentiate from GI or ENT source
- ROS: fever, SOB, CP, wt loss, epistaxis (granulomatosis polyangiitis, coagulopathy)
- Identify history/RFs for COPD, PE, TB, CHF, cancer, autoimmune dz, coagulopathy

Physical Examination

- Assess airway 1st; if compromised, proceed directly to stabilizing airway
- Pulmonary: May show signs of COPD (wheezing, prolonged expiration), PNA (rhonchi), edema (crackles)
- Cardiac: Eval for signs of CHF or valve dz (murmurs, S3/S4)
- Skin: Evaluate for evidence of bleeding &/or telangiectasias

Evaluation

- Labs: CBC, PT, PTT; type & screen. Consider AFB, BNP, D-dimer, UA (Goodpasture, granulomatosis polyangiitis) based on clinical scenario
- Imaging: CXR if unstable; chest CT if stable (much more helpful); ± bronchoscopy

Treatment

- Airway: HOB >45°; lean to side of bleeding (if known-protects the nonbleeding lung), suction (large bore), supplemental O_2 PRN
  - If intubation necessary: Double suction, large-bore ETT (consider advancing ETT into unaffected lung; double-lumen ETT if skilled operator), urgent bronchoscopy
- Definitive management: Minor hemoptysis can usually be managed conservatively; but if massive, requires bronchoscopy or IR embolization; surgical resection if all else fails

Disposition

- Healthy, minimal bleeding: Get CXR; if negative: Home w/ outpt f/u
- High-risk pt, minor bleeding: Get CT, consider admit for observation & bronchoscopy
- Massive: ICU, consult pulmonology, interventional radiology, thoracic surgery

ABDOMINAL PAIN

Approach

- Assess nature of pain: Location, chronicity, constant or intermittent, relation to eating, associated sxs such as fever, nausea, vomiting, dysuria, change in bowel habits
- Always ask about previous abdominal surgeries
- Labs depend on presentation. Consider CBC, BMP, UA, LFTs, lipase, lactate. Strongly consider hCG in women of childbearing age
- Need for imaging is strongly influenced by age & likelihood of surgical pathology
- Always consider thoracic/cardiac sources of pain—esp ACS in the elderly
- Somatic pain: occurs w/ irritation of parietal peritoneum, sharp & localized
- Visceral pain: results from stimulation of autonomic nerves, dull & poorly localized, often earliest manifestation of dz process
- Referred pain: felt distant to source due to converging peripheral afferent nerve fibers that enter spinal cord. Consider abdominal pain as source of back or shoulder pain

Abdominal Pain Differential	
Location	**Differential**
RUQ	Biliary colic, acute cholecystitis, cholangitis, acute hepatitis, liver abscess, hepatic congestion due to heart failure, perforated duodenal ulcer, RLL pneumonia, PE
LUQ	Gastritis/PUD, splenic enlargement/rupture/infarction, LLL pneumonia, PE
Epigastric	Gastritis/PUD, pancreatitis, MI, peri/myocarditis, GERD, AAA
Lower quadrants	Ruptured ectopic pregnancy, ovarian cyst/torsion, PID/TOA, endometriosis, kidney stone, incarcerated/strangulated hernia
RLQ	Appendicitis, Meckel diverticulum, mesenteric adenitis, psoas abscess
LLQ	Diverticulitis, Colitis
Diffuse	Early appendicitis, mesenteric ischemia, gastroenteritis, peritonitis, AAA, SBO, large bowel obstruction/volvulus, spontaneous bacterial peritonitis, IBD, colitis, DKA, sickle cell pain, IBS, anaphylaxis, colon ischemia, constipation

UPPER QUADRANT PAIN

Biliary Disease

Biliary Etiologies	
Dx	**Definition**
Cholelithiasis	The presence of gallstones in the gallbladder
Biliary colic	Intermittent obstruction of gallbladder outlet by gallstones
Cholecystitis	Inflammation of the gallbladder, usually due to obstruction in cystic duct by stone
Choledocholithiasis	Obstruction of the CBD by a stone
Cholangitis	Infxn of the CBD, often precipitated by stone obstruction

Biliary Colic

Presentation

- Pain occurs when gallstones cause obstruction of gallbladder outlet or cystic duct opening leading to intermittent epigastric &/or RUQ pain, +n/v, classically a/w fatty meals
- Pain may radiate to the back or to the R scapula (referred)
- Sxs generally resolve completely b/w episodes (min–h) as obstruction resolves
- Mild RUQ tenderness but no fever or Murphy sign

Evaluation

- Nl labs in biliary colic (AST, ALT, alk phos, bilirubin, lipase)
- RUQ US is highly sens & spec for stones

Treatment

- NSAIDs, antiemetics, opioids if needed. Elective cholecystectomy

Disposition

- If pain controlled, D/C home w/ surgery f/u to consider cholecystectomy
- If persistent pain, consider possibility of impacted stone in GB neck/developing cholecystitis

Pearls

- Acutely, biliary colic presents w/ diffuse upper abd pain before localizing to the RUQ
- RFs for gallstones (cholesterol or pigment): female gender, increasing age & parity, obesity, hemolytic dz, SCD, congenital anomalies, rapid weight loss

Cholecystitis

Presentation

- Persistent RUQ pain (+/– radiation to the back/shoulder), may be accompanied by fever, tachycardia, n/v
- Usually a/w cholelithiasis, but may be acalculous in minority of cases
- In elderly, delayed presentation w/ fever & poorly localized abd pain
- RUQ tenderness; Murphy sign (arrest of inspiration w/ RUQ palpation), or Sonographic Murphy sign (maximal pain from pressure of US probe w/ visualization of gallbladder)

Evaluation

- CBC (elevated WBC + L shift), LFTs (may be mildly elevated, but are often nl), bili & lipase (usually nl)
- RUQ US: Features of chole—presence of stones, thickened gallbladder wall (>3 mm), pericholecystic fluid
- HIDA scan: May be considered if US equivocal; high sens/spec for cystic duct obstruction
- CT scan: Not preferred imaging modality. Less sensitive than HIDA for biliary obstruction (*Abdom Radiol* 2024;49(2):384–398). Helpful to evaluate for cx (eg, perforation, gallstone ileus)

Treatment

- Symptomatic mgmt & supportive care as w/ biliary colic
- 2nd- or 3rd-gen cephalosporin (to cover coliforms) plus anaerobic coverage (metronidazole) or piperacillin-tazobactam, broaden coverage if septic
- Surgical c/s for cholecystectomy; may do percutaneous drain if poor surgical candidate

Disposition

- Admit for IV abx & (in most cases) surgical mgmt

Choledocholithiasis & Cholangitis

Presentation

- Choledocholithiasis: RUQ pain lasting longer than biliary colic pain; may be a/w jaundice later
  - Mild RUQ tenderness but no fever or Murphy sign
  - Can have palpable gallbladder (Courvosier sign)—late finding
- Cholangitis: Charcot triad: RUQ pain, jaundice, fever. Low sensitivity, high spec (*ANZ J Surg* 2017;232–238)
  - Reynolds pentad: Charcot triad + shock & MS chgs (severe cholangitis)
  - A/w cholelithiasis, malignancy, stricture leading to obstruction

Evaluation

- Labs: ↑ LFTs early, ↑ bilirubin ↑ alk phos late, ↑ lipase in biliary pancreatitis, ↑ WBC & + BCx in cholangitis
- RUQ US can be suggestive, CBD >6 mm
- CT is more sensitive & can evaluate for cx
- ERCP is diagnostic & can be therapeutic if obstructing stone is found

Treatment

- If cholangitis suspected, broad-spectrum abx for gram-negative enterics (eg, *E. coli, Enterobacter, Pseudomonas*): piperacillin/tazobactam OR ertapenem OR ceftriaxone/cefepime + metronidazole

Disposition

- Admx to medicine for ERCP w/ surgery & GI consultation

Pearls

- Always consider predisposing causes—gallstones (req. cholecystectomy), malignancy (req. resection vs biliary stenting)

Pancreatitis (*Am J Gastroenterol* 2024;119(3):419–437)

Etiology

- Gallstones (40–70%), alcohol (25–35%), idiopathic, hypertriglyceridemia (TG >1,000), hypercalcemia, drugs (thiazides, furosemide, sulfa, ACE-I, protease inhs, estrogen, APAP, steroids), obstructive tumors, viral infxn, trauma, post-ERCP, ischemic. A/w smoking

Presentation

- Epigastric pain radiating through to the back, constant, a/w nausea, vomiting
- Often h/o prior pancreatitis, gallstones, alcohol abuse
- May be ill appearing, tachycardic, epigastric ttp, guarding, ↓ bowel sounds (adynamic ileus)

Evaluation
- ↑ Lipase >3 × nl (amylase is less sensitive & spec), can be nl in chronic pancreatitis
- Check serum triglycerides in absence of gallstones/EtOH hx
- If severe: ↑ WBC, ↑ CRP, ↑ BUN, ↑ Hct, ↑ Cr
- CT scan: Not required for dx if pain & ↑ lipase; should be obtained to r/o cx (fluid collection, pseudocyst, necrosis, abscess), esp after 48–72 h if no improvement
- MRCP: alt to CT, advantage of ↑ sens for choledocholithiasis & pancreatic duct eval
- Abd US: Used to evaluate for gallstones, CBD dilatation, or pseudocyst
- CXR: Pleural effusions & pulmonary infiltrates a/w severe dz

Treatment
- Moderate IV fluids (LR preferred; 1.5 cc/kg/h w/ boluses for hypovolemia); aggressive hydration a/w worse outcomes (*NEJM* 2022;387:989–1000)
- Early enteral nutrition if tolerated. No e/o benefit w/ NPO
- IV analgesia, antiemetics
- Prophylactic abx have little benefit; use for infected necrosis
- Delayed cholecystectomy for gallstone pancreatitis
- IR drainage for persistent or infected fluid collection

Disposition
- Admx for supportive care if severe or not tolerating PO
- Early cholecystectomy for mild gallstone pancreatitis
- Delayed cholecystectomy w/ necrosis

Pearls
- Be aware of fluid shifts—pleural effusions, abdominal compartment synd

LOWER QUADRANT/PELVIC PAIN

Appendicitis

History
- Classically, dull vague periumbilical pain → migrates to RLQ, localizes & becomes sharp
- Nausea, vomiting, anorexia, fever
- Greatest incidence at 10–30 y but can occur at any time

Physical Exam
- RLQ (McBurney point) tenderness, localized rebound, & guarding
- Psoas sign: RLQ pain w/ active R hip flexion against resistance or R hip extension
- Obturator sign: RLQ pain w/ internal rotation of the flexed R hip
- Rovsing sign: RLQ pain w/ palpation of the LLQ

Evaluation
- Labs: Leukocytosis (not sens or spec); Check hCG in women; Consider CRP in children
- Abd CT (95% sens, 94% spec; *Cochrane Syst Rev* 2019;2019(11):CD009977)
- US: Less sens than CT but high spec. Consider esp in children & young (thin) adults
- MRI is a useful modality in pregnancy & children
- In cases w/ strong clinical c/f appendicitis & low suspicion of alternate etiology, may be reasonable to proceed to OR w/o imaging
- Alvarado score places pts in low risk (1–4 points), intermediate risk (5–6) & high risk (7–10) groups. High sens (99%), but low spec (*J Traum Acute Care Surg* 2018;84:946–950)

Alvarado Score for Acute Appendicitis (*Ann Emerg Med* 1986;15(5):557–564)	
RLQ tenderness	+2
Elevated temp >37.5 °C	+1
RLQ rebound tenderness	+1
Migration of pain to RLQ	+1
Anorexia	+1
Nausea or vomiting	+1
Leukocytosis >10k	+2
Leukocyte L shift	+1

- Pediatric Appendicitis Score for children—uses hx, PE, & labs to risk stratify

Management
- Abx: 2nd/3rd-gen cephalosporin (cefoxitin, cefotetan, CTX) or cipro PLUS metronidazole OR piperacillin-tazobactam
- Surgery c/s & admx

- Uncomplicated appendicitis—traditionally surgically removed though mounting evidence for non-op tx w/ abx (*Cochrane Sys Rev* 2024;4(4))
  - There may be slightly higher rates of tx failure w/ abx & ~31% of pts will require appendectomy w/i 1 y
- Appendectomy for perforated appendix, older pts, pts w/ appendicolith

Pearl

- Pts at extremes of age are more likely to have atypical presentations & present w/ perforation

Hernia

Definition

- Defect in the abd wall that allows protrusion of abd contents
- Incarcerated hernia: Cannot be reduced
- Strangulated hernia: Incarcerated hernia w/ vascular compromise (ischemia)

History

- Bulging mass in abd wall (eg, umbilical, epigastric, ventral), inguinal region, scrotum, or inner thigh (femoral); worse w/ ↑ intra-abd pressure
- Inguinal hernias are either direct or indirect; medial or lateral to the inferior epigastric vessels, respectively

Physical Exam

- Bulge &/or palpable defect in abd wall or groin
- Strangulated: tenderness, fever, skin discoloration, or associated peritonitis

Evaluation

- If concern for strangulated hernia, consider CBC, lactate, pre-op labs
- CT scan required if concern for strangulated hernia

Management

- Attempt reduction w/ generous analgesia/anxiolysis, pt in Trendelenburg, steady pressure
- If easily reduced, D/C w/ analgesic, stool softener, & surgery f/u
- If not reducible or if strangulated, c/s surgery for operative intervention

Pearl

- Be cautious about reducing a hernia that has been irreducible by the pt for more than 12 h & is difficult to reduce in the ED as bowel may be compromised

Diverticulitis

Definition

- Inflammation of colonic diverticula—most common location is sigmoid
- Complicated diverticulitis: associated perforation, obstruction, abscess, or fistula

Presentation

- LLQ pain, guarding, fever, nausea, change in bowel habits
- Urinary sxs due to bladder inflammation (fecal uria, pneumaturia, pyuria, c/f colovesicular fistula), stool per vagina (c/f colovaginal fistula)
- Complicated diverticulitis may have peritonitis, septic sx

Evaluation

- Clinical Dx if mild sxs & typical presentation
- Labs: ↑ WBC, ↑ CRP
- CT to confirm dx or if c/f complicated diverticulitis. May see wall thickening, pericolonic stranding, abscess, fistula, or contained free air if microperforation, sens & spec 94–99% (*Ann Intern Med* 2022;175(3):379:271)

Treatment

- Mild & w/o comorbidities: No abx (*Dis Colon Rectum* 2020;63(6):728–747; *Ann Intern Med* 2022;175(3): 399–415)
  - There is little evidence for low fiber/residue diet in sx control & preventing recurrence (*Nutrients* 2018;10(2):137)
- Mild & w/ significant comorbidities: Consider (1) PO amoxicillin-clavulanate OR (2) metronidazole + (cipro OR TMP/SMX) for 10 d
- Severe: NPO, IV fluids, IV ampicillin–sulbactam OR piperacillin–tazobactam OR ceftriaxone/metronidazole OR quinolone/metronidazole OR carbapenem
- Most complicated diverticulitis can be managed medically +/– IR drainage
- Surgery is required if medical therapy fails, peritonitis, free air is present, or for large abscess that can't be drained percutaneously. Elective surgery may be recommended for cx & recurrent dz (≥2 episodes)

Disposition

- If mild & uncomplicated, D/C w/, antiemetic, analgesia & PCP or general surgery f/u +/– abx. If severe, admit

Pearl

- Consider diverticulitis in older pts w/ urinary sxs but unremarkable or equivocal urine sediment
- Pts should undergo colonoscopy 6–8 wks after recovered (*Gastroenterology* 2015;149(7):1944–1949)

Diffuse Pain

Abdominal Aortic Aneurysm

Definition

- Dilation of the abd aorta (true aneurysm, involves all layers of the vessel wall)

History

- Older pt w/ low back pain, abd pain, or flank pain (may mimic renal colic), syncope/ hypotension
- Rupture into RP can temporarily tamponade, intraperitoneal rupture is rapidly fatal, can rupture into GI tract (aortoenteric fistula, p/w massive GIB) or IVC (aortocaval fistula)
- RFs: smoking, HTN, CAD, PVD, age ≥65 y, male, FH, cigarette smoking

Physical Exam

- Pulsatile mass (often not present), early satiety due to duodenal compression, flank pain due to ureteral obstruction
- Ruptured/leaking AAA: hypotension, abd tenderness, decreased femoral pulses, mottling
- Thromboembolic cx: occlusion of iliac, femoral, or popliteal arteries, microemboli causing livedo reticularis or cyanotic toes

Evaluation

- Abd CT (preferably CT angiography) if hemodynamically stable
- Bedside US may reveal enlarged aorta (+free fluid if ruptured/leaking)

Treatment

- Stable, nonruptured: Urgent surgical or endovascular repair may be required if symptomatic, >5.0 cm, or rapidly growing
- Ruptured/leaking: Immediate surgical repair, allow permissive hypotension (SBP 90s)

Disposition

- Direct to OR/IR if unstable

Pearls

- Larger the AAA the greater the risk for rupture
- 50% mortality for AAA if ruptured at presentation (*Eur J Endovasc Surg* 2008;35(5):558)

Small Bowel Obstruction

Definition

- Mechanical obstruction of nl intestinal transit from intraluminal or extraluminal compression leading to proximal small bowel dilation
- RFs: 90% due to adhesions (most common), hernias, neoplasms (*Am J Surg* 2000;180(51):33–36)
- Can be complete or partial, simple or closed loop (obstructed in 2 locations)

History & Physical Examination (*Eur J Surg* 1998;164:777–784; *Scand J Gastroenterol* 1994;175:109–113)

- Diffuse, colicky abd pain, n/v, abd distension, h/o abd surgeries (+LR = 2.7–3.9, –LR = 0.2–0.4)/prior obstructions/hernia, obstipation (not passing gas), constipation (+LR = 3.7–8.8, –LR = 0.6–0.7)
- Diffuse abd tenderness (+LR = 2.6–5, –LR = 0.4–0.7), distension (+LR = 5.6–16.8, –LR = 0.3–0.4), high-pitched bowel sounds (early), no bowel sounds (late)

Evaluation (*Radiology* 2015;275(2):332)

- Supine & upright abd x-rays (50–85% accurate): mx air–fluid levels, >3-cm small bowel dilation, more than 3-mm of small bowel wall thickening
- Bedside US (92–93% sens & spec): >2.5-cm dilated bowel, back & forth peristalsis (*Eur J Radiol* 2021;(136):109565)
- Abd CT (95% sens & spec) can be diagnostic & used to characterize the obstruction (level, cause, cx)

Treatment

- NPO, bowel rest +/– NGT placement for gastric decompression
  - Mounting evidence for selective NGT insertion based on sx + etiology (*Am J Surg* 2022; 223(6):1179–1182)
- IV fluids & correction of electrolyte abnormalities, analgesia, antiemetics
- Broad-spectrum abx if concern for peritonitis, perforation, or sepsis
- Surgical consultation—many cases managed conservatively

Disposition
- admx
- Direct to OR if high risk (eg, closed-loop obstruction, impending perforation, e/o bowel ischemia)

Large Bowel Obstruction/Volvulus

Definition
- LBO: Mechanical obstruction of the large bowel (most commonly caused by cancer)
- Volvulus (twisting of the large bowel on itself)—most common at sigmoid & cecum
- Other causes of obstruction: intussusception, fecal impaction, cx of diverticulitis, IBD, extrinsic tumor, foreign body, fecal impaction

History & Physical Examination
- Insidious onset of diffuse, colicky abd pain, distention, constipation/obstipation, n/v (emesis is late finding), change in bowel habits, weight loss

Evaluation (*Radiology* 2015;275(3):651)
- Abd x-rays (supine, upright, decubitus): Dilated large bowel (84% sens, 72% spec), differentiated from small bowel by haustral markings, air–fluid levels, often cannot identify underlying cause
- Abd CT (sens 96%, spec 93%): Can be helpful to distinguish from pseudo-obstruction or megacolon (no transition point), identify cause, assess for ischemia

Treatment
- NPO, bowel rest, gastric decompression w/ NGT placement
- IV fluids & correction of electrolyte abnormalities analgesia, antiemetics
- Broad-spectrum abx if concern for peritonitis, perforation, or sepsis
- Surgical consultation for operative reduction (particularly for cecal volvulus, perforation, closed-loop obstruction, or peritonitis)
- GI consultation for endoscopic reduction &/or stenting (particularly for sigmoid volvulus, obstructing mass)

Disposition
- Admit to hospital

Pearls
- Sigmoid volvulus most common in ill, debilitated, elderly pts, or pts w/ psychiatric/neuro disorders & h/o constipation
- Cecal volvulus common in young adults, classically marathon runners

Perforated Viscus

Definition
- Perforation of hollow viscus leading to abd free air, intraluminal spillage

History & Physical Examination
- Acute onset, constant, severe abd pain, worse w/ movement, +/– fever, n/v
- May be consequence of perforated ulcer, bowel obstruction, diverticulitis, cancer, or other primary GI pathology
- Acute peritonitis: rigidity, tap tenderness, rebound, hypotension, sepsis

Evaluation
- Supine & upright abd x-rays: May show free air under the diaphragm
- Abd CT: Definitive study, but not required if clinical suspicion high

Treatment
- Immediate surgical c/s
- Broad spectrum abx to cover polymicrobial infxn (enteric GNR, GPC, anaerobes)

Disposition
- Surgical admx

Pearls
- Findings may be masked in pts who are elderly or chronically immunosuppressed

Mesenteric Ischemia

Definition
- Insufficient perfusion to the intestine, can result in bowel necrosis, high mortality
- Classified as acute or chronic
- Etiologies (*Curr Gastroenterol Rep* 2020;22(4):17): arterial embolism (~50%, typically SMA), arterial thrombosis (~25%, a/w severe atherosclerosis), nonocclusive mesenteric ischemia

(~20%, low cardiac output state), mesenteric venous thrombosis (5–10%, a/w clotting disorders)

History
- RFs: age >60, recent MI, AF, vascular dz (coronary, peripheral), CHF (↓ forward flow)
- Chronic: May have h/o prior abd angina: postprandial pain, food aversion, weight loss
- Acute presentation w/ abd pain, anorexia, vomiting, bloody stools
- Classic triad: severe pain, bowel emptying (diarrhea or vomiting), & embolic source
- Clinical course often acute pain, followed by improvement & then worse pain & peritonitis

Physical Exam
- Ill appearing, pain out of proportion to exam, tachycardia, fever. Late signs include peritonitis, shock

Evaluation
- Early surgical eval
- Labs (low sens/spec): ↑ WBC, AG acidosis, ↑ lactate
- CT angiography: test of choice: high sens, spec
- Abd CT (lower sens/spec): colonic dilation, bowel wall thickening, pneumatosis intestinalis, portomesenteric venous gas

Treatment
- Resuscitation w/ IV fluids, broad spectrum abx (3rd-gen cephalosporin & metronidazole)
- Surgical & IR consultation for revascularization +/– OR for resection of nonviable gut
- Anticoagulation for venous thrombosis & embolic dz, heparin infusion

Disposition
- Surgical admx vs IR/OR

Pearls
- Maintain high index of suspicion, particularly in pt w/ RFs
- Do not rely on negative CT to rule out ischemia—angiography is key

Colon Ischemia (Ischemic Colitis)

Definition
- Nonocclusive microvascular dz of the colon, caused by hypoperfusion & reperfusion injury
- Watershed areas (splenic flexure & sigmoid colon) particularly susceptible to ischemia from systemic hypotension

History & Physical Examination
- Sudden pain over affected colonic segment (typically L, R a/w increased mortality) w/ urge to defecate, passage w/i 24 h of bloody stool, diarrhea
- H/o recent surgery or illness
- Tenderness over affected colon usually mild, peritoneal findings suggest perforation

Evaluation
- Labs: WBC, BUN, Cr, LDH, lactate may be high, but are all nonspec
- Abd CT: nonspec mesenteric fat stranding, bowel wall thickening, abnl colon wall enhancement, thumbprinting, edema
  - Colonic pneumatosis & portomesenteric venous gas suggest transmural infarct

Treatment & Disposition
- Supportive care, bowel rest, hydration, pain mgmt, abx for severe dz
- GI consultation for colonoscopy, surgery if peritonitis or perforation

Spontaneous Bacterial Peritonitis

Definition
- Infxn of ascitic fluid (usually in pts w/ advanced cirrhosis)

History & Physical Examination
- Fever, abd pain, altered mental status, diarrhea, hypotension (in severe cases)
- Stigmata of liver failure, ascites

Evaluation
- Labs: ↑ WBC, ↑bili, ↓ PLTs increase likelihood of dz
- Paracentesis in suspected cases (before abx given): >250 PMN/mm^3 in the absence of intra-abd source of infxn or malignancy is diagnostic
  - Threshold for SBP in pts on peritoneal dialysis is lower—100 WBC/μL
- Send broad ascites labs to assess for alternative dxs (inc secondary peritonitis); culture, gram stain

Treatment

- Abx: cefotaxime 2 g IV q8h or ceftriaxone 2 g q24h. Ciprofloxacin 400 mg IV bid if allergic. Carbapenem if nosocomial, recent abx or long-term prophylactic abx
- Albumin 1.5 g/kg at dx shows survival benefit if bili >4 mg/dL or e/o renal dysfxn (*Clin Gastroenterol Hepatol* 2013;11(2):123)
- Pressors as needed for hypotension

Disposition

- Medical admx

Pearls

- Caused by bacteria that translocate from gut. 70% GNR (*E. coli, Klebsiella*), 30% GPC (*S. pneumoniae, Enterococcus*)
- Occurs in 20% of pts w/ cirrhosis
- Clinical signs unreliable; have low threshold for paracentesis in pts w/ ascites. Delayed paracentesis >12 h a/w higher mortality (*Am J Gastroenterol* 2014;109:1436)

Inflammatory Bowel Disease

Definition

- UC: Chronic inflammation of the colonic mucosal later
- CD: Transmural inflammation that may involve any portion of the GI tract

Inflammatory Bowel Disorder (Ulcerative Colitis & Crohn Disease)		
	Ulcerative Colitis	**Crohn Dz**
Clinical features	Fever, bloody diarrhea, tenesmus, urgency, painful BMs	Fever, abd pain, diarrhea (less often bloody)
GI involvement	Exclusively colon (primarily rectal), continuous lesions limited to submucosa, friable mucosa; irregular, shallow ulcers; pseudopolyps; crypt abscesses; loss of haustral markings	Colon & jejunum, but can extend to esophagus; transmural involvement; cobblestone mucosa; granulomas; skip lesions
GI cx	Toxic megacolon (>8 cm, usually transverse colon), stricture, colon cancer	Strictures, fistulas, perianal dz

History

- Women > men, typically present in 2nd or 3rd decade, weight loss, vomiting, abd pain/diarrhea (grossly bloody in UC) that flares w/ emotional stress, infxns, w/d from steroids

Physical Exam

- Diffuse abd tenderness (focal RLQ tenderness common in CD), ~20% of pts have extraintestinal sxs, perianal dz (seen in CD); fissures, fistulas, abscesses

Common Extraintestinal Features	
Arthritic	Ankylosing spondylitis, tendinitis, arthritis
Intra-abdominal	Primary sclerosing cholangitis, pancreatitis, nephrolithiasis, liver dz (autoimmune or fatty)
Dermatologic	Pyoderma gangrenosum, erythema nodosum, oral ulcers
Ophthalmic	Uveitis, episcleritis
Hematologic	Iron deficiency anemia, anemia of chronic dz, coagulopathy

Evaluation

- Labs: low H/H (from chronic blood loss + inflammation), increased WBC & PLTs, hypokalemia (from diarrhea), mildly elevated AST/ALT, elevated ESR/CRP
- Plain abd x-ray: if c/f perforation, obstruction, or toxic megacolon (dilated colon >6 cm)
- Abd CT: May r/o cx (eg, abscess, obstruction, fistula) or non–IBD-related dzs
- Outpt colonoscopy: If dx not known & once acute flare resolved

Treatment

- IV fluids, bowel rest, GI &/or surgical c/s, steroids, abx if concern for infxn
- TNF inhs, +/– azathioprine, +/– other antibody therapy
- Methotrexate, 5 ASA agents (mesalamine, sulfasalazine) may be recommended

Disposition

- Admit for severe dz or acute cx

NAUSEA AND VOMITING

Approach

- Common sxs of many dz processes (eg, intra-abd, genitourinary, metabolic derangements, toxic ingestions, neuro, cardiac)
- Careful attention to ROS, PMH, previous abd surgeries, content/color of vomit, timing & duration, associated sxs (diarrhea, abd pain, HA), substance use, medications
- Labs: Consider CBC, BMP, UA, LFTs, lipase, hCG
- Treat cause, antiemetics (eg, ondansetron, metoclopramide), IVF if poor PO

Nausea & Vomiting Differential			
Abdominal/GU	**Toxicologic**	**Neurologic**	**Metabolic/Other**
Obstruction (gastric outlet, small or large bowel), ileus, esophageal	Alcohol intoxication or w/d	Vertigo (cerebellar, vertebrobasilar, vestibular)	Systemic infxn
Infxns (hepatitis, appendicitis, cholecystitis, pyelonephritis)	Other drugs of abuse	Meningitis/ Encephalitis	Dehydration
Gastroenteritis, food poisoning	Drug tox (ASA, Tylenol, digoxin)	Increased ICP	Hypoglycemia, hyperglycemia
Gastritis/ulcers, pancreatitis	Chemotherapy or medication-related	Intracranial bleed	Hyponatremia, uremia, thyroid
Bowel ischemia, perforation	Caustic ingestions, organophosphates	Migraine	Acidosis (DKA, AKA, HHS)
Torsion (testicular or ovarian)	Cannabinoid hyperemesis	Tumors	Cardiac ischemia
Kidney stones	CO poisoning	Motion sickness	Pregnancy

Gastroenteritis

- **Definition:** Inflammation of the GI tract causing vomiting & diarrhea usually due to infxns (viruses, bacteria, bacterial toxins, parasites), medications, or diet
- **History:** vomiting (usually 1st) & diarrhea, crampy abd pain; may have fever
- **Physical Exam:** nl exam or mild diffuse abd ttp, tachycardia, dehydration
- **Evaluation:** Consider BMP if clinical concern for significant electrolyte derangement. Stool culture if systemically ill, fever, recent abx, exposure to treatable pathogen
- **Management:** Supportive care, antiemetics. IVF, electrolyte repletion. Home when tolerating PO. Abx & antimotility agents generally not indicated
- **Pearls:** Viral & bacterial toxins (food poisoning) are most common, typically resolve w/o tx in 48 h, may be confused w/ early appendicitis

GASTROINTESTINAL BLEED

Approach

- Hemodynamically unstable pts need 2 large-bore IVs (14–18 gauge), early tfx of blood (consider 1:1:1 tfx). Do not be reassured by nl initial H/H in acute bleeding
- Consideration of anticoagulant reversal, no clear role for TXA (*Lancet* 2020;395(10241):1927)
- ROS, PMH, previous GIB, alcohol/smoking/drug use, liver dz, meds (ASA, AC)
- Labs: CBC, BMP, LFTs, lipase, coagulation studies, lactate, type & screen. BUN/Cr ratio >30 suggests upper GI source (high sens, low spec)
- Imaging: not routinely indicated, consideration of CTA if suspected LGIB & active bleeding
- Consideration of endoscopy &/or colonoscopy w/ GI consultation
- Mimics of GI bleed: epistaxis, ingestion of iron/bismuth/charcoal, red food/drink, GU bleed

GI Bleed Differential	
Location	**Differential**
UGIB (bleeding proximal to the ligament of Treitz)	PUD, gastritis, esophagitis, gastropathy, variceal bleed (esophageal or gastric), Mallory–Weiss tear, aortoenteric fistula, gastric cancer
LGIB (bleeding distal to the ligament of Treitz)	Diverticulosis, angiodysplasia, colon cancer, ischemic bowel, IBD, infectious diarrhea, FB, Meckel diverticulum, anal fissure, hemorrhoids

Upper GI Bleed

Approach

- Unstable pts require emergent GI consultation for endoscopy, consideration of intubation & balloon tamponade, admx to ICU
- NG tube w/ aspiration/lavage not routinely indicated
- Glasgow–Blatchford score predicts need for tfx or urgent endoscopy. A score of 0 identifies low-risk pts who can safely be discharged w/ outpt f/u (*JAMA* 2012;307:1072; *Lancet* 2000;356:1318)

Criteria for Glasgow–Blatchford Score of 0	
Hemoglobin	>12 g/dL (men) or >11.9 (women)
Systolic BP	>109 mmHg
Heart rate	<100
BUN	<18.2 mg/dL
No melena, syncope, heart failure, or liver dz*	—

*Modified Glasgow–Blatchford score eliminates qualitative factors.

Bleeding Peptic Ulcer Disease (PUD) & Gastritis

Definition

- Gastritis: Inflammation of the stomach lining
- Peptic ulcer: Defect through the gastric or duodenal mucosa into the deeper layers
- Caused primarily by *H. pylori* infxn, NSAIDs, (15–30%), alcohol (*NEJM* 2016;374:2367)

History

- LUQ/epigastric pain; bloody or coffee ground emesis; dark, tarry stool (melena), brisk upper GI bleed may appear as hematochezia

Physical Exam

- Epigastric tenderness, melena, or heme-positive stool

Evaluation

- Labs: CBC, LFTs/lipase, coags, BMP (elevated BUN); *H. pylori* testing via biopsy, urea breath testing, serology, or stool antigen

Treatment

- IVF resuscitation, PRBC if Hgb <7 or hypotensive; Emergent EGD if hemodynamically unstable
- High dose PPI before endoscopy reduces bleeding (*NEJM* 2007;356(16):1631)

Disposition

- If ongoing bleeding, Blatchford >0: Admit for EGD

Variceal Bleeds

History

- Bright red hematemesis, diffuse abd pain, h/o portal HTN, cirrhosis

Physical Exam

- Stigmata of liver failure (jaundice, spider angiomas, ascites, caput medusae), ill-appearing, hypotension, tachycardia, melena or hematochezia (w/ large volume bleeding)

Evaluation

- Labs: CBC, LFTs, coags, type & cross

Treatment

- Place 2 large-bore IVs, initiate IV fluid resuscitation, PRBC if Hgb <7 or active bleeding
- Octreotide bolus & drip; IV PPI, consider vasopressin (splanchnic constriction)
- Abx prophylaxis w/ ceftriaxone (quinolone if allergic) increases survival
- Emergent EGD if hemodynamically unstable, may need emergent TIPS if still bleeding
- Balloon tamponade w/ Minnesota or Blakemore tube if exsanguinating (after intubation)

Disposition

- Admx, consider ICU as pts can decompensate quickly

Pearls

- Always consider airway mgmt in large-volume UGI bleeding. Variceal bleeding can rapidly cause airway compromise + aspiration

Mallory–Weiss Tear

Definition

- Tears in the mucosal membrane of the distal esophagus caused by vomiting. A/w heavy alcohol use

History
- Specks of bright red blood in emesis or mild hematemesis after forceful retching

Physical Exam
- Usually nl, mild tachycardia

Evaluation
- Upright CXR if hemodynamically unstable to evaluate for subcutaneous or mediastinal air for Boerhaave synd (complete esophageal rupture)

Treatment
- Antiemetics, PO challenge

Disposition
- D/C w/ outpt EGD; Admit if unstable, severe bleeding, or concerns for Boerhaave

Pearl
- Boerhaave synd can result from emesis, but usually pts are ill-appearing w/ shock & require broad-spectrum abx & surgical mgmt. Consider water-soluble swallow study if high suspicion

Aortoenteric Fistula

Definition
- Fistula b/w the aorta & GI tract, most commonly in duodenum
- Primary are rare (usually due to untreated AAA), secondary are often related to aortic repair

History
- H/o AAA, aortic graft (usually >5 y), may have sentinel bleed or large-volume GIB
- May also have signs of infxn (often due to graft infxn)
- Classic triad: GI bleeding, abd pain, palpable mass

Physical Exam
- Rapid GIB, hemodynamic collapse

Evaluation
- CBC, type & cross, emergent surgical c/s, CT angiography if stable

Treatment & Disposition
- Large bore IVs, blood tfx if indicated
- Surgical repair (mortality directly related to time to OR), admit to surgical ICU

Lower GI Bleed

- Bright red or maroon blood per rectum (hematochezia), rarely may be melenic
- If unstable (shock index [HR/SBP] >1): Consider CTA, emergent surgical/GI consultation, consideration of brisk UGI source
- Disposition: Likely admit vs observation if not clear anorectal source

Diverticular Bleeding & Colonic Angiodysplasia
- **Diverticular bleeding:** most common cause of LGIB, caused by bleeding diverticula
- **Angiodysplasia:** enlarged, fragile blood vessels, usually in cecum or proximal ascending colon (10–20% of LGIB)
- **History:** painless rectal bleeding often preceded by strong urge to defecate
  - RFs: older age, smoking, NSAID use, EtOH, heart dz, obesity
- **Physical Exam:** nl abd exam, BRBPR, no etiology found on rectal exam
- **Evaluation:** Labs: CBC, LFTs, coagulation panel, type & cross
- **Treatment:** IV fluid resuscitation, blood tfx if indicated
  - Can be self-limited, may require endoscopic hemostasis or IR embolization
- **Disposition:** Likely admit for colonoscopy

Colorectal Cancer
- **History:** Recurrent blood in stool, change in bowel habits inc appearance of stool, anorexia, weight loss
- **Physical Exam:** Pale or heme-positive stools
- **Evaluation:** Labs: CBC, LFTs, coags; CT if concern for obstruction or significant bleeding
- **Treatment:** IV fluid resuscitation, blood tfx if indicated; surgical consultation if significant bleeding (rare)
- **Disposition:** If stable, D/C for outpt colonoscopy, oncology w/u

DIFFICULTY SWALLOWING

Definition

- Dysphagia is difficulty swallowing, odynophagia is pain w/ swallowing
- Common in elderly & pts w/ neuro dzs or head/neck malignancies

Approach

- Hx & physical: time course, sudden or progressive, localization (oropharyngeal vs esophageal), solids &/or liquids, associated pain, weight loss, vomiting, reflux sxs
- ROS, PMH, hx, or FH of GI disorders or neuro disorders or head/neck malignancy
- Labs: CBC, BMP
- Studies (based H&P & differential): Barium swallow/EGD for structural/mechanical lesions; motility studies, CT neck

Difficulty Swallowing Differential	
Dysphagia	**Differential**
Solids (mechanical obstruction)	Esophageal ring (intermittent), eosinophilic esophagitis (intermittent), esophageal cancer (progressive), oral/pharyngeal abscess, neck cancer
Solids & liquids (motility disorder)	Spasm (intermittent), scleroderma (progressive), achalasia (progressive), neuro (eg, myasthenia, ALS, brainstem stroke)
Odynophagia	Reflux esophagitis, infxn (eg, candida, herpes), radiation, chemotherapy

Esophageal Food Impaction/Foreign Bodies

Definition

- Food or FB stuck in esophagus (70% lodge at the lower esophageal sphincter)
- Can lead to significant morbidity or mortality from esophageal perforation & sepsis

History

- Sensation of food (often meat) or FB stuck in the esophagus, retching, unable to swallow secretions. Often a/w underlying conditions inc esophageal stricture, esophageal ring, eosinophilic esophagitis, etc

Physical Exam

- Odynophagia, neck/CP, respiratory distress (wheezing, stridor), drooling, retching

Management

- Airway eval, neuro eval
- Assessment of urgency of removal (dangerous object, time, completeness of obstruction)
- Radiographic eval for localization & cx
  - XR of chest, neck, &/or abd (may show dilated esophagus w/ air fluid level or FB)
  - CT when perforation suspected
- Medical mgmt: glucagon (no data to support its use), effervescents, benzos
- GI consultation for endoscopic removal (preferred), +/– surgery if needed
  - Necessary for dangerous objects (batteries, sharp) or FB doesn't pass w/i 12–24 h

Disposition

- If tolerating PO, D/C w/ outpt EGD

DIARRHEA

Definition

- Frequent, watery stools. Specifically, >3 loose stools/24 h
- Acute ≤7 d, prolonged 7–13 d, persistent 14–29 d, chronic >29 d

Approach

- Hx: duration, frequency, volume; bloody, mucus present; recent travel, hospitalization, or abx; associated sxs (fever, vomiting, etc), PMH (HIV, IBD, etc), meds
- Labs: Consider BMP for electrolyte derangements; consider CBC if c/f HUS. *C. diff* PCR & infectious stool studies indicated only in severe illness or high-risk pts (see below); other stool studies (WBC, osmotic gap, calprotectin, etc) not routinely indicated in the ED

Diarrhea Differential	
Causes	**Differential**
Infectious	<u>Acute</u> Viruses: Norovirus, rotavirus, adenovirus, CMV

	Preformed toxins (food poisoning <24 h): *S. aureus, B. cereus* Toxins formed after colonization: *E. coli* (ETEC), *C. difficile, C. perfringens* Invasive bacteria (generally +fecal WBC, +blood): *E. coli (EIEC, EHEC), Salmonella, Shigella, Campylobacter, Yersinia, V. parahaemolyticus* Parasites: *Giardia* (–blood), *E. histolytica* (+blood), *Cryptosporidium* <u>Chronic</u> Giardia, *E. histolytica, C. difficile*
Medications • ↑ secretion • ↑ motility • ↑ cell turnover	Abx, antacids, lactulose, sorbitol, GLP-1 RA, chemotherapy, colchicine, gold
Inflammatory • Fever • Hematochezia • Abd pain	IBD, radiation enteritis, ischemic colitis, diverticulitis
Malabsorption • Chronic • ↓ sx w/ fasting • ↑ osmotic gap • ↑ fecal fat • Vitamin deficient	Bile salt deficiency (cirrhosis, cholestasis, ileal dz, bacterial overgrowth), pancreatic insufficiency, mucosal abnormalities (celiac sprue, tropical sprue, Whipple dz), lactose intolerance
Secretory • nl osmotic gap-↓ sx w/ fasting • Nocturnal sx	Hormonal (VIP, carcinoid tumor, medullary cancer of the thyroid, Zollinger–Ellison, glucagon, thyroxine), laxative abuse, neoplasm
Motility	IBS, scleroderma, hyperthyroidism, diabetic autonomic neuropathy

Infectious Diarrhea

History
- Diarrhea ± blood/fever, recent ingestion of meats/poultry/dairy/shellfish/sea food/unrefrigerated food, sick contacts, recent travel (last 6 mos), abx use
- Invasive bacterial enteritis is a clinical Dx: fever, blood in stool, tenesmus, abd pain

Physical Exam
- Dehydration, mild abd tenderness. If invasive: heme-positive/bloody stool, fever

Evaluation
- Labs: Increased WBC (*Salmonella, C. Diff*), low WBC (*Shigella*), eosinophilia (parasites), may see hypokalemia & metabolic acidosis
- Stool culture, fecal WBC & O&P appropriate if ill appearing, severe diarrhea, extremes of age, chronic, immunocompromised, or for public health concerns
- Consider *C. difficile* in pts w/ recent abx use or hospitalization, or w/ chronic unexplained sx. Testing w/ antigen or NAAT assay +toxin immunoassay

Treatment
- IVF if needed, electrolyte repletion
- Abx for high-risk pts (immunocompromised, pregnant, advanced age), severe illness (fever, hypovolemia, severe pain), bloody diarrhea
  - Avoid abx if c/f STEC as can precipitate HUS
- Abx: Fluoroquinolone or azithromycin (recent travel, ill appearing, fever, immunocompromised), OR metronidazole (*C. difficile, Giardia, E. histolytica*)
- Antimotility agents may be used for traveler's diarrhea, avoid if bloody diarrhea or fever

Disposition
- Admit if unable to keep up w/ volume loss or toxic

Pearl
- Significant abd pain is not common & should be evaluated further

Diarrhea Epidemiology	
Pathogen	**Most Common Cause of …**
Norovirus	Infectious diarrhea in adults
Campylobacter	Bacterial diarrhea
Staphylococcus aureus	Toxin-related diarrhea
Giardia	Parasitic diarrhea in US (backpackers, freshwater)
Enterotoxigenic *E. coli*	Traveler's diarrhea

Diarrhea Pathogen Characteristics	
Pathogen	**Characteristics**
Campylobacter	Duration 5–7 d. Fever, vomiting, abd pain RFs: D care, food (dairy, meats, poultry), exposure to young dogs & cats, summer months Cx: Bacteremia, meningitis, cholecystitis, pancreatitis, reactive arthritis
Salmonella	Duration 2–7 d. Fever, vomiting, abd pain RFs: Food (dairy, meats, eggs), exposure to turtles, comorbidities (esp SCD) Cx: Enteric fever (*S. typhi*), bacteremia, meningitis, osteomyelitis, Reiter synd
Shigella	Duration 2–5 d. High fever, abd pain, no vomiting. Marked bandemia RFs: D care, swimming pools, summer & fall Cx: HUS, febrile szs in infants
Yersinia	Duration up to 1 mo. Fever, vomiting, abd pain RFs: Food (pork), winter Cx: Appendicitis, terminal ileitis, intussusception, toxic megacolon, cholangitis
Preformed toxin mediated (*Staphylococcus, Bacillus*)	Duration 1–2 d. Onset w/i 6 h of ingestion RFs: *Staphylococcus* (dairy, meats, custard, mayonnaise); *Bacillus* (reheated rice)
Enterotoxic *E. coli*	Duration 3–5 d. Fever, vomiting, abd pain RFs: Foreign travel
Enterohemorrhagic *E. coli*	Duration 3–6 d. Fever, no vomiting, abd pain RFs: Ground beef Cx: HUS. Abx may increase risk of HUS
Clostridium perfringens	Duration 1 d. No fever, vomiting, abd pain RFs: Food (meats, pork, vegetables)
Clostridium difficile	Variable duration. Fever, no vomiting, abd pain RFs: Hospitalization, abx use, hx of prior *C. diff* Cx: Fulminant colitis (2–3%), toxic megacolon (colonic dilation >6 cm), bowel perforation
V. parahaemolyticus	Duration 5–7 d. No fever, vomiting, abd pain RFs: Seafood (esp raw)
Giardia	Duration >7 d. No fever, vomiting, or abd pain RFs: Contaminated water (backpackers) Cx: Chronic diarrhea
Entamoeba	Duration 7–14 d. No fever, vomiting, no abd pain RFs: Contaminated water Cx: Liver abscess

Irritable Bowel Syndrome

- **Definition:** Disorder of the colon: Causes cramping, bloating, diarrhea, constipation (F > M)
- **History:** Recurrent abd pain ≥1 d/wk over the last 3 mos + 2 or more of the following: Pain related to defecation, change in frequency of stools, change in form of stools. No constitutional sxs, GIB, or FH of IBD (*NEJM* 2017;376(26):2566–2578)
- **Physical Exam:** May have mild lower abd tenderness, heme-negative stools
- **Treatment:** Fiber for constipation, antimotility for diarrhea, antispasmodics for pain
- **Disposition:** D/C, outpt mgmt
- **Pearl:** Dx of exclusion. Unlikely if age of onset >35 or associated constitutional sxs

CONSTIPATION

Definition

- Reduced frequency of stool (<3/wk), &/or difficult passage of hard stool, chronic: >3 mos

Approach

- Hx: duration, severity, character of stool, pain, fever, medication use, prior episodes, dietary chgs, associated sx (anorexia, n/v, bloody stool, weight loss), meds

Common Causes of Constipation	
Etiology	**Differential**
Functional	Slow transit (dietary, dehydration, immobility), pelvic floor disorders, IBS
Obstruction	Cancer, stricture, rectal FB, pseudo-obstruction, megacolon
Medication	Opiates, anticholinergics, iron, CCBs, AEDs, antidepressants, etc
neuro	Parkinson dz, MS, spinal cord lesion, stroke
Metabolic	DM, hypothyroid, hypokalemia, hypercalcemia, pregnancy

Simple Constipation (Including Stool Impaction)

History
- Poor diet, decreased fluid/fiber intake, decreased mobility, constipating medications
- Alarm sxs: sudden change in bowel habits, blood mixed in stool, weight loss, FH of colon cancer

Physical Exam
- Firm stool in the rectal vault, palpable stool on abd exam, minimal abd ttp

Evaluation
- Abd CT if need to r/o obstruction or to confirm dx in high-risk pt

Treatment
- Manual disimpaction if needed
- Docusate, mag citrate, enema (esp in elderly), bisacodyl (oral or suppository), PEG
- Natural bulking agents (eg, psyllium) when constipation resolves

Disposition
- Home

Pearl
- Simple constipation is a dz of exclusion; always consider anatomic or functional causes of obstruction

Rectal Foreign Body

Physical Exam
- FB in rectum on exam or anoscopy, peritonitis if perforation

Evaluation
- Abd x-ray or CT to eval location/shape & r/o pneumoperitoneum

Treatment
- Removal w/ forceps traction while the pt bears down. Impacted object may cause proximal vacuum suction; can pass Foley around object to break vacuum seal & use balloon to pull back on object
- Removal in OR if unsuccessful or if sharp object w/ risk of perforation

Disposition
- Home if removed

Pearl
- Procedural sedation may be needed to sufficiently dilate anus to remove FB in ED

JAUNDICE

Definition & Approach
- Yellowing of the eyes & skin as a result of elevated bilirubin (>2.5 mg/dL)
- Unconjugated bilirubin not albumin bound can cross blood–brain barrier leading to adverse neuro effects ranging from subtle AMS to encephalopathy & death
- Hx: duration, abd pain, fever, recent travel, h/o liver dz or alcohol abuse/IVDU
- PEx: Mental status, abd tenderness, hepatomegaly, petechiae, caput medusae, spider angiomata, asterixis, ascites
- Labs: CBC, BMP, LFTs, PT/INR, lipase, ±ammonia if MS chgs, paracentesis if ascites & MS chgs, constitutional sx, pain, or new jaundice
- Imaging: RUQ US or CT abd/pel

Jaundice Differential		
Hyperbilirubinemia	**Predominant Bilirubin Form**	**Differential**
Prehepatic: Increased bilirubin production or impaired bili uptake or conjugation	Unconjugated (indirect)	Hemolysis, hematoma resorption, prolonged fasting, Crigler–Najjar synd, Gilbert synd, CHF, portosystemic shunt

Hepatocellular: Intrinsic liver pathology (significant transaminase elevations)	Mixed, mostly conjugated	Infectious hepatitis, autoimmune, alcoholic (AST: ALT >2:1), hepatotoxic drugs (eg, tylenol, amiodarone, statins), metabolic disorders (Wilson, Reye), hemochromatosis, α_1-antitrypsin deficiency, ischemic ("shock liver"), nonalcoholic fatty liver dz
Intrahepatic (nonobstructive) or extrahepatic (obstructive)	Conjugated (direct)	Int: Cholestatic jaundice of pregnancy, Dubin–Johnson synd, Rotor synd, primary biliary cirrhosis, sarcoidosis, GVHD
Impaired excretion of conjugated bilirubin (significant alk phos elevation)	Conjugated (direct)	Ext: Cholecystitis, choledocholithiasis, cholangitis, pancreatitis, carcinoma (ampulla, gallbladder, pancreas, CBD), biliary stricture, sclerosing cholangitis

Viral Hepatitis			
Dz	**Transmission**	**Serologic Pattern**	**Comments**
Hepatitis A	Fecal–oral, contaminated food/water	Acute: IgM anti-HAV Prior: IgG anti-HAV	Incubation 2–6 wks, self-limiting, tx is supportive, no chronic carrier state. Vaccine preventable
Acute Hepatitis B	Bloodborne, sexual, perinatal	IgM anti-HBc: Acute HBeAg: Active infxn HBsAg: May appear before sxs	Incubation 1–6 mos, 70% acute infxns subclinical, 30% jaundice, 1% fulminant failure, acute tx is supportive, <10% persist to chronic hepatitis B. Vaccine preventable
Chronic Hepatitis B[a]	Bloodborne, sexual, perinatal	IgG anti-HBc HBsAg in serum >6 mos	Major cause of hepatocellular cancer. Vaccine preventable
Acute Hepatitis C	Bloodborne, sexual	HCV viral load	Incubation 2 wks–5 mos, 75% acute infxns subclinical, 25% jaundice, 50–80% persist to chronic
Chronic Hepatitis C	Bloodborne, sexual	HCV & anti-HCV	Major cause of cirrhosis (20–30%), 2–3% of pts w/ cirrhosis develop HCC
Hepatitis D	Bloodborne, sexual	Anti-HDV	Occurs only in association w/ hepatitis B, faster progression to cirrhosis
Hepatitis E	Fecal–oral	IgM anti-HEV	Self-limiting, mortality 10–20% in pregnancy

[a]Implies secondary, neonatal hep B transmitted from mother results in chronic dz in up to 90% (Derived from Dienstag JL, Delemos AS. Viral hepatitis. In: Bennett JE, ed. *Mandell, Douglas and Bennett's Principles and Practice of Infectious Diseases.* 8th ed. Saunders; 2015:1439–1468.)

Cirrhosis

Definition

- Fibrosis & nodular regeneration resulting from hepatocellular injury
- Major etiologies: viral hepatitis (esp HCV), alcohol use disorder, non-EtoH steatohepatitis

History

- Abd pain, jaundice, pruritus, abd distension

Physical Exam

- Liver: enlarged palpable liver or shrunken nodular liver
- Signs of liver failure: jaundice, spider angioma, palmar erythema, gynecomastia, asterixis, encephalopathy
- Signs of portal HTN: splenomegaly, ascites, caput medusae

Evaluation
- New onset: LFTs, BMP, CBC (for anemia, thrombocytopenia), INR (to evaluate liver synthetic function), abd US if pain, tenderness, or fever present to r/o acute biliary dz or if concern for Budd–Chiari, paracentesis if new-onset ascites
- Exacerbation/decompensation of known cirrhosis: CBC, BMP, INR, ammonia. Paracentesis to r/o SBP if fever, abd pain, AMS, GIB, significant leukocytosis.
- MELD score & Child Pugh classification are used to predict prog of pts w/ cirrhosis.

Treatment
- Outpt mgmt focused on slowing progression & evaluating for liver tpx
- ED care: Directed at evaluating for cx (hepatorenal, hepatopulmonary, SBP, variceal bleeding) + treating sx
- Hepatic encephalopathy (failure of liver to detoxify ammonia & other agents): Protein restriction, lactulose (goal 2–4 stools/d), rifaximin. Work to find provoking cause (eg, infxn, constipation, electrolyte abnl)

Disposition
- Admit if decompensated (increasing ascites/edema despite compliance w/ outpt regimen), pulmonary edema, renal failure, hypotensive, encephalopathic, febrile

Pearl
- Cxs: Portal HTN (ascites, varices), encephalopathy, hepatorenal synd, hepatopulmonary synd, infxns (relative immunosuppression), HCC

Acute Liver Failure

Definition
- American Association for the Study of Liver Diseases definition: (1) INR >/1.5, (2) neuro dysfxn, (3) no prior e/o liver dz, (4) course /<26 wks
- Etiologies: viral hepatitis (A, B, E), drugs (APAP), acute ischemic injury in critically ill pts, neoplastic infiltration, acute Budd–Chiari, mushroom ingestion, Wilson dz, CHF w/ hepatic congestion

History & Physical Exam
- Hx: Toxic ingestion, nausea, vomiting, malaise, confusion, substances, travel, pregnancy
- Ex: Jaundice, abd tenderness, enlarged liver, encephalopathy, pulmonary edema, GIB (decreased clotting factors, DIC)

Evaluation
- Labs: CBC (anemia, thrombocytopenia), PT/INR (elevated), BMP (electrolytes, renal function), APAP level, viral serologies, VBG, lactate, blood cx, abd US w/ Doppler

Treatment
- Closely monitor hemodynamics. Intravascular hypovolemia common 2/2 low SVR & fluid shifts
- Treat underlying causes (eg, APAP ingestion w/ NAC)
- If etiology unclear, low threshold for NAC regardless of APAP level
- Low threshold for broad-spectrum abx if H&P or labs c/f infxn
- Coagulopathy/GIB: Vit K, FFP, PCC, PLTs, cryoprecipitate if active hemorrhage
- Cerebral edema: lactulose, +/– ICP monitoring, hypertonic saline/mannitol, avoid fever & agitation
  - CNS cx inc brainstem herniation, are the most common cause of death in ALF
- Transplantation improves survival but not universally available
  - Pts w/ ALF should be managed in tpx centers

Disposition
- Admit medicine. ICU if fulminant, hypotensive, or otherwise unstable

ANORECTAL DISORDERS

Approach
- Nature: pain, duration, consistency of stools, bleeding, fevers

Differential	
Bleeding	Cryptitis (inflammation of epithelial pockets), hemorrhoids, anal fissure, proctitis (inflammation of the rectal mucosa), cancer, STIs
No bleeding	Anorectal abscess, anal fistula, anorectal FB, proctalgia fugax (idiopathic severe brief rectal pain), pilonidal dz, rectal prolapse

Anal Fissure

- **Definition:** superficial tear of the anoderm that begins just below the dentate line
- **History:** h/o passage of hard stools, sharp pain w/ defecation, blood on toilet paper
- **Physical Exam:** Visible fissure, painful. If not midline, eval for IBD, cancer, HIV, STDs
- **Management:** sitz baths (warm baths 15 mins 3×/d), high-fiber diet, lidocaine jelly, topical nitroglycerin ointment or nifedipine gel, topical diltiazem gel

Hemorrhoids

Definition

- Dilated or bulging veins of the rectum & anus. Internal hemorrhoids may prolapse & become incarcerated (irreducible) or strangulated (ischemic). External hemorrhoids may thrombose, leading to acute pain & bleeding

History

- Bright red–coated stool/toilet paper/dripping into the bowl, pain w/ defecation, h/o hard stools, constipation, prolonged sitting; bleeding hemorrhoids are usually painless

Physical Exam

- External hemorrhoids are visible on eversion of the anal orifice, thrombosed hemorrhoids are tender & dark, internal hemorrhoids may be palpable & are visible w/ anoscopy

Evaluation

- CBC only if significant blood loss suspected or concerning underlying condition

Management

- Outpt w/ stool softener (docusate, senna), sitz baths (15 mins TID & after BMs), suppositories for symptomatic relief
- Acute thrombosis (<48 h since onset of pain) can be excised at bedside in ED
- If prolapsed hemorrhoid is incarcerated w/ signs of strangulation, c/s surgery

Pearl

- Hemorrhoidal bleeding rarely a cause of significant anemia

Rectal Prolapse

- **Definition:** Protrusion of some or all of the rectal layers through the anus
- **History:** Most common among women, multiparous, elderly, & those w/ chronic constipation
- **Physical Exam:** protruding full-thickness rectal wall w/ concentric rings (hemorrhoids contain only mucosa & there are radial sulci between bundles)
- **Management:** For nonstrangulated, gentle manual reduction w/ analgesia & sedation as needed, granulated sugar to reduce edema; If strangulated, c/s surgery

FEVER

Background

- Body temp elevation due to chg in hypothalamic set point
- Defined as temp ≥100.4 °F/38 °C but rarely exceeds 105.8 °F/41 °C
- Caused by response to bacteria, viruses, inflammation; ↑ metabolic rate, meds
- Distinct from hyperthermia (failure of thermoregulation, can exceed 41 °C)

Approach

- Careful hx inc origin, provocation/palliation, max temp and how this temp was obtained, time of onset, duration, and associated sxs (N/V, diarrhea, cough, abd pain, rash, AMS)
- Eval directed by pt hx & sx localization
- Assess VS for significant abnormalities that may indicate serious infxn (↓ BP, ↑ HR)
- If immunosuppressed (chemotherapy, immunotherapy, transplant, HIV/AIDS, elderly, malnourished, chronic steroids, DM), more intensive eval & testing: CBC, Chem, UA & cx, CXR; consider blood cx & admission
- Intermittent/relapsing fever: Ddx vector-borne dzs, endocarditis, Still dz

Fever Differential	
Pathophysiology	**Differential**
Cardiac	Endocarditis (1), myocarditis (1j)
Pulmonary	PNA (2b), bronchitis (2b), empyema, TB (2b), PE (1b)
GI	Intra-abd abscess, cholangitis (3a), diverticulitis (3a), appendicitis (3a), hepatitis (3g), cholecystitis
GU	UTI (6a), pyelonephritis (6b), PID (7e)
Neurologic	Meningitis (5d), SAH, TBI, dysautonomia
ENT	Pharyngitis (13b), sinusitis (13), otitis, Lemierre's
Toxicology	NMS (10l), malignant hyperthermia (10l)
Environmental	Hyperthermia (10k), drug-induced, vector-borne & zoonotic dzs (4h), parasitic infxns (4l), RMSF (8a)
Infectious	Mononucleosis (4f), TB (2b), HIV (4g), rheumatic fever, viral infxns (4f)
Hematologic	DVT (1b), PE (1b), sickle cell (11e)
Orthopedic	Osteomyelitis (19k), septic arthritis (12c)
Oncologic	Malignancy (11), neutropenic fever, tumor lysis synd
Immunologic	Autoimmune, Mediterranean fever, vasculitis, sarcoid

BACTERIAL INFECTIONS

ENDOCARDITIS (*JAMA* 2018;320(1):72–83)

History

- RFs: IVDU, congenital or acquired valvular dz, prosthetic valves, HD, indwelling venous catheters, cardiac surgery, bacteremia, immunosupp inc HIV, previous endocarditis, poor dentition
- Dx difficult 2/2 nonspecific sx (lethargy, weak, anorexia, low-grade temp), or negative w/u

Findings

- Fever +/– back pain, new murmur, CHF, splenomegaly, petechiae
- Classic physical exam findings
  - Roth spots: Exudative, edematous retinal lesions w/ central clearing
  - Osler nodes: Violaceous tender nodules on toes & fingers
  - Janeway lesions: Nontender, blanching, macular plaques on soles & palms
  - Splinter hemorrhages: Nonblanching, linear, reddish-brown under nails
  - Septic emboli (pulmonary, splenic, renal, other)
- If SOB, consider acute pulm edema from valve rupture; confirm w/ B-lines on POCUS

Diagnosis

Modified Duke Criteria	
Classification	**Requirements for Dx**
Definite	Microorganism on culture or histology of vegetation/cardiac abscess OR Clinical criteria: 2 major, 1 major & 3 minor, or 5 minor
Possible	1 major & 1 minor, or 3 minor
Criteria	**Evidence**
Major	≥2 positive BCx, endocardial involvement, vegetation, new valvular regurgitation
Minor	Predisposing cardiac dz, IVDU or other RFs, fever, vascular phenomena (septic infarcts, ICH, Janeway lesions), immune phenomena (glomerulonephritis, Osler nodes, Roth spot), positive BCx not meeting major criteria

Evaluation

- 3 sets of BCx: Typically *Staph aureus* or *Strep* species; other causative organisms inc *Enterococcus*, HACEK (*Haemophilus, Aggregatibacter Cardiobacterium hominis, Eikenella, and Kingella*) organisms, and *Candida* (more common in IVDU and those w/ prosthetic valves). Up to 10% never have organism identified
- Echo looking for vegetations or valve ring abscesses (TEE more sens than TTE)
- EKG (heart block suggestive of intracardiac abscess), CXR, CBC, Chem, coags, ↑ ESR/CRP (nonspecific)

Treatment

- Immediate abx in suspected cases (see table on **Antimicrobial Treatment of Bacterial Endocarditis**), preferably after BCx
- Hemodynamic stabilization (more likely w/ valve rupture and resulting acute heart failure)
- Consider cardiac surgery consultation for valve rupture, valve ring abscess, removal of implanted device, or infxn refractory to IV abx

Disposition

- Majority should be admitted to cardiology floor w/ continuous telemetry & IV abx
- if hemodynamic compromise, admit to ICU

Pearls

- Mortality: in-hospital 15–20%, 40% at 1 y
- Worse prognosis if involves aortic valve, DM, *S. aureus* (30–40%)
- Left-sided endocarditis (mitral 41%, aortic valve 31%) most common
- IVDU: Tricuspid valve endocarditis; rheumatic heart dz – Mitral more common than aortic valve

Antimicrobial Treatment of Bacterial Endocarditis	
Hx	**Antibiotic**
Native valve	MRSA: Vancomycin 25–30 mg/kg loading dose → 15 mg/kg IV BID + CTX 2 g IV QD
Prosthetic valve (irrespective of post op period)	Vancomycin 25–30 mg/kg loading dose → 15 mg/kg IV BID + gentamicin 1 mg/kg IV q8h (for synergistic effect w/ vancomycin against enterococcus) + cefepime 2 g IV q8h + rifampin 300 mg PO/IV TID (can be removed in renal failure)
IVDU	Same as native valve except: cefepime 2 g IV q8h replaces CTX (to cover for pseudomonas)
PCN Allergy	Vancomycin 25–30 mg/kg loading dose → 15 mg/kg IV BID OR daptomycin 8–10 mg/kg q24h + ciprofloxacin 400 mg IV BID

SKIN AND SOFT TISSUE

Cutaneous Abscess (*Emerg Med Clin North Am* 2018;36:723–750; *NEJM* 2014;370:1039)

History

- Careful hx, associated sxs (fever, N/V/D, AMS), progression
- Often spontaneous but RFs include skin trauma, insect bites, venous insufficiency, edema, folliculitis, h/o IVDU/skin popping, prior skin infxns

Findings

- Focal, circumscribed area of pain, redness, tenderness, fluctuance; usually w/o fever or systemic tox

Evaluation

- Assess VS for significant abnormalities that may indicate serious infxn
- Check blood sugar if diabetic
- Blood work rarely needed unless appear systemically ill or immunosuppressed: CBC, Chem, CRP, CPK, UA & UCx, CXR; consider blood cx & admission
- Consider static or dynamic POCUS to localize fluid collection
- Culture/Gram stain only if systemically ill or failed initial tx
- Most commonly *Staph* species

Treatment

- No abx indicated in healthy hosts (although higher cure rate, lower rates of subsequent I&Ds, skin infxns at new sites, & infxns in household members (*NEJM* 2016;374:823) but if >2 cm, cellulitis, systemic illness, immunosupp, failed I&D, use the following abx: TMP-SMX DS 2 tablet BID, doxycycline 100 mg BID ×7 d
- I&D w/ regional nerve or field blocks +/− IV procedural sedation/analgesia
- Create elliptical incision to prevent premature wound closure, deep enough to drain cavity. Follow tension lines to minimize scarring.
- Break up loculations in abscess cavity w/ hemostat
- Consider loop drainage for larger abscesses to allow for ongoing drainage, removal in 7–10 d

Disposition

- D/c home w/ wound care instructions, f/u, and return precautions
- Warm soaks TID × 2–3 d after removal of packing to allow continued wound drainage

Pearls

- Do NOT routinely perform I+D in pt w/ HS

Cellulitis (*JAMA* 2016;316:325)

History

- See cutaneous abscess in the previous section
- Infxn of the deep dermis and subcutaneous fat

Findings

- Warm, blanching erythema, tenderness to palpation, mild to moderate swelling
- May lead to dilated/edematous lymphatics (peau d'orange), bulla formation or linear streaking/lymphangitis
- ± distal skin disruption (eg, tinea pedis b/w toes w/ cellulitis of anterior shin)

Evaluation (See cutaneous abscess previous section)

- Mark border w/ permanent ink, inc writing time & date
- R/o abscess and foreign body w/ POCUS
- Consider imaging if concerned for foreign body
- Consider Doppler vascular studies if cellulitis in single limb (especially posterior calf/medial thigh) and a/w diffuse swelling
- Most often caused by *Strep pyogenes* or *S. aureus* (inc MRSA); can be from metastatic seeding

Treatment

- Pain control w/ NSAID/APAP; if severe pain, consider necrotizing infxn
- Typically aim to treat Strep & MSSA but antibiotic choice depends on presence of purulence and systemic sxs (purulence increases likelihood of MRSA)
- Antibiotic regimens
  - Mild (Meets 0 SIRS criteria – Temp <38 °C >36 °C, HR >90, RR >20, WBC >12 or <4):
    - Nonpurulent: Cephalexin 500 mg PO QID or cefadroxil 1 g PO BID or Cefuroxime 500 mg PO BID or Dicloxacillin 500 mg PO QID or Clindamycin PO 450 mg TID (if PCN allergy)
    - Purulent: TMP-SMX DS 1 tablet BID (2 tabs BID if >100 kg or trauma induced) or doxycycline 100 mg PO BID
  - Moderate (Meets 1 SIRS criteria; Consider if age >75, DM, ESRD, low-grade immunosupp [<20 mg])
    - Nonpurulent: Cefazolin 1 g IV q8h (2 g if >100 kg) or CTX 1 g IV QD (2 g if >100 kg), or Clindamycin 600 mg IV q8h (if PCN allergy)

- Purulent: Cefazolin 1 g IV q8h (2 g if >100 kg) or CTX 1 g IV QD (2 g if >100 kg) AND TMP-SMX DS 1 tablet BID (2 tabs BID if >100 kg or trauma induced) or doxycycline 100 mg PO BID
- Severe (≥2 SIRS criteria; Consider if ANC <500/active chemo, high-grade immunosupp [>20 mg])
  - Nonpurulent/Purulent: Vancomycin 15 mg/kg IV q12h or linezolid 600 mg q12h
  - NSTI: Linezolid 600 mg q12h (or vancomycin 15 mg/kg IV q12h and clindamycin 600 mg IV q8h) and piperacillin/tazobactam 4.5 g q6h
- If LE cellulitis, recommend rest/elevation × 48 h, and crutches if needed

Disposition
- Mild: D/c w/ PO abx & 24–48 h f/u, strict return instructions
- Moderate/Severe: Admit for IV abx, consider surgery consultation if concern for NSTI or wound debridement

Pearls
- Mimics: Stasis dermatitis (more likely if bilateral), hematoma (consider if h/o trauma), gout/septic arthritis (consider if over joint), herpes (vesicular and dermatomal)
- There's no evidence to support the practice of giving 1 dose of IV abx prior to a course of outpt abx
- If water exposure: Add levofloxacin 750 mg PO QD+/– doxycycline 100 mg BID (if seawater exposure) +/– Metronidazole 500 mg q8h (if c/f anaerobic)
- Consider the 2nd-generation glycopeptides (dalbavancin, oritavancin) in pts who are at high risk of being lost to f/u given it is dosed once weekly

Erysipelas (*Prim Care* 2018;45:433–454)

History
- Skin infxn of the upper dermis & superficial lymphatics
- Well-demarcated, erythematous plaque a/w burning, tenderness, pruritus 48 h later
- RF: Lymphatic edema/obstruction, extremes of age, obesity, DM, CHF, postop, nephrotic synd

Findings
- Painful, superficial, indurated, raised; erythema w/ sharply demarcated border
- Distinguish from cellulitis given fast onset, sharp demarcation and raised edges
- Irregular erythema w/ lymphangitis, may see desquamation, dimpling, vesicles, LAD
- Mostly found on lower extremities, sometimes on face, typically malar or "butterfly" pattern

Evaluation
- No labs/imaging indicated unless toxic appearing
- Most often caused by *Strep pyogenes*

Treatment
- See cellulitis antibiotic regimens in the previous section
- Compression stockings if lower extremity is affected

Disposition
- D/c home w/ PO abx & analgesics, instructions to elevate affected area, 24–48 h f/u, & strict return instructions

Pearls
- Infxn involving the ear "Milian's ear sign" unique to erysipelas b/c ear does not contain deeper dermis tissues

Staphylococcal Scalded Skin Syndrome (SSSS) (*World J Pediatr* 2018;14:116–120)

History
- Prodromal sore throat → conjunctivitis, fever, malaise → painful red skin w/ sloughing
- Typically occurs in young children <5 y
- Rare in adults, a/w chronic illness, immunosupp, & renal failure

Findings
- Tender, erythematous cellulitis followed by acute exfoliation: Bullae, vesicles → large sheets of skin loss resulting in scalded-appearing skin
- Positive Nikolsky sign (epidermis separates when pressure applied)
- No mucous membrane involvement (vs TEN)
- General malaise, fever, irritability

Evaluation
- None indicated unless systemically ill

Treatment
- Similar to diffuse burns (IVF, antipyretics, topical wound care, burn consult, abx)
- Vancomycin is antibiotic of choice

Disposition
- Admit for burn care/IVF; consider ICU
- Prognosis: Children (<5% mortality) often w/o significant scarring; adults (60% mortality)

Pearls
- Caused by exfoliative exotoxins of *S. aureus*, inc MRSA
- Separation of epidermal layers vs more severe TEN (necrosis at level of basement membrane)
- Prognosis: Children (<5% mortality) often w/o significant scarring; adults (60% mortality)

Toxic Shock Syndrome (TSS) (*J Infect* 2017;74:S147–S152)

History
- Prodromal sxs, pain at site of infxn (out of proportion to findings), fever, GI upset, myalgia, confusion, lethargy
- Commonly, no source found but RFs include recent surgery, infrequently changed packing (tampons, nasal packing), disruption of skin

Findings
- Clinical dx w/ findings from all organ systems
- Staph TSS: Temp >38.9 °C, rash (diffuse macular erythroderma inc palms/soles), desquamation (1–2 wks after onset), hypotension, multisystem involvement (≥3 GI, muscular, mucous membranes, renal, hepatic, hematologic, CNS), negative blood/throat/CSF cultures (BCx may be positive for *S. aureus*
- Strep TSS: Culture positive for Strep (blood, CSF, tissue biopsy, throat, vagina, sputum); hypotension, multisystem involvement (≥2 renal impairment, coagulopathy, hepatic involvement, ARDS, generalized erythematous macular rash, soft tissue necrosis)

Evaluation
- CBC w/ differential, Chem, LFTs, coags, UA, cultures (blood, urine, throat, sputum, CSF)

Treatment
- Source control: Remove tampon/packing if still in place; drain abscesses if present; surgical debridement of necrotizing fasciitis or myositis; burn care
- Aggressive resuscitation, pressors if needed
- Abx regimen
    - Empiric tx: (See severe cellulitis antibiotic regimens in the previous section) + Clindamycin 600 mg IV q8h (to suppress bacterial toxin synthesis)
    - Abx may not have impact (toxin-mediated process)
- IVIG (blocks T-cell activation by superantigens) may be added if no clinical response to aggressive supportive therapy in 1st 6 h of tx

Disposition
- ICU admission

Pearls
- Rate ↓ w/ ↓ in use of superabsorbent tampons
- Caused by inflammatory response to superantigen from toxin-producing gram-positive organisms (*S. aureus, S. pyogenes*)
- *Strep:* Usually after surgery or trauma; scarlet fever-like rash; 30–44% mortality, fulminant. BCx positive ~60% of cases.
- *Staph:* More indolent, 0–20% mortality. BCx positive <5% of cases.

Necrotizing Soft Tissue Infections (*Infect Dis Clin North Am* 2021;35:135–155)

History
- Sudden onset of pain, erythema, warmth, and edema that is rapidly progressive
- RF: DM, IVDU, obesity, EtOH abuse, nutritionally compromised

Findings
- Cellulitis, skin discoloration/ecchymosis or gangrene, edema, spectrum of sensation from anesthesia to pain out of proportion
- Can have hemodynamic instability, crepitus (subcutaneous air due to gas-forming organisms)
- Bullae, crepitus, and skin necrosis are rare but should trigger emergent surgical debridement
- Can progress to involvement of deeper layers, causing myositis or myonecrosis

Evaluation

- Clinical dx
- CBC w/ differential, Chem, CRP, coags, type, & screen
- If obtaining imaging, CT preferred as plain radiographs are less sens in eval of gas w/i soft tissue

LRINEC Score	
Points	**Lab Indicators**
4	CRP ≥150 mg/L
1	WBC 15–25/mm^3 (2 points if >25 mm^3)
1	Hgb 11–13.5 g/dL (2 points if <11 g/dL)
2	Na <135 mmol/L (135 mEq/L)
2	Cr >1.6 mg/dL
1	Glucose >180 mg/dL
Score of ≥6	Sens 92.9%, spec 91.6% for necrotizing fasciitis

(From *Crit Care Med.* 2004;32(7):1535–1541.)

Treatment

- Early surgical consult for debridement (definitive tx)
- Hemodynamic support
- Early & broad spectrum IV abx
  - Vancomycin 25–30 mg/kg loading dose → 15 mg/kg IV q12h + Clindamycin 600–900 mg IV q8h OR linezolid 600 mg IV q12h AND
  - Cefepime 2 g IV q8h + Metronidazole 500 mg IV q8h
    OR
  - Piperacillin/tazobactam 4.5 g IV q6h
    OR
  - Imipenem/cilastatin 1 g IV q8h
- Consider IVIG (in conjunction w/ abx) after debridement (*Clin Infect Dis* 2021;72:293)

Disposition

- Surgical debridement and ICU admission

Pearls

- Mortality 16–46%, fatal if untreated
- Mostly *S. pyogenes* (group A), Clostridium, *S. aureus*, or mixed gram + & – bacteria, anaerobes

---

GENITOURINARY

Fournier Gangrene (*Urology* 2018;114:8–13; *Nat Rev Urol* 2017;14:205–214)

History

- Prodromal fever, lethargy prodrome → rapidly progressing scrotal swelling, pain, erythema, warmth, possible purulent drainage
- RF: Men (10:1), >50 y/o, diabetic, chronic EtOH abuse, immunocompromised, recent h/o instrumentation/surgery, urethral strictures or calculi, hemorrhoids, perirectal abscess, malignancies

Findings

- Intensely tender, swollen, warm scrotum w/o clear fluctuance, pruritic genitalia
- Fever, chills, systemic sxs (tachycardia, ↓ BP), ± crepitus, drainage

Evaluation

- CBC w/ differential, Chem, CRP, coag, T&S, BCx, UA, UCx
- CT will show extent of infxn & necrosis

Treatment

- Urology & general surgery consult for wide debridement & drainage
- Hemodynamic support & resuscitation w/ IVF & pressors
- Early & broad spectrum IV abx (see necrotizing soft tissue infxns antibiotic regimens in the previous section)
- Consider IVIG (in conjunction w/ abx) after debridement (*Clin Infect Dis* 2021;72:293)

Disposition

- Surgical debridement & ICU admission

Pearls
- Mortality 3–67%; early surgical debridement most strongly correlated w/ outcome
- Polymicrobial (*E. coli,* Proteus, Enterococcus, *Bacteroides,* & other anaerobes) necrotizing infxn of perineum, scrotum, & penis characterized by obliterative endarteritis of the subcutaneous arteries resulting in gangrene
- Rapid destruction of fascial planes w/ deep-space infxn often vastly greater than skin involvement would suggest

Bartholin Gland Cyst (*BJOG* 2020;127:671–678)
History
- Severe localized pain caused by obstructed Bartholin duct
- Difficulty walking & sitting secondary to pain
- Fever & signs of systemic tox are rare

Findings
- Painful, tender, cystic mass on inferior lateral margin of vaginal introitus at 4- and 8-o'clock positions often w/ purulent drainage from sinus tract

Evaluation
- Culture for chlamydia/gonorrhea; typically w/ mixed vaginal flora (*Bacteroides, E. coli, S. aureus,* gonorrhea, chlamydia)

Treatment
- I&D through mucosal surface, place Word catheter ×48 h
- Sitz baths TID for the 1st 2–3 d to assist drainage
- Gyn f/u for consideration of marsupialization to prevent recurrence

Disposition
- D/c w/ wound care instructions, 2-d wound care f/u

Pearl
- Recurrence rate still 5–15% after marsupialization; consider gyn malignancy

HAND

Paronychia (*Am Fam Physician* 2017;96:44–51)
History
- Pain & swelling lateral to nail edge; abscess beneath eponychial fold
- Often secondary to contaminated nail care instruments, nail biting, hang nail, or trauma

Findings
- Purulent collection lateral to nail bed w/ minimal surrounding erythema
- Most commonly *S. aureus, S. pyogenes, Pseudomonas* or *Proteus.*

Evaluation
- No labs necessary

Treatment
- Digital block w/ 1% lidocaine w/ or w/o epinephrine in each web space of affected digit
- #11 blade scalpel to lift cuticle from nail on affected side & express purulent material
- Only treat w/ oral abx (see cellulitis antibiotic regimen in the previous section) if associated cellulitis

Disposition
- D/c w/ wound care instructions, 2-d f/u
- Warm soaks to finger TID × 2–3 d to allow complete drainage

Pearls
- If recurrent or chronic paronychia, consider *Candida* infxn
- If vesicular, consider herpetic whitlow, and do not I&D
- If neglected, may spread to pulp space of finger (felon), deep spaces of hand (such as tendon)

Flexor Tenosynovitis (*J Hand Surg* 2019;44[11]:981–985)
History
- Infxn of the flexor tendon sheath commonly from direct penetrating trauma to the volar aspect of the digit

Findings

- Kanavel signs (4): flexed posture of digit, fusiform swelling, tenderness over flexor tendon sheath, pain w/ passive extension
- Most commonly *S. aureus* (75%)
- Systemic sxs may be present

Evaluation

- Clinical dx
- U/S may reveal fluid along tendon sheath

Treatment

- IV abx: ampicillin/sulbactam 3 g q8h, linezolid 600 mg q12h, or vancomycin 25–30 mg/kg loading dose → 15 mg/kg IV
- Operative drainage and irrigation of tendon sheath indicated for advanced/delayed presentation, ≥3 Kanavel signs, failure to respond to IV abx

Disposition

- Consultation w/ hand surgeon for surgical mgmt
- Delayed mgmt can lead to digit necrosis, tendon rupture, digit amputation, sepsis

Pearls

- Surgical emergency

NEUROLOGIC

See section "CNS Infections" in Section V: Neurology.

OPHTHALMOLOGIC

Periorbital/Preseptal Cellulitis (*Dis Mon* 2017;63[2]:30–32)

History

- Recent infxn of sinuses/periorbital skin, trauma to periorbital area, insect bites

Findings

- Unilateral eyelid swelling, erythema, warmth, discoloration of skin
- Injected sclera, conjunctival ecchymosis
- No pain w/ extraocular movements, no proptosis, nl pupillary rxn & vision

Evaluation

- Clinical dx but if uncertain obtain CT scan of orbits to look for posterior extension

Treatment

- Empiric abx coverage: Augmentin 875 mg PO BID or cefdinir 300 mg PO BID AND clindamycin 300 mg PO TID or TMP-SMX DS 1 tablet BID

Disposition

- D/c w/ close ophthalmology f/u except if <1 y/o or systemically ill → admit/tx as below

Pearls

- Infxn of soft tissue of eyelids & periocular region anterior to orbital septum
- Most often caused by *Staph*, *Strep*, & *anaerobes;* rarely *H. influenza* since widespread vaccination
- Distinguish from orbital cellulitis: No pain w/ EOM or proptosis in periorbital cellulitis

Orbital Cellulitis/Postseptal Cellulitis

History

- Orbital pain increased w/ extraocular movements, ↓ vision
- Recent infxn of sinuses/periorbital skin, trauma to periorbital area, insect bites

Findings

- Fever, HA, rhinorrhea, malaise
- Proptosis & ophthalmoplegia are cardinal signs
  - Unilateral eyelid swelling, erythema, warmth, discoloration of skin
  - Injected sclera, chemosis
  - Tenderness on gentle globe palpation, ↑ IOP
  - ↓ visual acuity, relative afferent pupillary defect, visual field abnormalities

Evaluation
- CBC w/ differential, CTV/MRIV of orbits (venous phase helps detect cavernous sinus thrombosis), BCx

Treatment
- Immediate broad spectrum IV abx: Vancomycin 25–30 mg/kg loading dose → 15 mg/kg IV q12h + Ampicillin/Sulbactam 3 g IV q6h
- Urgent ophthalmology consult

Disposition
- Admission for abx

Pearls
- Infxn of soft tissues of orbit posterior to orbital septum
- Most common: *Strep, Staph, H. influenzae,* polymicrobial
- Consider fungal etiologies (mucor, aspergillus) in pts w/ comorbidities
- Cx: Meningitis, brain abscess, death, cavernous sinus thrombosis (bilateral involvement, rapidly worsening, congestion of veins of face or conjunctiva)

Otolaryngologic

Ludwig Angina (*Am J Emerg Med* 2021;41:1–5)
History
- Fever, malaise, neck swelling, trismus, "hot potato" voice, drooling, pain w/ tongue movement, stridor
- RFs: Recent dental infxn, mandible fractures, tongue piercings, DM, HIV, alcoholism

Findings
- Swelling of submandibular/sublingual space; hard/"board like"/woodiness on palpation

Evaluation
- CBC w/ differential, Chem, BCx, coags, T&S
- CT scan of head & neck w/ IV contrast

Treatment
- If severe swelling and threatened airway threatening, fiberoptic nasotracheal intubation may be the best initial approach w/ cricothyrotomy as backup
- Emergent consultation w/ otolaryngologist for surgical intervention
- Broad spectrum IV abx
- Immunocompetent:
  - Ampicillin/Sulbactam 3 g IV q6h OR
  - CTX 2 g IV q24h + Metronidazole 500 mg IV q8h
- Immunocompromised (increased risk of pseudomonas)
  - Cefepime 2 g IV q8h + Metronidazole 500 mg IV q8h OR
- Piperacillin/tazobactam 4.5 g IV q6h OR
  - Imipenem/cilastatin 1 g IV q8h
- Low-threshold for Vancomycin (25-30 mg/kg loading dose → 15 mg/kg IV q12h) OR linezolid 600 mg q12h if concerned for MRSA

Disposition
- Admit to ICU

Pearls
- Rapidly spreading bilateral cellulitis of submandibular space a/w displacement of tongue causing life-threatening airway obstruction
- Polymicrobial, inc *Strep, Staph, Fusobacterium, Bacteroides*

Rectal

Pilonidal Cyst (*Emerg Med Clin North Am* 2016;34:251)
History
- Painful, tender abscess in midline pit b/w upper part of the gluteal clefts, often in obese or hirsute individuals
- More prevalent in males; fever & systemic tox very rare

Findings
- Painful, localized abscess in natal cleavage/midline sacrococcygeal region, 4–5 cm superior to anal opening; often w/ surrounding erythema

Evaluation
- No labs necessary unless systemically ill or immunosuppressed
- Consider static or dynamic POCUS to localize fluid collection
- Culture/Gram stain only if systemically ill or failed initial tx
- Mixed flora: *Staph* or *Strep* species, anaerobic cocci, mixed aerobic, & anaerobic flora

Treatment
- Same as for cutaneous abscess, I&D
- abx (Mild cellulitis abx regiment + Metronidazole 500 mg PO TID) if overlying cellulitis, immunosuppressed or systemically ill
- For definitive mgmt, surgical referral for excision of follicle & sinus tract after acute episode subsides

Disposition
- D/c w/ wound care instructions, 2-d wound care f/u

Pearl
- Thought to be caused by hair penetrating into subcutaneous tissues

Anorectal Abscesses (Perianal and Perirectal Abscesses) (*Emerg Med Clin North Am* 2016;34:251)

History
- Pain & swelling in rectal area w/ defecation, sitting, or walking
- High fever & signs of systemic tox are rare
- RFs: IBD, obesity, DM, hemorrhoids, rectal trauma

Findings
- Rectal exam essential to ensure abscess localized outside of anal sphincter/identify upper pole of abscess
- Perianal abscess: palpable mass close to anal verge
- Perirectal abscess: few outward exam findings, may have tenderness and induration more lateral to anal verge

Evaluation
- Lab studies unnecessary unless systemically ill or immunocompromised
- CT pelvis for large abscesses, MRI if concern for small abscess or fistula

Treatment
- ED I&D of small, superficial perianal abscesses outside the anal verge w/ visible indurated area
  - I&D extremely painful, procedural sedation often needed
  - Pack w/ Vaseline gauze ×48 h, Sitz baths TID for 1st 2–3 d to assist drainage
- Large, complex perianal abscesses and all perirectal abscesses require a general surgery consult for eval for operative intervention
- Abx regimen
  - Uncomplicated
  - Metronidazole 500 mg PO q12h + cefpodoxime 400 mg PO q12h
  - Complicated (surrounding cellulitis, systemic sxs, failure to improve, immunocompromised, prosthetic device/valve, incomplete I&D)
  - Metronidazole 500 mg IV q12h + CTX 1 g IV (2 g if >100 kg or severe infxn)
  - If suspect MRSA, add vancomycin 15 mg/kg IV q12h

Disposition
- Home w/ wound care instructions, 2-d wound care f/u
- Admit diabetic & immunocompromised for IV abx

Pearls
- 50–75% treated w/ I&D or spontaneous drainage will develop chronic anal fistula
- Typically mixed flora (*E. coli* species, *Enterococcus, Bacteroides* species, *S. aureus*)
- Consider adding stool softeners

Figure 4.1 Anorectal abscess locations.

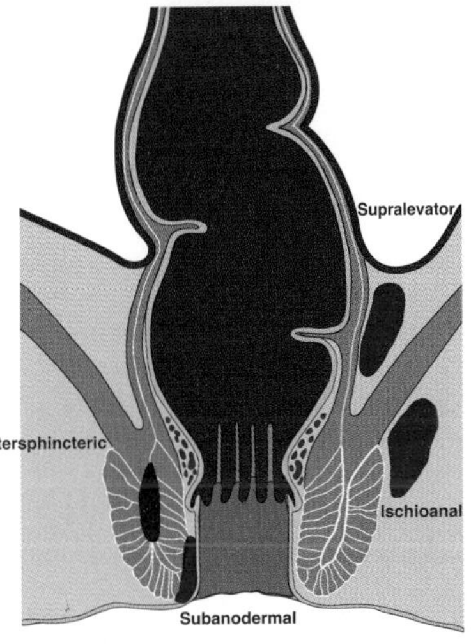

DIARRHEAL ILLNESSES

See Infectious Diarrhea in Section III: Gastrointestinal.

SYPHILIS (*TREPONEMA PALLIDUM*) (*Lancet* 2017;389:1550–1557)

History

- Primary syphilis: Chancre – painless, usually solitary, indurated, clean-based, ulcerative lesion 2–3 wks after sexual contact
- Secondary syphilis: Painless, 1–2-cm, macular rash involving palms & soles but can vary in appearance (thus the "great imitator"). May be a/w malaise, myalgia, HA (syphilitic meningitis), sore throat.
- Latent dz
- Tertiary syphilis: Late neurosyphilis (general paresis, tabes dorsalis), cardiovascular syphilis (aneurysm of ascending aorta, AV insufficiency, CAD), gummatous syphilis (reactive, granulomatous processes)

Findings

- Primary syphilis: chancre, ± nontender LAD
- Secondary syphilis: painless rash may be a/w fever, LAD, HSM, hepatitis
- Tertiary syphilis: General paresis causes progressive dementia, szs, psychiatric synds. Tabes dorsalis "lightening" radicular pains, ataxia, Argyll Robertson pupil (small, do not react to light but accommodate), loss of reflexes, impaired vibratory sense

Evaluation

- Treponemal test (eg, RPR, VDRL) → nontreponemal assay to confirm (eg, FT-ABS, TP-PA)
- Reactive CSF VDRL is diagnostic of neurosyphilis

Treatment

- Early (primary, secondary, or early latent): benzathine PCN G 2.4 million units IM ×1
  - If PCN allergy: Doxycycline 100 mg PO BID × 14 d
- Late/unknown duration latent syphilis: Benzathine PCN G 2.4 million units I × 3 wks
  - If PCN allergy: Doxycycline 100 mg PO BID × 28 d

- Neurosyphilis: PCN G 3–4 million units IV q4H × 10–14 d
- After tx 30–50% pts have Jarisch–Herxheimer rxn (fever, myalgia, worsening skin rash). Will self-resolve, can tx w/ IVF, antipyretics

Disposition
- Pts w/ neurosyphilis, ocular syphilis, or cardiovascular syphilis should be admitted for abx

Pearls
- Increases risk of HIV infxn; HIV incidence up to 20% in the decade after syphilis dx
- Spread through direct lesion contact, small proportion through blood transfer

---

TETANUS (*CLOSTRIDIUM TETANI*) (*Lancet* 2019;393:1657–1668)

History
- Acute-onset hypertonia, painful muscular contractions → generalized muscle spasms/rigidity, dysphagia
- 3–21-d incubation period
- RFs: Inadequate vaccination status, chronic wound, IVDU

Findings
- Autonomic dysfxn (BP ↑ or ↓), dysrhythmias, cardiac arrest
- Spasms of muscles near site of injury +/– resulting fractures/dislocations, cephalic tetanus, lockjaw, risus sardonicus (characteristic grimace), tetanic sz, respiratory failure

Evaluation
- Clinical dx

Treatment
- Heavy sedation (benzos, propofol, opioids) & paralysis supported by artificial ventilation
- Wound debridement to eradicate spores/necrotic tissue
- Abx: 7–10-d course
  - Recommended: Metronidazole 500 mg IV q6h
  - Alternative: PCN G 4 million units IV q4h
- Human tetanus immunoglobulin 500 units IM ×1 hastens clinical improvement
- Magnesium sulfate can be used to treat autonomic dysfxn and muscle spasms

Disposition
- ICU admission

Pearls
- *C. tetani* is obligate anaerobe, gram-positive spore forming bacillus, resistant to heat, desiccation, & disinfectants

Prevention
- Vaccination: DTaP (diphtheria, tetanus, pertussis, inactivated) vaccine given at 2/4/6 mos, booster at 15–18 mos & 4–6 y; Tdap booster at 11–12 y
- PEP:
  - Clean & debride wound as needed
  - Tx as below:

Tetanus Postexposure Prophylaxis Guide		
Wound	**Vaccination Hx**	**Prophylaxis**
Minor, clean	<3 doses of tetanus toxoid or unknown immunization status	Td vaccine booster
	>3 doses of tetanus toxoid	Td vaccine booster if ≥10 y since last dose
All other wounds	<3 doses of tetanus toxoid or unknown immunization status	Td vaccine booster + Tetanus immune globulin (250 IU IM)
	>3 doses of tetanus toxoid	Td vaccine booster if ≥10 y since last dose

- Pts who have not completed primary immunization series should repeat Td booster in 4–8 wks & 6–12 mos

---

ANTHRAX (*BACILLUS ANTHRACIS*) (*Pathogens* 2020;9:370)

History/Findings
- Contact w/ infected goats, sheep, cattle, horses, swine, 1–6-d incubation period
- Most commonly cutaneous infxn, also respiratory or GI; not human to human

- Cutaneous: Incubation 1–12 d; starts as small papule → vesicle containing serosanguineous fluid (1–2 d) → vesicle rupture leaves painless necrotic lesion w/ surrounding edema → massive edema
- Ulcer base develops 1–5 cm black eschar; after 2–3 wks separates & leaves scar
- Inhalational: Incubation 1–6 d; initial nonspecific sxs & cough × 2–3 d → sudden-onset respiratory distress (dyspnea, stridor, cyanosis, ↑ CP, diaphoresis) → rapid-onset shock & death in 24–36 h
- GI: From ingestion of infected meat; incubation 2–5 d; local oral/tonsillar ulcer, dysphagia & respiratory distress → abd pain, hematemesis, massive ascites, diarrhea
- Injectional: Characterized by skin lesions seen in "skin popping" drug users, may progress rapidly & require surgical debridement or may disseminate

Evaluation
- CBC, BMP, LFTs, EKG, CXR, CSF
- CDC requires positive test in 2/3: Laboratory Response Network (specialized Anthrax lab that is collaboration b/w CDC, FBI, US Army) PCR, direct identification via specialized IHC, rapid antianthrax antibody test (can be performed w/i 1 h, but not all labs have)
- Samples to send: Cutaneous (swabs from lesion), inhalational (BCx, CSF/pleural fluid if applicable), GI (same as Inhalational but also send stool/OP swab)
- CXR (inhalational): Mediastinal widening, pleural effusion, e/o ARDS

Treatment
- Systemic anthrax w/ meningitis: Cipro 400 mg IV q8h + meropenem 2 g IV q8h + linezolid 600 mg IV q12h + antitoxin (raxibacumab, obiltoxaximab, anthrax immunoglobulin) +/– Dex 10 mg IV q6h
- Systemic anthrax w/o meningitis: Cipro 400 mg IV q8h OR meropenem 2 g IV q8h + doxycycline 100 mg IV q12h
- Cutaneous/PEP: Doxycycline 100 mg PO BID, Cipro 500 mg PO BID, levofloxacin 750 mg PO QD, clindamycin 600 mg PO × 60 d
- Anthrax vaccine on days 0/14/28 for PEP

Disposition
- Admit +/– ICU if inhalation/GI/injectional

Pearls
- Large, aerobic, gram-positive, spore-forming, nonmotile, pyogenic *B. anthracis*
- Found in animals in South & Central America, Southern & Eastern Europe, Africa, Asia, Caribbean, Middle East
- Death from respiratory failure, overwhelming bacteremia, septic shock, meningitis
- Mortality variable: Cutaneous <1%, inhalational 45–92%, GI 25–60%, injectional 34%

PLAGUE (*YERSINIA PESTIS*)

(*Clin Microbiol Rev* 2020;34:e00044–19; *J Clin Microbiol* 2017;56:e01519–17)

History
- Contact w/ rat flea; 99% cases in SE Asia (Vietnam), rarely Southwest United States
- Acute onset high fevers, LAD, myalgias, SOB, CP, hemoptysis, sore throat, GI sx

Findings
- Bacilli spread to lymph nodes → supportive lymphadenitis, producing bubo → spread to other organs (spleen, liver, lungs, skin) & septic shock if untreated
- Bubonic (85–90%): Incubation 1–8 d; buboes emerge in groin, axilla, or cervical regions w/ f/C/HA, N/V, AMS, cough → buboes visible in 24 h, severely painful
- Septicemia (10–15%): Result of hematogenous dissemination of bubonic plague
- Pneumonic (1%): From inhalation of aerosols or hematogenous dissemination; productive cough w/ blood-tinged sputum, rales, decreased breath sounds

Evaluation
- Presence of painful bubo + isolation of organism in culture (Gram stain of bubo aspirate, lymph node aspiration, blood, sputum, CSF)
- CXR (pneumonic): Bilateral alveolar infiltrates, consolidation

Treatment
- Isolate pts for 1st 48 h after tx; if pneumonic plague, isolate for 4 d
- Streptomycin 1 g BID × 10–14 d OR gentamicin 5 mg/kg IV/IM QD × 10–14 d
- Alternative regimens: Doxycycline 100 mg PO/IV BID, chloramphenicol 25 mg/kg IV QID, levofloxacin 500 mg PO/IV QD

- PEP: Doxycycline 100 mg PO BID × 7 d or Cipro 500 mg PO BID × 7 d; use insecticides, reduce rodent populations

Disposition
- Admission +/– ICU

Pearls
- *Y. pestis:* Gram-negative nonmotile nonsporulating coccobacillus; can remain viable for days → weeks in water, moist soil, grain, buried bodies
- Mortality variable: Untreated bubonic 50%, Septic/pneumonic ~100%; tx reduces mortality to 10–15% overall

BOTULISM (*CLOSTRIDIUM BOTULINUM*)

(*Continuum* 2018;24:1459–1488; *Toxins* 2020;12:509)

History
- 6 h after exposure → descending paralysis, CN dysfxn (diplopia, dysphagia, ptosis) progresses to ventilatory failure
- Neurotoxin blocks ACh release at neuromuscular jxn & autonomic ganglions (nicotinic receptors)
- 4 main etiologies: Infant, foodborne, wound, iatrogenic; also potential for bioterrorism
- Infant: Consumption of dust, soil, or honey containing spores → colonize GI → release toxin in vivo
- Foodborne (adult): Ingestion of food contaminated w/ preformed toxin, usually a/w home-canned goods, home-aged or fermented foods, & prison "brew"
- Wound: Spores infiltrate skin wounds, germinate, & release tox into the bloodstream
- Iatrogenic: Recipient of high doses of botulinum injections "botox" for cosmetic use

Evaluation
- Clinical dx, confirmed w/ mouse bioassays through culture
- Descending & symmetric weakness, flaccid paralysis, respiratory arrest, autonomic dysfxn; CN affected 1st
- Infant: Weak cry, poor sucking, flaccid/hypotonic muscles
- Foodborne (12–36 h) & wound (several days): Autonomic dysfxn, descending symmetric motor paralysis, nl sensorium, euthermic
- Collect serum, stool, wound, & food samples for CDC testing

Treatment
- Antitoxin (equine derived), available exclusively from CDC
- Administer antitoxin 1 vial IV to adults & children
- Infants need only supportive care, no antitoxin
- Respiratory support inc mech ventilation, as necessary
- Contact CDC Botulism center (404-639-2206/3311) for antitoxin, BabyBIG from CA

Disposition
- ICU
- Recovery of strength may take ~4 mos; may require respiratory support for months

Pearls
- Not contagious
- Inhalational or gastrointestinal form could be used as weapon
- Foodborne (Infantile) form is most common and classically a/w honey

VIRAL INFECTIONS

HUMAN IMMUNODEFICIENCY VIRUS (HIV)

(*EM Reports* 2012;33:16; *Emerg Med Pract.* 2016;18:1–16)

History
- Acute HIV: Flu-like sxs, inc fever, fatigue, night sweats, pharyngitis, diarrhea, myalgia/arthralgias, HA
- Transmitted through sexual contact (70%), IVDU, and mother-to-child transmission (possible during pregnancy or birth)

Findings

- Fever, generalized maculopapular rash, oral ulcers (thrush), lymphadenopathy

Evaluation

- 3rd-generation HIV testing: HIV antibodies (3–4-wk postexposure)
- 4th-generation HIV testing: HIV antibodies +p24 antigen (2–3-wk postexposure)
- PCR to quantify viral load, CD4 count
- CBC: Leukopenia, thrombocytopenia; ↑ LFTs

Treatment

- Immediate initiation of antiretroviral therapy – counseling, urgent referral to ID clinic
- PEP
  - Men/women of child-bearing age on birth control/postmenopausal women: Tenofovir/emtricitabine 200–300 mg PO QD + dolutegravir 50 mg PO QD
  - Women of child-bearing age not on birth control/pregnant women: Tenofovir/emtricitabine 200–300 mg PO QD + raltegravir 400 mg PO QD

Disposition

- D/c (unless systemically ill) w/ ID f/u for antiretroviral tx

Pearls

- Undetectable viral load = Untransmittable (U = U)
- Untreated HIV → AIDS (CD4 <200)
- Routine HIV screening recommended in all individuals ages 13–64 once in their lifetime and all pregnant persons
- Routine opt-out HIV screening in the ED increases HIV detection and his cost effective

Organ Involvement of AIDS	
Organ	**Manifestation/Etiology**
Constitutional	Fevers: Bacterial, MAC, CMV, PCP, TB, lymphoma, drug rxn, endocarditis
Dermatologic	Kaposi sarcoma, lymphoma, VZV, HSV, HPV, *Molluscum contagiosum*
Ophthalmologic	CMV retinitis
Oral	Oral hairy leukopenia, Kaposi sarcoma, thrush, aphthous ulcers
Cardiac	Dilated cardiomyopathy, endocarditis, myocarditis, CAD, pericardial effusion, LVH
Pulmonary	PCP PNA, TB, fungal PNA (aspergillosis, *Cryptococcus,* etc), CMV
GI	Oral candida, hairy leukoplakia, esophagitis, enterocolitis, GIB (CMV, Kaposi, lymphoma), proctitis, hepatitis, diarrhea (*Cryptosporidium, Isospora*)
Renal	Nephropathy (drugs), HIV-associated nephropathy
Hematologic	Anemia (chronic dz), leukopenia, thrombocytopenia
Oncologic	NH & CNS lymphoma, Kaposi sarcoma, cervical cancer
Endocrine	Hypogonadism, metabolic synd, adrenal insufficiency, HIV wasting synd
Neurologic	Meningitis: *Cryptococcus*, bacterial, viral, TB, histoplasmosis Neurosyphilis: Meningitis, CN palsy, dementia Mass (toxoplasmosis), AIDS dementia, myelopathy, peripheral neuropathy, HIV encephalopathy, progressive multifocal leukoencephalopathy

Complications of AIDS	
CD4 Count	**Cx**
<500	Kaposi sarcoma, lymphoma, oral hairy leukopenia Candidiasis: Oral, esophageal, vaginal Recurrent bacterial infxns Pulmonary & extrapulmonary TB HSV, VZV
<200	PCP PNA, *Toxoplasma, Bartonella, Cryptococcus, Histoplasma,* Coccidioides, HIV encephalopathy
<50–100	CMV, MAC Disseminated *Bartonella,* invasive aspergillosis CNS lymphoma, PML

Opportunistic Infection Prophylaxis		
Infection	**Indication**	**Prophylaxis**
TB	Positive IGR or + PPD (>5 mm) or high-risk exposure	INH + rifampin + Vit B6 × 3 mos
PJP PNA	CD4 <200 or thrush	TMP-SMX DS 1 tab PO QD or Dapsone 100 mg PO QD or Atovaquone 1500 mg PO QD or Pentamidine 300 PO q4wk
Toxoplasmosis	CD4 <100 AND + toxoplasma serology	TMP-SMX DS 1 tab PO QD or Dapsone 200 mg PO QD + pyrimethamine 75 mg PO QD + leucovorin 25 mg PO qwk

Viral Hepatitis

Hepatitis C Virus (*Clinical Infectious Diseases* 2023. ciad319)

History
- Bloodborne pathogen, increasing incidence w/ opioid epidemic
- High-risk populations: IVDU, blood tfxs prior to 1992, born 1945–1965

Findings
- Chronic infxn – cirrhosis, HCC, liver failure

Evaluation
- Universal serology screening for all adults ≥18 y and all pregnant persons
- Confirm by viral RNA; ~25% (15–45%) naturally clear infxn spontaneously

Treatment
- Direct acting antivirals: Glecaprevir/pibrentasvir for 8 wks or sofosbuvir/velpatasvir for 12 wks (>95% cure rate)
- Cure = sustained virologic response at 12 wks following tx completion

Disposition
- Refer to ID or hepatology for tx
- Ensure linkage to care for high-risk individuals

Pearls
- Universal ED screening improves HCV detection and linkage to care

Hepatitis A, B, D, and E Viruses
See Section III: Gastrointestinal.

Infectious Mononucleosis (*Am Fam Physician* 2015;91:372–376)

History
- 4–6-wk incubation period → 1–2-wk prodrome: Fatigue, malaise, myalgias, low-grade temp → Acute sxs: Fever, pharyngitis, lymphadenopathy, HA, rash

Findings
- Low-grade temp, pharyngitis, tonsillitis
- LAD: Tender & firm for 1–2 wks, most often postcervical nodes, but can be generalized
- Rash: Papular erythematous on UE, erythema nodosum, erythema multiforme
- Splenomegaly: Severe abd pain uncommon, may indicate splenic rupture
- May have petechiae, jaundice, hepatomegaly, periorbital edema

Evaluation
- CBC: ↑ WBC, ↑ atypical lymphocytes, ↓ platelets; ↑ LFTs (bilirubin, AST, ALT); positive monospot test
- Consider rapid strep if clinical ambiguity

Treatment
- Supportive, rest, analgesics, antipyretics
- Consider corticosteroids if airway edema

Disposition

- Admission rarely indicated; close PCP f/u
- Advise to avoid contact sports or vigorous exercise × 1 mos to prevent splenic rupture

Pearls

- Represents atypical syndromic response to EBV (ie, most cases of mono caused by EBV, but most EBV infxns do not result in mono)
- Secondary etiology: CMV
- Transmission through saliva: EBV infects epithelial cells of oropharynx & salivary glands
- B lymphocytes become infected → allows viral entry into bloodstream
- Self-limited; usually spontaneous resolution in 3–4 wks, complete in several months

---

INFLUENZA (*Lancet* 2017;390:697–708; *Nat Rev Dis Primers* 2018;4:3)

Epidemiology

- Two main virus subtypes: Human influenza A and B
  - Influenza A is more prone to epidemics/pandemics due to antigenic shift (2 or more different strains of a virus combining to form a new subtype)
  - H1N1 is a type of Influenza A virus
- Spread primarily person to person via respiratory droplets; masking and social distancing can significantly reduce spread
- Typical incubation time is 2–4 d; medial viral shedding time is 5 d

History

- Classic sxs: Fever, myalgias, fatigue, nonproductive cough, sore throat, URI sxs
- Inquire about recent sick contacts
- RFs for severe dz: Age <2 or >65, chronic dz (CVD, Chronic lung dz such as COPD/asthma, CKD, DM, SCD, Cirrhosis), immunocompromised states (malignancy, autoimmune dz, AIDS), close quarters (prisons, group homes, nursing homes)

Findings

- Often febrile and fatigued
- May have associated tachypnea, hypoxemia, and dyspnea in severe dz

Evaluation

- Gold standard diagnostic: Influenza A & B PCR (>95% sens)
- CXR: Typically benign except pt w/ primary influenza PNA (bilateral opacities) or bacterial superinfxn (lobar infiltrate)
- Consider CPK given risk of myositis/rhabdomyolysis
- Consider EKG, troponin, and cardiac U/S to screen for pericarditis and myocarditis

Treatment

- Strict isolation precautions (inc contact/droplet isolation precautions)
- Empirically treat admitted and high-risk pts w/ Oseltamivir 75 mg PO BID × 7 d
  - Oseltamivir tx reduces duration of sx by 1 d if given w/i 48 h of sx onset (*CDC.* 2011; 60(1):1–2)
- Consider abx (inc MRSA coverage) if procalcitonin ≥0.2, CXR w/ lobar infiltrate, or pt being admitted to ICU

Disposition

- Dispo based on dz severity, but majority of pts can be safely discharged

Pearls

- Rapid influenza testing is specific, but not sens, so don't use to r/o illness

---

COVID-19 (SARS CoV-2) (*NEJM* 2020;383:1757–1766; *NEJM* 2020;383:2451–2460)

Epidemiology

- Spread person to person, inc by asymptomatic and presymptomatic carriers, primarily via respiratory droplets and aerosols; proper ventilation, social distancing, masking, and vaccination all significantly reduce spread

History

- Classic sxs: Cough, fever, dyspnea, URI sxs, myalgias, fatigue, dysosmia/dysgeusia, GI sxs
- Cx: SIRS, ARDS, myocarditis, thrombosis (DVT, PE, limb ischemia, stroke), encephalopathy, MIS-C, bacterial coinfxn

- RFs for severe dz: age >55, CVD, chronic lung dz (COPD/asthma), CKD, DM, HTN, immunocompromised state (malignancy, autoimmune dz, AIDS), obesity, smoking.

Findings
- Often febrile
- Tachypnea and hypoxemia are a markers of severe dz

Evaluation
- Gold standard diagnostic: SARS-CoV-2 RT-PCR; antigen (rapid) tests have ↓ sens; serology (IgG antibody detection) detects prior infxn
- CXR or Chest CT helpful in evaluating severity of PNA
- Consider troponins &/or cardiac U/S if concern for myocarditis

Treatment
- Mild–mod dz managed outpt w/ supportive care
- Severe dz: Hospitalization
  - Respiratory support: Nasal cannula → high flow nasal cannula → mech ventilation (ARDSnet low tidal vol strategy) +/– prone positioning → add on NM blockade → inhaled pulmonary vasodilators → ECMO
- Dexamethasone: Mortality benefit in pts on O_2 or mech ventilation; Dose: 6 mg × 10 d PO or IV (*NEJM* 2021;384[8]:693; *JAMA* 2020;324[13]:1330)
- Remdesivir: Improves time to recovery in pts on low-flow O_2; Dose: 200 mg IV × once, then 100 mg IV × 5–10 d (caution w/ renal/hepatic dysfxn) (*NEJM* 2002;383[19]:1813)
- Monoclonal antibody tx—(eg, bamlanivimab-etesevimab)—may benefit when given early on to pts w/ RFs for severe dz and when there is a match b/w the mAb and circulating variant
- High-titer convalescent plasma tx: ↓ Risk of severe dz if given w/in 72 h of illness to older pts (age ≥75, or age ≥65 w/ comorbidities) (*NEJM* 2021;384[7]:610)
- MIS-C: Consider IVIG, aspirin, &/or glucocorticoids for pediatric pts
- Prophylactic dose A/C to prevent thromboembolic cx
- Consider abx if procalcitonin ≥0.2, CXR w/ lobar infiltrate, or pt being admitted to ICU

Disposition
- D/c w/ rapid f/u if mild–mod dz
- Admit for severe dz: Respiratory distress, hypoxia or e/o cx

Pearls
- Prolonged sxs of COVID-19, or "post-COVID syndrome," may persist for >12 wks

---

EBOLA VIRUS DISEASE (*Annu Rev Pathol* 2017;12:387–418; *Lancet* 2019;393:936–948; *Nat Rev Dis Primers* 2020;6:13)

History
- Fever, chills, myalgias, malaise → 5 d later GI sxs (severe watery diarrhea, nausea/vomiting, abd pain) +/– bleeding, chest pain, SOB, HA, confusion
- 2–21-d incubation period
- Recent travel to country w/ outbreak (primarily West Africa, reference CDC website for most up-to-date recommendations)

Findings
- Fever, abd tenderness
- Diffuse erythematous maculopapular rash may develop day 5–7

Evaluation
- CBC (leukopenia, lymphopenia, late elevated neutrophils, thrombocytopenia), ↑ amylase, ↑ AST/ALT, ↑ PT/PTT, ↑ fibrinogen, UA (proteinuria)
- RT-PCR assay specific for Ebola

Treatment
- Supportive care of cx (hypovolemia, electrolyte abnormalities, hematologic abnormalities, hypoxia, MSOF, septic shock, DIC): Volume repletion, pressors as needed, pain control, nutritional support

Disposition
- Admit under strict contact isolation, prevent contact or splashes w/ blood & body fluids, equipment, and surfaces
- Pts w/ fatal dz typically die day 6–16 from cx (see previous section)

Pearls

- Can be confused w/ more common dzs (malaria, typhoid, PNA, meningitis)
- Enters through mucous membranes, breaks in skin, or parenterally

SMALLPOX (VARIOLA) (*Viruses* 2020;12:138)

History

- Incubation 10–14 d while spreading hematogenously (regional lymph nodes, blood vessels) → nonspecific sxs → skin chgs 2–3 d later
- +/– High fever, HA, rigors, malaise, myalgias, N/V, abd pain, back pain

Findings

- 2 types: Major (30% mortality), minor (<1% mortality)
- Skin exanthem on face/hands/forearm → trunk/lower extremities
- Macules → papules (day 2) → vesicles (day 5) → umbilicated pustules (day 8); pustules form scabs after 8–14 d; death in 2nd wk from toxemia (mortality 25%)

Evaluation

- Clinical dx: Classic centrifugal distribution w/ lesions all in same stage of development

Treatment

- Isolation, hemodynamic support, skin care, vaccination (before rash appears)
- Contact CDC for antiviral tecovirimat 600 mg BID ×14 d (no trials in humans)
- PEP: Vaccination w/i 3 d

Disposition

- Isolation in negative pressure w/ airborne & contact precautions ×17 d
- Pts most infectious on day 3–6 after onset of fever, remain infectious until all scabs separated

Pearls

- Variola virus: Highly infectious by aerosol, environmentally stable, prolonged infectivity
- Transmitted through respiratory droplets, bodily fluids
- Last occurrence in Somalia in 1977; routine vaccination stopped in 1972

MALARIA (PLASMODIUM SPP.)

See section on mosquito-borne dzs.

PARASITIC INFECTIONS: PROTOZOA

Gastrointestinal Protozoal Infections				
Infection	**Epidemiology**	**Symptoms**	**Diagnosis**	**Treatment**
Amoebiasis (*E. histolyticum*)	Low- and middle-income countries w/ poor sanitation	Acute diarrhea, dysentery, amebic colitis, amebic liver abscesses	Stool O&P, PCR	Metronidazole, then intraluminal agents (iodoquinol or paromomycin)
Giardiasis (*G. lamblia*)	Worldwide, untreated water, anal–oral sex	Nausea, vomiting, bloating, weight loss	Stool O&P	Metronidazole
Blood and Tissue Protozoal Infections				
Infection	**Epidemiology**	**Symptoms**	**Diagnosis**	**Treatment**
Chagas (*T. cruzi*)	Texas, Mexico, Central and South America; vector—triatomines/reduviid bugs	Acute phase: fever, localized swelling (eyelid edema) Chronic phase (10–20 y): organomegaly, cardiomyopathy, megaesophagus, megacolon	Acute phase: Thin and thick blood smears Chronic phase: Serology	Benznidazole, nifurtimox

Sleeping sickness (*T. brucei*)	Sub-Saharan Africa; vector – tsetse fly	Fever, encephalopathy, coma	Serology, CSF/blood microscopy	Based on subtype and dz stage: pentamidine or eflornithine, suramin or melarsoprol
Leishmaniasis (Leishmania spp.)	Tropical and subtropical areas of Asia, Africa, Middle East, Latin America; vector – sand fly	Cutaneous: painless ulcerative papules Visceral: hepatosplenomegaly, pancytopenia	Histology, serology	Sodium stibogluconate, amphotericin B, miltefosine, local cutaneous therapy

ROUNDWORMS (NEMATODES)

Gastrointestinal Roundworm Infections				
Infection	**Epidemiology**	**Symptoms**	**Diagnosis**	**Treatment**
Ascariasis (*A. lumbricoides*)	Tropics/subtropics	Intestinal discomfort, obstruction, pulmonary sxs (Löffler synd)	Stool O&P	Albendazole, mebendazole
Hookworm (*A. duodenale, N. Americus*)	Tropics/subtropics	Abd pain, diarrhea, anemia, chronic protein def	Stool O&P	Albendazole, mebendazole
Whipworm (*T. trichiura*)	Tropics/subtropics, esp. children	Chronic abd pain, malnutrition, dysentery, rectal prolapse	Stool O&P	Albendazole, mebendazole
Strongyloidiasis (*S. stercoralis*)	Tropics/subtropics	Abd pain, diarrhea, pulm sx	Stool O&P	Ivermectin
Trichinellosis (*T. spiralis*)	Consumption of undercooked meat	GI sx, muscle pain, periorbital edema	Serology, muscle biopsy	Albendazole, mebendazole
Pinworm (*E. vermicularis*)	Worldwide, #1 helminth infxn US, esp. children	Perianal itching	"Tape test"	Albendazole, mebendazole
Blood and Tissue Roundworm Infections				
Infection	**Epidemiology**	**Symptoms**	**Diagnosis**	**Treatment**
Loa Loa	Central, W. Africa	Migration across eye, pruritic, arthralgias, encephalopathy, Calabar swellings	Blood microscopy	Diethylcarbamazine (DEC), albendazole
River blindness (*O. volvulus*)	Sub-Saharan Africa, Latin America	Dermatitis, blindness	Skin biopsy, serology	Ivermectin, doxycycline
Lymphatic filariasis (*W. bancrofti*)	Tropics/subtropics	Lymphedema, hydrocele	Blood microscopy	DEC, albendazole, ivermectin

FLUKES (TREMATODES)

Fluke Infections				
Infection	**Epidemiology**	**Sx**	**Dx**	**Tx**
Schistosomiasis (Schistosoma spp.)	Sub-Saharan Africa, Middle East, SE Asia, Latin America	Acute: fevers, chills, myalgias (Katayama fever) Chronic: abdominal sx (chronic abd pain, hepatosplenomegaly) or urinary sx (dysuria, hematuria)	Microscopy (stool/urine), serology	Praziquantel
Fascioliasis (*F. hepatica*)	Worldwide, areas of sheep/cattle domestication	Acute: fever RUQ pain Chronic: biliary obstruction, cholangitis	Stool microscopy, serology, RUQ US, CT	Triclabendazole
Clonorchiasis (*C. sinensis*) and **Opisthorchiasis** (*O. viverrini*)	E and SE Asia, respectively	RUQ pain, cholecystitis cholangitis, cholangiocarcinoma	Stool microscopy, serology, RUQ US, CT	Praziquantel

TAPEWORMS (CESTODES)

Fluke Infections				
Infection	**Epidemiology**	**Sx**	**Dx**	**Tx**
Cysticercosis (*T. solium*)	Latin America, Sub-Saharan Africa, Asia	Neurocysticercosis, HAs, szs	Neuroimaging, serology	Albendazole or praziquantel w/ steroids
Taeniasis (Taenia spp.)	Worldwide, areas of pork consumption	Asymptomatic to mild GI distress	Stool O&P	Praziquantel, niclosamide
Echinococcosis (Echinococcus spp.)	Worldwide, areas of sheep grazing	Abdominal pain, hepatomegaly, liver dysfxn, jaundice	Imaging, serology	Albendazole, surgery (PAIR)
Diphyllobothriasis (*D. latum*)	Worldwide, areas of undercooked fish consumption	Diarrhea, megaloblastic anemia (B12 deficiency)	Stool O&P	Praziquantel

ECTOPARASITES PEDICULOSIS (HEAD LICE) (*Am Fam Physician* 2019;99[10]:635–642)

History
- Common in children (ages 5–13 y)
- Transmission via head-to-head contact

Findings
- Pruritus of scalp, excoriations

Evaluation
- Visual inspection, wet combing most sens for detection

Treatment
- Permethrin 1% lotion or shampoo (10 mins application); reduced efficacy in the setting of rising resistance
- Malathion 0.5% lotion (8–12-h application); strong odor

- PO ivermectin, 2 doses 7 d apart; high efficacy, used w/ failure of topicals
- Environmental decontamination of bedding and clothing in hot water

Disposition
- Return to school following tx

PTHIRIASIS (PUBLIC LICE) *(Am Fam Physician* 2019;99[10]:635–642)

History
- Transmission via sexual contact
- Incidence decreased w/ grooming of pubic hair

Findings
- Pruritus of areas of pubic hear, red papules

Evaluation
- Visual inspection

Treatment
- 1st line: permethrin 1% lotion/shampoo or pyrethrins
- 2nd line, in case of tx failure: malathion or ivermectin (repeat dose in 7 d)
- Evaluate and treat other STIs

Disposition
- Dc w/ tx for partners

MITES: SCABIES (*S. SCABIEI*) (*J Am Acad Dermatol* 2020;82:533–548)

History
- Persistent pruritus, worse at night; Sometimes multiple family members involved
- Common in overcrowding, poor hygiene, elderly, homeless
- More common in winter (survive longer on fomites, more crowded living)

Findings
- Small, pruritic, erythematous papules typically found in web spaces b/w fingers & toes, flexor aspects of wrists, under armpits, around umbilicus, under knees, around nipples, genital region
- Burrow from mites: elevated thin red or gray line
- Secondary skin infxns may also be present

Evaluation
- Clinical dx; Other Dx tests (skin scrapings, shave biopsy, tape test, etc) may increase certainty but negative results do not r/o

Treatment
- Permethrin 5% cream ×2 applications 1 wk apart OR oral ivermectin 200 mcg/kg ×2 applications 2 wks apart
- 2nd line: crotamiton 10% cream, lindane 1% lotion
- Symptomatic relief, tx 2° infxns & household members, clean clothes/linens

Disposition
- D/c w/ instructions for household to be treated, decontaminate clothing, bedding
- Exclude from school until treated, topical permethrin usually effective w/i 12 h

Pearls
- Caused by female mite, *S. scabiei*
- Delayed type IV hypersensitivity rxn to mite proteins (from saliva, feces, eggs, mite itself), sxs initially develop 3–4 wks after exposure, then 1–2 d after reexposure
- Skin-to-skin contact, indirect contact through bedding or clothing

TICKS

See "Zoonoses" in the section that follows.

DERMATOPHYTOSES

See "Fungal Exanthems" in Section VIII: Dermatology.

Cutaneous Candidiasis/Intertrigo

See "Fungal Exanthems" in Section VIII: Dermatology.

Systemic Fungal Infections				
Infection	**Geography**	**Sx**	**Dx**	**Tx**
Aspergillosis	Ubiquitous	Fever, cough, dyspnea, hemoptysis	Serum PCR, histopath, culture	Voriconazole, amphotericin B
Blastomycosis	Great Lakes, St Lawrence River Basin, Mississippi River Basin, Ohio River Basin	Fever, cough, dyspnea, cutaneous lesions	Urine Ag, histopath, culture	Itraconazole, amphotericin B
Cryptococcosis	Ubiquitous	Fever, HA, type B sx	Serum Ag, CSF Ag, histopath, culture	Amphotericin B + flucytosine
Coccidiomycosis (Valley Fever)	SW USA, MX, Central America	Fever, cough, arthralgias, erythema nodosum	Serology, histopath, culture	Fluconazole, itraconazole, amphotericin B
Histoplasmosis	Mississippi River Basin, Ohio River Basin	Fever, cough, weight loss	Urine Ag, serology, culture	Itraconazole, amphotericin B

ZOONOSES

Rabies (*Curr Infect Dis Rep* 2016;18:38; *Nat Rev Dis Primers* 2017;3:17091)

History
- Exposure to rabid (agitated, drooling, unprovoked attack) mammal (bats most common in US; dog most common in developing countries)
- Nonspecific prodrome: Fatigue, loss of appetite, HA, anxiety, irritability, fever 2–10 d

Findings
- Encephalitic (80%, brain) & paralytic (20%, spinal cord) rabies
- Encephalitic: Hypersalivation, sweating, piloerection, hydrophobia, impaired consciousness → quadriparesis → death
- Paralytic: Weakness in bitten limb → quadriparesis, facial weakness, urinary incontinence → neurologic progression → death
- Dog-acquired cases: Hydrophobia, aerophobia, encephalopathy
- Bat-acquired cases: Sxs at exposure site, abnl neuro findings (tremor, myoclonus, CN palsy)

Evaluation
- Neutralizing antirabies virus AB in serum (if not vaccinated), RABV antigen in tissues, RABV RNA in saliva or CSF
- CSF: Pleocytosis, ↑ protein; Ab titer diagnostic regardless of vaccine status
- Imaging (CTH, MRI) used to evaluate for other causes of encephalopathy

Treatment
- Palliative care given universally fatal w/i 14 d of initial sxs
- No proven medical tx has been shown to be effective
- Therapeutic coma (ketamine, benzos) & antiviral therapy (amantadine, ribavirin) rarely a/w survival

Disposition
- ICU admission if neuro or resp sxs
- Notify public health department & animal control center
- Identify others at risk & initiate PEP if indicated

Pearls
- Caused by *Lyssavirus* in family *Rhabdoviridae*
- Incubation period is variable (typically 20–90 d but ranges from days to 1 y)

- Rabies PrEP
  - 2 doses, days 0 and 7
  - Eliminates need for rabies immune globulin (RIG) and reduces PEP vaccine course
  - Simplifies PEP in resource-limited settings, partial immunity if delays in PEP
- Rabies PEP
  - Wound care (soap, water, irrigation w/ povidone–iodine solution), debridement of devitalized tissue, secondary closure, update Tetanus vaccination
  - If domestic dog or cat bite, determine vaccination status of animal from owner. If animal can be observed, start PEP only if animal develops sxs
  - Assess rabies risk & need for human RIG & HDCV
  - RIG: 20 IU/kg; as much as possible at exposure site, remaining administered at distant site (eg, deltoid)
  - HDCV: 1-mL dose in deltoid in ED. F/u doses given days 3, 7, 14
  - HDCV 5th dose on day 28 if immunocompromised
  - Do not stop rabies immunization b/c of mild rxn to vaccine doses
  - Rabies cases from nonbite exposures > from known bite exposures; consider prophylaxis for any contact w/ high-risk animals (eg, bats, skunks, raccoons, coyotes, foxes)

Tick-borne Diseases

Lyme Disease (*Borrelia burgdorferi*) (*Nat Rev Dis Primers* 2016;2:16090; *J Emerg Med* 2017;52:815–824)

History

- Exposure to wooded & nonwooded endemic areas b/w May & September
- *I. scapularis* (deer tick) attachment (tick must be attached for ≥36 h to cause infxn)
- Incubation period 3–31 d
- Erythema migrans (typical "bull's eye" rash w/ central clearing, but can be uniform or enhanced central erythema w/o clearing; can last 3–4 wks if untreated), malaise, fatigue

Findings

- Progression can result in cardiac conduction dz, neurologic sequelae, and arthritis
- Lyme carditis: AV block +/– myopericarditis
- Lyme meningitis: Does not present as classic bacterial meningitis
  - Early: HA, Bell's palsy, radiculoneuritis
  - Late: Neurocognitive dysfxn (ie, encephalomyelitis)

Evaluation

- Testing not recommended for pts w/ only erythema migrans
- For pts w/ nonerythema migrans presentations: enzyme immunoassay (EIA) → immunoblot (if EIA positive); Both must be positive to confirm dx.
- ECG to assess for HB, consider CSF in pts w/ neurologic involvement

Treatment

- Tick removal: Using forceps or tweezers, grasp the tick as close to skin as possible, pull upward w/ steady pressure, disinfect site, save tick for identification.
- Abx regimens

Antibiotic Regimens for Treatment of Lyme Disease	
Sxs/Findings	**Treatment**
Asymptomatic exposure (>36 h attached, <72 h since removal)	Doxycycline 200 mg PO ×1
Erythema migrans, Arthritis, Bell's palsy, 1st-degree AV block <300 ms	Doxycycline 100 mg PO BID ×10–21 d or Amoxicillin 500 mg PO TID ×14–21 d or Cefuroxime 500 mg PO BID ×14–21 d
1st-degree AV block >300 ms, 2nd/3rd-degree heart block myocarditis, meningitis	CTX 2 g IV qd × 14–28 d or PCN G 4 mil units IV q4h × 14–28 d

- Avoid doxy in pregnant, breastfeeding, children <8 y/o; use alternatives above

Dispositions

- D/c w/ abx regimen and PCP f/u unless has concerning cardiac/neurologic sequelae

Pearls
- Most common tick-borne dz in US; 90% of cases in MA, CT, RI, NY, NJ, PA, MN, WI, CA
- Deer tick tiny (head of pin) vs dog tick (larger, more, common, don't transmit Lyme)
- Only 1/3rd recall h/o tick bite → if high suspicion, treat as exposed
- Consider concomitant basesiosis, anaplasmosis, ehrlichiosis

Rocky Mountain Spotted Fever (Rickettsia Rickettsii) (*J Emerg Med* 2018;55:42–50; *Dis Mon* 2018;64:185–194)

History
- Tick exposure (multiple ticks can carry bacterium) in spring/early summer
- Incubation period 2–14 d
- Sudden high fever, malaise, myalgia, HA, photophobia, anorexia, N/V, abd pain
- Rash 2–5 d after fever

Findings
- Temp >102 °F, may be ↓ BP on presentation
- Petechial rash typically starts at wrist & ankles (but may be diffuse at onset) → moves out (palms & soles) then in (arms, legs, & trunk) but spares face
- By end of 1st week, rash is maculopapular w/ central petechiae
- Multiple systems can be involved: Cardiac (myocarditis), pulmonary (cough, PNA), GI (abd pain, N/V, hepatomegaly), renal (ARF), CNS (meningismus, photophobia, confusion), ocular (conjunctivitis, retinal hemorrhage, arterial occlusion), muscular (CK elevation)

Evaluation
- IFA assay most used but cannot distinguish b/w rickettsial dzs and Ab not detectable until 7–10 d after dz onset
- CBC (thrombocytopenia, anemia), Chem (hyponatremia, ↑ BUN), LFTs, coags, blood cx
- CXR if appear toxic or abnl lung findings
- CT or MRI for AMS may show infarction, edema, meningeal enhancement
- CSF may show pleocytosis, nl glucose, elevated protein

Treatment
- Supportive care and resuscitation: Intubation if indicated, resuscitation w/ fluids, PRBC + platelets, dialysis if indicated
- Abx Tx should begin before laboratory confirmation
- Abx regimen: Doxycycline 100 mg IV/PO BID for at least 3 d after the fever subsides, consider doxycycline 200 mg IV loading dose for seriously ill pts
- Children/pregnant & breastfeeding women should still receive doxycycline

Disposition
- Most require hospitalization, consider ICU admit given risk of rapid progression

Pearls
- *R. rickettsii* obligate intracellular bacterium spread by ticks to human endothelial cells causing small, medium vessel vasculitis
- Found in US (primarily MD, VA, NC, SC, OK, TN, AR), western Canada, western & central Mexico, & South America

Ehrlichiosis and Anaplasmosis (*Clin Lab Med* 2017;37:317–340; *Dis Mon* 2018;64:181–184)

History
- Exposure/travel to endemic area b/w May & September +/– reported tick bite
- 5–14-d incubation period
- Fever, myalgia, HA, malaise, cough, chills, +/– rash

Findings
- Fever +/– LAD +/– maculopapular/petechial rash on UE &/or trunk

Evaluation
- CBC (↓ WBC, ↓ plts), ↑ AST/ALT, ↑ ESR; BCx not helpful
- Clinical dx in acute setting; Confirm dx w/ IFA

Treatment
- Abx regimen: Doxycycline 100 mg IV/PO BID × 10 d
- If allergy, rifampin 300 mg PO BID × 10 d

Disposition
- Admit if requires IV supportive tx

Pearls
- Obligate intracellular gram-negative bacteria; *Anaplasma* infects granulocytes (HGA) & *Ehrlichia* targets monocytes (HME); distinct epidemiologically but same clinical picture
- HGA—Ixodes scapularis & Ixodes pacificus; found in NE & Midwest US in summer
- HME—Lone star tick; found in SE & south-central US, April–September
- Presence of rash more suggestive of HME
- Consider concomitant Lyme dz and basesiosis

Babesiosis (*Int J Parasitol* 2019;49:165–174; *Expert Rev Anti Infect Ther* 2020;18:625–636)
History
- Exposure/travel to endemic area b/w May & September +/– reported tick bite
- Incubation period 1–4 wks
- Healthy host usually asymptomatic; affects elderly, immunocompromised, asplenic
- Fever, chills, weakness, fatigue, myalgias, HA, photophobia, AMS, cough, SOB, N/V, anorexia, abd pain, arthralgias

Findings
- Fevers, jaundice, hepatosplenomegaly, pharyngeal erythema, retinopathy

Evaluation
- CBC (hemolytic anemia, ↓ platelets), ↑ LFTs, ↑ LDH, ↓ haptoglobin, ↑ reticulocytes, UA (proteinuria or hematuria)
- Wright or Giemsa peripheral blood smear; If negative, PCR

Treatment
- Resuscitation, symptomatic tx, airway mgmt
- Abx regimens
  - Mild: Azithro 500 mg PO ×1, 250 mg QD + Atovaquone 750 mg PO q12h for 7–10 d
  - Severe: Azithro 500 mg IV + Atovaquone 750 mg PO q12h for 7–10 d
  - Alternative regimen: Clindamycin 600 mg PO/IV TID + quinine 650 mg PO TID
- RBC exchange tfx if parasite load >10%, severe anemia, end-organ dysfxn

Disposition
- Admit for ongoing supportive therapy & abx
- Most pts recover in 1–2 wks, fatigue may continue for months

Pearls
- Protozoan parasite *Babesia* transmitted by *I. scapularis* (or less commonly blood tfx from infected individual)
- Peak in May–October; found in Europe & US (MA, NY, RI, CT, upper Midwest, Northwest)
- Consider concomitant Lyme dz, anaplasmosis, ehrlichiosis

Mosquito-borne Diseases

Malaria (Plasmodium spp.) (*Nat Rev Dis Primers* 2017;3:17050; *Lancet* 2018;391:1608–1621)
History
- Travel to Central/South America, Sub-Saharan Africa, India, Southeast/Southcentral Asia, Middle East, Caribbean; incubation period 7–30 d, sxs may present months later
- Paroxysmal chills, sweats, & high fevers q48–72h
- +/– fatigue, myalgias, malaise, cough; less common: anorexia, N/V, diarrhea, HA

Findings
- Fever, hypotension, tachycardia +/– jaundice, pallor, splenomegaly, icterus
- Severe malaria: AMS, ≥2 szs, pulm edema, HD unstable, >40 °C, DIC, severe anemia, renal failure, hypoglycemia, hyperparasitemia, acidosis, hyperbilirubinemia
- Cerebral malaria: AMS, meningitis, szs, encephalopathy

Evaluation
- Labs looking for end-organ damage: CBC, Chem, LFTs, hemolysis labs, UA, blood
  - Classic triad: Thrombocytopenia, ↑ LDH, atypical lymphocytes
- Parasite-based confirmation: Thick & thin blood smear, rapid antigen tests
- CXR (if signs of pulm edema)

Treatment
- Resuscitation, symptomatic tx, airway mgmt
- Abx regimens

Antimalarials Guide		
Severity	**Chloroquine Resistance**	**Treatment**
Uncomplicated Malaria	Resistant	ACT PO × 3 d OR Atovaquone 250 mg–Progaunil 100 mg PO qd × 4 d
	Sens	Chloroquine 600 mg PO ×1→ 300 mg PO at 6/24/48 h OR Hydroxychloroquine 620 mg PO ×1 → 310 mg PO at 6/24/48 h
Severe Malaria	N/A	Artesunate 2.4 mg/kg/dose IM/IV at 0/12/24 h → PO/IV based on parasitemia/ability to tolerate PO OR Quinine 16.7 mg/kg × 1 8.35 mg/kg q8h

  - Consider adding primaquine 30 mg QD × 14 d if concerned for *P. vivax* or *P. ovale*
  - Tx regimen dependent on geography (Chloroquine resistance), species, & severity of dz
  - Monitor QT interval when giving antimalarials
- Prophylaxis regimen often recommended; depends on region of travel
  - Use DEET & insect repellent, bed nets w/ permethrin, long-sleeved clothing

Disposition
- Admit if suspected or confirmed case, especially if child, pregnant, or immunodeficient
- ICU if end-organ damage or signs of cerebral malaria
- Thin & thick blood smears should be performed qwk × 4 after d/c to ensure resolution

Pearls
- *Plasmodium (ovale, vivax, malariae, falciparum)* cause malaria, transmitted through bite of infected female *Anopheles* mosquito, causing systemic infxn of erythrocytes
- *P. falciparum* most severe: Can cause cerebral malaria, pulm edema, renal failure, anemia; highest occurrence in Sub-Saharan Africa
- *P. vivax* & *P. ovale* produce dormant form in liver, usually causes uncomplicated malaria
- 2 million deaths annually, majority in kids <5 y/o, ~90% in rural Sub-Saharan Africa
- Sickle cell trait, thalassemia, Hemoglobin C dz, & G6PD deficiency are protective

Yellow Fever (*J Clin Microbiol* 2018;56:e00827–18; *Curr Infect Dis Rep* 2019;21:42)

History
- Travel to endemic area (Sub-Saharan Africa, South America)
- Incubation 3–6 d
- Mild form sudden fever HA → more severe cases w/ high fever, chills, HA, myalgias, lumbosacral pain, anorexia, N/V, dizziness → 10–25% have severe recurrence 2 d later w/ multiple organ systems involved (GI, renal, cardiac, hematologic)

Findings
- High fever, relative bradycardia, epigastric tenderness
  - Severe cases: ↑ fever, somnolence, jaundice, hematologic cx (eg, hematemesis, melena, petechiae, epistaxis)
- Late: shock, confusion, coma, DIC, hemorrhage
- Liver is the most affected organ: Hepatocellular damage (steatosis, necrosis); bleeding
- Kidneys can also affected: Renal insufficiency, albuminuria, ATN
- Cardiac: Fatty infiltration of myocardium → myocarditis & arrhythmias

Evaluation
- CBC (leukopenia, thrombocytopenia), ↑ LFTs, abnl coags, ↑ BUN/Cr, ↓ fibrinogen (DIC), ↓ ESR
- ELISA for viral IgM, confirm w/ rise in viral titer btw acute and convalescent samples

Treatment
- Resuscitation: supportive care and symptomatic tx
- No approved antiviral meds
- Prevention: Extremely effective live attenuated vaccine available

Disposition
- Admit for supportive care +/– ICU if end-organ damage

Pearls
- *Flavivirus* transmitted by *A. aegypti* mosquito during tropical wet & early dry season
- Mandated reporting to WHO & local health dept

Dengue Fever (*Lancet* 2019;393:350–363; *Nat Rev Dis Primers* 2016;2:16055)

History
- Travel to endemic areas: Mostly SE Asia, Central America, Western Pacific, sometimes from Eastern Mediterranean, Africa
- Sxs begin after 3–7-d incubation
- Abrupt, high fever × 1–7 d, biphasic, w/ HA, vomiting, myalgia, joint pain
- Rash: Characteristically bright red blanching petechiae, usually 1st on lower limbs & chest → morbilliform, maculopapular & sparing palms & soles → desquamation

Findings
- Classic DF: Fever, rash, LAD, hemorrhage (petechiae, purpura, epistaxis, GIB, menorrhagia)
- DHF: High fever, hepatomegaly, hypotension, DIC; begins w/ sudden ↑ in temp & flu sxs
- DHF w/ shock synd occur during 2nd infxn by different dengue virus

Evaluation
- CBC (↓ plat), Chem (↑ BUN), ↑ LFTs, DIC panel, CXR, CTH (if AMS)
- Clinical dx; Confirm w/ IgM immunoassay or ELISA of viral protein antigen

Treatment
- Aggressive supportive therapy, IVF, fluid status important 2/2 to plasma leakage, blood tfxs for severe bleeding

Disposition
- Admit +/– ICU for supportive tx

Pearls
- Caused by dengue virus (*Flavivirus*) infxn, transmitted by *A. aegypti* mosquitoes
- Called "break-bone fever" due to acute onset severe HA, muscle & joint pains
- Benign acute febrile illness that can cause bleeding or DIC in small # of cases but can lead to lethal DHF

West Nile Disease (*Infect Dis* 2016;48:571–586)

History
- Outdoor exposures in area of outbreak during summer months, 2–14-d incubation
- Most infxns asymptomatic; Symptomatic pts have fever, HA, malaise, myalgia, GI sxs, rash
- <1% have neuroinvasive dx (meningitis, encephalitis, flaccid paralysis)

Findings
- Low-grade fever, hepatomegaly, splenomegaly, generalized LAD
- Rash: Erythematous maculopapular
- CNS: AMS, confusion, coma, meningismus, papilledema, CN abnormalities, flaccid paralysis, sz, ataxia, tremor, involuntary movements

Evaluation
- CBC (↓ WBC, ↓ lymphocytes, anemia), Chem (↓ Na), ↑ LFTs; ↑ lipase
- CSF: Mild ↑ protein, mild ↑ leukocyte, nl glucose; Obtain IgM serologies
- Brain MRI may be nl or show signal abnormalities in brainstem, basal ganglia, thalamus, anterior spinal cord
- Clinical dx; Confirm w/ ELISA of viral IgM Ab

Treatment
- Resus inc airway mgmt if severe neuro cx; Supportive care
- Limited evidence for interferon & IVIG in case series & reports

Disposition
- Admit for supportive tx, may need rehabilitation from neuro cx

Pearls
- *Flavivirus* transmitted by several types of mosquitoes to horses, dogs, birds; crosses the blood–brain barrier to infect nervous system
- Has been reported throughout the world
- Excellent prognosis unless elderly or w/ other comorbid factors

Eastern Equine Encephalitis (*Open Virol J* 2018;12:80–98)

History
- Outdoor exposure to area of outbreak in summer or early fall
- Fevers, chills, malaise, weakness, HA, myalgias → N/V confusion, coma

Findings
- Similar to any other encephalitis: fever, tachycardia, tachypnea
- Neuro: Papilledema, sz, nuchal rigidity, focal neuro abnl, CN abnormalities, spastic paralysis

Evaluation
- CBC (↑WBC), Chem (↓ Na)
- CTH/MRI brain: Punctuate/intraventricular hemorrhage, focal edema, meningeal enhancement
- CSF: CSF shows ↑ protein, ↑ RBC, ↑WBC
- Immunoassay of CSF/serum, viral isolation from CSF/blood/tissue

Treatment
- Resus inc airway mgmt, supportive care +/– IVIG, corticosteroids, & anticonvulsants

Disposition
- Admit to ICU; will need extensive rehab

Pearls
- *Arbovirus* transmitted subcutaneously by mosquito; birds serve as primary reservoir; virus causes acute inflammatory process mainly involving meninges
- Primarily found in North America (east of MS river; MI, MA, NY, NJ, NC, SC, FL, LA, GA); wooded areas near freshwater swamps, marshes; less commonly Central/South America
- Very poor prognosis

Chikungunya (*Lancet Infect Dis* 2017;17:107–117; *J Clin Invest* 2017;127:737–749; *Viruses* 2017;9:368)

History
- Incubation period 1–12 d → Sudden onset fever w/ joint pain, HA, photophobia, rash

Findings
- Polyarthralgia (can last months–years), joint swelling, fever, transient maculopapular rash

Evaluation
- Detect viral RNA via RT or serologies, r/o other possible culprits (eg, dengue)

Treatment
- NSAIDs for joint pain, supportive care

Disposition
- Admit if needing IV meds

Pearls
- Caused by alphavirus transmitted by *Aedes* mosquitos
- Found in tropical/subtropical regions (African, Indian Ocean Islands, Asia)

Zika Virus Disease (*Clin Microbiol Rev* 2016;29:487–524; *Emerg Infect Dis* 2016;22:1185–1192)

History
- 2–14-d incubation period → asymptomatic or mild dx (fever, arthritis/arthralgia, rash, conjunctivitis, HA, myalgia)

Findings
- Fever, maculopapular rash, conjunctivitis

Evaluation
- Detect viral RNA via RT or serologies

Treatment
- Supportive care

Disposition
- Home

Pearls
- Caused by Flavivirus transmitted by *Aedes* mosquitos
- Found in Southern US, Central America, South America, Southeast Asia
- Temporal & geographic relationship w/ neurologic cx in adults such as Guillain–Barré synd, meningoencephalitis, as well as a/w fetal loss and microcephaly (*Lancet* 2016;388:898)

ALTERED MENTAL STATUS

Approach (*Emerg Med Clinics of N Amer 2016;34(3):649; World J Emerg Med 2012;3(4):270*)

- **Definition:** Any transient or fixed change in cognition &/or arousability inc but not limited to disorientation, memory impairment, behavioral chgs, hallucinations, coma
- "AMS" can describe a wide spectrum of clinical severity & be 2/2 diverse causes
- **Approach:** Dictated by clinical severity of AMS; if unconscious or severely altered:
  - Immediate IV access, Tele, ABCs, O_2 for hypoxia (caution if hx severe COPD)
  - Bedside Gluc measurement: If low, give immediate 1–2 amps $D_{50}W$
  - If concern for narcotic o/d and respiratory depression: Naloxone 0.4–2.0 mg IV/IM/IN
  - If h/o ETOH abuse or malnutrition: empiric thiamine 100 mg IV (can give $D_{50}W$ 1st if hypoglycemia; replete thiamine before prolonged dextrose 2/2 risk of Wernicke's (*J Emerg Med 2012;42(4):488*))
- **History:** Start by assessing baseline MS, degree of change, acuity/timing of change, circumstances surrounding AMS (Δ meds, intoxication/substance use, trauma), PMH
  - Eyewitness accounts helpful: Contact eyewitness if not p/w pt
- **Exam:** Assess for focal neuro sxs (if present, consider CVA, ICH, space-occupying lesion), pupil exam (toxidrome, ↑ ICP/herniation), full skin exam (rash/wounds; diaphoresis may suggest tox; dehydration), asterixis (CO_2 or NH_3 excess), clonus
- **Evaluation:** All pts should get CBC, Chem 10, LFTs, UA, tox screen, ECG, ± hCG; Consider CXR, TSH, VBG, NH_3, drug levels, CO (esp if unwitnessed at home), head CT, CTA head/neck, LP, BCx, troponin, CT A/P

Organic Causes of Acute Altered Mental Status	
Category	**Differential**
Intracranial	**Ischemia:** CVA (can cause AMS if large ± swelling, brainstem) **Hemorrhage:** Epidural (if trauma), SDH (can be atraumatic), SAH (traumatic or aneurysmal), IPH (2/2 neoplasm, HTN, AVM) **Seizure (complex):** Sz, postictal, or consider nonconvulsive status **Space-occupying lesion:** Neoplasm, abscess (esp IVDU, HIV) **Other:** HTN encephalopathy, PRES, concussion (traumatic), diffuse axonal injury (traumatic), anoxic brain injury (esp if s/p ↓ O_2 or ↓ BP)
Metabolic	**Metabolic:** Acidosis, ↑ CO_2, ↓ O_2, electrolyte Δ (Na, Ca), uremia, NH_3 **Endocrine:** ↓ Gluc, ↑ Gluc (HHS, DKA), adrenal, thyroid (↑/↓) **Nutritional:** Wernicke, B_{12} deficiency
Infectious	Sepsis, occult infxn (esp in elderly: PNA, UTI, skin), fever-related delirium, meningitis/encephalitis, neurosyphilis, HIV
Substances	**Depressants:** Opioids, antipsychotics, sedative-hypnotics (eg, benzos), antihistamines, anticholinergics, alcohols (inc toxic alcohols) **Stimulants:** Sympathomimetic agents, hallucinogens, w/d states
Medications	Psychotropic meds most often at fault, but always consider polypharmacy **Serotonin syndrome** (SSRI, NSRI, linezolid, triptans, dextromethorphan, meperidine, methadone, tramadol, MDMA) **Neuroleptic malignant syndrome** (antipsychotics)
Trauma	ICH (see above), systemic inflammatory response, fat embolism, occult trauma (eg, abuse/neglect)
Environment	CO, cyanide, hypo-/hyperthermia

Physical Exam Clues in the Patient with Altered Mental Status		
Exam Finding		**Etiology**
VS	↑ Temp	Infxn, thyroid storm, toxic ingestion (drug o/d, w/d), environmental
	↓ Temp	Environmental, hypothyroidism, sepsis, hypoglycemia
	↑ RR	Metabolic acidosis (DKA), stimulant, aspirin OD, pulmonary dz
	↓ RR	Narcotic o/d, CNS insult
	↑ HR	Fever, sepsis, dehydration, thyroid storm, OD (stimulant, TCA, aspirin, theophylline, anticholinergic), acidosis
	↓ HR	Heart block, ingestion (BB, CCB, digoxin), ↑ ICP
	↑ BP	HTN emergency, preeclampsia, adrenergic stim (drug o/d, w/d), PRES, ↑ ICP, pain
	↓ BP	Shock, sepsis, hemorrhage, toxin, GIB, adrenal crisis, dehydration

Eyes	Miosis	Opioid ingestion, clonidine
	Mydriasis	Sympathomimetic or anticholinergic toxidrome
	Asymmetric	Intracranial process w/ mass effect or herniation
	Papilledema	↑ ICP

Delirium *(Am J Emerg Med 2020;38(2):349)*

- **Definition:** Acute state of temporary or fluctuating disturbance of attention, awareness, and cognition (eg, confusion, perception disturbances, reduced attention, hypo/hyperactivity), not from preexisting neurocognitive disorder or coma *(BMC Med 2014;12:141)*
- Can have many causes (see table above); w/u & tx dependent on causal etiology
- Confusion Assessment Method (CAM): Eval of (1) AMS and fluctuating course, (2) inattention, (3) disorganized thinking, (4) altered level of consciousness
  - Must have both 1 AND 2 and either 3 OR 4, spec 85%, sens 93% *(JAMA 2010;304(7):779)*
  - Other quicker assessment tools (sens >90%): Single question to identify delirium (SQiD), Ultrabrief 2-item bedside test (UB-2), Delirium triage screen (DTS)
- Delirium (vs dementia or psych) suggested by: Age <12 or >40, visual hallucinations (vs auditory), acute onset, exam abnormalities
- **Treatment:** Goal to control agitation and avoid oversedation
  - Options include benzos (can worsen delirium, useful only in delirium 2/2 sedative w/d), typical or atypical antipsychotics, ketamine
  - Nonpharmacologic strategies: Hearing/vision adaptations, reorientation, social support, early mobilization, sleep hygiene, family/pt support, avoid polypharmacy and high-risk meds (Beers list) *(Am J Emerg Med 2019;37(9):1734)*
- **Dispo:** Admit all pts not at baseline MS or w/ recent unexplained AMS; delirium in ED may independently predict 6-mo mortality *(Ann Emerg Med 2010;56(3):244–252)*

Dementia

- **Definition:** Progressive, unremitting decline in cognitive function due to a variety of causes (Alzheimer', vascular, Lewy-body, etc), classically marked by decline in short- & eventually long-term memory, but advanced cases may have behavioral chgs (hypo or hyperactive, agitation, personality chgs) or even nonverbal
- Much more subacute than delirium, though can predispose pts to delirium from otw occult pathology (eg, UTI, PNA) due to poor cognitive reserve; 50% of elderly pts w/ delirium have some degree of underlying dementia *(Ann Emerg Med 2010;56(3):261–269)*
- Important to screen for elder abuse (e/o physical trauma, neglect); EA is underdiagnosed but esp important in pts w/ dementia 2/2 inc risk of caregiver fatigue

Dementia Differential	
System	**Differential**
Degenerative	Alzheimer, Parkinson, Huntington, Pick dz
Vascular	Multi-infarct dementia
Infectious	Neurosyphilis, Creutzfeldt–Jakob dz, HIV
Inflammatory	Lupus, demyelinating dz
Neoplastic	Primary CNS tumor, metastatic dz, paraneoplastic synds
Traumatic	TBI, SDH, anoxic brain injury
Toxic	Alcohol, medications, heavy metals
Metabolic	B_{12}/folate deficiency, thyroid, Wilson dz, lipid storage dz
Psychiatric	Depression
Hydrocephalus	NPH, noncommunicating hydrocephalus

HEADACHE

Approach *(Semin Neurol 2019;39:20)*

- Must differentiate life-threatening HA (minority) from benign HAs (majority)
- **History:** Essential to describe timing/acuity of onset, location, quality, radiation/movement, severity, & associated sx (fever, photophobia, emesis, vision chg, eye pain, neck pain, focal neuro sx, chg in speech or cognition, sinus congestion), circumstances surrounding onset (trauma, med chgs, environment)
- **PMH:** Always ask about HA hx (if present: obtain detailed info regarding how current HA is similar/different), IVDU, immunosupp, current/recent meds (eg, A/C, abx)

- ***Red flags*** requiring neuroimaging: Sudden/rapid onset (<1 min to peak), exertional onset, trauma, worst of life, AMS, 1st severe HA >age 50, fever, neck stiffness/meningismus, sz or syncope at onset, immunosupp, daily HA, no similar prior HAs, abnl neuro exam, papilledema, worse w/ Valsalva/cough/recumbent positioning (↑ ICP)

Headache Differential	
Pathophysiology	**Differential**
Primary HA	Migraine, tension, cluster, trigeminal neuralgia, analgesia rebound
Trauma	ICH (SAH, SDH, EDH, IPH), postconcussive synd
CNS infxn	Meningitis, encephalitis, abscess
Vascular	HTN emergency, aneurysm/AVM growth, cerebral venous sinus thrombosis, carotid/vertebral art, dissection, temporal arteritis, preeclampsia, RCVS; HA rarely presenting complaint w/ CVA
Neoplastic	Malignancy (primary, met., paraneoplastic), benign (meningioma)
CSF d/o (↑↓ ICP)	Hydrocephalus, pseudotumor cerebri, dural leak/post-LP (↓ CSF)
Otolaryngologic	Sinusitis, TMJ synd, mastoiditis
Ophthalmologic	Glaucoma, myopia/presbyopia/hyperopia/astigmatism
Environmental	CO poisoning (Section X: Environmental), noxious aerosols

PRIMARY HEADACHE SYNDROMES (*Emerg Med Clin North Am* 2009;27(1):71)

Migraine Headache & Variants

History, Physical Examination, & Evaluation

- HX: Slow in onset (over h), unilateral throbbing or pulsatile, often w/ N/V (>50%), photo/phono phobia; visual or sensory aura/prodrome may precede HA (15%); duration 4–72 h, recurring, often functional disability 2/2 HA, variants discussed below
  - Classically have migraine hx; beware of assuming migraine if 1st time & age >35
- EXAM: Nl neuro exam (except in migraine variants)
- DX: No studies or c/s routinely indicated unless need to exclude other cause (eg, CT, LP, MRI) as in the case of severe or prolonged sx (see Migraine Variants)

Treatment

- Parenteral preferred due to gastric stasis, delayed absorption (*Headache* 2007;47(10):1443)
- Abortive (*Headache* 2016;56(6):911): Most effective if given w/i 15 mins of onset; often involves combo tx w/ IVF, NSAIDs (ketorolac), APAP, dopamine antagonist antiemetic (check QTc; common options: prochlorperazine, droperidol, metoclopramide; additional options include triptans & DHE (both c/i in preg & CAD)
  - Avoid opioids (↓ efficacy, ↑ recurrence, ↑ side effects) (*Acad Emerg Med* 2008;15(5):414–418)
  - Valproic acid as second line (*Ann Emerg Med* 2003;41(6):847–453)
  - Dexamethasone can ↓ rate of recurrence after discharge (*Acad Emerg Med* 2008;15(5):414–418)
- Prophylaxis: Indicated if >2/mo, duration >24 h, major lifestyle disruption, failure of abortive tx; Options include AEDs, BB, TCAs, CCBs, SSRIs, behavioral/environ chgs

Disposition

- Most pts able to return home w/i h; may need Observation Unit if protracted

Migraine Variants (*Cephalalgia* 2018;38(1):1)

- Migraine variants are rare but can resemble other concerning conditions; often strong h/o similar events in the past, but if not, requires involved w/u to r/o other more serious dx
- **Hemiplegic migraine:** HA a/w hemiplegia (± paresthesias, dysphasic speech); sxs may resolve w/i h to d; HA may be subtle but classically pts have h/o similar prior sx
- **Basilar migraine:** HA w/ vertigo, ataxia, N/V, tinnitus, AMS, dysarthria, diplopia
- **Abdominal migraine:** Paroxysmal mid-abd pain a/w N/V, often w/o HA; strong h/o prior similar episodes & +FH; ddx inc cyclic vomiting synd; more common in Peds
- **Ocular migraine:** Gradual loss of vision in one eye 2/2 transient vasospasm of retinal arteries; often h/o prior similar episodes & +FH; avoid triptans & DHE
- **Status migrainosus:** Migraine HA >72 h

Pearl

- Migraine HA are independent RF for ischemic CVA (RR 1.64) & silent CVA (avoid triptans/DHE) (*Neurol Sci* 2017;38(1):33–40)

Tension Headache

History, Physical Examination, & Evaluation

- **HX:** Dull, aching or throbbing "vice-like" pressure HA w/ gradual onset, bilateral frontal &/or occipitonuchal; absence of N/V or prodrome or functional disability (migraine characteristics); duration 30 mins to 7 d; a/w insomnia, stress, anxiety, or depression

- **EXAM:** Nl neuro exam, no true photophobia
- **DX:** No studies or c/s routinely indicated (unless need to exclude other cause)

Treatment
- NSAIDs or APAP, neck massage & heat, relaxation techniques, *not* narcotics
- Trigger point injection or occipital nerve block if MSK tenderness
- Some efficacy of migraine meds (metoclopramide, chlorpromazine, triptans)

Disposition
- Most pts can go home w/i h; if chronic HA, refer to HA specialist

Cluster Headache

History, Physical Examination, & Evaluation
- **HX:** Sudden-onset unilateral, paroxysmal, sharp, stabbing severe temporal/periorbital HA that may awaken from sleep; ± ipsilateral lacrimation, flushing, rhinorrhea or nasal congestion, conj injection or Horner synd (30% of pts); occur in clusters of short (15–180 mins) episodes (1 QOD to >8/d) for up to 6–8 wks; more common in young men
- **EXAM:** Nl neuro exam or +Horner; may have +lacrimation, flushing, conj injection
- **DX:** No studies or c/s routinely indicated (unless need to exclude other cause)

Treatment
- Abortive: High-flow O_2 (12–15 L/min) by mask (*Neurology* 2004;63(3):593)
  - Medications: Sumatriptan (CI in pregnancy or CAD) (*Neurology* 2000;54(6):1382), DHE, dopamine antagonist antiemetics, octreotide, intranasal lidocaine, NSAIDs
- Prophylaxis: Corticosteroid as transitional tx (*Ann Neurol* 2004;56(4):488), ± verapamil (*Neurology* 2000;54(6):1382) or valproic acid

Pearl
- Make sure to distinguish from acute angle-closure glaucoma

Trigeminal Neuralgia (*Am Fam Physician* 2009;79(11):1001)

History, Physical Examination, & Evaluation
- **HX:** Sudden, unilateral paroxysmal pain in sensory distribution of CN V (usually maxillary (V2) or mandibular (V3) branches); ± brief facial spasm or tic ("tic douloureux"); may be triggered by light touch or vibration, shaving, face washing, chewing, cold, talking
  - 2 categories (classic and symptomatic): Classic has no established etiology, no neuro deficit; symptomatic a/w structural abnlty (MS, tumor, skull base abnl)
- **EXAM:** No e/o CN dysfxn or other neuro abnlty
- **DX:** Can be treated w/o w/u if characteristic hx; MRI to r/o other causes if atypical features present (neuro deficit, age <40, bilateral, no response to tx). Refer to neurology outpt f/u

Treatment
- Carbamazepine 100 mg BID, increase by 200 mg/d up to 1200 mg/d
- Alternatives include oxcarbazepine, baclofen, lamotrigine, pimozide

Pearl
- Most common cause is compression of the nerve root by an aberrant vessel

---

ACUTE SINUSITIS

See section *Sinusitis in Section XIII: Otolaryngology/Dental/Ophthalmology*

HYPERTENSIVE HEADACHE

See section on *Hypertensive Emergencies in Chapter I: Cardiology*

History, Physical Examination, & Evaluation
- **HX:** Untreated HTN or other precipitants (pregnancy, drug use, serotonin synd)
- **EXAM:** BP often >240/140 (unlikely w/ DBP <120); May have papilledema, encephalopathy, ± focal neuro abnormalities or szs
- **DX:** Assess for e/o end-organ damage (HTN emergency): Head CT (r/o ICH, edema), MRI (assess for PRES, CVA), ECG, e/o aortic injury, pulm edema, renal failure

Treatment
- IV Anti-HTN: ↓ MAP by 25% over 1 h (Caution: ↓ BP too quickly could lead to ischemia)
- Common agents: Nicardipine gtt or Labetalol IV or gtt or IV Hydralazine

Cerebral Venous Sinus Thrombosis

Overview (*NEJM* 2005;352(17):1791–1798; *Pract Neurol* 2020;20(5):356)

- **Pathophysiology:** Thrombosis of the sinuses of the brain (eg, sagittal, straight, occipital, transverse) w/ or w/o thrombosis of the cortical veins of the brain
- Sinus thrombosis impairs CSF absorption causing ↑ ICP (eg, HA, AMS, vision chgs)
- Cortical vein thrombosis causes venous infarction & localized injury (eg, focal deficits)
- B/c of cerebral injury, secondary hemorrhage may develop (40% cases)
- Prothrombotic RF (trauma, hypercoagulable state [preg, OCPs, infxn, malignancy]) present in 85%; other causes include post-LP (2/2 downward traction on cortical veins from pressure chgs), sinusitis (cavernous thrombosis), otitis/mastoiditis

History, Physical Examination, & Evaluation

- **HX:** HA present >90%, often gradual over d but can be sudden/thunderclap; ± N/V, vision chgs, focal neuro deficits, worse w/ Valsalva, szs, prothrombotic RFs
- **EXAM:** Papilledema, focal neuro deficits ~40% (*J Stroke Cerebrovasc Dis* 2017;26:1848)
  - Cavernous sinus thrombosis will have CN III/IV/VI compromise, periorbital chemosis/ edema, & ↓ vision ipsilaterally
- Signs and sxs depend on location and extent of brain injury and effect on ICP
- **DX:** CBC, PT/INR, PTT, Upreg, ± D-dimer; MRI/MRV more Se than CTV but balance accuracy w/ urgency & desire to r/o other diagnoses (eg, SAH, IPH)
  - Non-con head CT shows spec signs (venous sinus or deep vein hyperdensity, dense triangle sign, ischemia, hemorrhagic transformation) but not sens (*Neuroradiol* 1985;27:145)
  - D-dimer may help r/o CVST if low pre-TP and isolated HA (weighted Se 94%, Sp 90%) (*J Thromb Haemost* 2012;10(4):582–589); Lower sens w/ longer duration of sxs (*Int J Neurosci* 2017; 127(6):534)

Treatment

- A/C (heparin) preferred even in presence of hemorrhagic infarcts
- Mgmt of ↑ ICP: Mannitol, hypertonic saline, elevating HOB
- Antiepileptics only for pts w/ sz (*J Thromb Haemost* 2010;8:877)
- Endovascular thrombolysis can be used, often reserved for those w/ worst prognosis or deterioration despite tx
  - TO-ACT trial: Endovascular tx vs A/C w/o benefit (*JAMA Neurol* 2020;77(8):966–973)

Disposition

- Admission to neurology; may warrant ICU care if e/o hemorrhagic conversion or AMS

Temporal Arteritis (Giant Cell Arteritis)

Overview (*World J Clin Cases* 2015;3(6):484)

- **Definition:** Granulomatous inflammatory vasculitis of medium/large arteries, usually affects branches of carotid, vertebral, distal subclavian, axillary arteries, thoracic aorta; causes ischemic sx by vessel occlusion

History, Physical Examination, & Evaluation

- **HX:** Unilateral HA, jaw/tongue claudication, malaise, low-grade fevers, visual impairment
  - RFs: Age >50 y/o (90% >60 y/o), F > M, h/o PMR (50% of pts) (*Lancet* 2008;372:234)
- **EXAM:** May have tenderness over temporal art. (↓ Se) or ↓ visual acuity (↓ Se)

Evaluation (*NEJM* 2014;371:50–57)

- ↑ ESR (Se ~84%), ↑ CRP (Se ~86%), combined Se of ESR & CRP may be >95%, but poorly spec in pts w/ other causes for elevation
- Duplex sonography: Assess for inflammatory edema of vascular wall, flow behavior, Se ~85%, Sp >90% (*NEJM* 1997;337(19):1336)
- Temporal art. bx: High Se for even low levels of inflammation *if present at site of bx* (requires 1.5–2.0-cm segment); given focality of dz, may need repeat bx or imaging if high pre-TP & 1st-bx neg
- CTA &/or MRA: Can assess for other etiology of sxs (CVA); Not used to make dx, but may serve as adjunct if –bx &/or assess extent of dz if +bx

Treatment

- High-dose corticosteroids (*Rhematol* 2010;49:1594): Induction w/ 15 mg/kg IV methypred ×3 d then prednisone 1 mg/kg/d (do not wait for bx results if vision sx) ~2–4 wks, long taper
  - Symptomatic relief in 24–48 h (*Curr Cariol Rep* 2014;16:498)
- C/s neurology, ophthalmology, rheumatology if concern for dx & to arrange f/u

Disposition

- Admit for visual deficits; otw can be discharged on steroids w/ f/u

Pearls
- Failure to diagnose & treat may result in permanent blindness
- 75% of pt w/ visual deficits in 1 eye will develop contralateral deficits w/i 3 wks
- 20× higher risk of thoracic aortic aneurysm

Idiopathic Intracranial HTN (Pseudotumor Cerebri)

Overview
- Pathophysiology: Unclear etiology; due to obstructed venous/CSF outflow rather than ↑ CSF production, ↑ ICP w/o hydrocephalus or mass lesion and nl CSF composition

History, Physical Examination, & Evaluation (*Cephalgia* 2015;35(3):248–261)
- **HX:** Gradual onset, global, daily/constant HA (>90%) or retrobulbar pain, ± N/V, ↓ vision (~70%; may be transient), intracranial noises (~60%); sx can be worst in morning
  - RFs: Young obese females, recent weight gain; some meds (tetracyclines, retinoids)
- **EXAM:** Nl neuro exam (except possible CN VI palsy), check vision & for papilledema
- **DX:** Can be clinical dx (sx, papilledema); ocular US for optic nerve sheath diameter >5 mm (LR+ 12.4, LR– 0.05); LP for opening pressure (>25 cm H_2O in lateral decubitus) confirms dx; Neuroimaging may be nl or show signs of ↑ ICP (empty sella, swelling of optic disc)

Treatment (*J Neurol Neurosurg Psychiatry* 2018;89:1088)
- Neuro c/s (± ophthalmology) if new dx or refractory to tx
- Weight loss remains most effective tx
- Diuretics to decrease ICP: Acetazolamide 1 mg PO QD
- Refractory cases may need VP shunt or optic nerve fenestration to preserve vision
- Use of steroids controversial & may worsen weight gain

Dural Leak/Post-LP Headache

Overview (*Postgrad Med J* 2006;82(973):713)
- **Definition:** HA caused by ICP caused by loss of CSF from recent dural injury (eg, due to LP, myelogram, spinal anesthesia, vigorous coughing)

History, Physical Examination, & Evaluation
- **HX:** Occipital HA radiating to shoulders/neck, worse w/ sitting/standing (± alleviated w/ supine); worsened by activities that ↑ ICP (eg, coughing, sneezing, Valsalva); usually present 48–72 h postdural injury (but can be >1 wk); ± N/V, LBP, photophobia, tinnitus
- **EXAM:** Nonfocal neuro exam; HA improved w/ lying flat, worse w/ sitting up
- **DX:** None spec, clinical dx; evaluate for other causes of HA, if indicated
  - If obtained, LP may show ↓ opening pressure and slightly ↑ CSF protein/lymphocytes, brain imaging may show dural enhancement or e/o sagging, descent of brain stem

Treatment
- As much as 85% will resolve w/o tx; tx indicated for severe or prolonged (>72 h) sx
- Epidural blood patch (clot seals defect): 70–98% success (*Br J Anaesth* 2003;91(5):718)
- Caffeine (PO/IV) may be helpful, limited data, acts as cerebral vasoconstrictor
- Surgical closure of dural gap is last-resort effort if blood patch &/or other options fail

Pearls
- Minimize risk of post-LP HA w/ small caliber spinal needle (24–27G), bevel alignment w/ dural fibers, atraumatic needles, minimized number of attempts, replacement of stylet
- Factors not proven to influence: Volume of CSF removed, bed rest after LP, IV hydration, positioning, original opening pressure
- Severe cases can precipitate sz & SDH (2/2 ↓ ICP → brain pulled → bridging vein strain)

Intracranial Neoplasm

Overview (*Lancet* 2018;392(10145):4432)
- **Definition:** Any of a spectrum of neoplasms (benign or malignant), each w/ distinct pathology, epidemiology, natural hx, mgmt, & prognosis; often cause acute sx due to mass effect of tumor, vasogenic edema, sz, or secondary hemorrhage
- Tumors either extraparenchymal (meningioma, pituitary neoplasm) or intraparenchymal
  - Intraparenchymal most commonly glioma (eg, oligodendroglioma, mixed glioma, astrocytoma), primary CNS lymphoma, or metastatic non-CNS primary cancer
  - DDx of brain mass also includes infxn, inflammatory d/o, vascular lesion

History, Physical Examination, & Evaluation

- **HX:** Subacute onset, often daily morning HAs (2/2 ↑ ICP), ± N/V, focal deficits, chgs in personality or speech, sz; alleviation w/ NSAIDs/APAP does not help r/o dx
- **EXAM:** Look for signs of herniation:
  - Uncal (most common): ↓ mental status, blown ipsilateral pupil, contralateral weakness, decerebrate posturing
  - Subfalcine: Contralateral LE weakness
  - Central: AMS, yawning, Cheyne–Stokes breathing, miosis. Decorticate → decerebrate.
  - Tonsillar (posterior): Bradycardia, nystagmus, coma, respiratory arrest
  - Upward: Ataxia, dysarthria, somnolence, patchy loss of brain stem reflexes
  - Cushing reflex (due to ↑ ICP): HTN, bradycardia, irregular breathing
- **DX:** Neuroimaging w/ CT, usually f/b MRI (w/ gadolinium contrast); In those suspected w/ pituitary tumors, check lytes, cortisol, TSH
  - Tx & prognosis depend on tumor phenotype & grade

Treatment (glioma)

- Dexamethasone 4 mg TID (dose varies) for peritumor edema (*Neuro Oncol* 2015;17:448)
- Antiepileptic tx if sz, routine ppx not recommended (*Neurology* 2000;54:1886)
- C/s NSGY (consideration of resection), Neuro-oncology

Disposition

- Admit all pts w/ new dx of intracranial neoplasm; or transfer to facility w/ NSGY
- Prognosis heavily dependent on phenotype & grade (mos to y)

CNS INFECTIONS

Meningitis (*Infect Dis Clinic N Amer* 2008;22(1):35)

Overview

- **Definition:** Inflammation of the meninges overlying the brain due to either infectious (bacterial, fungal, viral) or noninfectious etiology; sx & tx differ widely based on etiology
- Bacterial meningitis rare in developed nations; common bacteria include *S. pneumoniae, N. meningitidis, H. influenzae type b, L. monocytogenes (infants, elderly, pregnant, immunocomp), staph* (VPS, trauma, NSGY); seeding of subarachnoid space 2/2 hematogenous spread (eg, from resp tract) or direct spread (eg, sinusitis, acute OM)
- Viral meningitis caused by enteroviruses (most common), HSV, other less common are mumps, HIV, CMV, VZV (more common in immunocompromised pts)
- Other infectious causes of aseptic meningitis: TB, syphilis, Mycoplasma, Chlamydia, Coccidioides, Histoplasma, Cryptococcus sp.
- Causes of noninfectious aseptic meningitis include drugs (eg, antimicrobials, vaccines, NSAIDs), inflammatory dz (SLE, Behçet); rarely malignancy can p/w leptomeningeal dz

History

- Bacterial: Typically acute (<1 d), high-grade fever, HA, nuchal rigidity, ill appearing, AMS
  - RFs: Extremes of age, immunosupp (esp HIV, steroids, MM/blood ca), crowded living environment (dorms, shelters), splenectomy, ETOH abuse/cirrhosis, IVDU, recent illness (esp sinusitis/OM), dural defect (recent trauma, surgery; congenital, VPS)
  - Classic triad for bacterial etiology: Neck stiffness, fever, AMS (3 of 3 present <50%, 2 of 3 present >95%) (*Lancet* 2016;388(10063):3036–3047)
- Viral: Typically subacute (1–7 d), also w/ HA, fever, photophobia, neck stiffness; unless HSV, usually nl mental status; HSV usually w/ AMS
- Fungal/TB: Subacute (>1 wk), HA, low-grade fever, weight loss, night sweats, ± AMS

Physical Examination

- May have nuchal rigidity, disorientation/AMS, photophobia
  - Signs: Brudzinski (hip flexion elicited by passive neck flexion) & Kernig (flexing hip and extending knee elicits pain in legs/back): High Sp, low Se (5%) (*Cin Infect Dis* 2002;35(46)
- Petechial/purpuric rash suggests meningococcus (*N. meningitidis*)
- Expect subtle presentation in elderly or immunocompromised pts; may be AMS only

Evaluation

- LP is gold standard for dx but should not delay abx if high pre-TP for bacterial/HSV
  - See table for indications for CT prior to LP (risk for brain herniation if increased ICP and obstruction of CSF flow and equilibration (*CMAJ* 1993;148:961))
  - LP tubes: (1 & 4) cell count & diff, (2) gluc & protein, (3) Gram stain, cx ± HSV PCR
  - Gram stain Se depends on etiology: *S. pneumoniae* (Se >90%), *H. influenzae* (75%), *N. meningitidis* (50%), *L. monocytogenes* (33%); GS & Cx yield may ↓ by 40% if done after abx, improved by PCR (*Clin Infect Dis* 2004;39(9):1267; *Lancet* 2016;388:3036–3047)
- BCx, infectious w/u (CBC, CXR, UA, +/–CRP/procal); TCP suggests meningococcus

Treatment (*Clin Infect Dis* 2004;39(9):1267)
- Respiratory precautions if suspect bacterial
- Empiric abx based on suspected etiology (see table); acyclovir 10 mg/kg q8h if c/f HSV
- Early steroids may ↓ inflammatory cascade in *S. pneumo* meningitis; therefore, if proven or high pre-TP bacterial etiology, give dexamethasone 0.15 mg/kg w/i 20 mins of 1st abx (↑ favorable neuro outcomes & ↓ mortality) (*NEJM* 2002;347:1549)
- C/s NSGY in all pts w/indwelling hardware (eg, VPS): Removal improves tx success
- Postexposure ppx (if +*N. meningitidis*): Ciprofloxacin 500 mg PO × 1. Alternatives are rifampin 600 PO BID ×2 d, CTX 250 mg IM (peds or pregnancy)
- If viral (non-HSV): Supportive care only, prophylaxis not needed

Disposition
- Admit bacterial, HSV, fungal; Non-HSV viral: D/C vs observation based on sx severity

Indications for CT before LP (*IDSA Guidelines. Clin Infect Dis* 2004;39(9):1267)	
Age >60	Any neuro abnormalities: ↓ GCS*, CN abnlty, abnl visual fields, pronator drift, abnl language (eg, aphasia)
Immunocompromised	
h/o CNS/neuro dz	
Recent sz w/i 1 wk of presentation	Inability to follow 2 consecutive commands
Papilledema	Inability to answer 2 consecutive questions

*No clear data on precise GCS cut-off; some studies suggest CT for any GCS <13, while others suggest CT only if GCS <8. Others simply use "alert" or "not alert" (*NEJM* 2001;345:1727–1733).

Interpretation of LP Results		
CSF Test	**Normal**	**Implications of Abnormal Results**
WBC	<5 WBC <1 PMN	Bacterial: Marked ↑ WBC (usually >1,000), ↑ PMN Viral: Usually ↑ WBC but <500, mononuclear *Traumatic tap: If serum WBC nl, expect 1 WBC for every 700 RBC (limited data)**
RBC	None	↑↑ RBC: Traumatic LP (if T1 > T4) or SAH (T1~T4) ↑ RBC (& ↑ WBC): Consider HSV Xanthochromia indicates RBCs present >/4 h
CSF:Serum Gluc	0.6:1	↓ in bacterial/fungal meningitis or hyperglycemia
Protein	15–45 mg/dL	↑ in bacterial/fungal meningitis, syphilis, neoplasm, demyelination, bleed (SAH)
Opening pres**	<20 mmH_2O	↑ in bacterial, fungal, or TB
Gram stain	neg	Positive in 80% of bacterial meningitis (see above)

*Limited data from adult population. In infants 0–60 d, may be safe to use ratio of 1 WBC: 877 RBCs (*Ann Emerg Med* 2016;pii:S0196-0644(16)31223–31229).
**Can be elevated 2/2 noninfectious etiologies as well.

Common Bacterial Pathogens in Meningitis by Age with Empiric Antibiotics		
Age	**Common Pathogens**	**Empiric Antibiotic Regimen**
<1 mo	Group B strep, *E. coli, L. monocytogenes, Klebsiella*	Ampicillin *AND* (Cefotaxime *OR* Gentamicin)
1–24 mo	Group B strep, *S. pneumo, H. influenzae, N. meningitidis*	Vancomycin *AND* CTX
2–50 y	*S. pneumo, N. meningitidis*	Vancomycin 1 g *AND* CTX 2 g
>50 y	*S. pneumo, N. meningitidis, P. aeruginosa, L. monocytogenes*	Vancomycin 1 g *AND* CTX 2 g *AND* Ampicillin 150 mg/kg/d div q4h
Surgery/Trauma	*S. aureus, S. epidermidis, P. aeruginosa*	Vancomycin 1 g *AND* Cefepime 2 g

Encephalitis (*Infect Dis Clinic N Amer* 2008;22(1):35)

Overview
- **Definition:** Inflammation of brain parenchyma usually due to infxn (often viral); rarely autoimmune/paraneoplastic (*Lancet Neurol* 2016;15(4):391–404)
- Differentiated from meningitis by presence of AMS and/or focal neuro findings
- HSV (5–10% encephalitis) life-threatening (>70% mortality w/o tx) (*BMJ* 2012;344:e3166)

History & Physical Examination
- **HX:** Acute onset fever (>90% w/ HSV), HA (>80% w/ HSV), behavior chgs (>70% w/ HSV), hallucinations/altered awareness (>60% w/ HSV), confusion/impaired memory (25% w/ HSV); ± diffuse or focal neuro sx (weakness, ataxia, speech disturbance), sz, or e/o meningeal involvement (+photophobia, +neck stiffness) (*BMJ* 2012;344:e3166)
  - Absence of fever or HA strongly suggests against the dx of HSV encephalitis

- HSV encephalitis often preceded by nonspec viral prodrome (fever, malaise, N/V)
  - Assess for immunosupp, recent travel, tick/mosquito bites
- **EXAM:** AMS (may progress to coma), more likely to have focal neuro deficits than isolated meningitis (may progress to diffuse paralysis &/or ataxia); may have e/o concurrent meningeal involvement

Evaluation (*BMJ* 2012;344:e3166)

- LP: CSF ↑ WBC, ± ↑ RBC/xanthochromia, ± ↑ protein levels, nl Gluc, gram stain, cx
  - Important to send HSV PCR, but should not defer tx
- MRI: Imaging modality of choice & helps r/o CI to LP; Se 90% in HSV encephalitis
- EEG: Se 84%, Sp 32% for HSV encephalitis (may help guide need for AEDs)

Treatment

- If concern for HSV encephalitis: Acyclovir 10 mg/kg q8h IV, AEDs
- If low concern for HSV: Supportive ± anticonvulsants, steroids
- If concern for possible bacterial meningitis, tx w/ abx and steroids as above
  - Steroids may be beneficial in HSV encephalitis w/o bacterial meningitis (trials ongoing)

Disposition

- Admit if confirmed/suspected HSV, not at baseline neuro status (eg, AMS), immunosupp

Abscess

Overview (*NEJM* 2014;371(5):447)

- **Definition:** Begins as localized cerebritis that coverts to collection of pus surrounded by capsule (intraparenchymal, epidural, subdural, spinal); form by contiguous spread (sinus, mastoid, dental) or hematogenous seeding (PNA, endocarditis, bacteremia),
  - RFs: Immunosupp, IVDU, trauma/surgery, local infxn (mastoiditis, sinusitis, dental), & RFs for systemic infxn (eg, endocarditis, line infxn, bacteremia)
- Certain medical conditions predispose to certain pathogens: HIV (*Toxoplasma gondii, M. tuberculosis*), solid-organ tpx (nocardia, aspergillus, candida), postsurgical (staph)
- Common organism by etiol: Contiguous spread (strep, staph, anaerobes, polymicrobial); hematogenous spread (staph, strep, anaerobes)

History, Physical Examination, & Evaluation

- **HX:** HA (most common), ± low-grade fever; AMS/neuro sx often absent (*Neurol* 2014;82:806)
  - Up to 25% of pts may p/w szs
  - Assess for RFs & ROS suggesting possible source infxn
- **EXAM:** May have nl neuro exam depending on site of abscess & timing of presentation
- **DX:** ↑ WBC, ↑ ESR, BCx. CT w/ contrast ("ring-enhancing" lesion)
  - MRI useful for differentiating from other brain masses (*Surg Neurol* 2006;66:246)
  - LP not routinely performed 2/2 risk of brain herniation & low Se (25%)
  - NSGY consultation for diagnostic stereotactic aspiration for cx & decompression
  - Antitoxoplasma IgG can confirm toxoplasma dx in HIV pts (no need for aspiration)

Treatment

- Although diagnostic NSGY aspiration aims to decompress maximally, therapeutic NSGY aspiration (eg, if pathogen already known) indicated only for large abscesses or those w/ e/o IV abx failure (*J Neurosurg* 1980;52:217; *Neurosurg* 1995;36:76)
- Early IV abx w/ good CSF penetration, tailored to likely pathogen
  - Start broad-spectrum IV abx (table below)
  - Consider coverage for fungi, toxoplasmosis, tuberculosis in immunocompromised pts
- Low threshold to intubate and admit ICU (may progress rapidly)

Disposition

- Admit all pts; may require ICU

Pearls

- Mortality 15%, unless abscess ruptures into ventricular system (mortality 27–85%)
- Morbidity from residual neuro deficits, new sz from scar tissue or neuropsych Δ (30%)

Empiric Antibiotics for Brain Abscess (*NEJM* 2014;371(5):447)	
Standard	CTX* 2 g *AND* Metronidazole 500 mg ± Vancomycin 1 g
Transplant pts	CTX* 2 g *AND* Metronidazole 500 mg ± Vancomycin 1 g *AND* Voriconazole *AND* Trimethoprim-Sulfamethoxazole
HIV-positive pts	CTX* 2 g *AND* Metronidazole 500 mg ± Vancomycin 1 g *AND* Pyrimethamine *AND* Sulfadiazine Consider TB tx (INH, Rifampin, Pyrazinamide, Ethambutol)

*Meropenem can be substituted for cephalosporin if allergies present.

SEIZURE

Overview (*Am Fam Physician* 2012;86(4):334)

- **Definition:** Spontaneous or provoked abnl synchronous cortical electrical activity; recurrent unprovoked szs referred to as "epilepsy" (*Ann Emerg Med* 2014;63(4):437–447)
- **ILAE 2017 Classification** (*Epilepsia* 2017;58:512): Based on origin (focal, generalized, or unknown), degree of awareness (retained or impaired awareness), level of body movement (motor or nonmotor)
  - **Status epilepticus:** >5 mins continuous generalized sz activity or continued intermittent sz w/o return to baseline mental status (*Front Neurol* 2019;10:427)
  - **Epilepsy:** ≥2 unprovoked szs occurring >24 h apart OR 1 unprovoked sz and probability of further szs based on neuroimaging/EEG OR dx of epilepsy synd (*Epilepsia* 2014;55(4):475)
  - **Nonepileptic seizures:** Transient duration of sxs w/o electrical brain disturbance
- Szs can be separated into 3 categories of DDx: Nonepileptic, provoked (also called acute symptomatic sz, numerous etiol), and unprovoked (2/2 previous or progressive brain dz or unknown etiol)
- Lifetime risk of nonfebrile sz is 2–5% (*Ann Emerg Med* 2004;43(5):605–625)

Common Etiologies Provoking Seizure (*Epilepsia* 2010;51(4):671)	
CNS	Ischemia (eg, CVA), ICH, vascular malformations (aneurysm, AVM), Neoplasm (primary, met), sinus thrombosis, trauma, PRES, HTN enceph, inherited conditions (NF, Tub. sclerosis, Sturge–Weber, etc)
infxn	Febrile sz (peds), meningitis, encephalitis, brain abscess, HIV OIs, HIV enceph, neurocysticercosis, neurosyphilis, malaria
Toxic	W/D (ETOH, benzo, barb), OD (sympathomimetic, TCA, anticholinergic, SSRI/SNRI, bupropion, lidocaine, INH), Caffeine, tramadol
Metabolic	↑↓ Gluc, ↑↓ Na, ↓ Ca, ↓ Mg, ↓ O_2, uremia, liver failure, thyrotoxicosis
Obstetric	Eclampsia
Environmental	Heat stroke, stress, lack of sleep
Neonatal	CMV, congenital syphilis, rubella, inborn errors of metabolism (eg, PKU)

Common Types of Seizures (*Epilepsia* 2017;58:512)		
Location	**Type**	**Description**
Generalized onset	Motor (Tonic, clonic, tonic–clonic, myoclonic, atonic)	Abrupt LOC, often apneic; Rigid (tonic), rhythmic jerking (clonic), tonic phase f/b clonic phase (tonic–clonic, grand mal), loss of tone (atonic); Often a/w incontinence, tongue biting, trauma (eg, shoulder dislocation) F/b postictal state of depressed mental status lasting min–h; pts unable to recall event Affects all ages; In older adults, more likely 2/2 focal lesion that rapidly generalizes
	Nonmotor (Absence)	Abrupt LOC; Staring spells or rhythmic blinking; no incontinence Minimal postictal state, but pts unable to recall event School-aged children (usually resolves by adulthood)
Focal onset	Motor	Isolated unilateral motor (eg, convulsions, automatisms) or sensory (eg, loss or change), or autonomic activity Can be aware or impaired awareness, can progress to bilateral tonic–clonic
	Nonmotor	Autonomic (rising sensation in stomach, hot/cold), behavior arrest, cognitive (impaired speech), emotional, sensory (taste/smell) Can be aware or impaired awareness, can progress to bilateral tonic–clonic

Approach

- If actively seizing: Immediate IV access, roll pt into decubitus (avoid aspiration), suction airway, supplemental O_2, fingerstick Gluc, magnesium (if pregnant), antiepileptic agents (IV, IO, IM, IN)
- If not actively seizing: Assess return to baseline mental status, focal deficits

History

- Description of events before, during, & after sz: Prodrome, associated sxs (fever, vomiting, HA, trauma, photophobia, visual chg), any focal neuro sxs, AEDs given, type of sz (focal vs generalized; level of awareness) & duration, postictal state
  - Lateral tongue lac and incontinence: High Sp for epileptic sz (*Epilepsia* 2008;49(6):962)
  - **First-time Sz:** Assess possible causal etiologies (see above)
  - **Breakthrough Sz:** Assess similarities &/or differences from prior sz, typical sz frequency, last sz prior to presentation, any chgs in AEDs, outpt provider, factors that may lower sz threshold (stress, sleep, noncompliance, new meds, toxins, alcohol, infxn)
- Differentiate from syncope (may have myoclonic jerks, no incontinence or tongue biting, quick return to baseline mental status)
- May be difficult to differentiate from PNES (a/w childhood trauma/abuse, PTSD, hx of self-harm, high frequency and duration of szs, resistance to antiepileptic drugs, gradual onset, no postictal state, pelvic thrusting) (*Epilepsy Behav* 2011;20(2):308)
- Assess for sx of traumatic injury

Physical Examination

- Assess GCS, orientation, & memory (compare w/ baseline), neuro deficits
- Evaluate for e/o trauma (inc tongue biting) or ingestion; if persistent AMS & unwitnessed sz w/ e/o head trauma or fall, may need temporary C-spine immobilization until cleared

Evaluation (*Ann Emerg Med* 2004;43(5):605–625; *Neurology* 2007;69(21):1996)

- **If active seizing:** Defer eval until cessation of sz (see Approach)
- **First-time Sz & back to baseline:**
  - Labs: CBC, BMP (Gluc, Na, Ca), HCG; ± lactate, CPK (↑ lactate & ↑ CPK can help differentiate b/w unwitnessed convulsive sz & syncope w/ myoclonus or PNES but lactate superior to CK (*Intern Emerg Med* 2018;13(5):749))
  - PRN based on hx: Tox screen, LFTs, LP (if c/f infectious process, obtain CT prior)
  - ECG for syncope assessment for all pts w/ LOC
  - Neuroimaging: Obtain noncontrast CT in ED if feasible
    - May defer neuroimaging to outpt if: Age <40 y, nl neuro exam, no concern for intracranial path (no trauma, no hx malignancy or immunosupp, no fever, no HA, no A/C use), & good outpt f/u; preferred outpt study is MRI w/contrast
    - MRI w/contrast > CT for eval of tumors (esp in elderly, hx cancer), but can be done as outpt in most pts if CT neg
  - EEG: May be performed as outpt; urgently indicated only for persistent AMS, SE, dx of viral encephalitis, intubated/paralyzed, r/o nonconvulsive SE
- **Breakthrough sz:**
  - Labs: Electrolytes, UA, AED levels, ± CXR; ± lactate, CPK
  - Neuroimaging: Consider if different from prior sz, prolonged duration since recent sz, trauma, or other c/f intracranial pathology
  - Keep differential broad even if known sz d/o, esp if therapeutic med levels

Treatment

- Airway: Nasal trumpet, supplemental O_2, suction, positioning, may need to intubate if SE
- **Abortive meds:** Benzodiazepines 1st line (available IV, IM, IN, buccal, PR);
  - IV lorazepam vs IM midazolam: IM midazolam is noninferior & may be superior to IV lorazepam w/ regard to sz termination/need for rescue tx, & is quicker if no IV access (*Epilepsia* 2015;56(2):254; *NEJM* 2012;366(7):591)
  - IV lorazepam vs IV diazepam: IV lorazepam superior to IV diazepam w/ regard to sz termination/need for rescue tx (*Cochrane* 2014;(9):CD003723)
  - 2nd-line agent options are levetiracetam, fosphenytoin, or valproate (similar efficacy and incidence of adverse events (*NEJM* 2019;381(22):2103))
  - Special cases w/ alternative 1st-line tx: Pregnant (Mg 4 g IV/IO), INH tox (pyridoxine 1 g)
- If not seizing, tx w/AED depends on risk of recurrence: (*Ann Emerg Med* 2014;63(4):437)
  - 1st-time sz (provoked or unprovoked): No AED indicated if back to baseline mental status, no current or known h/o structural brain dz/injury
  - If h/o sz d/o & ↓ AED levels, load w/ AED (PO or IV; home agent preferred)
  - If h/o sz d/o & nl AED levels & no clear provoking trigger: Contact outpt prescriber to discuss ↑ outpt AED dose

IV Treatment of Status Epilepticus (*Epilepsy Curr* 2016;16(1):48)

Step	Antiepileptic	Dose
1	Lorazepam OR	2–4 mg (0.1 mg/kg), repeat q5–10min if sz persists
	Diazepam OR	5–10 mg (0.2 mg/kg), repeat q5–10min if sz persists
	Midazolam	5–10 mg (0.2 mg/kg), repeat q5–10min if sz persists

2	Phenytoin OR	1–1.5 g (10–15 mg/kg) over 20 mins
	Fosphenytoin OR	1–1.5 g (15–20 mg/kg) over 5–10 mins
	Valproic acid OR	25–45 mg/kg (absence sz)
	Levetiracetam	20–60 mg/kg IV
3	Phenobarbital	200–600 mg slow push, then 10–20 mg/kg if no resolution
4	General anesthesia w/ propofol, midazolam, or pentobarbital ± paralytics	

Disposition

- Provoked sz: Dispo depends on underlying cause; if underlying cause cannot be rapidly reversed & pt remains at risk for recurrent provoked sz, admx vs observation
- Unprovoked sz: Most can be safely discharged w/ close neuro f/u if nl mental status, exam, & w/u (above)
- If on long-term meds or 2nd sz, discuss w/ neurology regarding dose adjustments or starting a long term
- Explicit instructions to not drive, operate hazardous machinery or perform tasks where recurrent sz may cause harm; some states have mandatory reporting to DMV
- Admit all pts w/ 2+ sz in prehospital/ED or SE; may need ICU

Pearl

- Treat alcohol w/d sz w/ BZD, almost never responsive to phenytoin

VERTIGO

Definition (*Am Fam Physician* 2017;95(3):154)

- Dizziness traditionally classified into 4 categories: Vertigo, presyncope, disequilibrium, lightheadedness, but pts typically have difficulty describing sxs and no not reliably predict cause of dizziness (*CMAJ* 2011;183(9):E571)
- Vertigo: The sensation of disorientation in space combined w/ sensation of motion/ spinning
- May be due to benign (usually peripheral) or life-threatening (usually central) causes
  - Central comprise ~10% of cases; CVA comprises ~4% (*Mayo Clin Proc* 2008;83:765–777)
  - RFs for central vertigo: Older age, males, HTN, CAD, DM, AF, h/o CVA/TIA

Differential Diagnosis for Vertigo	
Peripheral	FB, cerumen impaction, acute otitis media, labyrinthitis, benign paroxysmal positional vertigo, Ménière dz, vestibular neuronitis, perilymphatic fistula, trauma, motion sickness, acoustic neuroma, ototoxic medications (eg, gentamicin, furosemide)
Central	Infxn (encephalitis, meningitis, cerebritis), vertebrobasilar art. insufficiency, subclavian steal synd, cerebellar or brainstem hemorrhage or infarction, vertebrobasilar migraine, trauma (temporal bone fracture, postconcussive synd), tumor (brainstem or cerebellum), MS, temporal lobe epilepsy

History & Physical Examination

- **HX:** Onset & duration of sxs; chgs w/ position & direction; associated sxs (HA, neuro sx, dysarthria, chgs in hearing, CP/LH, palpitations); circumstances surrounding onset (trauma, torsional neck inj, neck manipulation, new meds); PMH inc meds
  - Distinguish b/w vertigo & presyncope or light headedness
  - TiTrATE approach: **Ti**ming, **Tr**iggers, **A**nd a **T**argeted **E**xamination (*Neurol Clin* 2015;33(3):577), separates into episodic triggered, spontaneous episodic, or continuous
- **EXAM:** Assess for neuro deficits, nystagmus, cerebellar exam, gait, ± Dix Hallpike; listen for carotid bruits, otoscopy, cardiac murmurs
  - HINTS exam (head impulse, nystagmus, test of skew) useful for distinguishing central from peripheral cause of acute vestibular synd (*Stroke* 2009;40(11):3504)
  - Diagnostic value of HINTS exam in ED has been questioned as may pts do not meet criteria for use (continuous vertigo, nystagmus) (*Acad Emerg Med* 2021;28(4):387)
  - Dix–Hallpike maneuver: Used to diagnose BPPV, start in seated position, rapidly lie flat on back, extend pt's head back 45°, then immediately to L or R 45°, keep pt's eyes open, monitor nystagmus & sxs, repeat on other side (*NEJM* 2014;370(12):1138)

Historical & Exam Features of Central vs Peripheral Vertigo		
	Peripheral	**Central**
Timing	Acute onset (s) Can be intermittent or constant Often self-resolves (s–h) Present early in course	Gradual onset (min–h) Progressive & constant Present later in course
Intensity	Severe	Mild–mod
Nystagmus	Always present: Unidirectional, fatigable horizontal or rotatory (*never vertical or direction changing*)	May be absent, can be bidirectional. Vertical nystagmus almost always central in origin
Head Impulse (W/ pt sitting, head is thrust 10° to L/R w/ eyes fixed on examiner's nose)	Corrective saccade (rapid movement of both eyes)	No eye movement
Test of skew (pt looks straight ahead, then cover/uncover each eye)	No eye movement	Vertical deviation of covered eye after uncovering
Associated sxs	Intense N/V Provoked by movement/position ± hearing loss or tinnitus Nl brainstem/cerebellar exam	Mild nausea, often HA Not affected by movement Usually no auditory sxs May have abnl neuro exam

Evaluation

- ECG (r/o arrhythmia), Gluc & electrolytes, UA, HCG (if child-bearing age)
- Neuroimaging: Indicated if any neuro findings or c/f central etiology
  - Preferred modality is MRI; head CT PRN to r/o hemorrhage (eg, HA, trauma, A/C), CT has limited utility for cerebellum/brainstem
  - Consider CTA or MRA to evaluate for vascular dz (carotid, vertebrobasilar)

Treatment

- **Central:** Symptomatic relief (antiemetics, benzodiazepines); Neurology c/s, ASA (if ischemic CVA); NSGY (if hemorrhagic CVA) & A/C reversal
- **Peripheral:** Usually supportive care w/ antivertigo medications (diazepam 2–4 mg IV/5–10 mg PO, meclizine 25 mg PO, diphenhydramine, promethazine)
  - For BPPV, consider trying Epley maneuver (or modified self-Epley maneuver at home)
  - For acute bacterial labyrinthitis: ENT c/s, IV abx, usually need admission
  - For Ménière: Supportive medications, encourage decreased salt intake, diuretic (eg, HCTZ), close ENT f/u

Disposition

- Home once sxs improve w/ PCP/ENT f/u
- Admit if (a) central/CVA, (b) peripheral w/ refractory sx, (c) acute bacterial labyrinthitis

Pearl

- More than half of pts presenting to ED w/ a chief c/o "dizziness" or "vertigo" may have nonneuro processes (*Mayo Clin Proc* 2008;83:765–777)

Common Causes of Peripheral Vertigo	
Etiology	**Findings**
Benign paroxysmal positional vertigo (*Otolaryngol Head Neck Surg* 2008;139(5 suppl 4):S47; *Neurology* 2008;70(22):2067)	• Due to otolith disruption w/i semicircular canals (often posterior) • Most common cause of peripheral vertigo (lifetime prev 2.4%; annual rate of recurrence 15%) (*NEJM* 2014;370:1138–1147) • **Hx:** Brief (sec/min) spinning sensation, episodic (<1 min each), precipitated by chg in head position (eg, rolling over in bed), severe, a/w N/V • **Dx:** Dix–Hallpike causes sx & unidirectional nystagmus in >70% • **Tx:** Usually resolves w/o tx (median duration 7 d w/ horizontal canal, 17 d w/ posterior canal); Epley maneuver may cure sx in >70% w/ 1 cycle & almost 100% w/ successive cycles (*Cochrane Database Syst Rev* 2014;(12):CD003162)

Labyrinthitis • Viral • Acute bacterial • Toxic (*Prim Care* 2014;41(1):115)	• Inflammatory d/o of inner ear 2/2 infxn or external toxin • Distinguished from vestibular neuronitis by hearing involvement • **Viral/Serous:** Usually coexisting or recent URI/OM, may have hearing loss; usually nontoxic, may have mild fever; r/o VZV (Ramsay Hunt, a/w vesicular rash/facial nerve palsy) requiring IV acyclovir & admx; usual tx is supportive care (antiemetics, hydration), other etiol are CMV, rubella, mumps, measles • **Acute bacterial:** Coexisting OM ± cholesteatoma (esp if s/p abx) or meningitis; severe sxs, hearing loss; toxic, w/ fever; tx w/ IV abx, ± ENT c/s for myringotomy; admit (only cause of peripheral vertigo that usually needs admx) • **Toxic:** Due to medication ototoxicity; progressive sxs, often w/ hearing loss, tinnitus, NO nystagmus
Vestibular neuronitis (*Acta Otolaryngol* 1983;96(5–6):389)	• Noninflammatory d/o of vestibular system (poss 2/2 viral etiol) • **Hx:** Sudden onset, severe, isolated vertigo (no auditory sx); progressive over h & then gradually subsides, but may have persistent mild sxs for wk/mo; May have h/o prior infxn/toxin; ± nystagmus, abnl gait (fall to affected side) • **Tx:** Symptomatic tx (see above), reassurance • Resolves over d–mo
Ménière Dz (*J Vestib Res* 2015;25(1):1)	• Increased pressure w/i inner ear endolymphatic system, either due to known cause (metabolic, endocrine, trauma, meds, etc) or idiopathic • **Hx:** Classic tetrad: Episodic severe vertigo (a/w N/V, lasting min to h, often most severe sx), unilateral chgs in hearing, tinnitus, & sensation of ear fullness or pressure; sx followed nonspec fatigue & nausea × d, then prolonged sx-free remission • **Tx:** Supportive care, trigger avoidance, if severe may warrant trial of diuretics or steroids (limited supporting data)
Acoustic neuroma (also called vestibular schwannoma)	• Intracranial benign neoplasm arising from Schwann cells encasing vestibular or cochlear nerve; cause sx both by affecting signal transmission on affected nerve or by mass effect • **Hx:** Gradual onset, progressive unilateral sensorineural hearing loss (most common sx), ± tinnitus, HA, imbalance (rarely frank vertigo), facial weakness/numbness, a/w NFII • **Dx:** Unlike other causes of peripheral vertigo, dx requires neuroimaging (MRI w/ contrast) • **Tx:** Observation (if few sx), surgical excision, stereotactic XRT

CRANIAL NERVE DISORDERS

Facial Droop (*Ann Emerg Med* 2018;71(5):618)

- **Definition:** Unilateral weakness of the facial muscles, w/ or w/o other neuro deficits; either due to central (upper motor neuron) or peripheral (lower motor neuron) etiologies
- Strength of eye closure & eyebrow elevation helps differentiate central vs peripheral:
  - Central etiology *spares* forehead due to bilateral innervation → *w/u for stroke*
- Bedside fingerstick blood Gluc early b/c hypoglycemia can cause this

Differential Diagnosis for Facial Droop	
Location	**Differential**
Peripheral	Bell's palsy (idiopathic), facial nerve injury, postsurgical (parotidectomy), infectious (Lyme dz, mastoiditis, HSV, HIV, VZV [Ramsay Hunt synd]), acoustic neuroma, parotid malignancy, botulism, sarcoidosis
Central	CVA/TIA, intracranial bleed, Todd paralysis, Guillain–Barré synd, cerebral vasculitis/arteritis, MS, myasthenia gravis, progressive supranuclear palsy, infxn (meningitis, encephalitis, brain abscess), mass lesion, sarcoidosis, Lyme

Localizing the Lesion in Facial Droop					
Location	Upper Face	Lacrim*	Saliva* Taste**	± Associated sx	Common Causes
Cortex***	Intact	Intact	Intact	UE weak	Infarct
Subcortical***	Intact	Intact	Intact	UE weak	Infarct
Pons	Weak	Intact	Intact	UE weak/numb, ataxia, nystagmus, CN VI palsy	Infarct, glioma, MS
CPA	Weak	Intact	Intact	Tinnitus, face numb ataxia, nystagmus	Neoplasm, AVM, sarcoid
IAC proximal to geniculate gang	Weak	Change	Change	Tinnitus, hearing loss, nystagmus	Bell's palsy, acoustic neur., Ramsay hunt
IAC/FC distal to geniculate gang	Weak	Intact	Change	Tinnitus, hearing loss, nystagmus	Bell's palsy, acoustic neur., AOM
FN distal to SMF	Weak	Intact	Intact	None (except if trauma, parotid)	Head injury, parotid path

*Lacrimation and salivation innervated from nucleus superior salivatory nerve in pons via nervus intermedius (both) & chorda tympani (salivation only).
**Taste innervated from nucleus of fascia solitarius in pons via nervus intermedius & chorda tympani.
***Cortical and subcortical lesions contralateral to sx (all others ipsilateral).
IAC, internal auditory canal; FC, facial canal; FN, facial nerve; SMF, stylomastoid foramen.
NEJM 2004;351(13):1323–1331.

Bell's Palsy

History (*Otolaryng Neck Surg* 2013;149:S1)

- Acute onset (over h) painless unilateral facial droop not sparing the forehead, ± aching of ear (60%), taste disturbances (60%), hyperacusis (30%), dry eye, ± cheek/mouth paresthesias (but true sensory loss suggests central lesion)
  - RFs: Adult, diabetics, pregnancy, tick exposure, HTN, recent URI
  - Evaluate risk for more concerning pathology: RFs for TIA/CVA, sx of neoplasm, etc
- Accounts for ~50% of all facial palsies. Can be bilateral, but this requires further w/u
- Unclear etiology (proposed: ischemic mononeuropathy, HSV reactivation in geniculate g)

Physical Examination

- Paralysis *must include forehead;* inability to smile or close eye, drooling, hyperacusis
  - Assess for chgs in lacrimation, salivation, & taste (see above)
- Look for findings of spec etiology; eg, erythema migrans (Lyme), vesicles (HSV)

Evaluation

- Labs & imaging not routinely indicated if typical presentation
- If atypical presentation, other signs, systemic sxs: Neuroimaging & neuro c/s

Treatment (*Neurology* 2012;79(22):2209; *CMAJ* 2014;186(12)917)

- Artificial tears, tape eyelid before sleeping to prevent corneal injury (cannot close lids)
- Prednisone 60 mg QD × 5, then slow taper (NNT 11) (*Cochrane* 2010;3:CD001942)
- *No empiric abx/antivirals*, but consider in addition to steroids if concerned or severe: Acyclovir (HSV), doxycycline (Lyme)
  - No clear benefit of antiviral tx in Bell's (*Cochrane* 2009;4:CD001869)

Disposition

- Home w/ reassurance, neuro f/u if paralysis persists for months or worsening
- Prognosis: >70% complete recovery in 3–5 mos, severe sequelae <5% (*Acta Otolaryngol Suppl* 2002;(549):4)

Diplopia

Approach (*Semin Neurol* 2010;30:54)

- Binocular (sxs only w/ both eyes open) vs monocular (primary ophthalmologic)
- Hx: Timing of onset, direction of diplopia, presence of pain, other associated sxs

Differential Diagnosis for Diplopia	
Location	**Differential**
Binocular	Basilar artery thrombosis, aneurysm, vertebral artery dissection, ischemic neuropathy, IIH, entrapment, orbital myositis or mass, thyroid myopathy, Miller Fisher, MS, migraine, brainstem mass or infarct, cavernous sinus thrombosis, Wernicke, myasthenia gravis, botulism, meningitis
Monocular	Astigmatism, cataract, lens dislocation, dry eyes

Specific Cranial Neuropathies

- Oculomotor (CN III) palsy: Diplopia in all directions except lateral gaze to affected side
  - Exam w/ affected eye deviated down and out w/ dilated pupil and ptosis
  - If 2/2 microvascular ischemia (HTN, DM), pupil is classically spared
  - If 2/2 compression (aneurysm), pupil is classically dilated
- Trochlear (CN IV) palsy: Rotational diplopia that worsens on gaze down and toward nose
- Abducens (CN VI palsy: Diplopia that worsens on lateral gaze to affected side)
- Isolated mononeuropathy ddx: Demyelinating process, hypertensive or diabetic vasculopathy, compression from aneurysm, elevated ICP (most commonly CN VI)
- Mx cranial neuropathy ddx: Cavernous sinus infxn or mass (CN III, IV, VI), CNS infxn, malignancy, metabolic dz

INTRACRANIAL HEMORRHAGE

Overview (*Emerg Med Clin North Am* 2016;34(4):883)

Approach

- Immediate IV access; low threshold for intubation if GCS <8 or declining; assess for e/o herniation (give empiric hyperosmolar tx); emergent neuroimaging, NSGY/neurology c/s
  - Attend to concurrent life-threatening pathology (eg, ATLS, ACLS)
- Pts w/ ICH can decompensate rapidly 2/2 ↑ ICP

History & Physical Examination

- **HX:** Acuity/timing of onset, position, severity, duration, circumstances surrounding onset (trauma, exertion, Valsalva, cocaine), associated sx (HA, N/V, vision chgs, focal neuro sx, speech or behavior chg, fatigue, neck pain, sz, AMS), PMH (HTN, cancer, connective tissue d/o), FHx (ICH, aneurysm/AVM, PCKD), SHx (ETOH, cocaine), Meds (A/C, anti-plt)
- **EXAM:** VS; NIHSS (see section under Ischemic Stroke), GCS, motor/sensory & coordination, meningeal signs, e/o trauma
- Signs of impending herniation: ↓ GCS, asymmetric nonreactive pupil, decorticate or decerebrate posturing, Cushing reflex (↑ BP, ↓ HR)

Evaluation

- CBC, BMP, PT/INR, PTT, type & screen
- STAT noncontrast CT head to evaluate location & extent of bleeding
  - Based on type of ICH, CTA may help clarify vascular etiology (eg, AVM, aneurysm) or active contrast extravasation (spot sign)
- MRI useful for detecting underlying lesion (CVA, mass), but given timing, CT preferred
- NSGY consultation: If ↑ ICP & ↓ GCS, may need bolt, drain, craniotomy vs craniectomy

Treatment (*Stroke* 2015;46(7):2032)

- Reverse A/C: See section on A/C Reversal (Section XI: Hematology, Oncology, & Immunology)
- Optimize BP (SBP >90 and <140–160 mmHg): Nicardipine, Clevidipine, Labetalol, Esmolol gtt 1st line; Consider IV enalaprilat or labetalol if no need for continuous gtt
  - INTERACT2 trial: No improved outcome of death or severe disability w/ intensive BP tx (SBP <140 mmHg) compared to standard (SBP <180 mmHg), but intensive BP lowering appeared safe and secondary outcomes superior inc functional outcomes (*NEJM* 2013;368(25):2355)
  - ATACH2 trial: No improved outcome of death or severe disability w/ intensive BP tx (SBP <140 mmHg) compared to standard (SBP <180 mmHg), higher adverse events in intensive tx group (*NEJM* 2016;375:1033)
- Cerebral protection: HOB elevation to 30°
- Maintain homeostasis: Minimize ↑↓ Gluc, hyperthermia, ↓ BP, ↓ O_2, ↑ CO_2, szs
- Hyperosmolar therapy to decrease ICP if signs of herniation: Hypertonic saline/mannitol
  - Neither have been shown to improve mortality or functional outcome, but small studies suggest hypertonic saline may be superior (*Crit Care* 2018;22:37)

- Sz prophylaxis not universally recommended, give if clinical or EEG evidence or sz, consider continuous EEG in AMS/coma (*Stroke* 2009;40(12):3810)
- TICH-2 trial of TXA in ICH <8 h after onset did not show benefit of functional recovery at 90 d, but there was benefit of reduction of death at 7 d (not at 90 d) and less hematoma growth over 24 h w/ low risk of adverse events (*Lancet* 2018;391:2107)

Subarachnoid Hemorrhage

Overview (*Stroke* 2012;43:1711; *West JEM* 2019:20(2):203)

- **Definition:** Acute bleed into subarachnoid space b/w pial & arachnoid mater; can be traumatic (often focal) or atraumatic (eg, ruptured aneurysm, AVM; often generalized)
  - 85% of atraumatic SAH from ruptured aneurysm, but 30–50% of these may have had prior sentinel bleed (eg, leak); important to consider sentinel bleed in ddx of HA

History & Physical Examination

- **HX:** Classically sudden "thunderclap" HA, max pain w/i 1 h, "worst HA of life", ± neck pain, N/V, photophobia, syncope or AMS, focal neuro deficits, sz
  - Red flags: Exertional/Valsalva, neck pain, arrival by ambulance, LOC, N/V
  - RFs: Age >60, FH (4× risk), HTN, smoking, alcohol, cocaine, amphetamine use, PCKD, collagen/connective tissue d/o
- **EXAM:** Ranges based on severity; if sentinel bleed w/ low-grade, may have nl neuro exam, or if high grade w/ low GCS, may be obtunded; Assess for photophobia & nuchal rigidity; May have ocular motor palsy 2/2 aneurysm compression

Evaluation

- Ottawa SAH rule: If any one criterion present, suggests pt should get full w/u (Se 100%, Sp 15%) (*JAMA* 2013;310(12):1248)

Ottawa SAH Rule (*BMJ* 2010;341:c5204)		
Age ≥40	**Applies to:**	**Exclusion criteria:**
Neck pain or stiffness	Age ≥15	New neuro deficit
Witnessed LOC	New severe atraumatic HA	Prior aneurysm or SAH
Onset during exertion	Maximum intensity w/I 1 h	Known brain tumor
Thunderclap (peak pain w/i 1 s)		Chronic recurrent HA
Limited neck flexion on exam		

- Noncontrast head CT: In pts w/ low pre-TP (*low risk* by hx & *nl* neuro exam): Se 100% (–LR 0.01) if w/i 6 h, 89% if later (*BMJ* 2011;343:d4277; *Acad Emerg Med* 2016;23(9):963–1003)
  - Inclusion criteria: HCT >30%, isolated thunderclap HA w/o sz, syncope, or neck pain, CT must be 3rd gen or newer, read by attending radiologist w/ indication of thunderclap HA (*Stroke* 2016;47(3):750)
- LP (recommended if CT not definitive based on timing, interpretation, or pt factors): ↑ opening pressure (>20 cm H_2O), RBCs, Xanthochromia (100% Se if >12 h)
  - No established "lower limit" for RBCs: Mx "test thresholds" have been studied, inc visible xanthochromia (Se 31%, Sp 98%), RBC <1 K × 10^6/L in Tube 4 (pooled Se 76%, Sp 88%; +LR 5.7, –LR 0.21); Spectrophotometric bilirubin (Se 100%, Sp 95%; +LR 28.8, –LR 0.22) (*Acad Emerg Med* 2016;23(9):963–1003)
  - Use shared decision making, low diagnostic utility after CT if performed w/I 6 h (*J Emerg Med* 2016;50(4):696), if after 6 h, LP revealed aneurysm in 0.4% (*Acad Emerg Med* 2015;22(11):1267)
- CTA: Reaches sens of 98% for bleed, if neg CTA and NCHCT posttest probability of SAH <1% (*Acad Emerg Med* 2010;(4):444)
  - CTA w/ shared decision making can be used as alternative to LP after neg NCHCT if high risk for SAH (*Ann Emerg Med* 2019;74(19):e41)
  - Obtain CTA if SAH is diagnosed in order to localize aneurysm/AVM
- Conventional angiography: Gold standard for localizing aneurysm/AVM if CTA neg

Treatment

- See Approach above; early consultation to NSGY critical for aneurysm coiling/clipping
- Per guideline, goal SBP 140–160 mmHg (*Stroke* 2023;54(7):e314–e370)
- 70% of SAH will have vasospasm (usually 3–21 d, peak 7–10 d), causing delayed cerebral ischemia; nimodipine (60 mg q4h PO ×21 d) should be started w/i 96 h of SAH

Disposition

- Admit, may need ICU; prognosis dependent on severity, neuro s/s, GCS

Subdural & Epidural Hematoma

Overview

- **Definition:** Bleeding into the subdural or epidural spaces due either to trauma (EDH, SDH) or tearing of the bridging veins from rapid acceleration/deceleration injury (SDH), occasionally there is no h/o trauma present (SDH)
- Both cause sx as a result of mass effect on brain parenchyma & are NSGY emergencies

History, Physical Examination, Evaluation, & Treatment

- See section on EDH & SDH in Trauma chapter as well as General Approach above to ICH

Nontraumatic Intraparenchymal Hemorrhage

Overview (*Lancet* 2018;392(10154):1257)

- **Definition:** Hemorrhage often w/i the subcortical white matter or (less likely) brainstem, causing sx due to mass effect, vasogenic edema & localized inflammation
- Classified as either primary (HTN, amyloid angiopathy) or secondary (coagulopathy, AVM or AVF, aneurysm, neoplasm, CSVT, vasculitis, endocarditis, PRES, hemorrhagic conversion of ischemic infarct)
- Intraventricular hemorrhage and hydrocephalus are independent prognostic determinants (*Stroke* 1998;29(7):1352)

Characteristic Appearance & Location of Common Nontraumatic Etiologies		
Cause	**Typical Location**	**Typical Appearance**
HTN	Int capsule, thalamus, cerebellum/pons	Round, homogenous
CAA	Lobar (cortical/subcortical)	Round, homogenous
Coagulopathy	Lobar	Irregularly shaped
*Neoplasm	Variable; may be mx	Surrounding edema

*Common neoplasms: Primary CNS tumors, melanoma, lung, breast (*Semin Roentgenol* 2014:49(1):112–126).

History, Physical Examination, Evaluation, & Treatment

- See Approach above to ICH

Disposition

- Admit to neurology if no e/o aneurysm/AVM on CTA; often require ICU

ISCHEMIC STROKE

Overview (*Neurosurgery* 2019;85:S38)

Approach

- Requires immediate & rapid assessment; utility of thrombolysis is time limited
- Immediate IV access, Tele, supplemental O_2 if hypoxic, neuro c/s if tPA candidate
- Quick assessment of ABCs: If GCS <8 but RR & O_2 nl, weigh risk/benefits of sending pt to CT scan w/o intubation, intubate if concern for imminent deterioration
  - If possible, obtain pt advanced directive (goals of care) to guide resuscitation
- All pts need STAT fingerstick Gluc to r/o hypoglycemia as cause of sx
- Goal to R/O TIA, Sz, & ICH ASAP & provide lytics if w/i eligible time frame and identify LVO for possible thrombectomy

History

- Establish time of onset (if unwitnessed, establish time "last known well"), sx progression (stable vs improving), circumstances surrounding onset (recent health, trauma, sz, toxins), medical sx (CP, SOB, n/v)
  - Complaints may be vague (AMS, numb, weak, vision Δ, dysarthria)
- Assess RFs for ischemic CVA (HTN/HLD, DM, AF, CAD/PVD, CHF, Valve dz, hypercoagulable states, PFO [5–10% of pop w/ clinically significant PFO])
- Assess for other causes (see table), inc. recrudescence ("unmasking") of old CVA

Differential Diagnosis for Ischemic Stroke	
CNS	TIA, ICH, neoplasm, sz (Todd paralysis), recrudescence of prior CVA (eg, 2/2 infxn, metabolic, GIB; may not have known CVA hx), complex migraine, cerebral venous sinus thrombosis
Vascular	Aortic dissection, cervical arterial dissection (carotid, vertebral), endocarditis, HTN encephalopathy, PRES
Tox/Metabolic	↓ Gluc, ↑↓ Na, Wernicke encephalopathy, drug tox
Hematologic	TTP
Other	Bell's palsy, conversion d/o, cryptogenic (25%)

Physical

- Quick but detailed neuro exam using NIH Stroke Scale (see below) (*Stroke* 2018;49(3):e46)
  - Score >/6 has Se 87%, Sp 52% for LVO, >/10 Se 73%, Sp 74% (*Stroke* 2018;49(3):e111)
  - NIHSS has limited value in posterior circ and parietal stroke (*Arch Neurol* 2001;58(4):621)
- Check for arrhythmia, murmur, bruits, & rectal for occult blood if considering lytics

NIH Stroke Scale (*Stroke* 1994;25:2220)		
Variable	**Finding**	**Points**
Consciousness	Alert, keenly responsive	0
	Arouses w/ minor stimulation	1
	Arouses w/ repeat or painful stimulation	2
	Coma	3
Orientation (month, age)	Answers both correctly	0
	Answers one correctly	1
	Answers none correctly	2
Commands (close eyes, grip)	Performs both correctly	0
	Performs one correctly	1
	Performs none correctly	2
Best gaze	nl	0
	Partial palsy (no forced deviation)	1
	Total gaze paresis or forced deviation	2
Visual fields	No visual loss	0
	Partial hemianopsia	1
	Complete hemianopsia	2
	Bilateral hemianopsia (blind)	3
Facial palsy	None	0
	Minor paralysis (eg, flattened nasolabial fold)	1
	Partial paralysis (near total in lower face)	2
	Complete paralysis (total lower/upper face)	3
Motor arm (10 s drift)	No drift	0
	Drift but does not hit bed	1
	Some effort but drifts to bed	2
	No effort against gravity	3
	No movement	4
Motor leg (5 s drift)	No drift	0
	Drift but does not hit bed	1
	Some effort but drifts to bed	2
	No effort against gravity	3
	No movement	4
Ataxia (finger/nose, heel/shin)	Absent	0
	Present in 1 limb	1
	Present in 2 limbs	2
Sensory	nl	0
	Mild–mod loss ("pinprick feels less sharp")	1
	Severe–total loss	2
Language (writing if intubated) (*Naming objects, pictures*)	nl, no aphasia	0
	Some loss of fluency or comprehension	1
	Severe aphasia; fragmented	2
	Mute, global aphasia	3
Dysarthria (*Have pt read list of words*)	nl	0
	Slurs some words, but understandable	1
	Severe, unintelligible	2
Extinction/Inattention (*Bilateral stimulation*)	No abnlty	0
	Inattention or extinction to bilateral stimulation	1
	Profound hemi-inattention	2
Score <5 = minor, Score >20 = severe neurologic deficit		

Evaluation

- CBC, BMP, PT/INR, Troponin, UA, T&S, (+/– ESR if c/f GCA, tox screen, TSH)
- ECG: May reveal AF; cerebral T waves (deep symmetric precordial) suggest ↑ ICP (rare)
- Noncontrast CT: R/o hemorrhage & exclude other etiologies; eval for early e/o infarction (loss of grey–white differentiation, sulcal effacement, mass effect; hyperdense vessel segment)
- CT Angiography: R/o arterial dissection; localize thrombus and LVO & map vasculature limitations (eg, stenosis, tortuosity) to help guide potential EVT
- MRI: Highest Se & Sp for CVA in acute setting (initially ↑ DWI & ↓ ADC signal; after 6 h ↑ T2 FLAIR; after 16 h ↓ T1 signal), but often not immediately available
- Perfusion imaging: CTP (preferred, can be performed w/ CTA) or MRP, useful in assessing ischemic core (irreversible infarct) and tissue at risk (ischemic penumbra)
- In pts who present 6–24 h after LKW time w/ NIHSS >/6, obtain CTA w/ CTP, DW-MRI or MR-P to determine whether pt would be eligible for EVT
- Echocardiography: Eval for atrial/LV thrombus, mitral valve pathology, myxoma, PFO; diagnostic yield 4–10% (TTE) & 11–41% (TEE), but +findings often chg long-term mgmt; most useful in pts w/ abnl ECG or c/f embolic source (*Postgrad Med J* 2014;90(1066):434–438).
- Once CVA dx'ed: addx tests to evaluate RF (HgbA1c, Lipid panel) & guide 2° prevention

Transient Ischemic Attack

Overview (*Stroke* 2014;45(7):2160)

- **Definition:** Acute focal neuro dysfxn 2/2 ischemia from arterial occlusion (thrombotic or embolic) but completely resolving w/i 24 h (usually <1 h) & not a/w residual tissue infarction; signals ↑ CVA risk 2/2 shared underlying pathophysiology w/ CVA
- Etiologies: Often thromboembolic event (AF, PFO, atherosclerosis), small-vessel dz, or fixed large-vessel stenosis w/ transient ↓ BP
- Risk of CVA after TIA: >5% w/I 2 d, >10% w/i 90 d (*JAMA* 2000;284:2901)
- ABCD^2 Score may predict risk, should not replace clinical judgment or dictate f/u urgency

ABCD^2 Score: Stroke Risk after TIA						
Factor	**Criteria**	**Pts**	**7-d CVA Risk***		**7-d CVA Risk****	
Age	Age >60	1	0 pts	0%	<4 pts	2.3%
BP	1st BP >140/90	1	1 pt	0%	≥4 pts	10.2%
Clinical signs	Motor weakness ± speech	2	2 pts	0%		
	Isolated speech disturbance	1	3 pts	0%	**90-d CVA Risk****	
Duration	>60 mins	2	4 pts	2.2%	<4 pts	2.4%
	10–59 mins	1	5 pts	16.3%	≥4 pts	7.2%
Diabetes	Requiring meds/insulin	1	6 pts	35.5%		

*Original study (single-community, UK) (*Lancet* 2005;366(9479):29–36).
**Pooled meta-analysis of 29 cohorts (*Neurology* 2015;85(4):304–305). Up to 1/3 of pts w/ TIA-mimics may have ABCD^2 ≥4, and 1/3 of pts w/ true TIA have ABCD^2 <4. In addition, 1/5 pts w/ ABCD^2 <4 have >50% carotid stenosis, needing urgent f/u. Thus, score should accompany clinical judgement, eval of other CVA RFs (cervical arterial stenosis), and strong consideration should be given to ED neurology c/s to guide mgmt & urgency of f/u.

History & Physical Examination

- See Approach; If acute, emphasis should be placed on assessing degree of resolution

Evaluation

- If sx not fully resolved (NIHSS >0): W/u as acute CVA (noncontrast CT & CTA)
- If sx fully resolved (NIHSS = 0): May defer CT & obtain MRI/MRA w/i 24 h, unless c/f other etiologies (eg, partial sz 2/2 underlying neoplasm)
- Assess for etiology of TIA (echo, carotid imaging, Holter, MRI/MRA), usually as inpt

Treatment (*Stroke* 2021;52(7):e364–e467)

- Tx focuses on short- & long-term risk reduction
- ASA (325 mg QD) ± clopidogrel (75 mg QD) based on severity of intracranial stenosis
- BP control: In acute setting, may be reasonable to avoid active BP control for >24 h unless markedly elevated (>220/120) or concurrent medical condition requiring ↓ BP; if BP remains elevated after 1st several d, tx w/ goal BP <130/90
- High-intensity statin therapy regardless of LDL-C level
- Anti-coagulation if e/o Afib/Aflutter (VKA or NOAC); if CI to A/C, ASA ± clopidogrel
- Carotid revascularization: Recommended for high grade (>70%) & mod (50–69%, NNT 15; if not otw high surgical risk) stenosis no risk reduction if stenosis <50%; if able to undergo CEA, CEA preferred over CAS (*Cochrane* 2012;9:10:662–668)
- Lifestyle modifications: Screen for and treat DM, weight loss, diet/low-salt, exercise, ↓ ETOH, ↓ tobacco, sleep study, A1c <7%

Disposition

- Admit if 1st TIA, mx TIAs in short time, cardiogenic, or posterior circulation
  - In some stroke centers, select cases can be managed outpt (eg, recent full w/u)
- ABCD[2] is a useful data point but not well validated as a dispo tool

Pearl

- Recurrent TIAs w/ different sxs are likely cardiac emboli; if same sxs, likely cerebral

Ischemic Stroke

Overview

- **Definition:** Acute focal neuro dysfxn 2/2 ischemia causing tissue infarction, often due to acute arterial occlusion (embolic >25% thrombotic > vascular dissection, etc) or fixed stenosis w/ hypotension

History, Physical Examination, & Evaluation

- See Approach; If acute, initial assessment should not delay imaging & decision to provide lytic tx (apart from reviewing CIs)
- Sxs & exam findings will depend on arterial distribution affected (see table)
- Anterior circulation: Unilateral motor/sensory deficit (eg, numbness, weakness, facial droop, monocular blindness [amaurosis fugax], aphasia)
- Posterior circulation: Nonlateralizing sxs (eg, diplopia, dysarthria, dysphagia, ataxia)
- ASPECT (Alberta Stroke program Early CT) Score: 10-point scale used to quantify MCA territory ischemic burden, has been studied as screening tool for endovascular thrombectomy (EVT) eligibility (*North Am Ed* 2016;387(10029):1723)
  - Score 10: no ischemic chgs; score <6: high ischemic burden, may benefit from EVT
  - Score may worsen w/ time ("ASPECTS decay") so important to obtain repeat imaging when pt is transferred from OSH (*J NeuroIntervent Surg* 2015;7(1):22)

Common Ischemic Stroke Patterns	
Stroke Location	**Presentation**
Ophthalmic Art.	Transient painless monocular vision loss (often embolic from ICA)
Internal Carotid Art.	See ACA & MCA: profound motor & sensory deficits
Ant. Cerebral Art.	C/L hemiparesis & sensory loss (leg, perineum > arm, face) ± impaired judgment/confusion, ± incontinence (pelvic floor weakness), ± disconnection synd (↓ awareness of I/L body, 2/2 corpus callosum infarction)
Mid. Cerebral Art.	C/L hemiparesis & sensory loss (face, arm > leg, perineum) ± aphasia (if dominant hemisphere; Broca/receptive [frontal] or Wernicke/expressive [temporal]) or neglect (if nondominant)
Post. Cerebral Art.	Homonymous hemianopsia ± cortical blindness
	± Agnosia (object recognition), alexia (word recognition), prosopagnosia (face recognition), memory deficits
	± Prominent contralateral sensory chgs w/o paralysis (thalamus)
Lacunar Art.	Pure hemiplegia (pons/internal capsule), pure sensory (thalamus), clumsy hand & dysarthria synd (pons), unilateral leg paresis & ataxia (pons/internal capsule)
Common Posterior Fossa Syndromes (*QJM* 2013;106(7):607–615)	
Post. Inf. Cerebellar Art. (Lateral Medullary Synd, Wallenberg)	NO motor deficits Sensory: *Crossed* sensory loss on I/L face, C/L arm/leg Ataxia: I/L limb & truncal (veer/lean) ataxia Oculobulbar: Ocular (diplopia, nystagmus, ocular torsion), bulbar (dysarthria, dysphagia, hiccups, uvular deviation) Autonomic sx: Horner synd
Ant. Inf. Cerebellar Art. (Lat Pontine Synd)	I/L facial weakness & sensory loss I/L sensorineural hearing loss (labyrinthine art.) Ataxia, nystagmus
Basilar Art. (pontine)	Impaired or alternating responsiveness (may present w/ coma) Various B/L motor sxs, inc bulbar ± Visual impairment/cortical blindness
	• "Locked-in syndrome": Only ocular muscles remain intact

Treatment (*Stroke* 2018;49:e46; 2019;50:e344)

- Early Neurology C/S & imaging: Recommended door-to-physician, ≤10 mins; door-to-stroke team, ≤15 mins; door-to-CT initiation, ≤25 mins; door-to-CT interpretation, ≤45 mins

- ASA 325 mg PO/PR. May use clopidogrel, ticlopidine, or warfarin per neurology
- BP control: Labetalol (IV) & Nicardipine (gtt) 1st line, use short-acting IV agents
  - If TPA candidate: BP goal <185/110 (lysis contraindicated if >185/110 after 2 doses)
  - If not TPA candidate: Treat only if persistently >220/120, s/s other end-organ damage (eg, AMI), or alternative med condition needing BP control; lower ≤10–20%
- If arterial dissection or suspected cardioembolic stroke, may consider AC w/ heparin
- EVT (typically w/ tPA) (eg, Merci retrieval system): Recanalization w/ Merci retrieval 57%, in combo w/ IA tPA 70%; ICH risk 7–10% (*Stroke* 2008;39(4):1205)
  - Indications for EVT w/i 6 h from LKW: prestroke mRS 0–1, causative occlusion of ICA or MI, age ≥18, NIHSS ≤6, ASPECTS ≥6, tx can be initiated w/i 6 h
  - DEFUSE3 (*NEJM* 2018;378:708) and DAWN (*NEJM* 2018;378:11) trials showed benefit of EVT 6–24 h after LKW in pts w/ clinical deficits out of proportion to infarct size or based on perfusion imaging, respectively
- Lytic therapy (rtPA 0.9 mg/kg): In selected pts w/i appropriate timeframe & w/o CIs
  - Odds of favorable recovery decrease w/ time after sx onset (see table)
  - Risks of tPA: ICH (6% risk, clinically significant 1–2%), angioedema (1-5), systemic bleeding; ↑ 7 d mortality, but no ↑ mortality at final f/u (*Lancet* 2012;379(9834):2364–2372)
  - See table below for inclusion criteria, absolute & relative Cis
  - WAKE UP trial (*NEJM* 2018;379(7):611): MRI guided (acute ischemic lesion on DWI but no hyperintensity on FLAIR) tPA for pts w/ unknown onset of sxs and LKW >4.5 h, found improvement of neuro outcomes at 90 d in tPA group, but trial stopped early
  - Intra-arterial tPA (available at some stroke centers) may be preferred (w/ or w/o prior IV tPA) for proximal lesions (distal ICA, MCA, basilar), severe sx, CI to systemic tPA, or delayed presentation after sx onset up to 6 h
- For pts w/ minor noncardioembolic ischemic stroke who did not receive tPA, initiate dual anti-PLT w/i 24 h w/ ASA + clopidogrel (*NEJM* 2013;369:11)

Pooled Odds of Favorable Outcome After TPA			
Time of TPA administration after sx	**0–1.5 h**	**1.5–3.0 h**	**3.0–4.5 h**
Odds of favorable neuro recovery at 3 mo	**2.81**	**1.55**	**1.40**

Data pooled from 6 RCTs (*Lancet* 2004;363(9411):768–774); no change in mortality w/ different timing of tx.

Criteria for Thrombolysis in Acute Stroke
Inclusion Criteria
• Age >18 • Clinical Dx of acute ischemic stroke w/ measurable neuro deficit • Time of onset <3 h (well established), or <4.5 h in some centers • Consider in unknown time of onset w/ LKW >4.5 h and sx recognition <4.5 h w/ MRI DWI positive, FLAIR neg lesion (*NEJM* 2018;379(7):611)
Absolute CIs to Lysis
• CTH shows ICH or very large stroke (>33% of hemisphere) • High clinical suspicion for SAH (even w/ nl CTH) or endocarditis • Active internal bleeding (eg, GIB) • Bleeding diathesis (PLT <100K, heparin in past 48 h w/ elevated PTT, A/C w/ INR >1.7, DOAC use) • Stroke, intracranial surgery, or head trauma in past 3 mo • Abnl blood Gluc (<50 mg/dL) • Recent arterial puncture at noncompressible site • Prior ICH, AVM, aneurysm, or known intracranial neoplasm • Refractory HTN (SBP >185 mmHg & DBP ≥110 mmHg despite tx)
Relative CIs (weigh risk–benefit)
• Minor or rapidly resolving sxs • Witnessed sz at time of stroke onset • Recent LP or arterial puncture at noncompressible site • Acute MI in past 3 mos, post-MI pericarditis • Recent GI/GU hemorrhage in past 3 wks • Major surgery or serious trauma in past 2 wks • Pregnancy
Additional Relative CIs (for use *after 3 h & before 4.5 h*)
• Age >80 • NIHSS >25 (suggests large stroke) • Oral anticoagulant use (regardless of INR) • Combination of prior ischemic strokes & DM • CT shows multilobar infarct (hypodensity >1/3 cerebral hemisphere)

Disposition
- Admit all pts; Large strokes may need ICU (risk of edema, hemorrhagic conversion)

Pearls
- Inpt w/u includes carotid imaging, echo, Holter monitor, advanced serology (hypercoagulability, lipids, bleeding diathesis, ESR, ANA, TSH)
- NIHSS correlates w/ neuro outcome at 3 mos but poor predictor for posterior CVAs

NEUROMUSCULAR SYNDROMES

Myasthenia Gravis

Overview (*Neurohospitalist* 2011;1(1):16)
- **Definition:** Autoimmune d/o (Abs against *post*synaptic ACh nicotinic receptors) causing progressive weakness of incremental muscle groups, w/ intermittent crises marked by potential need for ventilatory support
- Epidemiology: Most commonly affects women in 20s–40s, men in 50s–70s (peak)
- Myasthenia crisis: Respiratory failure leading to mechanical ventilation
- DDx includes Lambert–Eaton myasthenic syndrome (LEMS) and botulism
  - LEMS: Auto-abs decrease release of ACh from nerve terminals leading to weakness, proximal > distal, paraneoplastic synd, weakness improves w/ activity, autonomic dysfxn, tx focused on underlying dz +/– IVIG
  - Botulism: Caused by *C. botulinum* toxin that irreversibly binds to presynaptic nerve terminal and inhibits release of ACh, blocks autonomic and motor function, no pain or sensory deficits, most often caused by ingestion of contaminated food, classically descending paralysis w/ bulbar and anticholinergic sxs, treat w/ antitoxin

History
- Gradual, symmetric, fluctuating proximal & ocular muscle weakness, worsens w/ activity
  - Common: Extraocular/ptosis (present in 50% initially), bulbar, limb (prox > distal); however, w/i 1 y most pts have generalized involvement
  - Sx least severe in morning; worsen w/ repetitive activity & throughout d
- Assess for triggers of crisis: Stress, infxn, pregnancy, surgery, med chgs (abx, steroids, BBs, CCBs, levothyroxine, lidocaine, stopping anticholinergics)
- If advanced dz: Obtain clear goals of care in case need for intubation

Physical Examination
- Proximal weakness & fatigability worse w/ repetitive activity, relieved by rest
- CN affected early (ocular: ptosis, diplopia; bulbar: dysarthria, dysphagia)

Grading Score for Motor Strength
5 = nl strength
4 = weak but able to resist
3 = moves against gravity but unable to resist
2 = moves but unable to resist gravity
1 = flicker but not able to move
0 = no movement

Evaluation
- Neuro C/S: if new onset, poor outpt f/u, or probable need for admx
- If new dx: AChR Ab test has high Sp, but poor Se, esp in localized dz; Tensilon (edrophonium) test (2 mg IV over 15 s; binds to AChE, blocking ACh hydrolysis)
  - If no adverse rxn but ptosis not improved, can give up to 10 mg total
  - Tensilon test may precipitate bradycardia, heart block, airway secretions—have atropine at bedside
  - Alternative is ice bag test: place ice bag over eyes for 2 mins, positive if ptosis improved by at least 2 mm (Se 94%, Sp 97% for ocular MG)
- If known dx: Differentiate MG crisis from cholinergic crisis (most pts on cholinergic meds)
  - Cholinergic tox: Lacrimation, salivation, perspiration, bronchorrhea, N/V, diarrhea, brady
- Measuring NIF (neg inspiratory force) and VC (vital capacity) can identify pts at risk of respiratory failure; NIF <20 cm H_2O &/or VC <1 L or <20–25 mL/Kg (less Se) suggests severe resp weakness (*Semin Neurol* 2003;23:97)

Treatment
- Ventilatory support as indicated (NIPPV, intubation)
- Plasmapheresis & IVIG: Tx for acute crisis (*Cochrane Database Syst Rev* 2012;CD002277)
- Corticosteroids given in crisis but can worsen sx initially; minimal short-term effect, immunosuppressants also used for chronic control
- Long-term txs include AChE-inh (pyridostigmine) & immunomod (steroids, etc), IV therapy not recommended in ED for myasthenic crisis given PLEX and IVIG highly effective
- Thymectomy can lead to remission or reduction of other chronic medications

Disposition
- Admit all pts w/ myasthenia crisis, may require ICU per respiratory status
- If no e/o crisis & good outpt f/u, can d/c w/ close outpt f/u

---

Amyotrophic Lateral Sclerosis (ALS)

Overview (*Lancet* 2011;377(9769):942)
- **Definition:** Degenerative dz of UMNs & LMNs
- Epidemiology: Age >40, M = F
- DDx includes poliomyelitis (affects anterior horn cells resulting in lower motor neuron dz), neuropathies (distal weakness that ascends), myelopathy (spinal cord pathology, p/w signs of upper motor neuron dz +/– bowel and bladder involvement)

History, Physical Examination, & Evaluation
- **HX:** Progressive motor weakness & atrophy, fasciculations, spasm; NO sensory loss
  - Assess pt goals of care regarding life-support interventions inc airway
- **EXAM:** UMN & LMN findings, initially distal; fasciculations 2/2 denervation; may have bulbar findings (dysphagia, dysarthria) in advanced dz, spasticity, ↑ DTRs, +Babinski
  - Bladder & bowel sphincters & ocular muscles often spared
- **DX:** If new onset, neuro c/s & consider MRI brain & spinal cord

Upper vs. Lower Motor Signs			
Motor Neuron	**Deep Tendon Reflexes, Tone**	**Atrophy, Fasciculations**	**Babinski**
Upper Motor	Increased	No	Present
Lower Motor	Decreased	Yes	Absent

Treatment
- Supportive care (respiratory support, antispasmodics)
- In pts w/ known dx, treat cx (DVT from immobility, asp PNA, UTI, decubitus ulcers)
- Chronic tx: riluzole (prolongs survival), may have PEG for nutrition

Disposition
- Depends on respiratory status, acuity

DEMYELINATING SYNDROMES

Guillain–Barré Syndrome

Overview (*NEJM* 2012;366:2294)
- **Definition:** Acute inflammatory demyelinating peripheral polyneuropathy, often in response to external infectious exposure (or vaccination) & characterized by loss of peripheral nerve reflexes and albuminocytologic dissociation
- Common associated pathogens: *Campylobacter* (~30%), EBV, CMV, HIV, *Mycoplasma*
- Slow recovery (can take mos in worst affected); 5% die from cx (sepsis, PE, dysautonomia)
- DDx: Neuromuscular dz, tick paralysis, spinal cord injury

History, Physical Examination, & Evaluation
- **HX:** Progressive ascending weakness; can start w/ numbness/paresthesias or pain in LEs, f/b symmetric b/l weakness over h–wks
  - Usually (2/3) heralded by recent URI or diarrheal illness d–wk prior to sx
- **EXAM:** Acute ascending symmetric weakness, sensory chgs, ↓ DTRs (however, 10% of early cases will have DTRs), 20% will have autonomic dysfxn & potentially-fatal arrhythmias; ± CNS (hallucinations, psychosis, vivid dreams) (*NEJM* 2012;366:2294–2304)
  - Miller Fisher variant = triad of ataxia, areflexia, ophthalmoplegia

- **DX:** Clinical dx; w/u generally to r/o other dx
  - CPK nl (acute myopathy may present similarly but nl sensation & ↑ CPK)
  - LP (can r/o lyme, lymphoma): Albuminocytologic dissociation (↑ protein, no WBCs or bacteria) only present 50% of cases in 1st wk, 75% by 3rd wk (*NEJM* 2012;366:2294–2304)
  - Assess NIF and FVC for respiratory status; FVC <20 mL/kg or NIF <30 cm H_2O associated w/ need for intubation (*Ann Neurol* 2010;67:781)
  - If abnl respiratory parameters obtain ABG

Treatment

- C/s neurology
- Hemodynamic stabilization: Tele (risk for arrhythmia; some pts may need PPM), rapidly titratable vasoactive agents as needed for dysautonomia
- Respiratory support as indicated (25% pts need intubation): Avoid succinylcholine for RSI
- Plasmapheresis & IVIG equally effective; combo not superior
- Steroids have limited effectiveness in speeding recovery

Disposition

- Admit until no e/o progression; ICU if respiratory compromise
- Prognosis: Full recovery can take mos & can be c/b mx dz (PNA, sepsis, PE, etc)

MULTIPLE SCLEROSIS (MS)

Overview (*Lancet* 2017;389(10076):1336)

- **Definition:** Progressive chronic immune-mediated demyelinating dz of the CNS
  - Generally follows relapsing-remitting (85–90%; may not have complete recovery b/w relapses) or primary progressive course (usually w/o relapses)
- Epidemiology: Relapsing-remitting presents young (30 y) & F > M (3:1); primary-progressive presents older (40 y) & F = M; ↑↑ risk if 1st-degree relative also affected
- Dx requires 2+ distinct episodes w/ differential neuro sxs &/or MRI findings (findings separated in time and space w/ no alterative Dx (*Ann Neurol* 2011;69:292))
- Neuromyelitis optica spectrum d/o: A/w serum aquaporin 4 IgG, distinct dz from MS w/ distinct tx (*Neurology* 2015;85:177)

History

- Acute episodes develop over h–d (also remit over same time course)
  - Look for precipitating factors for exacerbation (eg, infxn, hyperthermia)
- Sx can be highly variable: Vision, sensation, mobility/balance, cognition, sphincter control
  - See table for typical presentations, ocular sx common
  - Uhthoff phenomenon: Sxs worsen w/ ↑ body temp (exercise, hot bath, fever)

Typical and Atypical Multiple Sclerosis Presentations (*Lancet* 2017;389(10076):1336)	
Typical	**Atypical (Consider other etiology)**
Acute unilateral optic neuritis*	Bilateral optic neuritis
Diplopia (2/2 INO or CN VI palsy)**	Unilateral optic neuritis w/ poor recovery
Facial sensory loss or trigeminal neuralgia	Complete or fluctuating gaze palsy
Cerebellar ataxia, nystagmus	Intractable n/v or hiccups
Partial myelopathy	Complete transverse myelopathy
Sensory sx in a CNS pattern	Encephalopathy
Lhermitte's sign***	Subacute cognitive decline
Asymmetric limb weakness	Headache or meningismus
Urge incontinence, erectile dysfxn	Isolated fatigue or asthenia
	Constitutional sxs

*Optic Neuritis: Painful EOM, afferent pupillary defect, decreased visual acuity, ± papilledema.
**INO: Internuclear ophthalmoplegia (affected eye is able to abduct but not adduct; unaffected eye EOM nl) due to MLF lesion; ***Lhermitte sign: Electric-shock sensation travelling down spine w/ neck flexion.

Evaluation

- Neuro c/s indicated due to clinical benefit of early dx
- MRI Brain (Se 80% in pts w/ isolated synd): Multifocal T2 hyperintense white matter lesions (periventricular, juxtacortical, infratentorial) (*Brain* 2008;131:808; *Neurology* 1999;53:448)
- MRI Spine (Se 50% in pts w/ isolated synd; mostly c-spine): Indicated if sx localize to spinal cord or MRI Brain nondiagnostic
- LP: Indicated only if uncertainty based on MRI findings; may show pleocytosis (50%) & IgG oligoclonal bands (85–95%) (*J Neurol Neurosurg Psychiatry* 2013;84:909)

Treatment (*Lancet* 2018;391(10130):1622)

- Treat any reversible underlying triggers (eg, infxn, dehydration, fevers)
- High-dose corticosteroids are 1st line for acute relapses; may consider addition of 2nd-line plasmapheresis in fulminant cases (*Neurology* 2011;76(3):294–300)
- Supportive: Spasticity (baclofen, gabapentin), pain (gabapentin, TCA), fatigue (amantadine), bladder dysfxn (oxybutynin), bowel regimen

Disposition

- Admit all new-dx for further w/u
- Most pts admitted for relapses; can D/C if mild sx, nonprogressive, & close neuro f/u

Pearl

- Due to complexity of dx, rates of mis-dx pts (ie, w/o dz) may be as high as 10% (*Lancet* 2017;389(10076):1336–1346)

TRANSVERSE MYELITIS

Overview (*NEJM* 2010;363:564)

- **Definition:** Acute or subacute inflammation & varying demyelination of a limited length of spinal cord causing motor, sensory, & autonomic dysfxn w/ sx correlating to level affected
- Often >2 vertebral seg involved; MS-associated TM can be <2 seg & partial cord
- Epidemiology: All ages affected; bimodal peak (10–19 y & 30–39 y); M = F; unrelated to FHx
- Etiologies: Postvaccination (60% in children), postinfxn, systemic autoimmune dz, or acquired demyelination dz (eg, MS), neuromyelitis optica, idiopathic (15–30%)

History, Physical Examination, & Evaluation

- **HX:** Acute or subacute paraplegia, sensory chgs (w/ definitive spinal cord level), & sphincter loss (below level); onset over h to d; bilateral but often asymmetric, often w/ neuropathic back/midline pain
  - Ask about recent viral illness, immunization, FHx of MS, vision sx (NMO)
- **EXAM:** Symmetric or asymmetric weakness & sensory loss referable to a spinal cord level, hyperreflexia, +Babinski, +Lhermitte sign (+electric radiating back pain w/ neck flexion)
- **DX:** MRI entire spine w/ contrast; Neurology c/s; If confirmed by imaging, may need LP (+pleocytosis) to help differentiate etiology & prognosticate

Transverse Myelitis Diagnostic Inclusion and Exclusions (*Neurology* 2002;59(4):499)

Inclusion	Exclusion
Bilateral sensorimotor and autonomic spinal cord dysfxn (may be asymmetric)	Radiation to spine w/I 10 y
Clearly defined sensory level	Arterial distribution of clinical deficit c/w thrombosis of anterior spinal artery
Progression of sx b/w 4 h & 21 d after sx onset	Serologic or clinical e/o connective tissue dz (sarcoid, Sjögren, Behçet, SLE, etc)
Demonstration of spinal cord inflammation*	Brain MRI abnormalities suggesting MS**
Exclusion of other etiology (compressive, postradiation, neoplastic, vascular, metabolic)	CNS manifestations of infxn (syphilis, Lyme, HIV, HTLV-1, Mycoplasma, HSV-1/2, VZV, EBV, CMV, HHV6, enteroviruses)
	H/o clinically apparent optic neuritis**
	Abnl flow voids c/w AVM

*CSF pleocytosis, elevated IgG index = (CSF IgG/serum IgG)/(CSF albumin/serum), MRI w/ contrast enhancing spinal cord lesion.

**Does not exclude dz associated with transverse myelitis.

Treatment (*NEJM* 2010;363:564)

- Ventilatory support as indicated by level of cord involvement (upper C-spine or brain stem)
- Supportive care: Analgesia (TCA, carbamazepine), spasticity (baclofen, benzos), immobility (DVT ppx, PT, rehab), GU/bowel dysfxn (oxybutynin, bowel reg)
- High-dose steroids (1-g methylprednisolone QD IV) are 1st line, esp for postinfectious or demyelinating etiology (*NEJM* 2010;363:564)
- May consider plasmapheresis if fulminant or refractory to steroids; limited data

Disposition

- Admit to neurology
- Prognosis depends on etiology: Most recovery takes mos to y
  - MS-associated TM: Quicker & complete recovery; but ↑ risk of relapse c/w idiopathic, postviral, or postimmunization

DYSURIA

Definition (*Am Fam Phys* 2025;111:37)

- Feeling of pain or discomfort during urination; often UTI, also STI, irritants, skin lesions, chronic pain

History

- HPI: Onset/severity/location, frequency/hesitancy/urgency, itching, hematuria, abnl penile/vaginal D/C, genital lesions, perineal pain, pain w/ intercourse
- ROS: Fever, trauma, flank pain, abdominal or suprapubic pain, joint/back pain
- PMH: Prior GU procedures, STIs, DM, immunocompromise
- MEDS: Topical irritants
- SOCIAL: Recent intercourse, new sexual partner, smoking, illicit drugs

Physical Examination

- All: Abdominal exam, costovertebral angle tenderness
- Women: Consider pelvic exam if risk factors for STIs, vaginal sxs, postmenopausal
- Men: Should perform penile exam, testicular exam & prostate exam given risk of complicated dz

Evaluation

- Urine studies (clean catch UA ± Ucx, hCG if female, NAAT for G/C if risk factors); CBC/chemistries rarely indicated, unless suspected complicated dz (*see below*)
- Consider vaginal/urethral studies (smear w/ wet mount, genital cx), renal U/S, CT abdomen/pelvis if warranted
- Further studies may include urine cytology, voiding cystourethrography, cystoscopy, urodynamic testing, but not routinely performed in ED

Dysuria Differential

Pathophysiology	Differential
Structural	Kidney/bladder stone, BPH, urethral stricture/diverticula, endometriosis
Infectious	Vulvovaginitis, urethritis, cervicitis, prostatitis, epididymo-orchitis, balanitis, cystitis, pyelonephritis, STDs
Meds	Cyclophosphamide, ketamine, opioids, SGLT-2 inhs, topical hygiene products (vaginal spray/douche/lubricant)
Neoplastic/autoimmune	GU cancer (penile, vulvar/vaginal, prostate, bladder), Behçet, Reiter
Other	Instrumentation, urethral trauma, interstitial cystitis, atrophic vaginitis, pelvic irradiation

URINARY TRACT INFECTIONS

Definitions

- UTIs are classified according to the predominant clinical sxs, location of the infxn, & frequency of infxn
  - **Asx bacteriuria:** Absence of urinary sxs w/ presence of bacteria in urine
  - **Acute uncomplicated cystitis:** Acute urinary sxs w/ presence of bacteria in urine
  - **Acute uncomplicated pyelonephritis:** Fever, chills, flank pain in the absence of alternative dx & urologic abnlty w/ presence of bacteria in urine
  - **Complicated UTI/pyelonephritis:** Features of uncomplicated cystitis/pyelonephritis AND 1 or more of the following—pregnancy, diabetes, male gender, immunosupp (eg, chemo, AIDS), functional GU abnlty (indwelling catheter, neurogenic bladder), structural GU abnlty (renal stone, intestinal fistula, PCKD, kidney transplant pt)
  - **Recurrent cystitis:** 2 separate culture proven episodes of acute bacterial cystitis in last 6 mos or 3 episodes w/i 1 y

Asymptomatic Bacteriuria

Definition (*Clin Inf Dis* 2019;68:e83)

- Absence of urinary sxs w/ Ucx ≥10^5 CFU/mL of 1 or more species of bacteria irrespective of presence of pyuria

Evaluation

- USPSTF: Screen for asx bacteriuria w/ Ucx for pregnant women at 12–16-wk gestation given increased risk of pyelonephritis, preterm labor & low birth weight
- USPSTF: Do not screen for asx bacteriuria in men or nonpregnant women

- The IDSA recommends against routine screening for asx bacteriuria in diabetic women, older persons >65 y/o residing in the community or institutionalized residents of long-term care facilities, spinal cord injury, & pts w/ indwelling urethral catheters

Treatment
- Only treat asx bacteriuria in pregnancy
- IDSA: careful observation rather than tx of asx bacteriuria in older patients w/ fxnl or cognitive impairment and new fall or delirium if no systemic s/sx of infxn
- 3–7-d course of nitrofurantoin or cephalosporin (cephalexin, cefpodoxime, cefdinir, cefaclor)

Pearl
- Given the high LR of leukocyte esterase (4.2) & nitrites (4.2) on UA for bacteriuria, a single positive test result in an asx pregnant pt in the ED should be considered for tx pending culture data

Acute Uncomplicated Cystitis

Definition
- Acute urinary sxs (dysuria, urgency, frequency, suprapubic pain) w/ UA ≥10 WBC/mm^3 & Ucx ≥10^3 CFU/mL (but ≥10^5 CFU/mL also used to define UTI); absence of structural/functional urogenital tract abnormalities

Pathophysiology
- Occurs when uropathogen from bowel or vagina colonize periurethral mucosa & ascend through urethra & bladder
- Predominant uropathogens: *E. coli* (75–95%), *K. pneumoniae, P. mirabilis, E. faecalis, S. saprophyticus,* & *S. agalactiae* (group B Strep); rarely *P. aeruginosa*, Ureaplasma species

History
- Combination of dysuria, frequency, hematuria, fever, back pain, &/or self-dx all increase the probability of UTI, whereas their absence decreases its probability
- Vaginal D/C or irritation w/o the above sxs decreases probability of UTI
- Risk factors: Prior UTI, sexual intercourse (esp ≥3/wks in last 30 d), new sex partner (w/i 1 y), use of spermicide, stress incontinence in previous 30 d, diabetes mellitus

Physical Examination
- ±Fever; tenderness w/ suprapubic palpation
- GU exam if vaginal D/C or irritation present

Evaluation
- CBC/BMP rarely indicated
- Urine hCG, UA (*both* +leukocyte esterase AND +nitrite most specific; *either* +LE or +nitrite more sensitive, UA ≥10 WBC/mm^3)
- Routine Ucx is not indicated
- Probability of dz in pts presenting w/ 1 or more UTI sxs is ~50%

Treatment
- Spontaneous resolution may be observed in 25–42% of untreated women
- Symptomatic tx: NSAIDs, phenazopyridine
- Antibiotic regimens:

  1st-line
  - Beta-lactams (cephalexin 500 mg PO BID, cefuroxime 500 mg PO BID, cefpodoxime 100 mg PO BID) × 3–7 d
  - Nitrofurantoin 100 mg BID × 5 d
  - Trimethoprim-sulfamethoxazole 160/800 mg (1 DS tablet) BID × 3 d (if <20% resistance in community)
  - Fosfomycin 3 g in a single dose

  Alternative regimens:
  - Fluoroquinolones (ciprofloxacin 250 mg PO BID, levofloxacin 250 mg PO QD) × 3 d

Disposition
- Home

Pearls
- Probability of cystitis >90% in women w/ sxs of UTI in the absence of vaginal D/C or irritation, thus consider empiric tx w/o UA or w/ nl UA (neg LE & nitrites do not reliably r/o UTI)
- UTI in males is rare, consider STD, prostatitis, urinary retention, immunocompromise
- Increasing *E. coli* resistance to amoxicillin & trimethoprim-sulfamethoxazole

Acute Uncomplicated Pyelonephritis

Definition

- Infxn of upper urinary tract (renal pelvis & kidney) most commonly due to ascending lower UTI (see *Acute Uncomplicated Cystitis for Common Uropathogens*)

History

- Highest incidence 15–29 y/o females, followed by infants & elderly
- Combination of constitutional sx (fever, chills, malaise), lower urinary tract sx (dysuria, frequency, hematuria) & upper urinary tract sx (flank pain); n/v
- Risk factors: Same as cystitis

Physical Examination

- ±Fever, tachycardia, hypotension; CVA tenderness (~25% b/l)
- Mental status change (esp. in elderly)

Evaluation

- CBC may show leukocytosis, but can be nl
- Chemistries (esp BUN/Cr) if renal impairment suspected
- Urine hCG, UA (+leukocyte esterase AND + nitrite has best diagnostic utility, where *either* + LE or + nitrite helpful w/ high pretest probability pts, UA ≥10 WBC/mm^3)
- Ucx & sensitivities should always be performed (usually reveals ≥10^5 CFU/mL of single uropathogen)
- Routine BCx not indicated
- Diagnostic imaging usually not indicated; can be considered to r/o alternative dx. If complicated dz suspected, if sxs do not improve, or if recurrence → CTAP > U/S

Treatment

Outpt tx

- Cefpodoxime 200 mg PO BID for 10–14 d
- Trimethoprim-sulfamethoxazole 160/800 mg (1 DS tablet) BID × 14 d
- Ciprofloxacin 500 mg PO BID × 7 d
- Levofloxacin 750 mg PO QD × 5 d

Inpt tx

- CTX 1 g (2 g if >100 kg or severe infxn) IV QD
- Ciprofloxacin 400 mg IV BID
- Levofloxacin 750 mg IV QD
- If PCN allergy, gentamicin 5 mg/kg IV QD or aztreonam 2 g IV TID
- If suspected pseudomonas, cefepime 2 g IV TID OR piperacillin-tazobactam 3.375 g IV q6h
- If suspected enterococcus, vancomycin 20 mg/kg IV load OR ampicillin 2 g IV QID + gentamicin 1 mg/kg IV TID
- If ESBL isolate, imipenem 500 mg IV q6h over 3 h or meropenem 1–2 g IV q8h over 3 h

Disposition

- Home: Most cases in well-appearing, healthy ptv
- Observation: Consider for pt requiring IVF or antiemetics, but o/w well appearing

Complicated Cystitis/Pyelonephritis

Definition

- Features of cystitis/pyelonephritis AND "complicated" as defined above

Evaluation

(See Uncomplicated Pyelonephritis for Diagnostics)

- Consider urology consultation (esp w/ known or suspected structural/functional abx, recent urologic procedure, UG tract FB, obstructive uropathy, UTI in male)

Treatment (*Ann Intern Med* 2017;167(7):ITC49–ITC64)

- Outpt & inpt tx course is same as uncomplicated pyelonephritis w/ 1 exception (fosfomycin can be used for complicated cystitis but dosing is 3 g q48h × 3 doses)
- If pregnant, treat w/ beta-lactams (cephalexin 500 mg PO QID, cefuroxime 500 mg PO BID, cefpodoxime 200 mg PO BID) × 7 d OR fosfomycin 3 g q48h × 3 doses

Disposition

- Cystitis: Home if o/w well-appearing and excellent f/u in place
- Pyelonephritis: Admit

Catheter-Associated UTI

Definition (*J Hosp Med* 2020;15:552)

- **CAUTI:** Sxs or signs compatible w/ UTI w/ no other identifiable source of infxn w/ ≥10^3 CFU/mL uropathogen in pts w/ indwelling urethral, suprapubic, or intermittent straight catheter in urine sample obtained w/i 48 h of removal

- **Catheter-associated asx bacteriuria:** Presence of ≥10^5 CFU/mL uropathogen in a catheter urine specimen in a pt w/o sxs

History
- New onset or worsening fever, rigors, AMS, malaise, or lethargy w/o identifiable cause in pt w/ catheter
- Dysuria, frequency, urgency, hematuria, suprapubic pain, flank pain in those whose catheters were recently removed

Physical Examination
- ±Fever, tachycardia, hypotension, CVA tenderness, suprapubic tenderness
- Cloudy/malodorous urine should not be used to differentiate CAUTI & CA-ASB

Evaluation
- Obtain CBC, chemistries, urine studies inc Ucx & sensitivities
- If available, review previous Ucx and sensitivities
- Obtain BCx & diagnostic imaging if febrile, tachycardic, or hypotensive
- Consider urology consultation (esp w/ known or suspected structural/functional abx, recent urologic procedure, UG tract FB, obstructive uropathy, UTI in male)

Treatment
(See Complicated UTI for Antimicrobials)
- Screening for & tx of CA-ASB are not recommended except pregnant women
- 3-d regimen may be considered in CAUTI pts ≤65 y/o w/o upper tract sxs
- 5-d regimen of levofloxacin may be considered in CAUTI pts not severely ill
- 7-d regimen recommended for CAUTI pts w/ prompt resolution of sxs
- 10–14-d regimen recommended in those w/ delayed response

Prevention
- Strongly consider indication for catheter insertion, limit catheterization chgs, aseptic technique w/ placement, among others

Disposition
- Home if no signs/sxs of upper urinary tract or systematic infxn & excellent f/u in place; o/w admit

Pearl
- Classic s/sx may be absent in spinal cord injury or neurogenic bladder, evaluate for dysautonomia or neurologic chgs

MALE UROGENITAL TRACT INFECTIONS

Urethritis

Definition
- Urethral inflammation w/ infectious or noninfectious etiology (eg, Reiter's)
- Infectious causes include gonococcal (*N. gonorrhoeae*) & nongonococcal (*C. trachomatis, M. genitalium, T. vaginalis,* HSV, adenovirus, CMV, syphilis, enteric bacteria)

History
- Highest prevalence in adolescent, sexually active men
- Dysuria, urethral pruritus, mucopurulent or purulent urethral D/C; however, asx infxns are common
- Urinary frequency & urgency typically absent
- Sexual hx: Current sexual activity, type (oral, vaginal, anal), MSM, number of sex partners, condom use, h/o STDs (esp GC/*Chlamydia*)
- Systemic sxs? (fever, sore throat, arthritis, rash, back pain)

Physical Examination
- GU exam: Urethral meatus for skin lesions, erythema, D/C (inc milking urethra for D/C); testicular/epididymal exam in men, pelvic exam in women

Evaluation
- 1st-void ("dirty") UA (may reveal + LE & ≥10 WBC/hpf), urine hCG
- Gram stain of urethral secretions w/ ≥5 WBC/hpf (presence of gram-neg intracellular diplococci c/w gonococcal dz) & culture
- Urine NAAT for *N. gonorrhoeae* & *C. trachomatis* is most sens

Treatment
- GC & *Chlamydia* coinfection common, so therapy should be geared toward both
- Doxycycline 100 mg PO BID × 7 d AND CTX 500 mg in a single IM dose
  - If pregnant or poor f/u, azithromycin 1 g PO × 1 in place of doxycycline

- Abstain from intercourse for 7 d & until all sex partners (w/i previous 60 d) are evaluated or empirically treated

Disposition
- Home w/ PCP referral for counseling & further STD testing

Pearl
- GC & *Chlamydia* are reportable to state health department
- Consider concomitant HIV testing

Acute Bacterial Prostatitis

Definition
- UTI sxs w/ e/o prostate infxn
- Chronic if >3 mo of sxs
- Predominant uropathogens (*E. coli* in 50–90% of cases. *K. pneumoniae, P. mirabilis, Enterobacter, Serratia, E. faecalis, S. saprophyticus, P. aeruginosa, U. urealyticum*) or sexually transmitted organisms (*N. gonorrhoea, C. trachomatis, T. vaginalis*)

History
- Typical age 20–45 y/o; most common urologic dx in men <50 y/o
- Acute onset fevers, chills, malaise, frequency, dysuria, poor urine stream, feeling of incomplete bladder emptying, lower back/abdominal/pelvic pain, possible sexual dysfxn (ejaculatory discomfort & hematospermia)
- Risk factors: Recent urologic intervention/instrumentation, urethritis/cystitis, BPH, urethral stricture, phimosis, immunocompromised
- Sexual hx: Current sexual activity, type (oral, vaginal, anal), MSM, number of sex partners, condom use, h/o STIs (esp GC/*Chlamydia*)
- Systemic sxs? (fever, sore throat, arthritis, rash, back pain)

Physical Examination
- ±Fever; suprapubic abdominal discomfort
- Testicular exam should be performed to r/o epididymitis/orchitis
- DRE w/ warm, tender, swollen prostate (aggressive pressure on prostate may increase risk of bacteremia)

Evaluation
- Obtain Ucx, sensitivities, urine NAAT for G/C
- Obtain CBC, BCx, & diagnostic imaging if febrile, tachycardic, or hypotensive
- Consider postvoid residual measurement, as retention may not be evident
- Consider transrectal U/S or CT if prostate abscess suspected (poor response to abx)
- Prostate biopsy as an outpt

Treatment
- Systemically ill: CTX 2 g IV QD OR ciprofloxacin 400 mg IV BID OR levofloxacin 500 mg IV QD
- Clinically stable/STI not suspected: Cipro 500 mg PO BID, levofloxacin 500 mg PO QD, TMP/SMX 160/800 mg (DS) PO BID × 4–6 wk
- Clinically stable/STI suspected: Doxycycline 100 mg PO BID × 14 d AND CTX 500 mg in a single IM dose

Disposition
- Home w/ urology f/u in most cases
- Admit if systemically ill or known antibiotic-resistant pathogen

Pearls
- 10% men w/ acute bacterial prostatitis go on to suffer chronic prostatitis & 10% progress to chronic prostatitis/chronic pelvic pain synd
- Cx: Chronic prostatitis (5–10%), acute urinary retention, prostatic abscess (~2%), sepsis

Epididymitis/Orchitis

Definition

Epididymitis & orchitis are inflammation of the epididymis & testes, respectively, w/ or w/o infxn
- Can be acute (<6 wks), subacute (6 wks–3 mos), or chronic (>3 mos) based on sx duration

Pathophysiology
- Orchitis usually occurs when inflammation spreads from epididymis to adjacent testicle (epididymo-orchitis), but isolated orchitis w/o epididymitis can be seen w/ mumps
- Epididymitis can be sexually transmitted, caused by *N. gonorrhoeae* or *C. trachomatis*, or by ascending lower UTI by common uropathogens (*see Uncomplicated UTI*);

M. tuberculosis should be considered in high-risk pts, & fungal or viral causes found in pts w/ immunodeficiency

- Noninfectious causes of epididymitis include postinfectious inflammatory rxn to pathogens (ie, *M. pneumoniae,* adenoviruses), trauma, postprostatic biopsy, postvasectomy, exercise, prolonged sitting, vasculitides, meds (ie, amiodarone)

History

- Primarily affects young men aged 18–35 y, bimodal distribution 16–30 y & 50–70 y
- Testicular pain/swelling usually beginning posteriorly overlying epididymis; lower urinary tract sx may be present
- Risk factors: Unprotected intercourse (esp anal), MSM, increased number of sex partners, h/o STDs (esp GC/*Chlamydia*), structural/functional GU abnlty, urinary tract instrumentation

Physical Examination

- ±Fever; look for CVA tenderness/suprapubic pain as e/o other urinary tract dz
- Testicular exam: Palpation of epididymis/testes, tender, erythematous, swollen spermatic cord & testicular content, intact cremasteric reflex
- Prehn sign: Relief of pain w/ elevation of testes can be seen w/ epididymitis. Inguinal exam for hernia or swollen, tender nodes.

Evaluation

- 1st-void ("dirty") UA (+LE & ≥10 WBC/hpf suggests urethritis, favors dx); Ucx
- Cx & Gram stain of urethral secretions w/ ≥5 WBC/hpf (presence of gram-neg intracellular diplococci c/w gonococcal dz)
- Urine NAAT for *N. gonorrhoeae* & *C. trachomatis*
- Imaging: Testicular ultrasonography w/ color Doppler (Findings: Thickened epididymis w/ increased blood flow suggesting hyperemia, ±abscess)

Treatment

- Supportive: Rest, ice, NSAIDs, scrotal support
- If STI suspected: Doxycycline 100 mg PO BID × 10 d AND CTX 500 mg in a single IM dose
    - IF STI suspected & practices anal sex: Levofloxacin 500 mg PO QD × 10 d × 10 d AND CTX 500 mg in a single IM dose
- If STI not suspected: Levofloxacin 500 mg PO QD × 10 d
- Abstain from intercourse for 7 d & until all sex partners (w/i previous 60 d) are evaluated or empirically treated

Disposition

- Home

Pearl

- Pts <35 y/o likely to have an STD organism as etiology; >35 y/o more likely enteric pathogen

TESTICULAR TORSION

Definitions

- Twisting of the spermatic cord & its contents (venous plexus, spermatic arteries, vas deferens) → increased venous congestion → decreased arterial blood flow → ischemia
- Accounts for 10–15% of acute scrotal dz in children
- Bimodal age distribution: Neonates, puberty

History

- Sudden onset severe pain (±swelling) in scrotum w/ radiation into abdomen; pain may be intermittent; n/v
- Can present w/ abdominal pain/flank pain
- Bell-clapper deformity (tunica vaginalis w/ abnormally high attachment to spermatic cord) leaves the testes free to rotate, predisposing torsion

Physical Examination

- Ill appearing, very tender/swollen/elevated testicle that may lie horizontally or anteriorly rotated; presence of cremasteric reflex (elevation of testicle when stimulating the medial thigh) does not r/o dz
- Torsion of appendix testes: Similar presentation but exam w/ nl-appearing testes; tenderness localized to superior pole of testicle; may have nodular "blue dot" at superior pole of testicle due to cyanotic torsed appendage

Evaluation

- Labs: UA, Ucx, preop labs if surgery anticipated
- Imaging: Scrotal duplex U/S to assess flow to testicle (89% sens, 99% spec), but imaging should not delay time to OR
- If U/S neg but high suspicion, consider further discussion w/ urology for surgical exploration

Treatment

- C/s urology immediately if concern for testicular torsion as time to OR is critical for survival of testicle
- If delay to OR, may attempt manual detorsion in medial to lateral direction ("open book" technique)

Pearls

- Perform GU exam in every male pt w/ lower abdominal pain/flank pain and in infants w/ vomiting
- Clinical dx: Surgical exploration should not be delayed if high clinical concern
- >90% salvage rate if detorsion occurs <6 h
- Continuous pain >24 h suggests an infarcted testicle
- Torsion of appendix testes is benign condition (Tx w/ analgesia, scrotal support)

PHIMOSIS AND PARAPHIMOSIS

Definition (*Emerg Med Clin North Am* 2019;37(4):583–592)

Phimosis

- Inability to retract the distal foreskin over the glans penis; "ballooning" of the prepuce during urination; painful erection, preputial pain, weak urinary stream

Paraphimosis

- Inability to completely reduce foreskin distally back to natural position over glans penis. Entrapped foreskin forms constricting band, leads to pain & swelling.
- Associated w/ vigorous sexual activity & chronic balanoposthitis
- Occurs exclusively in uncircumcised males & is a urologic emergency
- Pediatric: Often seen w/ forceful retraction or forgetting to reduce foreskin after bathing/voiding; irritability may be the only sign in nonverbal children

Physical Examination

Phimosis

- Inability to retract foreskin proximally over glans penis

Paraphimosis

- Foreskin retracted behind the glans & cannot be replaced to nl position; proximal shaft is soft (unless there is accompanying infxn) w/ glans appearing erythematous/edematous → blue/black & firm

Treatment

- If significant manipulation is expected, you may perform a penile block. On the dorsal aspect of the penis in the 2 & 10 o'clock positions, deposit 1% lidocaine; subsequently complete a ring block by depositing anesthetic circumferentially around the proximal shaft.

Phimosis

- No acute intervention needed unless infxn suspected or causing urinary retention Consider topical steroids (0.05–0.1% betamethasone) × 4–6 wks for mild–moderate cases.
- Urology consultation for dorsal slit procedure if causing urinary retention

Paraphimosis

- Compress the foreskin & glans by snugly grasping it w/ the palm of the hand & apply pressure for several minutes
- Attempt manual reduction by placing index fingers on dorsal border of glans behind retracted prepuce & thumbs on glans; may facilitate w/ ice, EMLA, elastic bandage over glans or spreading hyperosmolar agents (such as sugar/dextrose) over glans to reduce swelling (will take 1+ h for osmotic reduction of edema)
- C/s urology if manual reduction unsuccessful

Disposition

- Phimosis: Home w/ urology f/u ± abx for accompanying infxn
- Paraphimosis: Home w/ urology f/u if skin is in the nl position; admit if not reduced by conservative methods

Pearls

- Educate parents/caretakers of children on importance of avoiding forcible retractions & of gentle reduction of foreskin after bathing & voiding
- Paraphimosis that is not immediately treated carries risk for necrosis & autoamputation

PRIAPISM

Definitions (*J Uro* 2022;208:43)

- Priapism is defined as a prolonged erection lasting generally >4 h in the absence of sexual stimulation
- Ischemic (low-flow) priapism is the most common subtype & is due to painful engorgement of the corpora cavernosa. This can lead to intracavernosal acidosis, sludging of blood, thrombosis of cavernal arteries, & impotence
- Nonischemia (high-flow) priapism is rare, painless, & is caused by increased arterial inflow to the penis as a result of traumatic arterial–cavernosal fistulas

History

- Painful, persistent erection lasting >4 h, not relieved by ejaculation
- Risk factors: Impotence agents (sildenafil), SCD, leukemia, urogenital malignancies, CVA, spinal cord injury, antihypertensives (hydralazine, prazosin, doxazosin), antidepressants (trazodone, fluoxetine, sertraline), antipsychotics (phenothiazines & atypicals), phosphodiesterase inhs, cocaine, toxins (scorpion, black widow, CO)

Physical Examination

- Obvious erection, generally involving only the corporal cavernosa & flaccid corpora spongiosum

Evaluation

- Labs: Preoperative labs if may need OR
- Consider sending blood gas from penile aspirate (acidic pH suggests low flow)

Treatment

- Perform penile nerve block: On the dorsal aspect of the penis in the 2 & 10 o'clock positions, deposit 1% lidocaine; subsequently complete a ring block by depositing anesthetic circumferentially around the proximal shaft
- To reduce flow/vasoconstriction
  - Intracavernosal phenylephrine injection: Using a 25G or 27G needle (or tuberculin syringe), inject 0.2–0.5 mg of phenylephrine 1 mg/mL solution into corporus q10–15min (maximum 4–5 doses) 2 cm distal to origin of shaft on dorsal penis at 2 or 10 o'clock position

  Note: Must dilute phenylephrine solution. Take phenylephrine 1% solution (10 mg/mL) & extract 1 mL (10 mg) from solution. Add this 1 mL to 9 mL of saline, which will give you 1 mg/mL of phenylephrine solution. You can then extract 0.2–0.5 mL (0.2–0.5 mg) of this for intracavernosal injection.

  Note: Pt should be on cardiac and BP monitor during phenylephrine injection
- If unsuccessful, aspiration/irrig technique:
  - Prep & drape penis in sterile fashion
  - At 2 or 10 o'clock position insert a 16–18G needle (also consider 18G dialysis butterfly access needle), & using a 10–30-mL syringe, slowly aspirate while milking corporus w/ other hand until return if bright red blood & detumescence occurs
  - If this fails, you can attempt to irrigate by injecting 20–30 mL of phenylephrine & NS solution (10 mg phenylephrine in 500 mL NS) as exchange for 20–30 mL aspirate
- C/s urology for refractory priapism (as may necessitate surgical decompression)
- Additional txs in SCD: IVF, O_2, pain control, consider exchange transfusion

Disposition

- Recommended to observe for at least 2 h to assess for recurrence
- Home: Once detumescence achieved. Recommended to D/C w/ 3-d course of oral alpha-adrenergic agent (pseudoephedrine)
- Admit: If priapism not responsive to tx

Pearls

- >12 h of priapism a/w onset of tissue demise w/ >24 h a/w permanent impotence
- Cx: Hematoma, infxn, systemic absorption of vasoactive agents (severe HTN), recurrence, impotence (this risk should be discussed w/ pt & is a possibility despite efforts & timeliness of therapy)

HEMATURIA

Definition

- Hematuria is blood in the urine. Called gross hematuria when visible vs microscopic hematuria when not visible & ≥3 RBCs/hpf in urine sediment
- Hematuria must be distinguished from pigmenturia (discoloration of urine). Pigmenturia can be caused endogenously by melanin, porphyrins, bilirubin, myoglobin, or hemoglobin or exogenously by meds (ie, warfarin, rifampin, phenazopyridine, phenytoin, etc), beets

History

- Onset (sudden vs chronic)? Dysuria/urinary frequency/renal colic? During entire or part of urine stream? (hematuria at beginning of urination → urethral; throughout urination → upper urinary tract or proximal bladder; end of urination → bladder neck or prostatic urethra)
- Painless hematuria should raise suspicion for genitourinary malignancy
- ROS (fever, weight loss, night sweats, rash, sore throat, abdominal pain, n/v, recent viral infxn or UTI; trauma; excessive exercises; pelvic radiation)
- PMH (kidney stones, HTN, cancer, congenital kidney dz, vascular dz, bleeding diathesis, SCD, hereditary spherocytosis)
- MEDS
  - Drugs that cause pigmenturia: Rifampin, phenazopyridine, phenytoin, azathioprine, deferoxamine, doxorubicin, riboflavin
  - Drugs that cause myoglobinuria: Amphotericin B, Barbs, cocaine, diazepam, EtOH, heroin, methadone, statins
  - Drugs that cause hematuria: NSAIDs, A/C, busulfan, cyclophosphamide, OCPs, quinine, vincristine
- Social (smoking, benzene, or aromatic amine exposure)

Physical Examination

- Evaluate for HTN, petechiae, arthritis, rash
- Assess for suprapubic & CVA tenderness; thorough GU exam inc prostate exam
- Postvoid residual if concern for urinary retention

Evaluation

Key question: Is this truly hematuria?

- Urine dipstick + blood (can be seen w/ hematuria, hemoglobinuria, myoglobinuria, or other pigmenturias); urine sediment necessary to confirm >5 RBCs/hpf as well as identify protein, RBC casts (suggests glomerulonephritis), & crystalluria (suggests urolithiasis)
- Other urine studies: Ucx, urine cytology
- CBC, BUN/Cr, coags (if isolated hematuria—erythrocytes in sediment, but no protein—suggests bleeding diathesis)
- Outpt imaging: CT urography (1st line), renal U/S, MRI. Cystoscopy if ≥35 y/o.

Disposition

- Large, gross hematuria may warrant continuous monitoring of Hct & urology eval. If microscopic, can obtain further outpt eval by nephrology or urology.

Hematuria Differential	
Pathophysiology	**Differential**
Structural	Urolithiasis, BPH, PKD, analgesic nephropathy, papillary necrosis, menstruation
Infectious	UTI, STDs, renal TB, malaria
Vascular	AVM, renal artery dz (thrombosis, dissection, malignant HTN), renal vein thrombosis, sickle cell crisis
Meds	Cyclophosphamide, anticoagulants
Inflammatory	Glomerulonephritis (poststrep, postinfectious, IgA nephropathy, lupus nephritis, Alport synd, thin basement membrane dz, etc), vasculitis (HSP, granulomatosis w/ polyangiitis, etc), transfusion rxn
Trauma/Other	Renal trauma, urethral or ureteral trauma, recent instrumentation, paroxysmal nocturnal hemoglobinuria, vigorous exercise
Neoplastic	Renal Ca, urethral Ca, bladder Ca, prostate Ca

FLANK PAIN

Approach to the Patient

History

- Onset (sudden vs progressive)? Location? Dysuria/hematuria/urinary frequency? Prior h/o similar sxs
- ROS (fever, rash, trauma, nausea, vomiting, weakness, abdominal pain), PMH (kidney stones, gout, cancer, AAA, congenital kidney dz, cardiac or vascular dz)

Evaluation

- CBC, BMP, UA, pregnancy test; Consider POCUS, renal US, or CT abd/pelvis

Flank Pain Differential	
Pathophysiology	**Differential**
Renal	Nephrolithiasis, urolithiasis, retroperitoneal hematoma, ruptured renal cyst, ureteral stricture
Infectious	Pyelonephritis, perinephric abscess, psoas abscess, pneumonia, discitis, vertebral osteomyelitis, epidural abscess
Vascular	Ruptured AAA, renal infarct, renal vein thrombosis, PE
GI	Biliary dz
Other	PCKD (ruptured cyst), renal malignancy, varicella-zoster
Trauma	Lumbar spasm, radiculopathy.

Urolithiasis (Nephrolithiasis and Ureterolithiasis)

Definition

- Urolithiasis denotes calculi (of mineral or organic solids) that form anywhere in the urinary tract; nephrolithiasis (kidney) & ureterolithiasis (ureter) more specifically denote location of calculi
- Kidney stones form when urine becomes saturated w/ stone-forming salts
- Types of calculi
  - Calcium oxalate stones (~80%): Predisposing conditions include hypercalciuria (hyperparathyroidism, sarcoidosis, type I RTA, hypercalcemia of malignancy, thiazides) & hyperoxaluria (CD other ileal dz)
  - Magnesium ammonium phosphate (struvite) stones (~15%): Requires combination of ammonia & alkaline urine. Source of ammonia from splitting of urea by urease-producing bacteria (*Proteus, Klebsiella, Pseudomonas, & Staphylococcus*)
  - Uric acid stones (~5–10%): Secondary to hyperuricosuria (gout, DM2, HTN)
  - Cystine stones: Secondary to inherited defects of tubular amino acid reabsorption
  - Drug-induced calculi: 2/2 metabolic abnormalities that favor stone formation or crystallization of drug or metabolites
- Stones lodged in ureter are typically found in 3 locations: Ureteropelvic junction, at the level of the iliac vessels, & ureterovesicular junction

History

- M:F, 2:1; Caucasian > Hispanic > Asian > African; peak incidence 20–50 y/o
- Renal colic (acute, spasmodic, unilateral flank pain radiating to groin/testes/labium) & visceral sxs (n/v/diaphoresis)
- Distal stones may cause lower abdominal pain & lower urinary tract sxs (dysuria, frequency, hematuria)
- PMH: FH nephrolithiasis, hyperparathyroidism, sarcoidosis, RTA, malignancy, Crohn, jejunoileal bypass, recurrent UTI, gout, DM2, HTN, structural urologic abnormalities
- Meds: Indinavir, loop/thiazide diuretics, laxatives, carbonic anhydrase inhs, ciprofloxacin, sulfonamides have been a/w drug-induced calculi

Physical Examination

- Fever? Tachycardic? Generally uncomfortable appearing, diaphoretic, cool/clammy skin
- CVA tenderness; lower abdominal/pelvic tenderness (if stone has migrated)
- Assess for midline spinal TTP, acute abdomen, etc, which suggest alternative dx

Evaluation

- UA (+RBCs, though sens 84%, spec 48% for stone; proteinuria, crystalluria), Ucx
- BUN/Cr; CBC usually nonspecific & not helpful
- Imaging
- Renal U/S (sens 45%, spec 94% for stones; sens 85–90%, spec 90–100% for hydro)
  - May be initial radiographic exam w/ high pretest probability or if CT not possible (pregnancy); esp useful for detection of hydronephrosis or ureteral dilatation; not sens stones <5 mm; can be done point-of-care

- CT abd/pelvis (w/o contrast: sens 96–98%, spec 100%)
  - Useful as initial radiographic exam, particularly w/ 1st presentation of suspected stone or low–moderate probability; able to make alternative diagnoses; modality of choice when available
  - Contrasted exam has similar sens for stones >3 mm w/ much superior sens for alternative diagnoses

Treatment
- IVF if pt appears dehydrated or has AKI
- Pain control: NSAIDs (ibuprofen 600 mg PO TID or ketorolac 15 mg IV if unable to take PO [caution in renal insufficiency]) & morphine 0.1 mg/kg × 1 then titrated for further relief
- Medical expulsive therapy: Tamsulosin 0.4 mg PO QD until stone passage (possible benefit shown for large but not smaller stones)
- Urology c/s: For concomitant infxn, renal insufficiency, refractory severe pain, or low likelihood of stone passage (>10 mm)

Disposition
- Home: Adequate pain control in ED, nl Cr; f/u w/ urology in 24–48 h if stone >5 mm
- Admit: Intractable pain, unable to tolerate POs, renal failure, infxn, renal transplant, single kidney, comorbid conditions (DM, baseline CRI), infected stone w/ obstruction

Pearls
- Presence or absence of hematuria alone cannot be used to diagnose or exclude nephrolithiasis
- Most stones ≤5 mm (70–98%) will pass spontaneously. Stones >5 mm have smaller chance (25–51%) of spontaneous passage & are more likely to need urologic intervention
- Send pts home w/ strainer, esp 1st-time stone formers for stone analysis
- Cx: Obstructed infected kidney (urologic emergency requiring urgent decompression), renal insufficiency, failed expulsion
- Very unlikely for unilateral obstructing stone to have AKI from obstruction, more likely prerenal from hypovolemia

ACUTE KIDNEY INJURY

Definition & Staging (*Lancet* 2025;405:241)
- AKI is defined as any of the following:
  - Increase in serum Cr by ≥0.3 mg/dL (≥26.5 μmol/L) w/i 48 h; or
  - Increase in serum Cr by ≥1.5 times baseline, which is known or presumed to have occurred w/i prior 7 d; or
  - Urine volume <0.5 mL/kg/h for 6 h
- AKI is staged for severity according to the following criteria:
  AKI Stage 1
  - Serum Cr: >/0.3 mg/dL increase w/i 48 h OR >/1.5–1.9× increase from baseline
  - UOP: <0.5 mL/kg/h for 6 h

  AKI Stage 2
  - Serum Cr: >/2–3× increase from baseline
  - UOP: <0.5 mL/kg/h for 12 h
- AKI Stage 3
  - Serum Cr: >/2–3× increase from baseline, Cr >/4, eGFR to <35 (if <18 y/o)
  - UOP: <0.3 mL/kg/h for 24 h, or anuria for >/12 h

History
- AKI is usually asx & diagnosed when labs reveal renal abnormalities
- Sxs may include decreased urine output, weight gain, fluid retention (peripheral edema, anasarca, ascites), fatigue, anorexia, n/v, pruritus, altered sensorium, thirst/orthostasis (prerenal)
- ROS (fever, rash, flank pain, hematuria)
- PMH: Baseline renal impairment, CHF, liver dz, SLE, multiple myeloma
- MEDS (ACEI/ARB, NSAIDs, aminoglycosides, other abx, cisplatin, amphotericin B, diuretics)

Physical Examination
- Assess volume status; myoclonus, pericardial or pl rub, rash, mental status, edema
- Stigmata of CHF, liver dz, collagen vascular dzs

Evaluation

- CBC, BMP (BUN/Cr ratio), serum osmolality; consider VBG w/ STAT potassium
- Urinalysis/sediment, urine lytes (urine Na, urine K, urine Cr, urine osmolality)
- $FE_{Na}\% = (\text{Urine Na} \times \text{Plasma Cr})/(\text{Plasma Na} \times \text{Urine Cr}) \times 100$
- Consider LFTs, BNP if indicated
- ECG for cardiac electrical instability from potential electrolyte abx
- Consider point-of-care cardiac, IVC, renal U/S
- Renal U/S w/ Dopplers (r/o obstruction, assess flow); consider CT abdomen if c/f pelvic mass
- Low threshold for renal biopsy

Differential Diagnosis of AKI	
Pathophysiology	**Differential**
Prerenal	**Hypovolemia:** Dehydration, hypotension/shock, hemorrhage, vomiting/diarrhea, diuresis, burns, pancreatitis, severe hypoalbuminemia **Altered Renal Hemodynamics:** Low cardiac output states (CHF, severe valvular heart dz, tamponade, massive PE, abdominal compartment synd), sepsis, anaphylaxis, Meds (NSAIDs, ACEI/ARBs), hepatorenal synd, renal artery stenosis
Intrinsic renal	**Renovascular Obstruction:** Renal artery atherosclerosis/thrombosis/embolism/dissection/vasculitis; renal vein thrombosis/external compression **Glomerular Dz:** Glomerulonephritis, vasculitis, malignant HTN, preeclampsia, DIC, collagen vascular dzs (SLE, scleroderma) **Intratubular Obstruction:** Multiple myeloma, uric acid, acyclovir, MTX, indinavir **Acute Tubular Necrosis:** Profound ischemia, infxn, radiocontrast, calcineurin inhs, abx (ie, aminoglycosides), antifungals (amphotericin B), chemo (ie, cisplatin), ethylene glycol, rhabdomyolysis, HUS/TTP **Interstitial Nephritis:** Allergic nephritis (β-lactams, fluoroquinolones, sulfa, NSAIDs), pyelonephritis, leukemia/lymphoma, sarcoid
Postrenal	**Ureter:** Calculi, clot, cancer (pelvic mass), external compression **Bladder Neck:** BPH, calculi, clot, cancer (pancreatic), neurogenic **Urethra:** Stricture, valves

Interpreting Laboratory Data in AKI/ARF						
	BUN/Cr	**FE_{Na}**	**$Urine_{Na}$**	**SpGrav**	**$Urine_{osm}$**	**Other**
Prerenal	≥20	<1%	<10 mmol/L	>1.018	>500	Hyaline casts
Intrinsic renal	10–20	>1%	>20 mmol/L	<1.015	300–500	• Muddy brown casts (ATN) • RBC casts (glomerular injury, tubulointerstitial nephritis) • WBC casts (interstitial nephritis) • Broad granular casts (CKD) • Eosinophiluria (allergic nephritis) • Uric acid crystals (urate nephropathy) • Oxalate/Hippurate crystals (ethylene glycol tox)
Postrenal	<10	>1%	—	—	<350	

Treatment

- *Prerenal:* Correct volume status/perfusion pressure (IVF, pressors, PRBCs if indicated, diuresis/inotropes if cardiorenal)
- *Intrinsic:* Eliminate nephrotoxins, treat underlying cause, consider glucocorticoids
- *Postrenal:* Transurethral or suprapubic catheter placement; may require ureteric stents or percutaneous nephrostomy tube placement
- Consider sodium bicarbonate if pH <7.2 or HCO_3 <15 mmol/L as bridge to dialysis

Indications for Emergent Dialysis and Renal Replacement
Therapy "A, E, I, O, U"
- **A**cidosis (pH <7.1)
- **E**lectrolyte imbalance (hyperkalemia, hypocalcemia, hyperphosphatemia)
- **I**ntoxication (lithium, salicylates, ethylene glycol, methanol, among others)
- **O**verload (volume overload)
- **U**remia (pericarditis, encephalopathy, neuropathy, bleeding)

Disposition
- Home: Mild prerenal azotemia may be adequately treated w/ hydration; pts w/ postobstructive ARF can be sent home if obstruction is relieved (ie, w/ bladder catheter) & no significant comorbidities
- Admit: Pts w/ uremia, significant electrolyte abnormalities, volume overload, severe metabolic acidosis, unexplained ARF

Pearl
Complications: Intravascular volume overload, hyponatremia, hyperkalemia, hyperphosphatemia, hypocalcemia, hypermagnesemia, metabolic acidosis, uremia, anemia, arrhythmias

EMERGENCIES IN DIALYSIS PATIENTS

Definition
- Common complaints & special considerations include:

Common Chief Complaints and Special Considerations in Dialysis Patients	
Chief Complaint	**Differential/Special Considerations**
Fever	PNA (healthcare associated), UTI, bacteremia, peritonitis (particularly w/ peritoneal dialysis), access-related infxn (hematogenous spread can lead to endocarditis, septic pulmonary emboli, septic arthritis, vertebral osteomyelitis, epidural abscess)
Dyspnea	Fluid overload/pulmonary edema, high-output cardiac failure (AV fistula), pl effusion (uremic, chronic fluid overload), anemia (decreased EPO production), PTX (after subclavian or IJ HC access), pericardial effusion (uremic), PE
CP	ACS, PE, AD, uremic pericarditis, uremic pleuritis
Syncope	Intradialytic hypotension, uremic autonomic neuropathy, dysrhythmias, other frequent causes of syncope
Hypotension	Intradialytic hypotension, dysautonomia, antihypertensives, pericardial effusion/tamponade, sepsis, anaphylaxis (oversulfated chondroitin sulfate contaminants in heparin)
Abdominal pain	Consider common causes of abdominal pain, uremic gastritis/colitis, peritonitis (particularly w/ peritoneal dialysis), abdominal wall hernias (from increased abdominal pressures w/ ascites)
HA/AMS	Dialysis dysequilibrium synd, uremic/HTN encephalopathy, hypertensive emergency, ICH, CVA, medication effects from altered pharmacodynamics (Benzos, morphine, meperidine, etc), hyponatremia
Skin chgs	Uremic pruritus, prurigo nodularis, calciphylaxis (cutaneous uremic arteriolopathy)
HD access sx	AV access "steal synd," AV fistula/catheter access vein thrombosis, AV fistula hemorrhage
Other	Electrolyte abnormalities (hyperkalemia, hyperphosphatemia, hypermagnesemia, hypocalcemia, hyponatremia), metabolic acidosis, uremic polyneuropathy (restless leg synd, paresthesias)

Approach to the Patient
History
- Should focus on assessing for common causes of respective chief complaints, w/ attention to special considerations unique to ESRD pt

Physical Examination
- Attention to abnl vital signs
- Pulmonary & cardiac exam inc assessment of friction rub, rhonchi, & rales
- Abdominal exam, esp in pts w/ PD catheters

- Extremity exam & JVP for signs of fluid overload
- Skin exam for e/o calciphylaxis
- Assess graft site for thrill & signs of bleeding, infxn, edema, & bruising; assess tunneled catheter site for e/o cellulitis or underlying abscess formation

Diagnostics

- ECG for cardiac electrical instability from potential electrolyte abx, ischemia
- CBC, BMP; consider blood gas w/ STAT potassium & to assess acid–base status
- Consider LFTs, BNP, cardiac markers if indicated
- Consider obtaining sample of PD dialysate fluid (cell count [WBC >100 cell/mm^3 suggest peritonitis], Gram stain, culture)
- Consider point-of-care cardiac & lung U/S & FAST exam to assess for effusion & ascites
- Imaging: Appropriate imaging for respective complaints; Doppler imaging of AF fistula site if concern for thrombosis

Treatment

- Refer to appropriate sections for tx of conditions noted above
- Special considerations:
  - **Peritonitis in PD patient:** Vancomycin 2 g AND cefepime/ceftazidime 1 g each added to 1 bag of dialysate infused into & allowed to dwell in the peritoneal cavity for 6 h
  - **Dialysis disequilibrium synd:** Exclude other causes, stop dialysis, Reduce ICP (HOB elevation >30°, consider hyperosmolar therapy [mannitol, hypertonic saline], euglycemia, euthermia, eunatremia, MAP >65, CO_2 40 mmHg, CPP 50–70 mmHg); renal c/s
  - **Clotted AV graft/fistula:** Immediate vascular surgery or IR consultation for consideration of catheter-directed thrombolysis, pharmacomechanical thrombolysis, surgical thrombectomy
  - **Clotted vascular access catheters:** C/s institutional policies; if feasible, attempt catheter-directed tPA via infusion of 2 mg tPA into occluded lumen & fill remainder w/ saline. After 15 mins, inject 0.3-mL saline to move the active enzyme toward the tip of the catheter. After another 15 mins, inject another 0.3 mL to move the active enzyme toward the tip of the catheter. After another 15 mins, try to aspirate catheter. If unsuccessful, send pt for catheter exchange.
  - **Vascular access hemorrhage:** Apply direct pressure for 10–15 mins; if peridialysis, consider protamine 1 mg per 100 U heparin received (or 10–20 mg if dose unknown) to reverse heparin A/C; consider DDAVP to treat platelet dysfxn; can try hemostatic agents (eg, gelfoam, surgicel) or figure-of-8-stitch (keep superficial over are of bleeding); vascular surgery consultation for uncontrolled hemorrhage

Disposition

- Depends upon presenting complaint, but often require admx

Pearls

- BP measurement over & use of AV fistula sites for blood draw/administering therapy is contraindicated
- BNP levels are not reliable in diagnosing fluid overload/HF in dialysis pts as basal BNP levels are typically elevated & increased BNP levels from baseline may not correlate w/ clinical HF
- Chronically elevated troponin common & a/w increased mortality; makes assessment of ACS challenging; however, the National Academy of Clinical Biochemistry (NACB) recommends a 20% change in troponin concentration from baseline for dx of AMI

VAGINAL BLEEDING

History

- Chronicity, pain, quality (dark vs clots vs bright red), quantity (number of pads/h, passage of clots and/or tissue), pregnant or postpartum, LMP, sexual hx, hx of STI, use of contraception, gravida & parity, trauma
- ROS: Sxs of anemia (light-headedness or presyncope, syncope, shortness of breath, fatigue), other bleeding, fever
- PMH (clotting disorder, hypo- or hyperthyroid, liver dz), meds (anticoagulants or antiplatelet tx, contraceptives, hormonal therapy), social hx (intimate partner violence)

Evaluation

- Exam: Pelvic exam; consider orthostatic VS (if c/f symptomatic anemia)
- Labs: CBC, urine hCG; quantitative hCG if pt is pregnant; type & screen (Rh); crossmatch (if heavily bleeding); consider coags; consider pelvic U/S (vs consider deferring to o/p setting if not pregnant)

Pearls

- Average pad holds 5–15 cc of blood
- Average tampon holds 5 cc of blood

Vaginal Bleeding Differential	
Pathophysiology	**Differential**
Nonpregnant: PALM-COEIN (*Int J Gynaecol Obstet* 2011;113:3)	**P**olyp, **A**denomyosis, **L**eiomyoma, **M**alignancy/hyperplasia, **C**oagulopathy, **O**vulatory dysfxn, **E**ndometrial, **I**atrogenic, **N**ot yet classified
1st trimester	Implantation bleeding, miscarriage, ectopic pregnancy, subchorionic hemorrhage, molar pregnancy
2nd/3rd trimester	Placenta previa, vasa previa, placental abruption, uterine rupture
Other	Postpartum hemorrhage, retained products of conception

Abnormal Uterine Bleeding (Nonpregnant)

Presentation

- History: Change in frequency, duration or amount of bleeding, bleeding b/w cycles, postmenopausal bleeding, PMH, parity, hx of STIs, A/C
- Exam: Ongoing bleeding; signs of anemia; vaginal or cervical lesions, D/C, mass

Evaluation

- Labs: Urine hCG, CBC, coags, consider STI testing, TSH
- Imaging: Consider pelvic US (often nonurgent, consider o/p)

Treatment

- Transfuse if unstable or Hgb <7, NSAIDs for pelvic pain/cramping
- Anovulatory bleeding: Combination OCP w/ 35 mcg of ethinyl estradiol and taper over 5 d (provided no CI to estrogen) or 10–20 mg medroxyprogesterone TID × 7 d
- For severe bleeding consider IV estrogen 25 mg every 4–6 h for 24 h (*Obstet Gynecol* 2013;122:176) provided no CI to estrogen (eg, venous thromboembolism)

Postcoital Bleeding

History

- Trauma during intercourse, vaginal D/C, intimate partner violence
- RFs: Cervical abnormalities (eval pap screening hx), STDs, postmenopausal

Physical Examination

- Ongoing bleeding; vulvar lesions, vaginal lacs, D/C, cervical lesions

Evaluation

- Labs: CBC, urine hCG, GC/*Chlamydia* & trichomonas testing

Treatment

- Abx: Treat STI appropriately (see *Vaginal Discharge* below)
- C/s: Gyn service if lac requiring extensive repair; social services if c/f intimate partner violence
- Referral to o/p Gyn if c/f malignancy (eg, cervical, vulvar)

PHYSIOLOGIC CHANGES OF PREGNANCY

- The maternal body adapts during pregnancy to accommodate the growing baby

Physiologic Changes of Pregnancy	
Organ System	**Associated Adaptions**
Cardiovascular	Increase in CO, HR, stroke volume Decrease in SVR BP drops in 1st trimester & then returns to baseline IVC compression can decrease venous return esp >20 wks (can lead hypotension, increase in LE edema)
Hematologic	Increased blood volume (plasma, RBCs, WBCs) Decreased Hct & hemoglobin Hypercoagulability
Metabolic	Increased body weight Decreased sens to insulin
Renal	Increased GFR & UOP Increased urinary frequency
Respiratory	Increased TV Decreased functional residual capacity Respiratory alkalosis (w/ metabolic compensation)
GI	Slower GI motility & reduced LES tone Inhibition of gallbladder contraction & biliary transportation Nausea & vomiting, constipation
Breast	Increased size Milk production

EARLY PREGNANCY COMPLICATIONS

Miscarriage (Spontaneous Abortion) (*Obstet Gynecol* 2018;132(5):e197–e207)

Definition
- Spontaneous pregnancy loss before 20 wks, most commonly w/i 1st trimester
- Early pregnancy loss defined as loss w/i 1st trimester; occurs in 10% of clinically recognized pregnancies
- Fetal demise if after 20 wks of gestation
- Pts w/ bleeding who do not miscarry often have nl pregnancies but increased risk of premature birth & low birth weight (*BJOG* 2010;117:245)

Presentation
- Vaginal bleeding ± passage of clots or tissue at <20 wks; abd pain/cramping
- Speculum & bimanual exam to assess for passage of blood/products of conception, eval for infxn, and determine whether cervical os is open or closed (If copious bleeding, remove products of conception from os w/ gentle traction to allow uterus to clamp)

Evaluation
- Labs: CBC, quant hCG, type, & screen (crossmatch if HD unstable)
- If products expelled, send to pathology
- Imaging: Pelvic U/S to determine location of pregnancy, confirmed IUP if intrauterine gestational sac PLUS yolk sac, fetal pole, or cardiac activity

Classification of Miscarriage
- Threatened: Os closed, mild cramping/bleeding, no passage of products of conception, may see viable fetus w/ heart tones
- Inevitable: Os open & effaced; products of conception in uterus being expelled; cramps, mod bleeding
- Incomplete: Os open or closed; some, but not all products have passed. Retained fetal or placental tissue
- Missed (embryonic demise): Os closed; pregnancy loss after development of embryo/ fetus

- Complete: Os closed; products of conception expelled, little cramping or bleeding, US w/ empty uterus

Treatment

- Supportive management; transfuse if HD unstable
- C/s Ob/Gyn if unstable or need for D&C
- Recent ACOG practice update suggests forgoing routine Rh testing and Rh immunoglobulin for pts w/ early pregnancy loss or abortion <12 wks, though can consider based on shared decision making (*Obstet Gynecol* 2024;144(6):e140–e143)
- Administer Rh immunoglobulin if ≥12 wks and Rh-neg (100 mcg for 12–18 wks, 300 mcg if >18 wks of gestation)
- Incomplete or missed: Expectant management, medical management (misoprostol alone or mifepristone-misoprostol regimen), or surgical evacuation; all require good counseling and strict return precautions; surgical management may be needed if expectant or medical management unsuccessful or contraindicated
- Medical management of early pregnancy loss a/w decreased time to expulsion and decreased risk of needing uterine aspiration (vs expectant management); giving mifepristone 24 h before misoprostol is superior to administering misoprostol alone for early pregnancy loss, but more regulatory restrictions are in place for mifepristone

Disposition

- Home: Stable pts w/ management plan in place; f/u w/ Ob/Gyn
- Admit: Uncontrolled bleeding or pts requiring immediate D&C

Pearl

- Threatened & missed abortions can only be distinguished by pelvic U/S; see *Table 1* in *Obstet Gynecol* 2018;132(5):e197-e207 for US findings diagnostic of or c/f pregnancy failure

Ectopic Pregnancy (*Obstet Gynecol* 2018;131(3):e91)

Definition

- Ectopic pregnancy—implanted pregnancy outside the uterus
- Heterotopic pregnancy (ectopic pregnancy & IUP) is rare but increased risk w/ assisted reproductive techniques (up to 1/100 IVF pregnancies)

Presentation

- Unruptured: Abd pain, cramping (often unilateral), amenorrhea
- Ruptured: Hypotension, tachycardia, abdominal pain, vaginal bleeding, syncope
- RFs: Prior ectopic, hx PID, tubal surgery, IUD, fertility tx, age >35 y, cigarette smoking
- Exam: Assess for HD stability, signs of peritonitis (if rupture has occurred). Speculum & bimanual exam may reveal pelvic tenderness and/or adnexal mass

Evaluation

- Labs: CBC, quant hCG, Hct, Rh screen, PT/PTT, type & crossmatch (if HD unstable)
- ACOG suggests if hCG used to help dx ectopic discriminatory level (hCG above which should see IUP on US) should be conservatively high (eg, 3500 mIU/mL); should not use hCG alone to dx ectopic
- Imaging is required: Pelvic US; if HD unstable, FAST exam to assess for free fluid
  - IUP is only definitively diagnosed by US visualization of a yolk sac or embryo (ectopic pregnancy can be accompanied by a "pseudosac" w/i the uterus that can be mistaken for IUP)
  - Identification of an IUP can rule out ectopic unless heterotopic is suspected (rare but more common w/ assisted reproduction)

Ultrasound Findings in Normal & Abnormal Pregnancy (*NEJM* 2009;361(4):379; *Ultrasound* 2018;26(3):153; *Obstet Gynecol* 2018;132(5):e197)			
Nl Pregnancy		**Abnl Pregnancy**	
Gestational Age (wks)	**Findings**	**Abnlty**	**Findings**
4–5	Gestational sac	Molar	Snowstorm pattern
5	Double decidua sign		Grape such as clusters w/i the uterus
5.5	Yolk sac		No definitive IUP

6	Embryonic pole	Miscarriage	Mean gestational sac diameter >25 mm w/o embryo
6.5	Fetal cardiac activity		Crown-rump length >7 mm w/o cardiac activity
			No embryo w/ heart beat either 2 or more wks following US w/ gestational sac and no yolk sac OR 11 d or more after US w/ gestational sac and yolk sac
		Ectopic	Extrauterine pregnancy +/– fetal pole +/– cardiac activity
			Adnexal mass (may be separate from ovary)
			Intrauterine pseudosac & absence of IUP
			Ring sign (hyperechoic ring around adnexal gestational sac)
			Free fluid

Treatment

- Supportive: 2 large-bore IVs, IVF resuscitation, monitor; tfx if HD unstable
- C/s: Urgent Gyn eval for consideration of medical (MTX) vs surgical tx
- Absolute CIs to MTX tx include unstable pts, ruptured ectopic, severe anemia, CIs to MTX due to other medications or medical hx; relative CIs include embryo w/ cardiac activity, high initial hCG, ectopic >4 cm, pt would decline blood tfx
- Most protocols advise checking baseline LFTs, renal function, and full blood count before considering MTX

Pregnancy of Unknown Location

- Diagnosed when + hCG but no pregnancy identified on TVUS
- If stable, discuss w/ & f/u w/ Ob/Gyn in 48 h for serial hCG/ pelvic US

Pearls

- Atypical presentations of ectopic pregnancy may mimic other dz such as appendicitis, UTI, or have nonspecific presentations such as LH, dizziness, vomiting

Hyperemesis Gravidarum (*JAMA* 2016;316:1392)

Definition: Nausea & vomiting that result in weight loss >5%, dehydration, ketonemia/uria

History: Pregnancy (1st trimester, usually improved by 20 wks), n/v, inability to PO

Physical Findings: Tachycardia, dehydration

Evaluation: Labs: electrolytes, UA; often have ketosis & electrolyte derangements

Treatment: IV fluids (w/ dextrose, thiamine), pyridoxine (vitamin B6), metoclopramide, pyridoxine-doxylamine, ginger

- Ondansetron use in 1st trimester is controversial; may ↑ risk of cardiac malformations (*Reprod Toxicol* 2019;83:14), but other studies suggest safe

Disposition: If tolerating PO, home w/ txs as above; admit if severe dehydration

Molar Pregnancy (*Obstet Gynecol* 2021;137(2):355)

- Form of gestational trophoblastic dz, benign placental tumor w/ malignant potential, can be complete or partial
- Presentation: Abnl bleeding, abdominal pain, uterine size greater than dates, absent fetal heart tones, hyperemesis gravidarum, ovarian enlargement, preeclampsia
- Evaluation: Abnormally high hCG level, US to establish dx (mixed echogenic pattern replacing placenta)
- Management: Ob/Gyn c/s for D&E, Rhogam if Rh-neg
    - Requires postevacuation monitoring of hCG to identify pts who develop malignant gestational trophoblastic neoplasia

Emergency Contraception (*Obstet Gynecol* 2015;126:e1)

- Therapy to prevent pregnancy after unprotected intercourse, none involve termination of preexisting pregnancy, no e/o adverse effects on developing fetus
- Oral: Inhibit ovulation – ulipristal acetate (30 mg, effective up to 120 h after intercourse), levonorgestrel (1.5 mg, effective up to 72 h after intercourse; maximally effective w/i 24 h); note levonorgestrel less effective among obese or overweight pts; impact of weight on ulipristal efficacy is limited
    - Adverse effects: Nausea, HA, irregular bleeding 1 wk–1 mo post-tx, no ongoing contraceptive benefit

- IUD more effective than oral emergency contraception; Copper IUD: Prevents fertilization, provides ongoing contraceptive benefit, effective if placed w/i 5 d; Levonorgestrel 52-mg IUD effective if placed w/i 5 d, noninferior to copper IUD for emergency contraception (*N Engl J Med* 2021;384(4):335)
    - Adverse effects: Cramping & bleeding
    - Consider concomitant STI testing & tx

Retained Products of Conception & Septic Abortion (*N Engl J Med* 2020;382(11):1029–1040)

History

- Retained products of conception: Pain, cramping, heavy vaginal bleeding, clots
- Septic abortion: Pain, cramping, bloody or purulent D/C, fever; infxn of products of conception that can spread to uterus → systemic infxn
- Relevant to know if hx uterine instrumentation (for spontaneous or induced abortion)
- Note that *both* cx can occur following either live birth, spontaneous abortion (ie, miscarriage) or induced abortion

Physical Examination

- VS: Hemodynamically stable vs unstable; fever?
- Pelvic exam: Eval for lacs, vaginal bleeding, retained tissue at cervical os, purulent D/C, uterine tenderness

Evaluation

- Labs: CBC, quant hCG, type & cross, coags; Bcx and lactate if c/f infxn
- Imaging: Pelvic U/S to eval for retained products of conception
- Septic abortion ultimately clinical dx but imaging (pelvic US or CT) can support dx

Treatment

- Supportive: Stabilize (see *Sepsis chapter*), correct anemia/coagulopathy
- If retained products of conception: As w/ miscarriage (see above), options include expectant management, medical management (misoprostol) or uterine aspiration; guided by pt stability, preferences
- If suspected infxn: Abx – gentamicin 5 mg/kg/d PLUS ampicillin 2 g q4h PLUS clindamycin 900 mg IV q8h OR metronidazole 500 mg q8h; OR clindamycin PLUS gentamicin PLUS PCN G (if c/f clostridium); OR piperacillin-tazobactam 4.5 g q8h
- C/s: Gyn service inc for consideration of D&C

COMPLICATIONS OF LATE PREGNANCY

Acute Fatty Liver

Definition: Disorder of the 3rd trimester that can result in hepatic failure & lead to complicated labor & fetal death, RFs include primiparous & twin gestation

- Differentiate from cholestasis of pregnancy which is characterized by jaundice & pruritus w/o systemic sxs, may have nl transaminases

Presentation

- Nausea, vomiting, malaise, RUQ pain, & jaundice in the 3rd trimester
- Can progress to DIC & hepatic encephalopathy
- DDx includes viral hepatitis, preeclampsia, HELLP synd, drug-induced hepatic failure

Evaluation: CBC (leukocytosis, low PLTs), coags (elevated), fibrinogen (low), BMP, LFTs, ammonia, uric acid, RUQ US (may be nl), fetal & maternal monitoring

Treatment: Supportive (manage airway, treat hypoglycemia, replace fluids & blood products), c/s OB, prompt delivery is only definitive tx

Disposition: Admit for stabilization & delivery

Pearls

- May be difficult to differentiate acute fatty liver from HELLP and preeclampsia w/ severe features but all involve supportive care and prompt delivery

Thromboembolic Disease

- Common cause of death in pregnancy
- Pregnancy is hypercoagulable state, other RFs are smoking, age >35 y, hypercoagulability, varicose veins, prior VTE, premature delivery, postpartum hemorrhage (*Obstet Gynecol* 2011;118(3):718)
- See VTE under cardiovascular section for more details

Preterm Labor

- Defined as uterine contractions w/ cervical chgs before 37 wks
- RFs: Substance use, hx of preterm delivery, multiple gestations, placental anomalies, infxn, extremes of age

- Management: Labs, fetal monitoring, US, OB consultation
- Goal of prolongation of gestation: Tocolytics (eg, indomethacin, nifedipine, terbutaline), fetal maturation therapy (corticosteroids), consider need for group B strep prophylaxis, bed rest, hydration

Premature Rupture of Membranes (PROM)

- Defined as rupture of amniotic & chorionic membranes before onset of labor (PPROM refers to premature PROM <37 wks)
- History & sterile exam: Gush of fluid, identification of amniotic fluid (nitrazine, ferning)
- Management: Testing for STI, assess for labor, US, fetal monitoring, OB consultation & admx, consideration of fetal maturation therapy, abx

Placenta Previa & Abruptio Placentae

History

- Placenta previa: Placental implantation adjacent to or over os. Presents as painless, bright red, vaginal bleeding usually after 20 wks. RFs: Multiple gestation, multiparity, advanced maternal age, previous placenta previa/C-section, smoking
- Abruptio placentae: Separation of implanted placenta b/w 20 wks & delivery. Presents as painful, dark red bleeding (80%), contractions; may also present w/ signs/sxs of DIC. RFs: Prior hx abruption, preeclampsia, HTN, abdominal trauma, cocaine, smoking
- Cx: Fetal distress or death, amniotic fluid embolism, fetomaternal tfx

Physical Examination

- Check fundal height, contractions, & uterine tenderness:
  - Firm/tender uterus = placental abruption until proven o/w
- AVOID SPECULUM & VAGINAL EXAM (can lead to hemorrhage if placenta previa)

Evaluation

- Labs: CBC, Chem 7, LFTs, PT/PTT, fibrinogen (r/o DIC), UA, type/crossmatch
- Imaging: Doppler U/S (fetal heart tones); abdominal U/S to assess placenta & signs of fetal movement, though may not always detect abruption

Treatment

- Supportive: Place on L side (uterus off IVC), 2 large-bore IVs, IVF, monitor pt & fetus
- Tfx: Blood products ± FFP (if HD unstable or signs of DIC)
- Medications: Rh immunoglobulin 300 mcg if Rh-neg, magnesium for fetal neuroprotection if emergent delivery under 32 wks
- C/s: Urgent Gyn eval for possible STAT C-section

Disposition

- Admit: All pts to the OB service even if HD stable for close monitoring.

Amniotic Fluid Embolism (*Obstet Gynecol* 2014;123(Pt 1):337)

Definition: Hypothesized to be due to release of amniotic fluid into maternal circulation, occurs during uterine contractions or manipulation or abruptio placentae (rarely can be spontaneous), triggers anaphylactoid response leading to maternal cardiovascular collapse that is rapidly fatal

Presentation

- Sudden-onset hypotension, hypoxia, coagulopathy
- Leads to DIC, ARDS, LV dysfxn, sz-like activity, syncope, cardiac arrest
- DDx includes PE, anaphylaxis, septic shock, eclampsia, HELLP, abruptio placentae, chronic coagulopathy

Treatment: Support oxygenation & ventilation (HFNC, intubation) and hemodyanmics (fluids, pressors), management of coagulopathy, STAT OB c/s

Disposition: Admit to ICU

Peripartum Cardiomyopathy (*J Am Coll Cardiol* 2020;75(2):207)

- Rare form of nonischemic CMP causing systolic heart failure that affects women at the end of pregnancy or in the mos following delivery
- RFs: African American race, preeclampsia, HTN, multigestation, age >30 y
- Sxs often confused for common sxs of nl pregnancy leading to delay in dx, diagnosed by echocardiography
- Cx include arrhythmia, thromboembolism, death
- Management depends on stage of pregnancy
  - During pregnancy: BB, loop diuretic, hydralazine/isosorbide mononitrate, digoxin, LMWH; note: ACE/ARB/spironolactone are contraindicated, consider early delivery, mechanical support devices for severe HF or cardiogenic shock
  - After pregnancy: BB, enalapril, spironolactone (safe during breastfeeding), AC if LV thrombus or severe LV dysfxn, consider ICD
- Outcomes include variable recovery (spectrum from complete recovery to persistent HF)

PREECLAMPSIA AND ECLAMPSIA

Definition (*Obstet Gynecol* 2020;135(6):e237)

- Chronic HTN: Systolic BP >140/90 before 20 wks of gestation
- Gestational HTN: BP >140/90 on 2 occasions after 20 wks of gestation w/o prior HTN dx
- Preeclampsia: Gestational HTN & either proteinuria, thrombocytopenia, or end-organ damage (eg, AKI, liver dysfxn, refractory HA), can be classified as mild to severe
- Preeclampsia w/ severe features: SBP >160 or DBP >110, PLTs <100k, renal insufficiency, impaired liver function, pulm edema, HA unresponsive to meds, visual sxs
- Eclampsia: Preeclampsia w/ szs or coma; generally 3rd trimester or postpartum

Approach to the Patient

History

- HA, visual disturbances, mental status chgs, n/v, abd pain, edema. PMH (prior preeclampsia, nulliparity, extremes of age, HTN, obesity, antiphospholipid antibody synd, DM, CKD, OSA, assisted reproductive technology)

Physical Examination

- HTN, abdominal tenderness, hyperreflexia, peripheral edema, papilledema, AMS

Evaluation

- CBC, BMP, Mg, LFTs, UA, LDH, uric acid, coags, type & cross, fetal/maternal monitoring
- Consider CT head to assess for CVT or ICH (esp if no hx of preeclampsia, refractory szs, AMS, or focal neuro sxs)

Treatment

- BP: Hydralazine, labetalol, or nifedipine (goal BP <140/90)
- Sz prophylaxis: Magnesium 2–6 g IV load + 1–2 g/h infusion; if do not have IV access can give 5 g IM in each buttock
- Szs: Magnesium (2–4 g IV q5–10 mins); refractory szs: AEDs
- Monitor for adverse effects of Mg (losing deep tendon reflexes, respiratory depression)
- C/s: Gyn for all pts; delivery is only definitive tx for eclampsia

Complications

- Maternal cx: Pulmonary edema, stroke, permanent CNS damage, renal insufficiency, death
- Fetal cx: Hypoxia, placental infarct, IUGR, abruptio placentae
- HELLP synd: Hemolysis, elevated liver enzyme levels, low PLTs (coags nl), increased maternal morbidity & mortality, p/w RUQ pain, n/v, malaise

Disposition

- Home: Mild preeclampsia (no e/o end-organ damage, BP controlled); OB f/u in 24 h
- Admit: Eclamptic & most severe preeclamptic pts need urgent delivery (pending BP & sz control) & ICU admx

EMERGENCY DELIVERY

(*Emerg Med Clin North Am* 2019;37(2):265)

Definition

- True labor: Regular uterine contractions of increasing intensity at decreasing intervals
- False labor (Braxton Hicks contractions): Uterine contractions that do not lead to cervical change
- 1st stage (cervical): Cervical dilatation & effacement (up to 12 h)
- 2nd stage (expulsion): Complete cervical dilatation, culminating in delivery (up to 2 h)
- 3rd stage (placental): Separation & delivery of placenta
- Precipitous delivery: Labor <3 h from onset of regular contractions to birth

Approach to the Patient

History

- Frequency & intensity of contractions, rupture of membranes (loss of fluid), bleeding, fetal movement; has pt had prenatal care for eval of cx of pregnancy, screening tests, etc; prior births & cx, estimated due date or LMP
- Sxs of labor: Contractions, back pain, abdominal/pelvic pain, urinary urgency

Physical Examination

- External exam: Assess for crowning or active bleeding; if fetus visibly crowning there is no time to transfer & need to deliver in ED
- Uterine fundal height: Palpated at the level of umbilicus at 20 wks & grows 1 cm/wk

- Sterile speculum exam: Confirm rupture of membranes by checking for ferning and/or nitrazine test
- Bimanual exam: Assess cervical effacement (paper thin) & dilatation (10 cm = complete), position, presentation (fetal part in canal), lie (relation of long axis to mother → longitudinal or transverse), & station (–3 to +3; 0 is at level of ischial spines); cord prolapse

Evaluation

- Abdominal U/S if placenta previa of concern, assess presentation, fetal heart tone

Normal Vaginal Delivery

- Basics of delivery
  - Supplies: Sterile gloves, PPE, 2 umbilical clamps/hemostats, scissors, bulb suction, towels, suture material, fetal resuscitation equipment
  - Place pt in lithotomy position; cleanse/drape perineum if possible; w/ contractions, ask pt to "bear down"
    - Head: One hand on occipital area & other on perineum, maintain fetal head in flexed position; palpate for nuchal cord, if present reduce over head
    - Shoulders: Rotate head & exert gentle pressure until anterior shoulder delivered; lift head upward to deliver posterior shoulders, attempt to guide posterior shoulder over perineum.
    - Body: Support head & catch body w/ the other hand. Suction mouth & nose
    - Cord: Clamp cord twice & cut, send cord blood for serology & Rh. Clamp cord 1–3 cm distal to navel. If infant vigorous, ACOG recommends delayed clamping 30–60 s after birth (*Obstet Gynecol* 2020;136(6):e100)
    - Placenta: Apply pressure above symphysis w/ minimal traction on cord (too much traction will cause uterine inversion); sudden gush of blood & lengthening cord will signify imminent placental delivery. Ensure placenta appears intact after delivery
    - Aftercare: Massage uterus ± oxytocin 10 U IV bolus, ideally prophylactic (can be given as 10 U IM if no IV access for ongoing hemorrhage); eval for lacs of cervix, perineum that require repair
    - Infant care: Suction mouth & nose, stimulate w/ warm blanket. BVM if no spontaneous respirations. If pulse <60 start CPR, neonatal resuscitation per PALS. Obtain Apgar scores at 1 & 5 mins

Complications of Delivery

- Cord prolapse: Manually place hand in vaginal vault, lift presenting part away from cord; place pt in knee–chest position (most effective) or deep Trendelenburg. Consider short-acting tocolytics (eg, terbutaline 0.25 mg IV or SQ) (*Am J Obstet Gynecol* 2021;225(4):357)
- Shoulder dystocia:
  - McRoberts (recommended initial maneuver): Hyperflexion of hips to abdomen w/ external rotation & slight abduction and apply suprapubic pressure
  - Rubin I maneuver: Downward pressure just proximal to symphysis pubis
  - Rubin II maneuver: Place fingers on fetal shoulder & push shoulder toward anterior surface of the fetal chest to decreased shoulder-to-shoulder dimension
  - Woods screw maneuver: Insert hand into vagina & apply pressure to anterior aspect of posterior shoulder to abduct/extend shoulder & free it
  - Delivery of the posterior arm: Insert hand into vagina, flex posterior arm of the fetus, bringing it across the chest. Deliver posterior arm hand first & then rotate fetus out
  - Gaskin position: Place mother in hands-and-knees position, increases pelvic outlet, and allows gravity to help open space
- Breech: Ideally OB present, or delivery in OR for c/s. If imminent, touch fetus as little as possible & let delivery happen spontaneously, do not pull on fetus which can entrap fetal head. If head becomes entrapped, uterine relaxant (eg, terbutaline) can be given; incomplete breech (1 or both feet deliver first) greater risk head entrapment, cord prolapse (vs complete breech)

Resuscitative Hysterotomy

- Perimortem delivery: >23 wks of gestational age (obvious gravid uterus), should initiate w/i 4 mins of maternal arrest
  - Vertical incision from epigastrium to pubic symphysis & extend through all layers to the peritoneal cavity
  - Uterus is exposed & incised at bladder reflection, retract bladder caudally
  - Incision extended to uterine fundus, w/ operator's hand used to palpate fetal parts & prevent damage. Infant extracted, clamp, & cut umbilical cord

POSTPARTUM COMPLICATIONS

Postpartum Hemorrhage (*Obstet Gynecol* 2017;130(4):e168–e186)

- Defined as EBL ≥1000 cc or loss of blood a/w signs & sxs of hypovolemia (primary PPH occurs in the 1st 24 h, secondary occurs up to 12 wks after delivery)
  - DDx: 4 T's (tone [uterine atony], trauma [lac, hematoma, uterine inversion, or rupture], tissue [retained or invasive placenta], thrombin [coagulopathy, DIC])
  - Uterine atony is most common etiology
  - Most effective strategy to prevent PPH is active management of 3rd stage of labor (administering oxytocin, controlled cord traction to deliver placenta, uterine massage)
    - Alternatives to oxytocin & 2nd-line agents: Carboprost (asthma is CI), methylergonovine (HTN, preeclampsia are CI), misoprostol, TXA
- Based on the WOMAN trial (*Lancet* 2017;389:1205), TXA reduces death due to bleeding in PPH when given w/i 3 h of birth, no increase in adverse events
- Ongoing PPH despite uterine massage and uterotonics may require intrauterine tamponade (eg. Bakri balloon, Foley catheter, or packing), uterine artery embolization; hysterectomy is last resort

Postpartum Fever

- Approach: Obtain through hx, evaluate breasts, wounds, urinary & respiratory tract, GU exam; obtain CBC, UA, BCx, +/– CXR, consider pelvic US or CT a/p

Differential Diagnosis of Postpartum Fever (*Obstet Med* 2014;7(3):98)		
Cause	**Dx**	**Treatment**
Endometritis	Common cause; clinical dx; p/w fever, abd or pelvic pain, uterine tenderness, foul smelling lochia	Clindamycin PLUS gentamicin is preferred tx
Pelvic abscess	CT > US	I&D, abx (as above for endometritis)
UTI	UA & culture, treat w/ abx	Abx
PNA	CXR	Abx
Wound infxn	Clinical exam, culture	Abx (cefazolin or vancomycin if cellulitis, otw as above for endometritis), debridement
Mastitis	Clinical dx; US to evaluate for abscess	Treat w/ abx to cover *S. aureus*, drain if abscess, continue breast-feeding
Thrombophlebitis	Suspect if fail to respond to abx for endometritis; CT	Abx (Clindamycin PLUS gentamicin ± ampicillin); A/C use recommended but controversial
PE/DVT	LENI, CT PE	A/C

NONINFECTIOUS PELVIC PAIN

History

- Acute vs chronic, gradual vs sudden onset, dyspareunia, vaginal bleeding or D/C, urinary sxs, n/v, LMP, PMH (STDs, recent procedure), meds (contraceptive devices, hormonal therapy), social (intimate partner violence)

Physical Examination

- Abdominal exam; pelvic exam (D/C or bleeding, masses, tenderness)

Evaluation

- Labs: UA, hCG, GC/*Chlamydia*, Wet mount
- Imaging: Pelvic US (eval for torsion; look for flow, mass, fluid)

Pelvic Pain Differential	
Pathophysiology	**Differential**
Nongynecologic	Appendicitis, diverticulitis, nephrolithiasis, UTI/pyelonephritis, IBD, IBS, hernia, SBO, perirectal abscess, aortic dissection, pelvic fx
Gynecologic	Ovarian torsion, ruptured ovarian cyst, adenomyosis, degenerating uterine fibroid, endometriosis, PID, TOA, mittelschmerz, dysmenorrhea, imperforate hymen
Pregnancy related	Ectopic pregnancy, miscarriage, corpus luteum hematoma, ovarian vein thrombosis, placental abruption, uterine rupture, endometritis

Ovarian Cyst

Definition

- Most common cause of gynecologic mass, usually benign, most common in reproductive y, can be a/w hemorrhage or torsion

Presentation

- Dull, vague, unilateral sensation of pelvic pain or dyspareunia; can be asx
- Rupture: Sudden, unilateral, sharp pelvic pain; may be following activity
- Exam: Lower quadrant abdominal tenderness, usually unilateral, adnexal tenderness/mass

Evaluation

- Labs: CBC, type & screen (crossmatch if HD unstable), hCG
- Imaging: Pelvic U/S to assess for size, complexity, torsion, presence of free fluid. POCUS if HD unstable

Treatment

- Supportive: IVF, transfuse if HD unstable & hemorrhagic
- Analgesia: NSAIDs, narcotics prn
- C/s: Gyn service if persistent pain, large-volume hemorrhage

Disposition

- Home if stable, pain well controlled and no c/f torsion; f/u w/ Gyn or PCP in 1–2 mos for repeat U/S to reassess size; prompt Gyn referral if mass c/f malignancy
- Admit if HD unstable

Ovarian Torsion

Definition

- Twisting of the ovary +/– fallopian tube on axis b/w utero-ovarian & infundibulopelvic ligament leading to venous & lymphatic obstruction initially which progresses to ischemia & necrosis; can progress further to hemorrhage, peritonitis, & infxn

Presentation

- Acutely onset unilateral lower abdominal/pelvic pain, n/v, can be intermittent
- RFs: Ovarian mass (most common when >5 cm), dermoid & other tumors, infertility tx, pregnancy (usually 1st half), most common in reproductive y
- Exam is nonspecific & variable; pelvic exam may reveal unilateral, adnexal mass ± tenderness

Evaluation

- Labs: hCG, preop labs
- Imaging: Pelvic US w/ Doppler is test of choice to eval for ovarian edema, mass, venous & arterial blood flow, free fluid; note torsion is clinical dx and may have nl flow
- CT findings in torsion inc asymmetric enlargement or enhancement, fallopian tube thickening, twisted vascular pedicle, fat stranding, uterine deviation.
- If low pretest probability & nl ovaries visualized on imaging, torsion is unlikely

Treatment

- Analgesia/antiemetics
- C/s Gyn service for urgent laparoscopy for definitive dx and tx (detorsion); attempts at salvage should be performed even if late dx, the ovary can sometimes recover given dual blood supply

VAGINAL DISCHARGE

Cervicitis

Definition

- Purulent or mucopurulent D/C from the endocervix & presence of cervical friability

History

- Purulent or malodorous D/C? Dyspareunia? Pruritus? Postcoital bleeding? Dysuria, urinary frequency or urgency? Vaginal hygiene; PMH STD; LMP; May by asx
- RFs: Multiple sexual partners, unprotected intercourse

Physical Examination

- External: Inspect for lesions, ulcerations, adenopathy
- Speculum: Vaginal wall inflammation; cervical inflammation; D/C; friability
- Bimanual: If cervical motion tenderness or uterine or adnexal tenderness, think PID

Evaluation

- Labs: GC/*Chlamydia* & trichomonas testing; wet mount; consider testing for other STIs inc HSV, HIV, syphilis, hepatitis

Treatment (*MMWR Recomm Rep* 2021;70(4):1–187)

- *N. gonorrhoeae:* CTX 500 mg IM × 1 if <150 kg (if wt ≥150 kg, give 1 g CTX); treat for chlamydial co-infxn unless already excluded
- *C. trachomatis:* Doxycycline 100 mg PO BID × 7 d
- *T. vaginalis:* Metronidazole 500 mg PO BID × 7 d (single 2-g dose rec for men, not women)

Pearls

- Educate pts on safe sex practices
- Advise pts critical to get their partners to get tested/treated
- If chlamydia, gonorrhea, or trichomoniasis dx, pt should have repeat testing in 3 mos even if partner treated (high rate of reinfxn)
- Empiric tx for both *N. gonorrhoeae* & *C. trachomatis*
- Encourage HIV testing outpt if not completed in ED
- Avoid alcohol on metronidazole; can cause disulfiram-like rxn (flushing, ↑ HR, ↓ BP)

Pelvic Inflammatory Disease & Tubo-Ovarian Abscess (*MMWR Recomm Rep* 2021;70(4):1–187)

Definition

- Spectrum of inflammatory disorders caused by ascending infxn leading to any of following: Endometritis, salpingitis, tubo-ovarian abscess, pelvic peritonitis
- Commonly a/w gonorrhea, chlamydia but only ~50% of pts w/ PID test positive for these organisms. Involves other bacteria (eg, GNR, anaerobes, *M. genitalium*)
- Cx include abscess, perihepatitis (Fitz–Hugh–Curtis), sepsis, chronic pain; increased risk of ectopic pregnancy, infertility

Presentation

- Lower abd pain, vaginal D/C or bleeding, dysuria, dyspareunia, nausea, ± fevers
- RFs: Age <25, multiple sexual partners, unprotected sex, h/o PID, IUD placement in the last mo, recent instrumentation of the cervix, douching, smoking
- Exam: Lower abdominal tenderness; must do pelvic exam—assess for cervical D/C, cervical friability, cervical motion tenderness, uterine tenderness, or adnexal tenderness

Evaluation

- Labs: Always check hCG; GC/*Chlamydia* & trichomonas testing, UA, CBC, ESR/CRP (not sens); recommend testing for additional STIs (as above for cervicitis)
- Abdominal CT or pelvic US if TOA is suspected (unilateral tenderness or palpable mass, systemically ill) or if c/f alternative diagnoses

Treatment

- Low threshold for empiric tx: Minimum criteria in sexually active young women or others at risk are pelvic or abdominal pain & either cervical, uterine, and/or adnexal tenderness
- Recommended outpt tx: CTX 500 mg IM × 1 + doxycycline 100 mg BID for 14 d + metronidazole 500 mg BID for 14 d
- Recommended inpt tx: CTX IV PLUS doxycycline PLUS metronidazole; or cefotetan IV OR cefoxitin IV PLUS doxycycline
- C/s Gyn if c/f TOA

Disposition

- Admit if toxic appearing, severe sxs, TOA, failure of outpt therapy (eg, not improved in 72 h), pregnant, immunocompromised, poor f/u w/i 72 h.
- Discharged pts need f/u in 3 d to ensure sx resolving. Partners should be tested/ treated.

Pearls

- PID can be difficult to dx; mild cases still can be a/w cx (eg, infertility)
- Given ↑ resistance to antibiotic regimens, CDC updates recommendations frequently
- PID in pregnancy is rare but does happen, requires admit; consider alternative diagnoses
- Pt(s) dx w/ PID should have repeat testing in 3 mos even if partner treated

Vaginitis (*MMWR Recomm Rep* 2021;70(4):1–187)

- Condition w/ sxs of abnl vaginal D/C, odor, irritation, itching, and/or burning

Vaginitis			
Etiology	**Cause**	**Evaluation & Dx**	**Treatment & Pearls**
Bacterial vaginosis	Not considered an STI; caused by alteration in vaginal flora w/ replacement of nl flora w/ anaerobic organisms (eg, *G. vaginalis*)	• Malodorous thin, whitish D/C • Fishy odor of vaginal D/C (accentuated w/ KOH, "whiff test") • Vaginal pH >4.5 • Clue cells on wet mount • NAAT also available • Commonly asx	• Treat all w/ sxs • Metronidazole 500 mg PO BID × 7 d OR metronidazole 0.75% gel intravaginally 5 g/d × 5 d OR clindamycin 2% cream intravaginally 5 g × 7 d • ↑ risk of STIs, PID & pregnancy cx
Candidiasis	Caused by *Candida* (usually *C. albicans*); recurrent infxns common, not considered an STI; classified as uncomplicated vs complicated (eg, severe, recurrent, immunocompromised)	• Pruritus, dyspareunia, external dysuria, thick curdy whitish D/C, vulvar/ vaginal erythema, & edema • Nl vaginal pH (<4.5) • Wet mount shows budding yeast or pseudohyphae • Vaginal culture if neg wet mount and sxs; or if c/f complicated vulvovaginal candidiasis	• Tx: Topical azoles (over the counter) generally 7 d OR fluconazole 150 mg PO × 1 • Fluconazole is contraindicated in pregnancy
Trichomoniasis	STI caused by *T. vaginalis*	• Green or yellow frothy D/C, vaginal pain • "Strawberry" cervix • Diagnosed by NAAT; wet mount low sens • Test for other STIs • May be asx	• Treated w/ PO metronidazole 500 mg BID × 7 d • Treat sexual partners • Retest in 3 mos • ↑ risk pregnancy cx

Definition *(Am Fam Physician* 2010;81(6):726–734)
- An eruption of one or more skin lesions

Approach
- HPI: Onset (timing, location); evolution (distribution, morphology); periodicity (constant vs waxing & waning, temporal associations); sxs (pain, pruritus, burning, fever, bleeding); new exposures or inciting events (topical or systemic exposures, recent travel, occupational exposures, sick contacts, animals, sexual hx)
- PMH/ROS: Be thorough as rashes can be 1st sign of a systemic process
- Meds: Current formulations/doses, new medications, supplements, illicit substances
- PEx: Determine distribution, shape (if applicable), morphology, & secondary chgs
  - Distribution: Localized/grouped/regional/generalized, central/peripheral, flexor/extensor surface, dermatomal, acral, intertriginous, follicular, mucosal, sun-exposed areas
  - Shape (if applicable): Annular (ring), round/nummular/discoid (coin), targetoid, arcuate (arc), linear, serpiginous, reticular (net-like/lacey), whorled (marble-like), polycyclic (coalescing circular/ring-shaped lesions)
  - Morphology & secondary chgs: See tables

Common Dermatologic Morphologies		
Flat	Macule	Flat circumscribed area of discoloration (compared to surrounding skin) <1.0 cm diam
	Patch	Flat circumscribed area of discoloration (compared to surrounding skin) >1.0 cm diam, or similarly sized confluence of macules
Raised	Papule	Raised solid lesion <1.0 cm diam; compared to nodule, papule is superficial; can be any color
	Plaque	Raised plate-like solid area >1.0 cm diam, or similarly-sized confluence of papules; can be any color
	Nodule	Raised, often-round, solid lump; compared to papule, nodule is larger & deeper (epidermal, epidermal–dermal, dermal, dermal–subdermal, subcut); can be any color
	Wheal	Raised variously-shaped, often-erythematous, edematous, pruritic area often >1.0 cm diam; compared to plaque, wheal is often w/ irregular & sharp borders
Fluid-filled	Vesicle	Raised fluid-filled lesion <0.5 cm diam; compared to pustule, vesicle fluid is clear; compared to cyst, vesicle is superficial, thin walled, & smaller
	Pustule	Raised fluid-filled lesion <0.5 cm diam; compared to vesicle, pustule fluid is purulent; coalescing groups of pustules are referred to as "lakes"
	Bulla	Raised fluid-filled lesion >0.5 cm diam; fluid can be clear or hemorrhagic
	Cyst	Firmly encapsulated cavity/sac filled w/ fluid or semisolid material; compared to vesicle, cyst is deeper & firmer
Vascular	Petechia	Numerous, uniform, small (pinpoint), nonblanching, red/purple, asx macules; 2/2 TCP
	Purpura	Irregularly shaped, circumscribed, nonblanching, macules or patches; occasionally painful; 2/2 blood extravasation, often a/w small-vessel thrombosis
Depressed	Eschar	Circumscribed depressed lesion covered by dry, adherent black necrotic tissue
	Erosion	Circumscribed minimally depressed lesion w/ open/exposed moist dermal tissue
	Ulcer	Circumscribed depressed lesion w/ open/exposed moist dermal or subcutaneous tissue

Common Secondary Changes	
Scaling	Thickened outer epidermis (stratum corneum), usually white
Crusting	Dried liquid debris (eg, serum, blood, exudates), usually yellow–brown
Lichenification	Thickening of epidermis w/ accentuated skin lines/markings
Excoriation	Superficial abrasions, usually due to scratching

Typical Manifestations of Common or Critical Acute Disseminated Rashes	
Viral Etiologies	
Acute HIV	Maculopapular **2–3 wks after initial infxn**; a/w constitutional sx
Dengue fever	Maculopapular/confluent macules w/ islands of sparing **a/w high fever, HA, retro-orbital & severe body pain**; lasts 2–3 d
Measles	Maculopapular, starts behind ears & face/neck, spreads to trunk & extremities (w/ palms/soles), ± confluence; a/w **fever, cough, coryza, conjunctivitis, Koplik spots; lasts 3–7 d,** leaves as arrived
Mononucleosis	Maculopapular; no palms/soles; a/w **fatigue, sore throat, fever**
Parvovirus B19	**Reddened ("slapped") cheeks** w/ circumoral pallor (lasts 1–4 d) –> generalized reticular/lacey rash, esp extensor surfaces (spares palms/soles) w/ progression to trunk/buttocks (can last 3 wks)
Pityriasis rosea	Small oval macular plaques distributed on lines of cleavage on trunk/prox extremities (spares face, palms, soles); often 1–3 wks after **herald patch** (single 2–4-cm plaque w/ fine scaling borders & depressed pale center); rash lasts 5 wks–5 mos
Roseola	Macules that start on neck/trunk **after defervescence** & spreads to face/extremities; lasts 1–2 d
Rubella	Maculopapular, starts on face/forehead then to trunk/extremities, ± coalesce; a/w **fever, HA, arthralgias; lasts ~3 d**
Varicella (Chicken pox)	Pruritic maculopapular –> vesicles –> crusting w/i 48 h **(all three stages present at same time);** trunk/face > extremities; ± mucous membranes; crusts fall off after 1–2 wks
Zika Virus	Pruritic maculopapular rash and nonpurulent conjunctivitis
Bacterial Etiologies	
Gonococcemia	Few scattered **hemorrhagic pustules** (often over joints) occurring after mucosal infxn; a/w **arthralgias & low-grade fever**
Leptospirosis	Initially warm & flushed, can develop transient petechia, later purpura; a/w fever, HA, myalgias, GI sx, **subconjunctival hem**; severe dz **(Weil synd)** a/w liver & kidney failure
Lyme	**Erythema migrans (bull's eye lesion)** in 20% of primary lyme; Secondary lyme, 3–10 wks after infxn, w/ small oval macules/patches, **a/w neuro, cardiac, msk cx**
Meningococcemia	Rapidly progressive **petechia & purpura**; **toxic appearing**; ±2–3 d prodrome of HA, URI sx (but 20% pts present w/ sepsis); mortality 10–15% w/ tx *(Intern Med 2016;55(6):567–572)*
Rocky mountain spotted fever (RMSF)	Numerous red macules w/ central petechia start on wrists/ankles, then palms/soles, then centrally to arms/legs/trunk; 10–15% may not have rash; **a/w abrupt fever, severe HA,** N/V, abd pain, myalgias
Scarlet fever	Diffuse fine erythematous **coalescent "sandpaper" eruption**; starts on neck & spreads to trunk/extremities, becomes macules coalescing into patches; flushed face w/ circumoral pallor; **a/w recent strep infxn;** lasts 7 d then fine desquamation
Staph scalded skin synd	**Widespread painful peeling of skin**; no mucous membranes; a/w malaise, fever
Secondary syphilis	Diffuse **macules, papules** (± pustules), **inc on palms/soles** & mucous membranes
Toxic shock synd	Diffuse erythematous **coalescent "sandpaper"** macules & patches, ± hemorrhagic bullae; mucous membranes involved**; a/w fever**, GI sx, confusion, multiorgan failure
Arthropod Bites	
Bed bugs	Painless pruritic red papules on **exposed areas**; occasionally wheals, hemorrhagic nodules, vesicles 2/2 bug proteases
Lice	Painless pruritic red papules & wheals, often concentrated in **high–hair-density areas (scalp/axilla/groin)** & sparing extremities
Scabies	Painless, intensely pruritic red papules, often **clustered**, classically affected interdigital web spaces of hands, spreads to genitals, buttocks, and trunk; eval for **intertriginous burrows**

Vascular/Hematologic	
HSP	Erythematous macules & papules becoming purpuric **(palpable purpura)** symmetrically on **lower extremities**; spares soles; **a/w abd pain & joint pain**
ITP	**Petechia**, esp in lower extremities & palette; can be asx
TTP	**Petechia, a/w fever, AMS**/neuro deficits, ± jaundice
DIC	**Petechia, purpura, hemorrhagic bullae**, acral cyanosis, localized necrosis/gangrene (inc. extremities); **a/w multiorgan failure**
Hypersensitivity Reactions	
Acute generalized pustular psoriasis	**Diffuse** small **sterile pruritic pustules on erythematous base**, a/w fever; trunk & intertriginous areas common (no mucous membranes); may have multiorgan dysfxn
Allergic contact dermatitis	***Poison ivy/oak:*** Wheals & **vesicles** (± bullae) **on exposed areas** **Topical (eg, hair dye): Vesicles** & papules w/ crusting, edema
Bullous pemphigoid	Acute or subacute pruritic, diffuse**, tense bullae** on nl, erythematous, or urticarial base **(-Nikolsky)**; many causal associations (diuretics, NSAIDs, captopril); bx dx
DRESS synd	Maculopapular, papulosquamous, pustular, bullous, or urticarial exanthem; a/w fever, LAN, **systemic sx; 2/2 drug**
Erythema multiforme	Diffuse erythematous macules/papules w/ **evolving morphology** (become **targetoid**, then polycyclic & annular configuration); trunk, extremities **(inc palms/soles), face (mucous memb ~70%)**
Erythema nodosum	**Painful**, round, oval, macular **nodules** (1–6 cm diam), can coalesce; symmetric & usually **anterior tibia** (also knees, ankles, thighs, forearms); self-resolves after 1–6 wks
Erythroderma	**Generalized erythema (>90% TBSA**; spares palms/soles), progresses to scaling & desquamation; pruritic; often w/ edema; LAN ± e/o high-output HF, hepatomegaly, splenomegaly
Morbilliform drug eruption	**Diffuse erythematous morbilliform** macules/papules (less commonly erythroderma, pustules, targetoid lesions), can coalesce & become edematous; trunk, extremities, face
Pemphigus vulgaris	Diffuse small or confluent painful **flaccid blisters & erosions** on erythematous base **(+Nikolsky)**; inc mucous membranes
SJS/TEN	Diffuse erythematous dusky confluent purpuric macules or patches, **rapidly evolve to coalesce & blister (+Nikolsky)**; often starts on trunk & spreads to extremities (inc palms/soles) & face **(inc mucous membranes);** eventually generalized sloughing
Scromboid	Diffuse macular or papular erythema w/ urticaria **<30 mins after ingesting scombroid** fish; **a/w HA, N/V**, palpitations
Serum sickness & serum sickness-like rxn	Diffuse urticarial or serpiginous macules & patches, **well-demarcated w/ intense red border** & central clearing; trunk, face, extremities (no palms/soles), **a/w arthralgias**
Sweet synd	**Tender, violaceous, well-demarcated** papules & plaques (± central pustules, bullae, or ulcers), can evolve to coalesce; commonly on upper body (inc face, mucous memb), **a/w arthralgias, fever, cancer, autoimmune dz, pregnancy**
Urticaria	Pruritic, erythematous, **migratory wheals**, ranging in size from a few mm to several cm in size; may be round or irregular in shape
Miscellaneous	
Guttate psoriasis	**Diffuse dewdrop**-like 1–10-mm salmon-colored papules w/ fine scaling; can coalesce; may be **preceded by URI or grp A strep infxn**
Photosensitive rash	Erythema or bulla (inc hemorrhagic) **at area of UV exposure**
Pityriasis versicolor	Noncontagious subacute **hypo- or hyperpigmented** macules & patches, often neck/trunk/UEs; 2/2 *malassezia* fungus, RFs are humidity, immunosupp, OCPs, poor nutrition

VIRAL EXANTHEMS

Measles (Rubeola; "First Disease")

Definition (*Lancet* 2017;390(10111):2490–2502)

- Highly contagious dz caused by the measles virus, spread by droplet contact
- Epidemiology: Usually nonimmunized or immunosupp (1° vaccine failure <0.2%); can occur in immunized adults (2° vaccine failure 5% >15 y after vaccination) esp if no herd immunity (though often milder); winter/spring common; incubation ~1 wk

History & Physical Examination

- Assess vaccination status
- Prodrome (lasts 3 d): Acute febrile illness; **4Cs: C**ough, **C**oryza (nasal mucosal inflammation), **C**onjunctivitis, **K**oplik spots (small irreg-shaped blue-white macules on buccal mucosa)
- Exanthem (lasts 3–7 d): Starts behind ears, on face/neck as discrete purple-red macules & papules; spreads to trunk & extremities (inc palms/soles), becoming confluent; disappears in same order as arrived

Evaluation

- Routine labs rarely indicated (CBC may show leukopenia)
- Lab confirmation: Measles serologies (enzyme immunoassay for measles IgG & IgM), throat or nasopharyngeal swab for viral isolation/RT-PCR. Contact lab specialist.

Treatment

- Supportive, c/s ID
- Two-dose Vit A may reduce mortality in children <2 y (*Lancet* 2017;390(10111):2490–2502)

Complications

- During/post-infxn: Otitis media (most common) & mastoiditis, keratitis, corneal ulcerations & blindness, croup, PNA (most common severe complication), myopericarditis, TTP, febrile sz, encephalomyelitis (1:1000 incidence ~2 wks after infxn; 2/2 autoimm demyelination; fever/sz/various neuro sx)
- Late cx (rare): Inclusion body encephalitis (mos after infxn; fatal), subacute sclerosing panencephalitis (y after infxn; fatal)

Disposition

- Home if no severe cx
- Notify public health department w/i 24 h

Rubella (German Measles; Three-day Measles; "Third Disease")

Definition (*Pediatr Rev* 2010;31(3):1279–1230)

- Contagious dz of childhood caused by rubella virus, spread by droplet contact
- Epidemiology: Usually children, but adults can get too (long-term vaccine failure <10%); winter/spring common; incubation 2–3 wks
- Rubella infxn in children/adults is distinct from congenital rubella synd (CRS), a severe teratogenic congenital infxn (not discussed here)

History & Physical Examination

- Assess vaccination status
- Prodrome: Malaise, low-grade fever, HA, sore throat, adenopathy, arthralgias
- Exanthem: Erythematous macules & papules begin on face/forehead, spread to trunk/extremities, may coalesce; typically lasts 3 d then resolves

Evaluation

- Routine labs rarely indicated (CBC may show leukopenia, TCP)
- Lab confirmation: Rubella serologies (enzyme immunoassay, latex agglutination, IFA), throat or nasopharyngeal swab for viral isolation/RT-PCR. Contact lab specialist.
  - Confirmation important in pregnant pts

Treatment

- Supportive

Complications

- During/post-infxn: Inflammatory arthritis (most common), encephalopathy (1:5000–1:30,000), transient TCP, hemolytic anemia (rare), GBS
- If pt is pregnant: Congenital rubella synd (highest risk in 1st trimester)

Disposition

- Home, avoid contact w/ pregnant women (severe congenital defects)
- Notify public health department w/i 24 h

Erythema Infectiosum ("Fifth Disease")

Definition

- Highly contagious dz caused by Parvovirus B19, spread by respiratory droplets
- Epidemiology: Mainly school-age children (2–14 y/o); winter/spring common; incubation 1–2 wks; transmission via blood products rare (virus lives in RBC precursor)

History & Physical Examination

- Prodrome: Malaise, low-grade fever, HA, arthralgias
- Exanthem: Intensely reddened face ("slapped cheek") w/ circumoral pallor (lasts 1–4 d), then generalized reticular/lacey rash, esp extensor surfaces (spares palms/soles) w/ progression to trunk/buttocks (can last 3 wks); rash uncommon in adults

Evaluation

- Routine labs rarely indicated; consider CBC, reticulocyte count, & haptoglobin in pts w/ hx hemolytic anemia (eg, hereditary spherocytosis) or hemoglobinopathies (ie, SCD)
- Lab confirmation: Serologic testing, DNA assays (direct hybridization)

Treatment

- Supportive
- If complicated (see below), can consider course of IVIG in consultation w/ hematology

Complications

- During infxn: Inflammatory arthritis (most common, esp adults), transient aplastic crisis (esp in pts w/ hemolytic anemias & hemoglobinopathies), pure red cell aplasia
  - Parvovirus temporarily shuts down RBC production during infxn
- In pregnant pts, risk of fetal loss 5–10%; greatest in 2nd trimester (*Birth Defects Res* 2017;109(5):311–323)

Disposition

- Home; CDC does not recommend avoidance of school or workplace

Roseola Infantum (Exanthema Subitum; "Sixth Disease")

Definition

- Dz of children 6–36 mos (95%) caused by HHV-6 & HHV-7, spread by salivary secretions
- Three stages of infxn: acute, latent, reactivation
- Epidemiology: Acute dz is most common viral exanthem in children <3 y (10–20% of all acute febrile illnesses in this age), no seasonality, incubation 1–2 wks; Reactivation can be severe in immunosupp (esp recent HSCT) (*Clin Microbiol Rev* 2015;28(2):313–335).

History & Physical Examination

- Prodrome: Abrupt high fevers (± febrile sz), HA, coryza, periorbital edema
- Exanthem: Begins after defervescence; erythematous macules; starts neck/trunk & spreads to face/extremities; clears in 1–2 d

Evaluation

- Routine labs rarely indicated (CBC may show leukopenia)
- Primary infxn w/ HHV-6 is difficult to confirm diagnostically

Treatment

- Supportive for primary infxn
- Reactivation in immunosuppressed: May tx w/ ganciclovir or foscarnet

Complications

- Primary infxn: febrile sz (most common complication)
- Reactivation infxn (most severe in transplant pts, esp recent HSCT): encephalitis, bone marrow suppression, pneumonitis, hepatitis, transplant failure, GVHD

Disposition

- Home

Herpes Simplex 1 and 2 (HHV-1 and HHV-2)

Definition

- Historically, HSV-1 a/w orofacial dz & HSV-2 a/w genital dz; now both can cause both dz; transmission by contact w/ active lesions, but also by resp droplets & infected secretions
- Three stages: Primary, latent (asx), reactivation; reactivation triggers include illness, fever, menstruation, sun exposure, psychological stress (but usually spontaneous)
- **Herpes gingivostomatitis:** Affects oral/perioral mucous membranes, usually 1° infxn
- **Herpes labialis:** Affects perioral skin & mucous membranes; difficult to distinguish 1° & 2° dz; latent virus lives in trigeminal ganglion; reactivation in >1/3 pts
- **Herpes genitalis:** Affects genitals & mucous membranes; difficult to distinguish 1° & 2° dz; 60–70% of primary infxn can be asx; reactivation is common (1-y reactivation of HSV-1 is 20–50%, HSV-2 70–90%); up to 25% of infected are asx carriers (*NEJM* 2016;375(7):666–674)

History & Physical Examination

- Herpes gingivostomatitis & labialis:
  - Prodrome: Malaise, fever, localized pruritus/tingling/burning, dysphagia if intraoral
  - Rash (gingivostomatitis): Oral/perioral vesicles, oral ulcers, gingivitis (lasts 1–2 wks)
  - Rash (labialis): Clustered vesicles on erythematous base, often outside of mouth at vermillion border (but can be on nose); ± LAN & sore throat; distinguish from aphthous stomatitis (canker sore), which are discrete painful intraoral lesions
- Herpes genitalis:
  - Prodrome: Malaise, fever, HA, tender LAN; localized burning/pain in genital region
  - Rash: Clustered vesicles on erythematous base, crusted ulcers if on dry skin
  - RFs: Number lifetime sexual partners, h/o STI/HIV

Evaluation

- Generally not needed in ED; if recurrent, determining HSV-1 vs HSV-2 guides prog & tx
- PCR (best), Tzanck smear (can't differentiate HSV-1 vs HSV-2), viral cx (slow), biopsy

Treatment

- Pain control, hydration
- Herpes labialis: Topical therapy (Docosanol 10% cream, penciclovir 1% cream, acyclovir 5% ointment, cidofovir 0.3 or 1% gel) & oral therapy (acyclovir, famciclovir, valacyclovir) may decrease sxs & time to healing; sunscreen may decrease relapses.
- Herpes genitalis: Tx differs for 1st infxn, recurrent infxn, & suppressive tx
  - 1st infxn: Acyclovir 400 mg TID, famciclovir 250 mg TID, valacyclovir 1 g BID (7–10 d)
  - Recurrent: Acyclovir 400 mg TID, famciclovir 125 mg BID, valacyclovir 1 g QD (5 d)
- Severe or disseminated dz: IV acyclovir 5–10 mg/kg q8h

Complications

- Bacterial superinfxn (eg, impetigo), keratitis (2/2 autoinoculation), disseminated dz (eg, meningoencephalitis, hepatitis, pneumonitis) esp in neonates & immunosupp

Disposition

- Home unless severe/disseminated (requires IV antivirals) or unable to tolerate PO
- Herpes genitalis pts should be counseled on safe sex & prevention

Varicella ("Chickenpox," HHV-3)

Definition (New Microbiol 2018;41(2):95–105)

- Primary infxn w/VZV; highly contagious (~90% transmission among household contacts; 10–35% w/ limited exposure); transmission by resp droplets or vesicle secretion
- Epidemiology: Mostly children (5–10 y/o), but can affect infants & adults (esp if from tropical regions, 2/2 childhood dz less common); mortality low, but ~4 × higher in infants & ~25 × higher in adults, inc most among immunocompetent; winter/spring common; incubation ~14 d

History & Physical Examination

- Prodrome (24–48 h before rash): Fever, malaise, HA, abd pain usually lasting 24–48 h before skin lesions. Rash & new lesion formation over 1–7 d.
- Exanthem: Pruritic macules, progress to papules & vesicles, crusting w/i 48 h; trunk/face > extremities; crusts fall off after 1–2 wks; may leave hypopigmented scars long-term
- Mucous membranes can be involved: Conjunctiva, genitals, oropharynx
- "Breakthrough varicella" in immunized pts is similar but mild (ie, <50 lesions)

Evaluation

- Routine labs rarely indicated (CBC may show lymphopenia & transaminitis)

Treatment

- Healthy children: Supportive (calamine lotion, colloidal oatmeal baths; AVOID salicylates 2/2 Reye synd)
- High-risk groups (infants, age >12, pregnant, any steroids, or any immunosupp, chronic skin or pulm dz, long-term ASA use, pregnant) or complicated dz: IV acyclovir
- Precautions: Put pts on airborne (neg pressure) & contact precautions until crusted
  - Pts should not be managed by providers w/o immunity or those who are pregnant

Complications

- Bacterial superinfxn (impetigo, cellulitis; most common); invasive bacterial infxns (PNA, arthritis, osteomyelitis, necrotizing fasciitis, sepsis) & varicella PNA; neuro (cerebellar ataxia [1:4000], encephalitis, myelitis); heme cx (TCP, purpura fulminans); vasculitis (inc intracranial); hepatitis
- In rare cases, maternal varicella in early gestation can result in a congenital varicella synd (microcephaly, mental retardation limb hypoplasias, cutaneous defects, etc); later in pregnancy, varicella can cause preterm delivery & neonatal varicella

Postexposure Prophylaxis
- Antivirals not recommended for PEP
- If eligible for VZV vaccine: Give vaccine w/i 3–5 d of exposure, if no e/o prior immunity
- If not eligible for VZV vaccine (allergy, immunosupp, pregnancy, infant): Varicella zoster immune globulin can prevent varicella or lessen severity, give w/i 96 h of exposure

Disposition
- Home for uncomplicated cases
- Admx for high-risk groups or those w/ cx

Herpes Zoster ("Shingles," HHV-3)

Definitions (*NEJM* 2013;369(3):255–263)
- Reactivation of VZV from sensory ganglia; 20–50% lifetime risk (if nonvaccinated)
- **Herpes zoster ophthalmicus:** (V1 branch of CN V) Rash on forehead, periocular, nose
- **Herpes zoster oticus (Ramsay Hunt synd):** (CN VII/geniculate ganglion) Rash on ear, hard palate, anterior 2/3 of tongue; can get ipsilateral facial nerve palsy; a/w variable other CN findings (tinnitus, hearing loss, N/V, vertigo, nystagmus, etc)
- Zoster sine herpete: Clinical features similar to VZV but w/o rash

History & Physical Examination
- RFs: Previous VZV infxn, age, immunosupp, neoplastic dz (esp hematologic)
- Prodrome (may be absent): 2–3 d of localized skin sensations (tingling, hot/cold sensation, pruritus, burning pain) prior to rash; can be a/w HA, photophobia, malaise,
- Exanthem: Grouped vesicles on erythematous base, eventually crusting; pain; distributed in dermatomal pattern, not crossing midline; overlap adjacent dermatomes in 20% cases
- Sensory chgs vary: Paresthesias (tingling), allodynia (pain), hyperesthesia (exaggerated), pruritus

Evaluation
- Clinical dx; testing may be indicated if rash is atypical or pt has comorbidities
- DFA for VZV Ag (~80% Se), PCR (lesion base) (95–100% Se)

Treatment
- Antivirals indicated if w/i 72 h of rash onset, but recommended even >72 h if new vesicles forming, cx present (inc eye), or pt RFs (immunosupp, elderly)
- Antivirals (valacyclovir, acyclovir, famciclovir) decrease course & neuralgic pain
  - Acyclovir 800 mg PO q4h 5 times daily × 7–10 d
  - Valacyclovir 1000 mg PO q8h × 7 d (may have better bioavailability than acyclovir)
  - Famciclovir 500 mg PO q8h × 7 d (may have better bioavailability than acyclovir)
- Corticosteroids: Data equivocal; may accelerate healing & possibly reduce pain; may not help prevent postherpetic neuralgia (*NEJM* 2013;369(3):255–263)
- Herpes zoster ophthalmicus: C/s ophthalmology
- Supportive care (NSAIDs/acetaminophen; may need opiates during acute rash)
- Postherpetic neuralgia: Tx disappointing (<50% pts have >50% reduction in pain); topical agents (lidocaine patch [NNT 2.0], capsaicin cream [NNT 3.3]), systemic tx (gabapentin [NNT 4.4], pregabalin [NNT 4.2], TCAs [NNT 2.6]); combo tx better than mono-tx (if tolerated); pain specialist c/s if considering opiates (*NEJM* 2014;371(16):1526–1533)

Complications
- Postherpetic neuralgia (pain >90 d after rash, can be long-term; ~20% incidence after VZV, risk inc w/ age); Bell's palsy; transverse myelitis, cerebrovascular dz; disseminated dz (pneumonitis, hepatitis, pancreatitis, CNS) esp in immunosupp
- Herpes zoster ophthalmicus: ~50% can have ocular comp (eg, iritis, episcleritis, keratitis)

Disposition
- Home unless disseminated

Pityriasis Rosea (associated HHV-6 and HHV-7)

Definition (*BMJ* 2015;351:h5233)
- Acute, self-healing exanthema of unclear etiology: May be viral (a/w HHV-6 & HHV-7), but can also be a/w drugs (esp if no herald patch & longer duration)
- Epidemiology: Mainly adolescents/young adults (age 10–35); a/w asthma, eczema, URIs

History & Physical Examination
- Const sx in only ~50%: Fever, HA, arthralgia, cough, N/V, LAN
- Herald patch present in 40–75%: Single oval plaque 2–4 cm diam w/ fine scaling borders & pale depressed center; precedes rash by up to 3 wks

- Exanthem: Numerous lesions similar in appearance to herald patch on trunk & prox. extremities but in characteristic lines of cleavage ("Christmas tree pattern"); spares face, scalp, palms, & soles typically; lasts 5 wks but can last up to 5 mos

Treatment

- Supportive (oatmeal baths & emollients may help): No recommended role for steroids, abx, or antivirals inc acyclovir. In severe cases, topical agents may be tried locally, & if improvement can then use widely.

Disposition

- Home ± dermatology f/u

Molluscum Contagiosum (Associated Poxvirus)

Definition (*Curr Opin Pediatr* 2016;28(2):250–257)

- Benign, self-limiting but long-lasting eruption 2/2 poxvirus; spread by fomite, skin-to-skin, sexual contact & auto-inoculation
- Can serve as marker or opportunistic infxn in pts w/ HIV

History & Physical Examination

- Exanthem: Nonpainful smooth tan dome-shaped papules (2–5 mm diam) w/ umbilicated center on face, trunk, extremities (but can see in axilla, groin, a/c fossa, etc); can last up to 12–18 mos

Treatment

- Self-limited & asx: No tx needed; can refer to dermatology for lesion eradication to dec risk of spread (cryotherapy, laser, curettage, imiquimod cream, trichloroacetic acid, or tretinoin), esp if numerous or HIV+

Disposition

- Home ± dermatology f/u

BACTERIAL EXANTHEMS

Refer to Section IV: Infectious Disease ("Soft Tissue Infections") for the following: Cellulitis, Erysipelas, Staph Scalded Skin Syndrome, Toxic Shock Syndrome, & Necrotizing Fasciitis

Scarlet Fever (Scarlatina, "Second Disease")

Definition

- Rash in children (3–12 y) 2/2 erythrogenic toxin-producing strains of group A β-hemolytic streptococci; transmitted via airborne droplets & fomites from ppl w/ dz & asx carriers; incubation 1–4 d; winter/spring common

History, Physical Examination, & Evaluation

- PRODROME: Acute-onset sore throat, fever, HA, vomiting, ± abd pain (can be severe)
- EXAM: Diffuse fine erythematous coalescent "sandpaper" eruption ("goosebump" appearance); starts on neck/axilla/groin & spreads to trunk/extremities (w/o palms/soles), becomes macules coalescing into patches; lasts 7 d then fine desquamation
- Characteristic features: Flushed face w/ circumoral pallor; inc intensity at flexor folds (Pastia lines: transverse red streaks in skin folds); strawberry tongue; beefy red pharynx & tonsils w/ or w/o exudate
- DX: Rapid strep test (Se 60–90%, Sp 90%), throat cx; CBC rarely indicated but usually leukocytosis w/ PMN predominance present

Treatment

- PCN VK QID × 10 d, benzathine PCN 1.2 million U IM × 1, or macrolide in PCN-allergic

Disposition

- Home

Impetigo

Definition (*Pediatr Rev* 2020;41(4):210–212)

- Highly contagious superficial infxn 2/2 S. aureus & group A β-hemolytic streptococci; transmitted via direct contact (inc autoinoculation) & fomites; summer common
- Two types: Nonbullous (majority of cases; represents host response to infxn), Bullous (caused by bacterial toxins, esp staph exfoliative toxins)
- Epidemiology: Affects mainly children (2–5 y; most common pediatric bacterial skin infxn)

History & Physical Examination
- Nonbullous impetigo: Begins as reddened macule or papule that becomes a vesicle; vesicle ruptures to form an erosion, & its contents dry to form honey-colored crusts; usually on face (cheeks or under lips) or extremities; self-limited over 2 wks
- Bullous impetigo: Begins as rapidly enlarging vesicles that form sharply demarcated bullae w/ little to no surrounding erythema; these rupture, forming yellow oozing crusts; usually moist intertriginous areas involved (neck fold, axilla, groin, perineum); self-limited

Evaluation
- Dx is clinical; gram stain & culture rarely indicated

Complications
- Cellulitis, lymphangitis, poststreptococcal GMN, TSS, SSSS, invasive bact infxns

Treatment
- Most will resolve spontaneously, but abx recommended
- Topical abx equally if not more effective than oral abx (mupirocin 2% ointment TID 3–5 d)
- Oral abx may be indicated in those who cannot tolerate topical tx or w/ extensive dz: Amoxicillin/clavulanate, dicloxacillin, cephalexin, macrolide for PCN-allergic pts

Disposition
- Home w/ instructions to prevent spreading

FUNGAL EXANTHEMS

Dermatophytoses

Definitions
- Superficial fungal infxns involving the stratum corneum, hair, or nails:
  - Tinea capitis: infxn of hair & scalp
  - Tinea corporis: infxn of smooth, hairless skin (except palms, soles, & groin)
  - Tinea cruris: infxn of groin, genitals, pubic area, or perineum
  - Tinea pedis: infxn of feet, commonly interdigital regions
  - Tinea manuum: infxn of hand, commonly interdigital regions
  - Tinea unguium (onychomycosis): infxn of the nail

Clinical Features and Treatment of Dermatophytoses

Dermatophytosis	Historical & Physical Examination	*Treatment

Tinea capitis	Hx: Often children 3–14 y; RFs: Poor hygiene, overcrowding, $\downarrow$ SES
	PE: Scalp w/ hair loss, scaling, pruritus
	Dx: Clinical; wood's lamp may reveal green fluorescence
		• Topical tx ineffective but selenium shampoo can reduce transmission
		• Systemic tx preferred:
		  • Terbinafine
		  • Itraconazole

Tinea corporis	Hx: RFs–occlusive clothing, minor skin trauma, freq skin-to-skin contact PE: Annular/polycyclic scaly plaque Dx: Clinical; KOH prep w/ septate & branching hyphae	

Tinea cruris	Hx: RFs include occlusion & humidity
	PE: Annular plaque & scaly raised borders; from inguinal folds; pruritic
	Dx: Clinical; KOH prep w/ septate & branching hyphae
		• Localized dz: tx w/ topical (azoles are fungistatic; allylamines & ciclopirox are fungicidal)
		• Extensive dz, immunosupp, hair follicles: systemic tx
		  • Terbinafine
		  • Fluconazole
		  • Itraconazole

Tinea pedis	Hx: RFs include communal bathing, locker rooms, pools PE: Scaling, erythema, & maceration of interdigital spaces; bacterial superinfxn causes erosions, pruritus, & malador ("athlete's foot")	
Tinea manuum	PE: Scaling of palms, interdigital region, & palmar creases	

Tinea unguium (Onychomycosis)	Hx: RFs include nail trauma (tight shoes), immunosupp, DM, communal bathing PE: Toenail varies from discoloration & thickening of proximal, distal/subungal, or superficial portions of nail plate	• Topical tx only for limited dz (<50% distal nailbed), may have poor cure rates: • Ciclopirox (not as monotx) • Systemic tx preferred: • Terbinafine (preferred) • Itraconazole

*Most tx regimens last from 2–6 wks. Onychomycosis can take mos to adequately treat, thus pts require f/u w/ their primary provider or dermatologist.

Disposition
- Home w/ primary care or dermatology f/u

Pearl
- Dermatophytid rxn: Delayed-type hypersensitivity rxn to fungal antigens in pts w/ dermatophytosis; pts p/w pruritic papules or vesicles on hands & feet; respond to tx of primary dermatophytosis infxn

Cutaneous Candidiasis/Intertrigo

Definition
- Fungal infxn by *Candida* species *(C. albicans);* predilection for colonizing skin folds (intertriginous areas) where the environment is warm & moist

History & Physical Examination
- RFs: Obesity, DM, occlusive clothes, immunosupp, poor hygiene
- Exanthem: Moist, red, shiny patch w/ scalloped borders & satellite macules & pustules, often in intertriginous areas (groin, axilla, pannus folds, gluteal fold, web spaces); can be pruritic, burning, or asx

Physical Findings
- Moist, red, shiny macules/patches w/ scalloped borders, adjacent satellite pustules

Treatment
- Keep dry, topical antifungals (various preparations: creams, lotions, powders, w/ or w/o mild steroid combinations)

Disposition
- Home

HIGH-RISK EXANTHEMS

Pemphigus Vulgaris

Definition (*Lancet* 2019;394(10201:882–894)
- Rare but potentially life-threatening acute progressive autoimmune (2/2 autoantibodies) bullous dz involving skin/mucosa; mortality 5–10% w/ tx
- Idiopathic, but a/w PMH/FH autoimmune dz

History, Physical Examination, & Evaluation
- HX: Subacute-onset (over d to wks) additive blisters on mucosa & skin (mucosa may precede skin by wks/mos); pain > pruritus; ask about PMH/FH autoimmune dz
- EXAM: Small or confluent flaccid blisters & erosions on erythematous base (+Nikolsky); diffuse, inc on mucous membranes (oropharynx, conjunctiva, anogenital)
- DX: Histologic dx (c/s derm for bx); labs to r/o other causes or cx

Treatment
- Supportive: Analgesia, wound care
- Steroids (1 mg/kg/d pred or equiv); c/s derm & ENT/ophthalmology based on location
- Role of steroid-sparing tx (MMF, azathioprine, cyclosporine, IVIG, plasma exchange, infliximab) in acute dz unclear, but may help reduce risk of relapse

Duration & Disposition
- Duration can be lifelong, or can remit (w/ tx) w/ risk of recurrence
- If rapid progression or extensive dz, admit; c/s derm on all cases in ED

Erythroderma (Generalized Exfoliative Dermatitis)

Definition (*Adv Skin Wound Care* 2015;28(5):228–236)
- Rare but potentially life-threatening acute generalized red rash, affecting >90% TBSA; more common in males; a/w high-output HF

- Idiopathic (25%) or 2/2 meds, malignancy, psoriasis, uncontrolled dermatitis, among others
- Common associated drugs: ACE inh, allopurinol, anticonvulsants, BBs, beta-lactam abx, CCBs, furosemide, minocycline, NSAIDs, sulfonamides, others

History, Physical Examination, & Evaluation

- HX: Subacute-onset (over d–wks) generalized rash w/ scaling, a/w malaise, chills ± fever; pruritic commonly; always ask about meds, recent infxn sx, PMH/FH inflamm dz & malignancy
- EXAM: Generalized erythema (>90% TBSA; spares palms/soles), progresses to scaling & desquamation; often w/ edema; LAN ± e/o high-output HF, hepatomegaly, splenomegaly
- DX: Elevated ESR, hypoalbuminemia, hyperglobinemia (2/2 antibodies), mild anemia; may see e/o heme malignancy necessitating additional w/u; c/s dermatology

Treatment

- Tx underling cause or d/c causal drug if known
- Supportive: Skin moisture, antihistamines, topical steroids; systemic steroids usually warranted (unless c/f SSSS or underlying h/o psoriasis); watch fluid balance (given risk of both dehydration & HF)

Duration & Disposition

- Resolution depends on cause & ability to control/remove it
- Admit, esp if rapid or unstable; c/s dermatology

Acute Generalized Exanthematous Pustulosis (AGEP)

Definition (*J Am Acad Dermatol* 2015;73(5):843–848)

- Rare but life-threatening immunologically mediated diffuse acute pustular exanthema, often w/ multiorgan dysfxn in ~17% (esp elderly)
- Often 2/2 drugs (90%), infxn (parvovirus B19, *C. pneumonia,* CMV), mercury, spider bites
- Common associated drugs: Beta-lactam abx, quinolones, sulfonamides, carbamazepine, terbinafine, diltiazem, hydroxychloroquine, others

History, Physical Examination, & Evaluation

- HX: Acute-onset (w/ h) diffuse pustular rash; often occurs w/i 48 h of starting drug (or longer if not 2/2 abx); pruritic; always ask about meds, recent infxn sx
  - May also have sx of systemic organ involvement: SOB, abd pain, N/V, skin infxn
- EXAM: Numerous small sterile pustules on erythematous base, a/w fever; trunk & intertriginous areas common (rarely mucous membranes); pruritic
  - Assess for systemic dz: Pl effusions/hypoxia, hepatic dysfxn, rarely systemic superinfxn & DIC
- DX: CBC w/ leukocytosis (± eosinophilia), LFTs, ± CXR; c/s dermatology for bx

Treatment

- D/C causal drug or tx underlying infxn
- Supportive: Moist dressings & antiseptic solutions; high-potency topical steroids may help pruritus, but no role for systemic steroids; ± empiric abx if unstable

Duration & Disposition

- 5% mortality, mostly 2/2 superinfxn
- Resolves d after causal drug stopped
- Admit (may need ICU)

Drug Reaction with Eosinophilia and Systemic Symptoms (DRESS)

Definition (*J Am Acad Dermatol* 2013;68(5):693)

- Rare but potentially life-threatening immune-mediated diffuse rash w/ multiorgan dysfxn
- Common associated drugs: Allopurinol, anticonvulsants, sulfonamides, others

History, Physical Examination, & Evaluation

- HX: Prodrome of pruritus & fever, f/b acute-onset (h to d) diffuse rash; occurs w/i 2–6 wks of starting drug
- EXAM: Diffuse erythematous morbilliform macules/papules (less commonly erythroderma, pustules, targetoid lesions), can coalesce & become edematous; trunk, extremities, face (can involve mucous membranes)
  - Eval for multiorgan dysfxn: Liver (>70% of pts; major source of morbidity/mortality), hematologic, lymphatic, renal, pulm (pneumonitis, ARDS), cardiac (myocarditis), gastroenteritis, meningoencephalitis
- DX: CBC w/ diff (WBC can be >50 k/L; Eos >1.5 k/L; +atypical lymphs), Chem 10 (Cr, lytes, LFTs), Troponin, CXR, dermatology c/s for bx

Treatment

- D/C causal drug
- Supportive: Antihistamines, tx underlying organ dysfxn
- Systemic steroids w/ gradual taper over 3–6 mos

Duration & Disposition

- 10% mortality, esp immunosupp
- Resolves mos after causal drug stopped
- Admit (may need ICU)

Stevens–Johnson Syndrome (SJS)/Toxic Epidermal Necrolysis (TEN)

Definition (*Am J Clin Dermatol* 2015;16(6):475–493)

- Acute generalized mucocutaneous desquamative eruption w/ various associated causes; immune-mediated but precise mechanism unknown
  - Mucous membranes a dz hallmark: 80% cases (1st sx in 30%); oropharyngeal, ocular (80% cases), anogenital, GI, endotracheal/bronchial; all w/ severe cx
- Differentiation b/w SJS & TEN depends on TBSA desquamated:
  - SJS: <10% TBSA w/ detachable epidermis w/ horizontal shear ("+Nikolsky sign")
  - SJS/TEN overlap: 10–30% TBSA w/ +Nikolsky
  - TEN: >30% TBSA w/ +Nikolsky
- Idiopathic (20%), but often a/w meds (most common cause), infxn (*M. pneumoniae,* HSV), less likely food additives, fumigants, malignancy
- Common associated drugs: Allopurinol, anticonvulsants, beta-lactam abx, nevirapine, piroxicam, sulfonamides, others

History, Physical Examination, & Evaluation

- HX: Flu-like prodrome (fever, malaise, HA, sore throat, rhinitis, myalgias) f/b acute-onset (over d) diffuse rash ± mucosal sx (dysphagia, etc); pain; always ask about meds (usually w/i 4 wks), recent infxn sx, PMH/FH inflamm dz & malignancy
- EXAM: Diffuse erythematous dusky confluent purpuric macules or patches, rapidly evolve to coalesce & blister (+Nikolsky); often starts on trunk & spreads to extremities (inc palms/soles) & face (inc mucous membranes); eventually generalized sloughing
  - Extent of TBSA w/ +Nikolsky dictates SJS (<10%) vs SJS/TEN (10–30%) vs TEN (>30%)
- DX: CBC, BMP, lactate & blood cx (esp if hypotensive), derm c/s for bx

Treatment

- Treat underlying cause or d/c causal drug
- Supportive: Analgesia, thermoregulation (28–32°; esp important if high TBSA), IVF, airway protection prn, nutritional support (helps healing) wound care (debridement, bacitracin)
- Limited high-quality data supports specific systemic tx modalities:
  - Systemic steroids are standard of care, but have unclear mortality benefit (*Ann Pharmacother* 2015;49(3):355–342)
  - High-dose (>2 g/kg) IVIG in conjunction w/ steroids may reduce hosp LOS by ~3 d, & dec mortality, benefit strongest in TEN & w/ Asian pts (*PLoS One* 2016;11(11):0167120; *Int J Dermatol* 2015;54(1):108–115)
  - Cyclosporine/TNF inhs may improve survival (*J Am Acad Dermatol* 2014;71(5):941–947, *J Clin Invest* 2018;128(3):985–996)

Complications

- Mostly from mucosal ulcerations in trachea & bronchi (resp distress), esophagus (GIB, malnutrition), eyes (uveitis, ulceration, blindness), GU (dysuria, retention)
- Sepsis can occur 2/2 superinfxn from skin breakdown

Duration & Disposition

- Mortality 5–30%; TEN prognosis predictable using SCORTEN (see table)
- All pts get admitted; TEN requires burn unit admx
- ED or early inpt c/s to ophthalmology, urology (early Foley), ± GI, pulm

Severity of Illness Score for TEN (SCORTEN) (*J Invest Dermatol* 2000;115(2):149–153)			
Point		**Points**	
1	Age >40	1	Epidermal detachment >10% TBSA on d 1
1	HR >120 bpm	1	BUN >28 mg/dL
1	Comorbid malignancy	1	HCO_3 <20 mEq/L
Score	**Mortality**	**Score**	**Mortality**
0–1	3.2%	4	58.3%
2	12.2%	≥5	90.0%
3	35.5%		

OTHER EXANTHEMS

Allergic/Urticarial Reactions

Definition

- Acute (can be chronic or recurrent) histamine-mediated exanthem, often due to IgE, direct mast cell activation, complement, or dysmetabolism of arachidonic acid (eg, NSAIDs)
- Triggers: Systemic exposures (foods, meds, insect stings, contact w/ external allergens, parasites), physical triggers (eg, cholinergic, exercise, pressure, aquagenic, cold, etc)
- Common associated drugs: ASA, ACE inh, beta-lactam abx, NSAIDs, sulfonamides, others

History, Physical Examination, & Evaluation

- HX: Acute-onset (over mins) diffuse urticaria, ± SOB, N/V, LH; pruritus (no pain); usually occurs w/i h of trigger
- EXAM: Diffuse or localized erythematous wheals, variably sized (mm to cm), round or irregular in shape, can be excoriated 2/2 pruritic nature; occur anywhere on skin
  - Assess for signs of anaphylaxis (wheezing, hypotension)
- DX: Clinical dx; if +myalgias, LFTs to r/o acute hepatitis

Treatment

- D/C causal drug or other trigger
- Antihistamines (H1 & H2), steroids for severe cases, epinephrine if anaphylaxis

Duration & Disposition

- Resolves h after trigger removed; no mortality risk (unless anaphylaxis)
- Home; RX EpiPen in case recurrence; F/U w/ allergy for allergen testing &/or desensitization

Serum Sickness & Serum Sickness–like Reactions

Definition

- Acute diffuse immune-mediated (type III hypersensitivity) rash, often 2/2 drug exposure
- Common associated drugs: Barbs, beta-lactam abx, fluoxetine, sulfonamides, thiazides, vaccines/antiserum, others

History, Physical Examination, & Evaluation

- HX: Fever, severe arthralgias, malaise, & acute-onset (over h) diffuse rash; pain > pruritus; usually occurs w/i 2 wks of starting drug
- EXAM: Diffuse urticarial or serpiginous macules & patches (though other morphologies possible), well-demarcated w/ intense red border & central clearing; trunk, face, extremities (no palms/soles); joint ROM limited 2/2 pain
- DX: Clinical dx, no testing indicated

Treatment

- D/C causal drug or other trigger
- Supportive: Antihistamines, NSAIDs for pain
- Steroids for severe dz

Duration & Disposition

- Resolves 2–3 wks after trigger removed; no mortality risk
- Home if pain controlled; F/U w/ allergy

Exanthematous (Morbilliform) Eruption

Definition

- Acute diffuse immune-mediated rash (type IV hypersensitivity) 2/2 drug exposure
- Common associated drugs: Allopurinol, anticonvulsants, beta-lactam abx, NSAIDs, sulfonamides, others

History, Physical Examination, & Evaluation

- HX: May have low-grade fever, f/b acute-onset (over h–d) diffuse rash; pruritus > pain; usually occurs w/i 2–6 wks of starting drug
- EXAM: Diffuse erythematous macules or papules (but can be pustular or bullous), becoming confluent; viral (morbilliform) appearance; trunk & extremities (no palms/soles & face)
- DX: Clinical; elevated CRP, CBC may have mild eosinophilia (if markedly elevated eosinophils, consider DRESS), LFTs nl (if elevated, consider DRESS)

Treatment

- D/C causal drug (if unknown, d/c all nonnecessary drugs); rarely, the causal medication can be continued through the rash if it is essential; discuss w/ dermatology
- Supportive care: Antihistamines
- Steroids for severe dz

Duration & Disposition

- Resolves ~2 wks after med d/c-ed; no significant mortality risk
- Home; f/u w/ dermatology

Fixed Drug Eruptions

Definition

- Acute but recurrent localized immune-mediated skin eruption 2/2 repeat drug exposure
- Common associated drugs: ASA, NSAIDs, quinine, sedatives, sulfonamides, tetracyclines, others

History, Physical Examination, & Evaluation

- HX: Rash w/o systemic sx; pruritic; occurs w/i h–d of starting drug; on repeat exposure, lesions occur in same location as prior (new lesions may be present as well)
- EXAM: Solitary or small group of erythematous or hyperpigmented oval macules evolving to plaques (may become brown); pruritus; common sites include lips, extremities, genitals
- DX: Clinical

Treatment

- D/C causal drug (hyperpigmented area may remain)
- Supportive: Antihistamines

Duration & Disposition

- Resolves d after med d/c-ed; no significant mortality risk
- Home; F/U w/ dermatology

Erythema Multiforme

Definition (*Am Fam Physician* 2019;100(2):82–88)

- Acute (but sometimes recurrent or persistent) diffuse immune-mediated rash which can have mucosal involvement
  - *Erythema multiforme major* – mucosal involvement
  - *Erythema multiforme minor* – no mucosal involvement
- Idiopathic, but can be a/w infxn (90% cases; esp HSV, *M. pneumonia,* HCV, EBV), meds, malignancy, XRT, inflamm dz
- Common associated drugs: Anticonvulsants, beta-lactam abx, NSAIDs, phenothiazines, sulfonamides, others

History, Physical Examination, & Evaluation

- HX: Prodrome (fever, malaise) present in EM major, f/b acute-onset (over d) diffuse rash (see exam); always ask about meds, recent infxn sx, PMH/FH inflamm dz & malignancy
- EXAM: Diffuse erythematous macules/papules w/ evolving morphology (become targetoid, then polycyclic & annular configuration); trunk, extremities (inc palms/soles), face (mucous memb ~70%)
  - Compared to SJS: Less purpuric, less truncal, less painful, less mucosa
- DX: Clinical & histopathologic dx (c/s derm for bx); labs inc HSV PCR/IgM (esp if recurrent episode), ± CXR to r/o causes & cx

Treatment

- Tx underlying cause or d/c causal med if known
- Supportive: Antihistamines, analgesia, ± oral anesthetic solutions/antiseptic rinses
- Topical steroids if mild, systemic steroids if severe dz (esp mucosal)
  - Consider long-term valacyclovir in pts if recurrent

Duration & Disposition

- Resolves w/i wks; no significant mortality risk, but can progress to SJS/TEN if offending agent not removed
- Home; f/u w/ dermatology & ophthalmology (if ocular involvement)

Erythema Nodosum

Definition (*World J Pediat* 2018;14(6):548–554)

- Panniculitis (inflam of subcutaneous fat) w/ unknown mechanism; thought 2/2 immune complex deposition in connective tissue
- Idiopathic ~30%, infxn ~30% (TB, recent Grp A strep infxn), sarcoidosis ~20%, inflamm dz, malignancy, pregnancy, drugs
- Common associated drugs: Sulfonamides, OCPs/estrogens, others

History, Physical Examination, & Evaluation

- HX: Prodrome (fever, fatigue, malaise, polyarthralgia (symmetric, additive, lg joint), HA, GI sx), f/b acute-onset (over d to wks) generally-localized rash, ± fever, fatigue, malaise, polyarthralgia (symmetric, additive, lg joint), HA, GI sx; painful; always ask about meds, recent infxn sx, PMH/FH inflamm dz & malignancy

- EXAM: Scattered tender erythematous or purple oval nodules (1–6 cm diam), can coalesce; symmetric & usually anterior tibia (also knees, ankles, thighs, forearms)
- DX: Clinical; labs prn for underlying dz (CBC, ESR/CRP, CXR [r/o TB, sarcoidosis])

Treatment
- Supportive: NSAIDs for pain
- Short course oral corticosteroids in severe dz

Disposition
- Most cases self-resolve w/i 6 wks, but EN may recur; no significant mortality risk
- Home; f/u w/ dermatology or rheumatology

Leukocytoclastic Vasculitis

Definition (*Neurol Clin* 2019;37(2):465–473)
- Acute, chronic, or intermittently recurrent immune-mediated (immune complex, ANCA) rash, sometimes w/ systemic organ involvement
- Idiopathic (~50%), or a/w recent infxn (viral [esp HBV/HCV], bacterial, parasites, fungi), inflam dz, meds (see table), illicits, malignancy
- Common associated drugs: Allopurinol, abx, anticoagulants (oral), anticonvulsants, NSAIDs, thiazide diuretics, thiouracil, others

History, Physical Examination, & Evaluation
- HX: Acute-onset (over dys) rash; ± systemic sx (fever, arthralgias, GI sx [diarrhea, abd pain], hematuria, hemoptysis); pruritic/burning; always ask about meds, recent infxn sx, PMH/FH inflamm dz & malignancy
- EXAM: Diffuse or localized tender palpable purpura or purpuric urticaria, can evolve to coalesce to form plaques or bullae; often lower extremities
  - Multiorgan involvement possible: MSK, GI, cardiac, lungs, ocular, kidneys
- DX: Clinical; labs to r/o systemic dz (CBC, ESR/CRP, Chem 10, UA, ± CXR)

Treatment
- Tx definitive cause (if known) or d/c causal drug
- Supportive (elevation of legs, compression stockings), antihistamines, analgesia w/ NSAIDs
- Colchicine (± dapsone) if no response to NSAIDs (0.6 mg BID); short-course steroids if still refractory

Duration & Disposition
- Resolves w/i 2 wks if 2/2 drug; if 2/2 underlying dz may persist or recur
- Home if no systemic indications for admx; refer to dermatology & rheumatology

Sweet Syndrome (Acute Febrile Neutrophilic Dermatosis)

Definition (*Rev Chil Pediatr* 2018;89(4):511–515)
- Rare presumed immune-mediated acute erythematous skin rash characterized histologically by dense neutrophilic infiltrates
- Idiopathic (~2/3 cases; F>M); malignancy (2nd most common cause; often undx'ed), inflam dz, infxn (esp URI, GI sx, others), meds, pregnancy
- Common associated drugs: Vaccines, G-CSF, TMP-SMX, minocycline, others

History, Physical Examination, Evaluation
- HX: Acute-onset (over h) rash w/ fever (may precede rash), a/w arthralgias, HA; painful
- EXAM: Tender, violaceous, well-demarcated papules & plaques (can get central pustules, bullae, or ulcers – esp if paraneoplastic), can evolve to coalesce; common esp on upper body (inc face, mucous memb)
- DX: Bx required for dx; elev ESR (>90%), CBC (WBC >8 k in 80%, +bands), anemia, low plts; LFTs, ± CXR; ± imaging to eval for malignancy dx

Treatment
- Supportive: Analgesia
- Systemic steroids for acute dz; mx agents used for suppressive tx

Duration & Disposition
- Rapid resolution w/ steroids (w/o tx may persist wks to mo); can recur
- Home if pain controlled & stable; f/u w/ dermatology

Photosensitive Reaction

Definition
- Any exanthem appearing in sun-exposed distribution after exposure to UV light
  - Drug-related causes: Exaggerated sunburn, photosensitive drug rxn (phototoxic, photoallergic), pseudoporphyria, phytophotodermatitis (rash following topical chemical and UV exposure)

- Common associated drugs: Diuretics, NSAIDs, phenothiazines, quinolones, sulfonamides, sulfonylureas, tetracyclines, others
- Not drug related: Porphyria cutanea tarda (PCT), inflamm dz (lupus, dermatomyositis)

History, Physical Examination, & Evaluation

- HX: Acute-onset (over h) rash localized to sun-exposed areas; h/o UV exposure (tanning booth, phototherapy, sunlight); always ask about meds (usually w/i 4 wks), recent infxn sx, PMH/FH inflamm dz
  - Phototoxic rxn: Onset min–h after UV
  - Photoallergic rxn: Onset 24–72 h after UV
  - Pseudoporphyria: Onset h after UV
- EXAM: Exanthem only present on sun-exposed area, morphologically diverse:
  - Phototoxic drug rxn: Exaggerated sunburn response (erythema, edema ± blistering)
  - Photoallergic drug rxn: Erythema ± eczematous chgs
  - Pseudoporphyria: Erythema, tense bulla (inc hemorrhagic) & erosions (as opposed to PCT, lacks chronic pigment, hair, or sclerodermal chgs)
- DX: Clinical; further testing prn to r/o PCT or inflamm dz (eg, porphyrins, ANA, etc)

Treatment

- Supportive: Sun protection (clothing, high-SPF sunscreen), cool compresses, wound care
- Topical steroids, systemic steroids for severe dz
- NAC may speed pseudoporphyria resolution

Duration & Disposition

- Resolution variable, but drug-induced pseudoporphyria may take mos
- Home; F/U w/ dermatology & rheumatology prn to exclude PCT or inflammatory causes

Dermatitis

- Class of skin inflammatory-mediated skin dz marked by similar s/sx: Erythema, pruritus, scaling, fissures, varying degrees of lichenification & blistering
- Usually chronic/subacute, but pts may come to ED if bad flare (esp if recent long remission)

Clinical Features and Treatment of Dermatitis		
Condition	**Presentation**	**Treatment**
Atopic dermatitis	Definition: Chronic, relapsing/remitting; mostly children (10–20% of kids; 1–3% of adults), most w/i 1st 1 y. RFs: Hx/FH atopy (asthma, allergic rhinitis, food allergies) Triggers: Temp, humidity, irritants, infxn, foods, allergens, stress Exam: Dry pruritic erythematous papulovesicular w/ excoriations & serous exudate ± lichenification; in kids often on face, neck, extensor surf; in adults often flexor folds	Skin hydration: Soaking baths f/b moisturizer w/i 10 mins Topical steroids: Low potency for maintenance, mid & high potency for flares Antihistamines: For pruritus; do not use topical agents 2/2 risk of skin sensitization Prevention: Avoid irritants F/U w/ derm: May need tx w/ topical calcineurin inhs
Contact dermatitis (allergic) Contact dermatitis (irritant)	Definition: Inflammatory rxn 2/2 direct contact w/ exogenous agent & subsequent type IV hypersensitivity rxn; in allergic CD, antigen reacts w/ proteins in skin to cause inflammation; in irritant CD, antigen chemically abrades or damages skin to cause inflammation Triggers: Latex, plant substances, metals (esp nickel), plant resins, soaps, detergents, fragrance, hair products, sunscreen, top meds Exam: Erythematous, papulovesicular w/ varying lichenification, fissuring, scaling, excoriation; often localized to exposed area	Avoid any suspected trigger Sx relief: Cold compresses, colloidal baths, emollients Topical steroids: Start w/ high-potency if localized (not on face, genitals), then transition to mid or low potency as sx improve Systemic steroids for severe or extensive dz Evaluate & tx superinfxn Antihistamines can be ineffective Refer to dermatology for patch testing

Nummular dermatitis	Definition: Morphologically unique type of atopic dermatitis; can occur older in adulthood; M > F RFs: Dry skin, atopy, skin injury/abrasion, poor vascular flow, Vit A containing meds Exam: Round/oval pink/brown pruritic papulovesicular rash w/ serous exudate, evolving to plaque (2–10 cm diam) w/ crust then scale; often on extremities (but can be torso)	See atopic dermatitis
Seborrheic dermatitis	Definition: Dz of the sebum-rich areas (scalp/face/trunk), possibly 2/2 abnl immune response to nl skin fungus (Malassezia); often in infants (cradle cap) & elderly, but also AIDS & Parkinson dz; 20% of pts have h/o dandruff; worse in winter Exam: Oily flaking patches of skin on scalp, face (nasolabial folds, eyebrows, ears), chest, flexural skin	Frequent bathing w/ keratolytic shampoos (eg, selenium, zinc-based), reduce oil Antifungal: Ketoconazole shampoo or creams Topical steroids: Low-potency creams (if not on scalp)
Xerotic dermatitis	Definition: Skin dz characterized by chgs 2/2 dry skin; common among elderly Exam: Dry skin w/ erythematous superficial cracks & excoriations, often on legs	Skin hydration: Soaking baths f/b moisturizer w/i 10 mins Topical Steroids: Low-potency & short duration
Pompholyx	Definition: Subtype of eczema 2/2 edematous fluid accumulation in areas w/ thick epidermis; affecting palmoplantar skin; acute, recurrent, or chronic Triggers: A/w atopic & contact dermatitis, drug rxns, stress, id rxn in pts w/ tinea pedis Exam: Nonerythematous pruritic vesicles or bulla on palms or soles	Topical steroids: High-potency Systemic steroids if severe F/U w/ derm: May need tx w/ topical calcineurin inhs

Topical Steroid Preparations by Potency (Generic)	
High Potency	**Upper-Mid Potency**
Clobetasol propionate[C,G,O,So]	Fluocinonide[C,G,O]
Betamethasone dipropionate[C,G,O,So]	Betamethasone valerate[O]
	Mometasone furoate[C,O]
Lower-Mid Potency	**Low Potency**
Triamcinolone acetonide[C,O,Sp]	Fluticasone propionate[C,L,O]
Hydrocortisone valerate[C,O]	Hydrocortisone 1%, 2.5%[C,L,O,Sp]
Desonide[C,L,O]	

Special Notes on Administration

(1) Vehicles: Ointment (O) most soothing for dry skin. Cream (C) most cosmetically acceptable. Lotion (L), gel (G) & solution (So) most ideal for scalp. Spray (Sp) in unique circumstances.
(2) Avoid high potency or prolonged upper-mid potency for pediatric pts (high absorption), skin folds inc genitals (causes striae), and face (causes atrophy/rosacea/ocular cx).

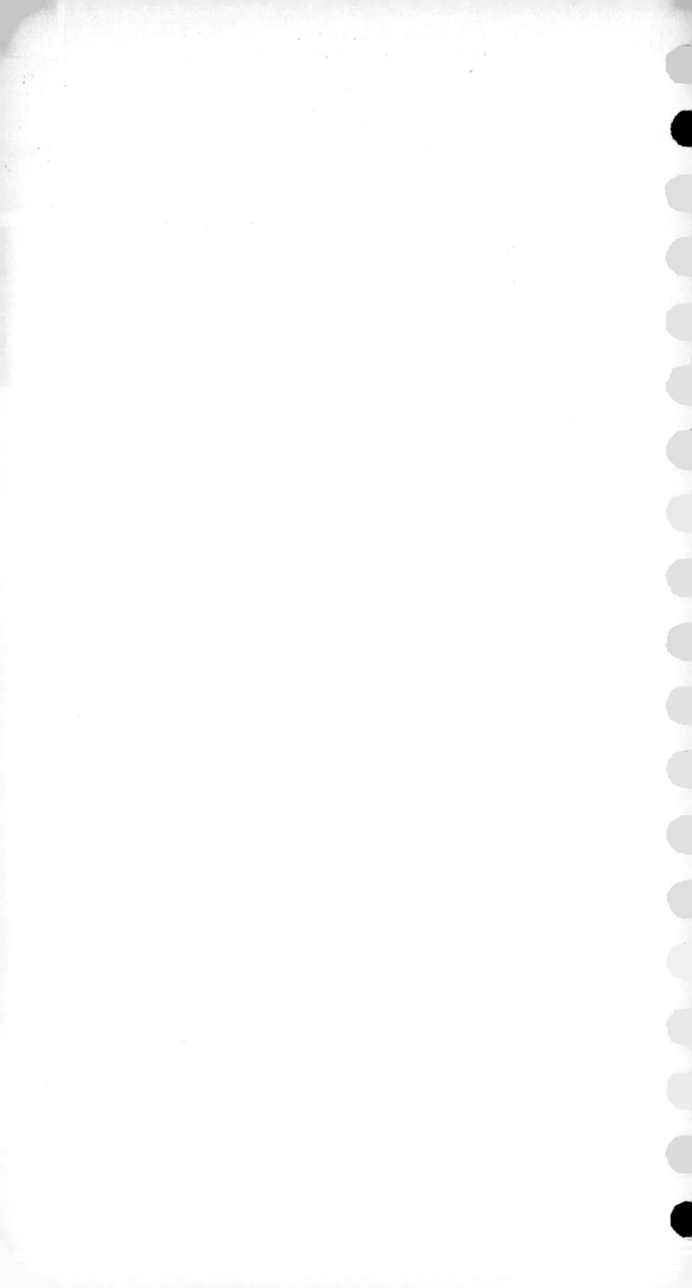

ACID–BASE DISORDERS

Approach to the Patient

Diagnostics

- BMP; consider LFTs, CBC, urine electrolytes, ABG/VBG, & serum osmolality
- Note: HCO_3 from ABG/VBG is calculated (not directly measured) & should be w/i 2 mmol/L of BMP total CO_2

Step-wise Approach

- **Step 1:** Is there an acidemia or alkalemia? (acidemia: pH <7.35; alkalemia: pH >7.45)
- **Steps 2 & 3:** Is the primary disturbance metabolic or respiratory? Is there compensation?

Assessing Primary Metabolic Disturbances & Physiologic Compensation				
Primary Disorder	**pH**	**pCO_2**	**HCO_3**	**Compensation Formula**
Metabolic acidosis	Low	Low	Low	$\Delta pCO_2{}^a = 1.2 \times \Delta HCO_3$
Metabolic alkalosis	High	High	High	$\Delta pCO_2 = 0.7 \times \Delta HCO_3$
Acute respiratory acidosis	Low	High	High	$\Delta HCO_3 = 0.1 \times \Delta PCO_2$
Acute respiratory alkalosis	High	Low	Low	$\Delta HCO_3 = 0.2 \times \Delta PCO_2$
Chronic respiratory acidosis	Nl or low	High	High or nl	$\Delta HCO_3 = 0.4 \times \Delta PCO_2$
Chronic respiratory alkalosis	Nl or high	Low	Low or nl	$\Delta HCO_3 = 0.4 \times \Delta PCO_2$

Note: Nl pCO_2 = 40 mm Hg; nl HCO_3 = 24 mEq/L

[a]Or calculate using Winter's formula: expected $pCO_2 = 1.5 \times HCO_3 + 8 \pm 2$ mm Hg

- **Step 4a:** Is there an anion gap?

  Anion gap acidosis: ($Na - [Cl + HCO_3]$) >14 (see chart)

  Note: Needs to be corrected for albumin; a fall in serum albumin 1 g/dL from the nl value (4.4 g/dL) decreases the anion gap by 2.5 mEq/L.

  $$\text{Corrected AG} = \text{AG} + (2.5 \times [4.4 - \text{albumin}])$$

- **Step 4b:** If an anion gap is present, is there an osmolar gap?

  Osmolar gap: Measured serum Osm – Calculated Osm >10 mOsm/L, where calculated Osm = (2 × Na) + glucose/18 + BUN/2.8 + Ethanol/4.6

- **Step 4c:** If no anion gap is present, what is UAG?

  Urinary anion gap: Urine Na + Urine K – Urine Cl

  Note: The UAG can help differentiate GI & renal causes of non-AG (hyperchloremic) metabolic acidosis, as base can be lost from gut or kidney (neg UAG: GI loss [ie, diarrhea, bowel fistula, ileostomy]; positive UAG: Renal loss, particularly RTA types I & IV)

- **Step 5:** What is the delta gradient (also known as the "delta–delta")?

  ($AG - nl\ AG$) – ($nl\ HCO_3 - HCO_3$), or simply **($AG - 12$) – ($24 - HCO_3$)**

  - If delta–delta >+6, suggests concomitant metabolic alkalosis or prior compensated respiratory acidosis
  - If delta–delta = 0, suggests uncomplicated AG metabolic acidosis
  - If delta–delta <–6, suggests concomitant hyperchloremic non-AG metabolic acidosis

Metabolic Acidosis	
Anion Gap Acidosis	**Nonanion Gap Acidosis**
"A CAT'S MUDPILE"	**"FUSED CARD TIP"**
Alcoholic ketoacidosis	**F**anconi synd
CO, cyanide	**U**reteroenterostomy
Aspirin	**S**mall bowel fistula
Toluene	**E**xcessive Cl^- (NaCl, ammonium Cl^-)
Starvation ketoacidosis	**D**iarrhea
Methanol, metformin, methemoglobinemia	**C**arbonic anhydrase inhs
Uremia	**A**ddison dz
DKA	**RTA**
Paraldehyde, phenformin, propylene glycol	**D**rugs (spironolactone, amiloride, cholestyramine, triamterene)
INH, iron	**T**oluene (chronic, secondary to RTA)
Lactic acidosis types A & B	**I**leostomy
Ethylene glycol, EtOH	**P**ancreatic fistula, parenteral nutrition, posthypocapnia

Causes of Osmolar Gap	
Toxic Alcohols	**Others**
*Methanol *Ethylene glycol *Propylene glycol Isopropyl alcohol	Acetone Mannitol Sorbitol Glycerol Ether trichloroethane

*A/w elevated anion gap

Causes of Low Anion Gap (<6)
Lab error Lithium tox Bromide tox Hypoalbuminemia Paraproteinemias (eg, mx myeloma) Severe hypercalcemia/hypermagnesemia

Metabolic Alkalosis	
Pathophysiology	**Differential**
NaCl responsive *(urine Cl < 10–15 mEq/L)*	• GI loss of H^+: Vomiting, NGT drainage, villous adenomas • Renal loss of H^+: Remote diuretic use • Chloride-wasting diarrhea (eg, laxative abuse) • Posthypercapnia: COPD, OHS, respiratory muscle weakness • Exogenous alkali administration w/ renal hypoperfusion: Citrate loads from blood tfxs, acetate loads from TPN, calcium-alkali synd (calcium supplements, milk, or antacids)

NaCl unresponsive *(urine Cl > 15 mEq/L)*	• Active diuresis
	• Bartter's (acts like loop diuretic), Gitelman's (like thiazide)
	• Severe hypokalemia or hypomagnesemia
	• Hypercalcemia/hypoparathyroidism
	• Mineralocorticoid excess of any etiology
	  • 1° hyperaldosteronism: Adrenal hyperplasia, aldosterone-producing tumor
	  • 2° hyperaldo: Renovascular dz, renin-producing tumor
	  • Exogenous mineralocorticoid, Cushing synd, licorice
	• Liddle synd

Respiratory Acidosis	
Pathophysiology	**Differential**
Central respiratory depression	Drugs (opioids, sedatives), brainstem infarct, high C-spine injury, obesity hypoventilation synd (ie, Pickwickian synd)
Nerve or muscular disorders	Paralysis, muscular dystrophy or other myopathies, myasthenia gravis, toxins (ie, organophosphate, botulism, tetanus, snake envenomations), Guillain–Barré, ALS
Airway issues	Upper airway obstruction, laryngospasm, bronchospasm
Respiratory issues	Asthma, COPD, CHF, PNA, ILD, aspiration, ARDS, inadequate mechanical ventilation
Chest wall trauma	Flail chest, PTX, hemothorax, diaphragmatic paralysis, kyphoscoliosis

Respiratory Alkalosis	
Pathophysiology	**Differential**
Cardiac, respiratory	Pulmonary edema, pulmonary embolus, restrictive lung dz, mechanical hyperventilation
Psychiatric, neuro	Hyperventilation synds (eg, anxiety, pain, stress), meningoencephalitis, tumor, trauma, CVA
Infxn	Fever, PNA, sepsis
GI	Liver failure
Meds, other	Salicylates, hyperthyroidism, high altitude, anemia, pregnancy

Treatment and Disposition
- Tx and dispo largely depend on severity & underlying etiology of the disorder
- Limited role for bicarbonate in the absence of hemodynamic collapse

ABNORMAL ELECTROLYTES

Hyponatremia

Definition

- Na <135, excess of water relative to serum sodium, usually from elevated ADH; generally not symptomatic at Na >125

History

- Most sxs are nonspecific: Fatigue, weakness, muscle cramps, thirst, or postural dizziness. Severe sxs include confusion, agitation, delirium, lethargy, somnolence, coma, or szs.
- Other important hx includes h/o CHF, cirrhosis, renal dz, cancer, adrenal or pituitary dysfxn, recent GI surgery, thiazide or loop diuretics use, alcoholism.

Physical Examination

- Assess fluid status:
  - Hypervolemia: Elevated JVP, peripheral edema, crackles, ascites, anasarca
  - Hypovolemia: Tachycardia, hypotension, dry mucous membranes, oliguria, poor skin turgor, IVC collapsibility on US
- Look for signs of severe hyponatremia: Lethargic, disoriented/abnl sensorium, depressed reflexes, hypothermic, pseudobulbar palsy, Cheyne–Stokes respiration

Diagnostics

- **Labs:** BMP, gluc, urine electrolytes (Na, Cr, Osm), serum Osm, albumin
- VBG w/ stat sodium & Osm may provide more rapid turnaround
- **Corrected $Na_{glucose}$ = Serum Na + (0.024 × [serum glucose – 100])**

Step-wise Approach to Hyponatremia

- **Step 1:** What is the serum osmolality? (*nl serum osm = 275–290 mOsm/kg*)

Causes of Hyponatremia by Serum Osmolality		
Hypertonic HypoNa	**Isotonic HypoNa**	**Hypotonic HypoNa**
Hyperglycemia Mannitol Glycerol Sorbitol IVIG	Lab/blood draw error Hyperparaproteinemia Hyperlipidemia Post TURP/hysteroscopy (irrig w/ osmotic agent)	Differential for etiology based on volume status

- **Step 2:** What is the pt's volume status? Hypervolemic, euvolemic, or hypovolemic?
- **Step 3:** What are the urine Na, urine Osm, & FeNa values?
  - **Fractional Excretion of Sodium (FeNa) = $(Na_{urine} \times Cr_{serum})/(Na_{serum} \times Cr_{urine})$**

Assessing Causes of Hypotonic Hyponatremia by Volume Status & Urine Analysis				
Volume Status	**Urine Na**	**Urine Osm**	**FeNa**	**Etiology**
Hypervolemic	>20		>1%	Renal failure
	<10		<1%	CHF, cirrhosis, nephrosis
Euvolemic		>100		SIADH[a], hypothyroidism, glucocorticoid deficiency
		<100		Psychogenic polydipsia (>12 L fluid/d), low solute (beer potomania, tea/toast diet, diluted infant formula)
		Variable		Chronic malnutrition (anorexia), pregnancy
Hypovolemic	>20		>1%	Renal losses: diuretic use, osmotic diuresis, salt-wasting nephropathy, mineralocorticoid deficiency, nonoliguric ATN
	<10		<1%	Extrarenal losses: vomiting, diarrhea, NGT drainage, 3rd spacing (pancreatitis, SBO), sweating

[a]Causes include PNA, asthma, COPD, SCLC, pneumothorax, trauma, CVA, ICH, tumors, HIV, hydrocephalus, antipsychotics/antidepressants, AEDs, chemo, vasopressin, postoperative, bath salts/amphetamines, hereditary, marathons

Treatment

- Rapid correction of chronic hyponatremia >10–12 mEq/L/d may result in osmotic demyelination synd (dysarthria, szs, quadriparesis due to focal myelin destruction in pons & extrapontine areas)
- Asx or mild sxs of hyponatremia: Correct serum Na at ≤0.5 mEq/L/h (max 10 mEq/L in 24 h) (*NEJM* 2023;389(16):1499–1509; *Nephrol Dial Transplant* 2024;39[10]:1583–1592)
  - There is emerging evidence for worse outcomes w/ overly slow correction (*JAMA Intern Med* 2025;185[1]:38–51)
- Severe manifestations of hyponatremia: Rapid correction serum Na at 2 mEq/L/h × 2–3 h OR until severe sxs resolve
  - Correct w/ 3% NaCl boluses
  - Severe sxs are more likely w/ acute development of hyponatremia

IV Fluid Management		
Total Body Water (TBW) = Weight (kg) × 0.6 (use 0.5 if female or elderly, 0.6 for infants)		
Rate of Infusion (cc/hr) = $\frac{1000 \times (\text{TBW} \times [\text{desired Na} - \text{serum Na}])}{(\text{Na [mmol/L]}_{\text{infusate}} \times \text{time [h]})}$		
Infusate concentrations: LR: 130 mEq/L	NS: 154 mEq/L	3% NS: 513 mEq/L

Requires checking serum Na* (& Glu) q1h

- Euvolemic hyponatremia
  - Asx: Free water restrict (500–1000 mL/d)
  - Symptomatic: See above
- SIADH
  - Free water restrict + treat underlying cause
  - Caution: If using hypertonic or nl saline esp if IVF Osm < urine Osm, serum sodium may worsen (higher Osm will draw out fluid)
  - Vaptans, urea, loop diuretics, & salt tabs are common outpatient therapies
- Hypovolemic hyponatremia
  - Volume replete w/ crystalloid, as above (once dehydration resolved, stimulation of ADH will decline & Na will correct)
- Hypervolemic hyponatremia
  - Free water restrict (0.5–1.0 L/d)
  - Severe hyponatremia: Consider diuresis + Na replacement w/ hypertonic saline

Disposition

- Home: Mild Asx hyponatremia
- Admit: Symptomatic, comorbidities, elderly. May require ICU admx if severe

Hypernatremia

Definition

- Na >145, usually from free water loss or sodium gain (eg, hypertonic fluid infusion)
  - Appropriate response to hypernatremia is increased free water intake stimulated by thirst & renal excretion of a minimal volume of maximally concentrated urine, regulated by ADH

History

- Mild sxs include increased thirst or polyuria
- Severe sxs: AMS (irritability, lethargy, confusion, delirium, coma)
- RFs: Elderly, infants, debilitated, confined (ie, those unable to access water freely). Endocrine pathology; cardiac, renal, liver dz; psychiatric disorder; Meds (see chart below)

Physical Examination

- Look for signs to assess pt fluid status:
  - Hypervolemia: Elevated JVP, peripheral edema, crackles, ascites, anasarca
  - Hypovolemia: Tachycardia, hypotension, dry mucous membranes, oliguria, poor skin turgor, IVC collapsibility on US
- Severe hypernatremia: Lethargy, muscle spasticity, tremor, hyperreflexia, szs, respiratory paralysis, ataxia

Diagnostics

- **Labs:** BMP, gluc, urine electrolytes (Na, Cr, Osm), serum Osm, albumin
- VBG w/ stat sodium & Osm may provide more rapid turnaround
- **Corrected $\text{Na}_{\text{glucose}}$ = Serum Na + (0.024 × [serum glucose – 100])**

Step-wise Approach to Hypernatremia

- **Step 1:** What is the serum osmolality?
  - Nl serum osmolality = 275–290 mOsm/kg

- **Step 2:** What is the pt's volume status? Hypervolemic, euvolemic, or hypovolemic?
- **Step 3:** What are the urine Na & urine Osm values?

Assessing Causes of Hypernatremia by Volume Status & Urine Analysis			
Volume Status	**Urine Na**	**Urine Osm**	**Etiology**
Hypervolemic	>20		**Increased Sodium Reabsorption:** Cushing dz, adrenal hyperplasia, exogenous steroids, mineralocorticoid excess
Euvolemic		<300	Complete DI (central & nephrogenic)[a]
		300–600	Partial DI (central & nephrogenic)[a]
		>600	**Exogenous Sodium Intake:** Hypertonic saline, sodium bicarb tablets, sea water ingestion, overconcentrated infant formula
Hypovolemic	>20	300–600	**Renal Water Losses:** Loop diuretic, osmotic diuresis (mannitol, urea, hyperglycemia)
	<20	>600	**Extrarenal Water Losses:** Vomiting, diarrhea, NGT drainage, szs, exercise, severe burns, fever, 3rd spacing **Decreased Water Intake:** Defective thirst mechanism, dementia, AMS, infancy, intubation, confinement

[a]Central DI: Congenital, trauma/surgery, tumors, hypothalamic dz, pituitary dz, hypoxic encephalopathy, anorexia, idiopathic. *Nephrogenic DI:* Congenital, drugs (lithium, amphotericin, demeclocycline, foscarnet, cidofovir), hypercalcemia, severe hypokalemia, protein malnutrition, polycystic kidney dz, sickle cell, Sjögren's, amyloid, pregnancy

Treatment

IV Fluid Management[a]
Free water deficit (liters) = TBW × ([current Na/desired Na] − 1)
Total body water (IBW) = Weight (kg) × 0.6 (use 0.5 if female or elderly; 0.6 for children)
Hourly maintenance rate of D_5W[b] (mL/h) = free water deficit (mL)/24 h

[a]Requires checking serum gluc & Na q1h initially, then spaced to q4–6h. Rate of Na correction should NOT exceed 10 mEq/L in 24 h to avoid cerebral edema. Goal urine output: >0.5 cc/kg/h

[b]Replace ongoing hourly water losses if known

- Hypervolemic hypernatremia
  - Treat underlying disorder
  - Replace free water deficit (as above)
- Euvolemic hypernatremia
  - Replace free water deficit (as above)
  - Treat underlying etiology
  - Central DI: Vasopressin 10 U SQ
- Hypovolemic hypernatremia
  - 1) Restore volume w/ crystalloid fluids first
  - 2) Then replace free water deficit using D_5W (as above) – add potassium IV to fluid replacement as needed once pt is urinating

Disposition
- Home: Mild hypernatremia
- Admit: Mod or severe hypernatremia, comorbidities, AMS

Hypokalemia

Definition
- K^+ <3.5 mEq/L (ie, decreased intake, shift into cells, loss); 98% of potassium is intracellular.

Hypokalemia Differential	
Pathophysiology	**Differential**
GI	Poor oral intake; diarrhea, vomiting, & NG tube drainage
Endocrine	High insulin levels, hyperaldosteronism, alkalosis, DKA, Cushing dz, hypomagnesemia
Renal	RTA (type 2), renovascular dz, Bartter synd, Liddle synd, Gitelman synd
Meds/toxins	Thiazide & loop diuretics, insulin, β-2 agonists, α-antagonists, amphotericin B, laxative abuse, exogenous mineralocorticoid use, massive blood tfxs, barium tox, toluene tox

History
- Usually not symptomatic until K^+ <3 mEq/L
- Nausea, vomiting, weakness, fatigue, myalgia, muscle cramps
- Pts at highest risk for electrocardiac cx of hypoK include those w/ acute ischemia, prolonged QT synd, & those taking digoxin

Physical Examination
- Paresthesias, depressed reflexes, proximal muscle weakness, ileus
- Severe hypokalemia: Hypoventilation, spasm, paralysis, rhabdomyolysis, myoglobinuria
- ARF, polymorphic VT, asystole

Diagnostics
- **Labs:** BMP, UA, urine electrolytes, urine Cr, urine Osm; consider blood gas, CPK, serum Osm
- Urine K^+ <15 mmol/d (spot Uk:Ucr <1.5) suggests extrarenal, whereas urine K^+ >15 mmol/d (spot Uk:Ucr >1.5) suggests renal etiology
- **ECG:** T-wave flattening/inversion, ST depression, U-waves, prolonged QT/QU interval; may also see PR prolongation, decreased voltage, QRS widening, atrial/ventricular dysrhythmias

Treatment
- ED
  - Potassium replacement: potassium chloride, potassium bicarbonate, potassium phosphate

(Decrease of 1 mEq/L = 200–400 mEq total body loss)
Mild (K^+ >2.8 mEq/L): 40 mEq K^+ PO q4–6h
Mod/severe: 40 mEq K^+ PO q4h (if tolerating oral) + KCl 10 mEq/h IV, recheck K^+ q4h

- Treat underlying cause
  - Replace Mg as needed (Note: Concurrent Mg & K^+ deficiency can interfere w/ K^+ repletion)
  - Goal K^+ = 4 mEq/L in pts at increased risk of cx (esp dysrhythmias)
- Home
  - Counsel pts to increase dietary intake of K^+ (nuts, avocados, wheat germ, vegetables [spinach, broccoli, cauliflower, beets, carrots], fruits [banana, kiwi, etc])
  - Discuss w/ PCP: Decrease diuretic dose; start/substitute for K^+-sparing med (β blockers, ACE-I, ARB, K^+-sparing diuretic)
  - Potassium replacement: KCl 20 mEq PO QD for prevention; KCl 40–100 mEq PO QD for tx

Disposition
- Home: Mild hypokalemia w/ close f/u to recheck labs
- Admit: Mod/severe hypokalemia, acid–base abnormalities, arrhythmia, severe sxs

Pearl
- Avoid dextrose-containing solutions (stimulate insulin & inward shift of K^+)

Hyperkalemia

Definition
- K^+ >5 mEq/L (ie, K^+ release from cells, decreased renal losses, iatrogenic)

Hyperkalemia Differential	
Pathophysiology	**Differential**
Endocrine/metabolic	Hypoaldosteronism, DKA, other acidoses
Renal	Renal insufficiency, end-stage renal failure, RTA (type 4), diabetic nephropathy, Gordon synd
Other	Tumor lysis synd, hemolysis, rhabdomyolysis, crush injury, burns, [a]pseudo-hyperK (hemolyzed sample, prolonged tourniquet w/ phlebotomy), exercise, hyperkalemic periodic paralysis
Meds	NSAIDs, ACE-I, ARBs, heparin, TMP/SMX, pentamidine, β-blockers, digoxin poisoning, K^+ sparing diuretics, exogenous KCl supplements, calcineurin inhs, succinylcholine, large-volume blood tfx

[a]Pseudohyperkalemia should be suspected in o/w asx pts w/o underlying causes. Repeated K+ should be obtained prior to initiating tx in such cases

History
- Weakness, muscle cramps, paresthesias, nausea, palpitations. Meds (see *Differential table*)

Physical Examination
- Assess fluid status
- Severe hyperkalemia: Flaccid paralysis, hypoventilation, PEA arrest, or asystole

Diagnostics
- Labs: BMP; consider blood gas w/ stat K^+, UA, urine electrolytes, urine Osm, CPK
- ECG: Early: Peaked & symmetric T-waves, flattened P-waves, PR prolongation, 1° AVB. Late: Widening/slurring of QRS → sinusoidal waveform → VFib or asystole

Hyperkalemia Treatment			
Intervention	**Dose**	**Onset**	**Mechanism**
Calcium gluconate OR Calcium chloride[a,b]	1–2 amps IV	Few minutes	Stabilizes cell membrane; used in pts w/ cardiac conduction abnormalities (no direct effect on K^+)
Bicarbonate	1–2 amps	15–30 mins (up to 2 h)	*Transient* shift of K^+ into cells in exchange for H^+ (may ↓ K^+ 0.47 mmol/L)
Albuterol (β-agonist)	10–20 mg inh or 0.5–2.5 mg IV	30–90 mins	*Transient* K^+ into cells (↓ K^+ 0.3–0.99 mmol/L)
Insulin + $D_{50}W$	5–10 U IV + 1 amp $D_{50}W$	15–30 mins, lasts 2–4 h	*Transient* K^+ into cells (↓ K^+ 0.45–1 mmol/L)
Sodium zirconium cyclosilicate	10 g PO	60 mins	Gastrointestinal cation exchange w/ K^+ out, Na^+/H^+ in (↓ K^+ 0.7 mmol/L in 4 h)
Patiromer	8.4 g PO	Unknown	Gastrointestinal cation exchange w/ K^+ out, Ca^{2+} in, typically for chronic use
Kayexalate[c]	30–90 g PO/PR	90 mins for PO, 30 mins for PR	Decreases total body K^+ by exchanging Na for K^+ in gut
Diuretics (furosemide)	≥40 mg IV	30 mins	Decreases total body K^+
HD (emergent)			Decreases total body K^+ (pts w/ cardiac cx or new/worsened renal failure)

[a]Standard teaching is not to use calcium in digoxin tox, however, more recent studies show that this is likely inaccurate (*J Emerg Med* 2011;40[1]:41–46)

[b]Calcium chloride contains 3 times more calcium ions, onset in seconds to minutes & lasts 30 mins, but much more caustic to veins than calcium gluconate

[c]May cause intestinal necrosis in pts w/ postoperative ileus; may also worsen pulmonary edema in pts w/ fluid overload; data on its efficacy at reducing total body potassium is poor. Avoid if other agents are available

Treatment
- Continuous cardiac monitoring
- Treating underlying cause
- Check electrolytes every 2–4 h until normalized

Disposition
- Home: Only if mild, stable hyperkalemia w/ good outpt f/u
- Admit: Most pts will require admx, nephrology consultation; some may require ICU admx for emergent dialysis

Pearls
- Think "ABCD" (albuterol, bicarbonate, calcium, dextrose/insulin, dialysis, diuretics)
- Combination therapy is proven more efficacious than any therapy alone
- HD is the most rapid & effective way of lowering plasma K^+

Hypocalcemia

Definition
- Ca <8.5 mg/dL (2 mmol/L) OR ionized Ca <4.5 mg/dL (1.1 mmol/L) (50% of Ca is bound to albumin, 40% is free, 10% complexed to anions)

Hypocalcemia Etiology		
Pathophysiology	**PTH**	**Differential**
Endocrine	↓	Hypoparathyroidism (familial, autoimmune, infiltrative, iatrogenic [surgery, neck irradiation]), DiGeorge synd, hypomagnesemia
Vit D deficiency	↑	Nutritional/sunlight deprivation; malabsorption; drugs (phenytoin, rifampin, ketoconazole, 5-FU/leucovorin); genetic; renal insufficiency (impaired production)
Renal	↑	Chronic renal failure, ARF (elevated phosphorus)
Neoplasm	↑	Osteoblastic metastases, tumor lysis (elevated phosphorus)
Other	↑	Pancreatitis, mx blood tfxs, rhabdomyolysis, burns, prematurity, pseudohypoparathyroidism, fluoride poisoning, calcium chelators, cinacalcet, foscarnet

History
- Weakness, muscle cramps, paresthesias, irritability, depression, tetany, AMS. Meds (see *Differential table*)

Physical Examination
- Paresthesias; Chvostek sign (tap over facial nerve causing facial twitching); Trousseau sign (inflate a BP cuff to 20 mm Hg above systolic BP over bicep × 3 mins to cause carpal spasm); may also see psychosis, szs, ↑ ICP, bronchospasm, laryngospasm

Diagnostics
- Labs: BMP w/ Ca/Mg/phosphorus testing. Check ionized calcium level, albumin, consider PTH level for continued inpt w/u:

Corrected Ca = measured serum Ca (mg/dL) + (0.8 × [4-serum albumin {g/dL}])

- ECG: Prolonged *QTc*, heart blocks, ventricular dysrhythmias, torsade

Treatment
- Asx: oral elemental Ca (1–3 g/d in divided doses) ± Vit D
- Symptomatic: (10% calcium gluconate [1–2 g IV over 20 mins] OR 10% calcium chloride [1–2 g IV diluted in 100 cc D_5W to decrease tissue irritation]), ±Vit D, ±Mg

Disposition
- Home: Asx, w/ oral regimen described above & PCP f/u in 5–7 d to recheck electrolytes
- Admit: Severe hypocalcemia, comorbid conditions, HD unstable

Hypercalcemia

Definition
- Ca >10.5 mg/dL; usually asx at levels up to 11.5 mg/dL

Hypercalcemia Etiology		
Pathophysiology	**PTH**	**Differential**
Excess PTH prod	↑	1° hyperparathyroidism[a] (adenoma, hyperplasia, rarely adenoCa, MEN), 2° hyperPTH (renal insufficiency), FHH
Vit D excess	↓	Sarcoidosis, TB, histoplasmosis, granulomatosis w/ polyangiitis, Vit D intoxication, lymphoma
↑ bone resorption	↓	Hyperthyroidism, immobilization
Neoplasm[a]	↓	PTHrP-producing solid tumors (squamous cell, renal bladder), lytic lesions (breast, myeloma), Paget dz
Other	↓	Meds (lithium, Vit A, thiazides, Ca-based antacids), massive dairy consumption (milk–alkali synd), TPN, endocrine d/o (adrenal insufficiency, VIPoma)

[a]Most common causes of hypercalcemia

History
- Polyuria, polydipsia, dehydration, nausea, vomiting, depression, confusion, coma, AMS; abdominal pain, anorexia, constipation, bone pain, Meds (see *Differential table*)
- May cause pancreatitis, nephrolithiasis, pathologic fractures. Suspect hypercalcemia in pts presenting w/ sxs consistent w/ these diagnoses

Physical Examination

- General weakness, epigastric tenderness, depressed deep tendon reflexes, coma

Diagnostics

- Labs: BMP w/ Ca/Mg/phosphorus testing, ionized Ca, lipase (if c/f pancreatitis), urine electrolytes, albumin (see corrected Ca equation above), consider PTH
- ECG: Shortened *QTc*, PR prolongation, QRS widening; rarely BBB, sinus bradycardia, or high-degree AV block

Treatment

- Address/treat underlying causes

Hypercalcemia Acute Treatment			
Intervention	**Dose**	**Onset/Duration**	**Effect**
Crystalloid IVF	4–6 L/d	Hours	Dilute and promote calcium excretion (Ca can drop 2 mEq)
Furosemide	20–60 mg IV q6h	Hours	Promotes calcium excretion; hold if c/f hypovolemia
Bisphosphonates (pamidronate, zoledronic acid, alendronate)	Variable	Days	Inhibit osteoclasts (esp useful in malignancy), caution in renal failure pt.
Calcitonin	4 IU/kg IM or SC q12h	Hours, lasts days	Peptide hormone analog, may develop tachyphylaxis
Denosumab	120 mg SQ monthly	Days	Monoclonal antibody, reduces bone resorption & osteoclast activity
Hydrocortisone	200–300 mg IV QD	Days	Useful only for Vit D toxic pts, mx myeloma, sarcoid & lymphoma pts
HD			Useful in renal failure pts

Disposition

- Home: Mild stable hypercalcemia. 1° hyperparathyroidism may require parathyroidectomy
- Admit: Mod, severe hypercalcemia, comorbidities, severe pain

Pearl

- Hypercalcemia = stones, bones, moans, abdominal groans, & psychiatric overtones

Hypomagnesemia

Definition

- Mg <0.7 mmol/L

Hypomagnesemia Differential	
Pathophysiology	**Differential**
Cardiac	CHF
GI	V/D, NGT suctioning, malabsorption, pancreatitis
Renal	Chronic renal failure (causing tertiary hypoparathyroidism), Bartter/Gitelman synd
Endocrine	Hyperaldosteronism, Vit D deficiency, hypercalcemia
Other/Meds	Alcoholism, pregnancy, thiazide & loop diuretics, aminoglycosides, amphotericin, gentamicin, pentamidine, tobramycin, PPI

History

- Weakness, AMS, muscle cramps, sz, choreoathetosis. Meds (see *Differential table*)

Physical Examination

- Tetany, Chvostek/Trousseau signs, papilledema, hyperreflexia

Diagnostics

- Labs: BMP w/ Ca/Mg/phosphorus testing, ionized Ca, albumin, consider PTH for continued inpt w/u
- ECG: Similar to hypokalemia & hypocalcemia (prolonged intervals, T-wave flattening, widening of QRS, U-waves)

Treatment
- Address underlying cause
- Magnesium replacement: 50% magnesium sulfate 2–4 g (16.6–33 mEq) IV over 30 mins. Oral forms may cause diarrhea (eg, magnesium citrate, milk of magnesia)
- Alcoholics: Consider thiamine; phosphorus & potassium replacement as needed

Disposition
- Home: Mild hypomagnesemia
- Admit: Severe hypomagnesemia w/ other associated electrolyte abnormalities (potassium, calcium), comorbid conditions

Pearl
- Most exogenously administered Mg is excreted in urine; full replacement takes days
- Hypomagnesemia leads to renal potassium wasting. Must correct Mg to correct K

Hypermagnesemia

Definition
- Mg >3 mEq/L

Hypermagnesemia Differential	
Pathophysiology	**Differential**
GI	Chronic constipation, bowel obstruction
Renal	Acute or chronic renal failure
Autoimmune/endocrine	DKA, adrenal insufficiency, hyperparathyroidism, hypothyroidism
Other/Meds	Hemolysis, lithium, exogenous Mg sources (antacids, laxatives, infusions for preeclampsia, Epsom salts), opioids, anticholinergics, tumor lysis synd, milk–alkali synd, rhabdomyolysis

History
- N/v, HA, lethargy, weakness, AMS; depends on level (renal insufficiency, GI motility disorder, adrenal insufficiency, hyperparathyroidism), Meds (see above)

Physical Examination
- Depends on level
  - Mg >4 mEq/L: n/v, cutaneous flushing, hyporeflexia, lethargy, drowsiness
  - Mg >6 mEq/L: Hypotension, bradycardia, areflexia, somnolence
  - Mg >10 mEq/L: Flaccid paralysis, respiratory failure, shock, coma, cardiac arrest

Diagnostics
- Labs: BMP w/ Ca/Mg/phosphorus testing, ionized Ca, albumin
- ECG: QRS widening, QT prolongation, prolonged AV conduction → complete block

Treatment
- Calcium:
  - Immediate: Calcium gluconate IV or calcium chloride (see *hypocalcemia*)
  - Continuous: 10% calcium gluconate 2–4 mg/kg/h if indicated
- Diuretics: Loop diuretics + aggressive hydration (improve Mg excretion)
- Dialysis: Particularly for pts in renal failure

Disposition
- Home: Asx, stable
- Admit: All need admx until sxs & lab values have normalized

Pearls
- Magnesium abnormalities are often seen w/ potassium or calcium abnormalities
- Check serial DTRs to assess tox in preeclamptic pts receiving Mg

Hypoglycemia

Definition
- Gluc <60 mg/dL; however, clinical hypoglycemia is any plasma gluc level low enough to cause sxs or signs c/w hypoglycemia (see below)
- Whipple triad: Sign/sxs of hypoglycemia, low plasma gluc, resolution of sx when plasma gluc is raised

Hypoglycemia Differential	
Pathophysiology	**Differential**
Medications[a]	Insulin, sulfonylureas (glyburide, glipizide, glimepiride), Meglitinides (repaglinide, nateglinide), EtOH
GI	Liver failure, postgastrectomy/gastric bypass

Renal	Acute renal failure
Endocrine	Hypothyroidism, insulinoma (inc MEN-1), hypopituitarism, adrenal insufficiency, insulin autoimmune hypoglycemia (Ab to insulin or its receptor)
Other	Sepsis, starvation, accidental/surreptitious/malicious hypoglycemia

[a]Most common cause of hypoglycemia

History
- Neurogenic/autonomic sxs: Agitation, tremor, diaphoresis, palpitations, pallor, hunger
- Neuroglycopenic sxs: Fatigue, HA, AMS, lethargy, somnolence, coma, sz
- Take detailed med hx (see *Differential table*); consider new meds, med dose chgs, incorrect use, intentional/accidental O/d, OTC/naturopathic meds, AKI
- Consider infectious causes (PNA, UTI, intra-abdominal infxns)
- Diabetics: Inquire about recent FSG values (if taken), last meal, dietary chgs, excess exercise
- RFs: Diabetes (esp on insulin), EtOH use, infants, elderly, s/p gastric bypass, critically ill

Diagnostics
- Labs: FSG, BMP; consider infectious w/u (CBC, UA, CXR)

*In o/w healthy, nondiabetic pts, consider LFTs, TSH, insulin, beta-hydroxybutyrate, proinsulin, & C-peptide (low in exogenous insulin, high in insulinoma or sulfonylurea OD) in consultation w/ an endocrine specialist

- Serial gluc testing may be necessary when prolonged hypoglycemia is expected esp in pts unable to communicate (eg, dementia, delirium, comatose, infants)

Treatment
- Gluc replacement
  - PO: Gluc paste/tablets (20 g), fruit juice, soft drinks, candy, a meal, etc
  - IV: 1 amp D_{50}; infusion may be needed
  - IM: 0.5–1 mg IM or SC glucagon (may cause n/v)

Disposition
- Home: Identifiable cause, does not need further monitoring
  - Prompt f/u w/ primary care or endocrinologist should be arranged
  - Pts should keep a gluc diary & should become concerned about the possibility of developing hypoglycemia when self-monitored gluc levels fall rapidly or are not greater than 70 mg/dL
- Admit: If c/f long-acting hypoglycemic agents, unable to tolerate POs, HD unstable

Pearls
- Beta blockers can mask adrenergic signs of hypoglycemia
- Should try to contact pt's primary physician or endocrinologist

HYPERGLYCEMIC EMERGENCIES (DKA/HHS)

Criteria for Diabetic Ketoacidosis (DKA) & Hyperosmolar Hyperglycemic State

	DKA (glucose >250 mg/dL)			HHS (glucose >600 mg/dL)
	Mild	Moderate	Severe	
Arterial pH	7.25–7.30	7.0–<7.25	<7.0	>7.3
Serum bicarbonate (mEq/L)	15–18	10–<15	<10	>18
Urine ketone	+	+	+	Small
Serum ketone	+	+	+	Small
Serum osmolality	Variable	Variable	Variable	>320 mOsm/kg
Anion gap	>10	>12	>12	Variable
Mental status	Alert	Alert/drowsy	Stupor/coma	Stupor/coma

Adapted from *Diabetes Care* 2009;32(7):1335–1343

Diabetic Ketoacidosis and Hyperosmolar Hyperglycemic State

Definition
- See *Criteria table* above for consensus diagnostic criteria. DKA characterized by uncontrolled hyperglycemia, metabolic acidosis, & increased ketone concentration. HHS characterized by profound hyperglycemia & serum hyperosmolality, nl arterial pH & bicarbonate, & AMS
- Marked by insulin deficiency & increased counterregulatory hormones
- HHS generally occurs in Type II diabetes; DKA generally occurs in Type I diabetes, but may occur in type II diabetes w/ stressors:

5 I's of DKA	
Etiology	**Cause**
Insulin deficiency	New-onset T1DM, failure to administer enough exogenous insulin
Infxn[a]	PNA, UTI, cellulitis, etc
Inflammation	Pancreatitis
Intoxication	Alcohol, drugs
Iatrogenesis	Glucocorticoids, thiazides, sympathomimetics, antipsychotics
Other	AMI, CVA, eating disorders

[a]Most common precipitating factor

History

- DKA often more acute in onset, HHS usually evolves over days to weeks
- Polyuria, polydipsia, n/v, dehydration, weight loss, abdominal pain, AMS
- Take detailed med hx (see *Differential table*); consider new meds, med dose chgs, incorrect use, intentional/accidental o/d, OTC/naturopathic meds, insulin pump
- ROS of contrib causes: Fever, chills, cough, abdominal pain, diarrhea, urinary sx, depression
- RFs: Insulin pump users

Physical Examination

- Pt may appear dry, Kussmaul respirations, lethargy, coma; abdominal tenderness (ileus)

Evaluation

- Labs: FSG, BMP (elevated anion gap acidosis, pseudohyponatremia, total body K^+ generally depleted despite nl/high value), Ca/Mg/Phos, urine/serum ketones, beta-hydroxybutyrate, UA, CBC, lactate, lipase, LFTs, serum osmolality, VBG, urine hCG, ECG; BCx, Ucx if clinically indicated

Equations
Anion gap (AG) = (Na – (Cl + bicarb))
Corrected AG = AG + (2.5 × [4.2 – albumin])
Calculated Osm = (2 × [Na^+]) + gluc/18 + BUN/2.8 + EtOH/4.6
Corrected $Na_{glucose}$ = Serum Na + [0.024 × (serum gluc – 100)]

- Imaging: CXR, abdominal CT, or U/S if c/f infxn and clinically indicated

Treatment

- Supportive: Continuous cardiac monitoring, 2 large-bore IVs
- Electrolyte monitoring: FSG q1h; BMP, Ca/Mg/phosphorus, VBG q2–4h

Acute Treatment	
Medication	**Dose/Frequency**
IV hydration[a,b]	Isotonic (LR or NS) bolus + 15–20 cc/kg/h (adjust for dehydration & cardiovascular comorbidities); usually 1–1.5 L during 1st hour → Continue isotonic infusion at 250–500 cc/h if corrected Na low → Δ IVF to ½ NS 250–500 cc/h if corrected Na nl or high → Δ IVF to D_5 NS or D_5½ NS at 150–250 cc/h when gluc ≤250 mg/dL
Insulin	Mod-Severe DKA or HHS – use IV insulin. Mild DKA – consider SQ insulin Dose: 0.1 U/kg/h in DKA, 0.05 U/kg/h in HHS → Goal: Fall in gluc by 50–70 mg/dL. Drop in gluc should not exceed 120 mg/dL/h HHS: → When gluc ≤250 mg/dL, reduce insulin dose by half until resolution to keep gluc b/w 250 and 300 mg/dL (to prevent cerebral edema) DKA → When gluc ≤250 mg/dL, reduce insulin infusion to 0.05 U/kg/h or administer 0.1 U/kg q2h SQ → After resolution of DKA, initiate long-acting insulin. Continue rapid acting for at least 2 h
Electrolyte repletion	Potassium: Goal to maintain K^+ 4–5 mEq/L → If K^+ >5.0 mEq/L: No supplementation required (continue to check q2h) → If K^+ is 3.5–5.0 mEq/L: Add 10–20 mEq K^+ per liter of IVF → If K^+ <3.5 mEq/L: Hold insulin & give K^+ 10–20 mEq/h HCO_3: If cardiac unstable or pH <7.0 Phosphate: Replete if <1 (20–30 mq/L Phos added to IVF)

[a]After volume resuscitation, choice of fluid replacement will depend on hemodynamics, hydration status, and electrolytes
[b]IVF volume should be used carefully considered in pts w/ cardiac or renal impairment
Adapted from *Diabetes Care* 2024;47(8):1257–1275

Disposition
- Home: Few if any
- Admit: Almost all pts will require admx, may need ICU monitoring

Pearls
- DKA w/ nl blood gluc can occur w/ SGLT2 inhs, pregnancy, or w/ very recent insulin use. Maintain a high index of suspicion for DKA in pts w/ RFs
  - Tx as above w/ insulin – early addition of dextrose-containing fluids to prevent hypoglycemia
- Consider increasing continuous insulin dose if gluc does not decrease sufficiently
- Pts w/ severe DKA hyperventilate in response to the metabolic acidosis, avoid intubation if possible as this takes away their physiologic compensation
- Cx: Hypoglycemia, hypokalemia, fluid overload, cerebral edema (more common in age <20), noncardiogenic pulmonary edema

THYROID EMERGENCIES

Hypothyroidism/Myxedema Coma

Definition
- Hypothyroidism is caused by insufficient production of thyroid hormone by the thyroid gland
- Hypothyroidism can be classified on the basis of its time of onset (congenital or acquired), the level of endocrine dysfxn (1° [thyroid] or 2° [pituitary or hypothalamic]), & its severity (subclinical, clinical, severe [myxedema coma])
- Myxedema coma is a rare expression of severe hypothyroidism. It typically occurs in pts w/ systemic illness superimposed on undiagnosed/untreated hypothyroidism

Hypothyroidism Differential	
	Cause
Endocrine	Hashimoto (autoimmune thyroiditis), subacute thyroiditis (de Quervain thyroiditis), postpartum thyroiditis, hypothalamic or pituitary failure, iodine deficiency or excess
Iatrogenic	Thyroidectomy or radiation therapy
Meds/toxins	Radioactive iodine, amiodarone, lithium, stavudine, interferon A, polybrominated/polychlorinated biphenyls, resorcinol (textile workers), thionamides, interleukin-2, tyrosine kinase inhs, checkpoint inh immunotherapy
Other	Congenital hypothyroidism (endemic iodine deficiency, thyroid gland dysgenesis, defective thyroid hormone biosynthesis); infiltrative dz

Factors Precipitating Myxedema Coma	
• Infxn (sepsis, PNA, UTI) • CVA • CHF • Hypothermia • GIB	• Metabolic disturbances (hypoglycemia, hyponatremia, acidosis, hypercapnia, hypercalcemia) • Meds (anesthetics, sedatives, opioids, amiodarone, lithium, w/d of L-thyroxine) • Ingestion of raw bok choy

History
- Hypothyroidism: Weakness, fatigue, myalgias, HA, depression, cold intolerance, weight gain, constipation, menorrhagia, dry skin, brittle hair, hoarseness, memory impairment
- Myxedema coma: Severely altered mental status/coma
- Meds (see Differential table)
- RFs: Postpartum women, family h/o autoimmune thyroid disorders, prior H&N surgery or irradiation, prior Grave dz s/p tx, other autoimmune disorders, Down synd, Turner synd

Physical Examination
- Hypothyroidism: Hypertension, bradycardia, obesity, goiter, periorbital puffiness, dry/coarse skin, cold skin, thinning of the lateral eyebrows, & delayed relaxation phase of the deep tendon reflexes
- Myxedema coma: Hypothermia & AMS are hallmark
  Vitals/Pulm/CV: Hypothermia, hypoventilation, hypoxia, hypotension, or bradycardia
  HEENT: Facial swelling, periorbital edema, macroglossia
  Neuro: Lethargy → comatose, cerebellar signs, poor memory, & cognition
  Psych: "Myxedema madness," disorientation, paranoia, depression, hallucinations, etc
  Other: SQ nonpitting edema (myxedema), pleural/pericardial/peritoneal effusions

Evaluation
- Labs: TFTs (TSH elevated) & free T4. Consider T3, antimicrosomal Ab, antithyroid peroxidase Ab, antithyroglobulin Ab, BMP (hyponatremia, hypoglycemia), CBC (anemia), creatine kinase (rhabdomyolysis), coags, cortisol
  - ↑TSH, ↓ free T4 confirms primary hypothyroidism of any cause
  - ↓TSH, ↓ free T4 consistent w/ secondary hypothyroidism disorders
    - ↑TSH, ↓ free T4, +antithyroid abs confirms Hashimoto/silent/postpartum thyroiditis
  - mild ↑TSH, nl free T4, & subtle sxs consistent w/ subclinical hypothyroid
- ECG: Myxedema-bradycardia, AV block, low voltage, flattened/inverted T-waves, prolonged QTc, atrial/ventricular dysrhythmias
- Bedside cardiac U/S: Pericardial effusion/tamponade may be seen in myxedema

Treatment (Only Start Empiric Treatment if Severely Symptomatic/Coma)
- Thyroid replacement: Start in ED if severely symptomatic/coma
- Levothyroxine: 200–400 μg IV × 1, then 50–100 μg QD; consider also giving synthetic T3 (b/c peripheral conversion impaired, but is more arrhythmogenic)
- Adrenal replacement: Hydrocortisone 100 mg IV × q8h (given c/f comorbid adrenal insuff)
- Additional supportive measures: Empiric abx, fluids/vasopressors, IV dextrose, passive rewarming, mechanical ventilation

Disposition
- Home: Discuss w/ PCP prior to starting any thyroid medications; usual starting dose of Levothyroxine 1.6 μg/kg PO QD (required repeat TFTs at 4–6 wks). Consider lower doses in elderly or those w/ cardiovascular dz
- Admit: All pts w/ severe hypothyroidism/myxedema; may require ICU admx

Hyperthyroidism/Thyrotoxicosis/Thyroid Storm

Definition
- Thyrotoxicosis is a disorder of excess thyroid hormone
- Hyperthyroidism specifically describes overproduction & secretion of excess of free thyroid hormones: Thyroxine (T_4), triiodothyronine (T_3), or both
- Thyroid storm is a rare, extreme expression of severe thyrotoxicosis
- Burch–Wartofsky score can be used to identify thyroid storm (*Endocrinol Metab Clin North Am* 1993;22:263–277)

Differential	
Thyrotoxicosis w/ Hyperthyroidism	
Endocrine	Graves dz[a], toxic multinodular goiter, toxic adenoma[b], TSH-secreting pituitary adenoma
Neoplasm	Metastatic follicular thyroid carcinoma, struma ovarii, choriocarcinoma (hCG secretion)
Other/Meds	Hyperemesis gravidarum (hCG), amiodarone, iodine/IV contrast
Thyrotoxicosis w/o Hyperthyroidism	
Thyroiditis (destruction of thyroid cells)	Early Hashimoto (autoimmune thyroiditis), painful thyroiditis (de Quervain's, a/w infxn), lymphocytic thyroiditis (postpartum thyroiditis), drug-induced thyroiditis (amiodarone, lithium), radiation thyroiditis
Other	Exogenous thyroid hormone, "Hamburger" thyrotoxicosis from food ingestions, infarction of thyroid adenoma

[a]Most common cause of hyperthyroidism caused by autoantibodies to & stimulation of TSH receptors
[b]Next most common causes of hyperthyroidism caused by autonomous overproduction of thyroid hormone
Adapted from *Lancet* 2012;379(9821):1156–1166

Factors Precipitating Thyroid Storm	
• Infxn (sepsis) • Sz • PE • Childbirth • Emotional stress	• Trauma (inc vigorous thyroid palpation), burns • Perioperative (stress from anesthesia, surgery) • Metabolic disturbances (hypoglycemia, DKA) • Meds (amiodarone, radioactive iodine tx, iodinated contrast, thyroxine/triiodothyronine OD, ASA OD, w/d of PTU/methimazole)

History
- Neck fullness, double vision, restlessness, anxiety, palpitations, sweating, heat intolerance, tremor, weight loss, loss of appetite, n/v, diarrhea, irregular menses, myopathy, periodic paralysis, lethargy, hair thinning/loss
- Thyroid storm: AMS (delirium, agitation, coma), sz, fever, tachycardia, n/v, diarrhea
- Meds (see *Differential table*; assess h/o hyperthyroidism)

Physical Examination

- Thyrotoxicosis: Diaphoresis, agitation, tremor, tachycardia, AFib, systolic HTN, widened pulse pressure, proximal muscle weakness, thyroid enlargement/ttp/nodularity, cachexia
- Graves: Pretibial myxedema, exophthalmos, lid lag, ophthalmoplegia, periorbital edema
- Thyroid storm: Hyperthermia & severe AMS are hallmarks
  - Vitals/Pulm/CV: Hyperthermia, hyperventilation, tachycardia
  - GI: Nausea, vomiting, diarrhea, diffuse abdominal pain (may mimic acute abdomen)
  - Neuro/Psych: AMS (delirium, agitation, coma), sz, disorientation, paranoia, psychosis

Evaluation

- Labs: Low TSH w/ elevated free T4 &/or elevated total T3; CBC/BMP/Ca/Mg/phosphorus, LFTs, UA, urine hCG; consider TSH receptor ab & antithyroid peroxidase ab for suspected Graves; consider thyroxine-binding globulin in pregnancy (to correct free T4)
- Imaging: Thyroid U/S. May require radioactive iodine uptake scan (+ in Graves/autonomous nodules)
- ECG: Tachycardia, supraventricular arrhythmias, AFib

Treatment (Only Start ED Treatment If Severely Symptomatic/Thyroid Storm)

- Thyrotoxicosis tx: Beta blockers (propranolol), antithyroid tx (methimazole/PTU), radioiodine, surgery
- Thyroid storm tx: β blockers → steroids + PTU or methimazole → iodine
  - Beta blockers: Propranolol or esmolol (improve hyperadrenergic activity & tachycardia). Consider decompensated heart failure prior to administration – can uncover occult dz
    - Propranolol 0.5–1 mg IV over 10 mins, then 1–2 mg boluses q3h
    - Propanolol 60–80 mg q4h if taking PO
    - Esmolol 250–500 μg/kg loading dose, then 50–100 μg/kg/min
  - PTU or Methimazole: Blocks hormone synthesis. PTU (also inhibits peripheral conversion of T4–T3)
    - PTU: Loading dose of 500–1,000 mg, then 250 mg q4h (*Thyroid* 2016;26[10]:1343–1421)
    - Methimazole: 20 mg q4h. Contraindicated in 1st trimester pregnancy
- Iodine: Blocks thyroid hormone release but give >1 h after methimazole/PTU (can potentiate thyroid storm if given before; similarly avoid iodinated contrast scans)
  - Potassium iodide (SSKI): 5 drops PO q6h
  - Lugol's solution: 10 drops PO TID
- Steroids: Hydrocortisone 300 mg IV bolus, then 100 mg IV × q8h (can decrease conversion of T4–T3)
- Consider plasmapheresis & therapeutic plasma exchange (Graves dz)
- Supportive care: Hyperpyrexia – APAP as needed; avoid aspirin (can increase T3 conversion)
- Treat underlying precipitant (often infxn)

Disposition

- Home: TSH low but no severe sxs: F/u w/ PCP or endo referral: Outpt meds ± surgery
- Admit: All pts w/ severe hyperthyroidism. Pts w/ thyroid storm require ICU admx

ADRENAL INSUFFICIENCY

Definition

- Condition in which the adrenal glands do not produce adequate amounts of steroid hormones
- Primary adrenal insufficiency (PAI) is due to pathology w/i the adrenal cortex that results in deficiency of all adrenocortical hormones (aldosterone, cortisol, androgens)
- Secondary and tertiary adrenal insufficiency result from pathology of the pituitary and hypothalamus respectively; only affect glucocorticoid production in the adrenal glands
- Dysfxn of the hypothalamic–pituitary–adrenal axis in critical illness = critical illness-related corticosteroid insufficiency (CIRCI)

Adrenal Insufficiency Differential	
	Cause
Infiltrative dz	Tuberculosis, CMV, fungal, histiocytosis, AIDS (opportunistic dz), syphilis, trypanosomiasis, amyloidosis, sarcoidosis, hemochromatosis
Vascular[a]	Hemorrhage, thrombosis, necrosis (meningococcemia, sepsis, APS)
Endocrine	Autoimmune adrenalitis (alone as Addison dz or as part of autoimmune polyglandular synds), pituitary failure
Neoplasm	Metastatic dz (lung, breast, kidney), lymphoma, pituitary tumor (primary or mets), craniopharyngioma, hypothalamic tumors
Meds	Glucocorticoid w/d, ketoconazole, fluconazole, etomidate, rifampin, phenytoin, megestrol, phenobarbital, troglitazone, mitotane, metyrapone
Other[a]	Trauma (esp head trauma, burns), postpartum pituitary necrosis (Sheehan synd), empty sella synd, pituitary radiation/surgery, adrenalectomy, congenital adrenal hyperplasia, adrenoleukodystrophy

[a]Causes of acute onset adrenal insufficiency

Adapted from *NEJM* 1996;335(16):1206–1212; *Lancet* 2014;383(9935):2152–2167

History
- Weakness, fatigue, anorexia, nausea, vomiting, postural dizziness & hypotension, craving for salt, cramping, abdominal pain, confusion, or somnolence
- Meds (see *Differential table*); also elicit if pt is on long-term steroids

Physical Examination
- Orthostatic hypotension, hyperpigmentation, vitiligo

Evaluation
- Labs: BMP (may see hypoglycemia, hyponatremia, hyperkalemia, acidosis, prerenal acute kidney injury from hypovolemia), CBC (may see mild normocytic anemia, lymphocytosis, & eosinophilia); random cortisol & ACTH level
  - In hypotensive pts, cortisol level <18 μg/dL suggests adrenal insufficiency
  - AM serum cortisol <5 μg/dL suggests adrenal insufficiency
  - High ACTH, high renin, & low aldosterone level supports a dx of PAI
  - 21-hydroxylase antibody testing is spec for autoimmune adrenalitis (eg, Addison's)
  - ACTH stimulation test is rarely used in the ED
    - ACTH stimulation test: Cortisol level <18 μg/dL 30–60 mins after ACTH stimulation test is suggestive of adrenal insufficiency
- Imaging: Consider head MR (assess pituitary), adrenal CT

Treatment (Only Start ED Treatment If Symptomatic/Hypotensive)
- IV hydration: Volume resuscitation w/ NS (LR w/ hypothetical risk of worsening hypoNa)
- Steroids (hydrocortisone preferred given glucocorticoid + mineralocorticoid effects)
  - Steroid dosing: Hydrocortisone 100 mg IV bolus, then 50 mg q6h
- Replete electrolytes as needed

Disposition
- Home: Stable, already on meds
- Admit: All pts w/ new-onset adrenal insufficiency; may require ICU admx if concomitant infxn or HD unstable

Pearls
- Adrenal insufficiency should be suspected in pts w/ shock w/ insufficient response to IVF + vasopressors
- Never delay tx for the sake of diagnostic w/u for suspected adrenal crisis
- Pts w/ known adrenal insufficiency + a febrile illness should be instructed to increase their home dose of steroid by 2–3 times until recovery to prevent possible adrenal crisis. Stress dose steroids can be given in the ED prior to dispo

DEHYDRATION

Approach
- Quickly determine etiology of volume depletion
- Prompt tx initiation to restore euvolemia may be life-saving

Dehydration Differential	
Pathophysiology	**Differential**
Cardiac	Arrhythmia
Endocrine	Adrenal insufficiency, DI, DKA, SIADH, thyroid dysfxn
Infectious	Encephalitis, fever, meningitis, Lyme dz, sepsis, syphilis
GI	Bowel obstruction, diarrhea, gastroenteritis, intestinal volvulus, vomiting, GIB
FEN/GU	Electrolyte disturbances, renal insufficiency
Neurologic	GBS, myasthenia gravis, ALS, stroke, migraine
Hematologic/oncologic	Metastatic dz
Toxic	Drug induced
Environmental	Hyperthermia
Psychiatric	Anorexia, bulimia, laxative abuse, psychosis

History
- Identify etiology of volume loss: renal loss (polyuria, diuretic use, nephropathies, aldosteronism), GI loss (diarrhea, emesis, melena/hematochezia), skin loss (burns, sweat), third-space sequestration (ascites, pancreatitis), or decreased intake (debilitated, institutionalized, NM d/o)

Types of Dehydration		
	Losses	**Mechanism**
Hypotonic	Na loss > water loss	Diuretics
Isotonic	Na loss = water loss	Vomiting, diarrhea
Hypertonic	Na loss < water loss	Fever, sweating, faulty thirst mechanism

Findings
- S/S of dehydration depend upon extent of tissue hypoperfusion

Degrees of Dehydration			
Degree	**Fluid Deficit**	**Sxs**	**Signs**
Mild	30 cc/kg (3%)	Thirst, fatigue	Slight ↑ HR, ↓ UOP
Moderate	50–60 cc/kg (5–6%)	Oliguria, weakness, LH	Postural hypotension (>20 mmHg), ↑ HR, flat neck veins, dry MM, skin tenting, delayed cap refill
Severe	70–90 cc/kg (7–9%)	AMS, cool extremities, sz, coma	Hypovolemic shock

Evaluation
- CBC (hemoconcentration), BMP (BUN/Cr ratio >20:1, abnl Na, K), abnl pH (met alkalosis vs acidosis), ECG abnl
- UA: Ketones, hyaline casts, spec grav >1.02 = severe dehydration. Spot U[Na] >30 mmol/L in renal causes; <30 mmol/L in extrarenal causes
- FENa: Differentiates oliguric/AKI etiologies: prerenal <1% vs ATN >1%

Treatment
- Initial fluid resuscitation w/ crystalloids (NS or LR; avoid NS if concern for hyponatremia), then tailor to electrolyte abnlty/pathology
- nl LV fxn: 2–3 L NS, follow clinical sxs, VS, UOP (goal of >0.5 mL/kg/h)
- Compromised LV fxn: 500 cc/h, watch pulmonary status (O_2 sat, SOB)
- Consider antiemetic if N/V contributes to dehydration

Composition of Resuscitation Fluids					
1 L Fluid	**Glucose (g/L)**	**Sodium (mEq/L)**	**Chloride (mEq/L)**	**Potassium (mEq/L)**	**mOsm/L**
NS	0	154	154	0	308
Ringer lactate	0	130	109	4	272
D_5W	50	0	0	0	278
D_5W ½ NS	50	77	77	0	432
3% NS	0	513	513	0	1026

Disposition

- Home: Once dehydration adequately addressed & pt is able to maintain hydration status
- Admx: Persistent hemodynamic instability, electrolyte repletion requirement, or on-going tx needs due to underlying etiology

Pearls

- Up to 30% of healthy pts are orthostatic w/o dehydration (βBs, autonomic dysfxn, DM)
- Oral rehydration w/ gluc to facilitate intestinal absorption of Na & water if pt tolerates, "recipe" is 2 tbsp sugar: 0.5 tsp salt: 1 quart water; ½ dilute apple juice also effective
- Healthy adults tolerating PO rarely require IV fluids; PO rehydration is usually adequate

BITES AND STINGS

Approach

- Treat anaphylaxis; give tetanus prophylaxis
- Consider x-ray for underlying fx or FB
- Assess for joint space violation, copious wound irrig/wash out; avoid closure in many cases
- 24–48-h wound check for high-risk bites, esp in kids or unreliable pts
- National Poison Control Center (PCC): (800) 222-1222

Human & Animal Bites

Human

History

- Human bites are unintentional ('love bites' vs nail-biting) or intentional (occlusive/ semicircular bites vs 'fight bites")
- Obtain time of injury, current immunization status, hx of immunocompromising conditions, known health conditions of biter if available (HIV, Hep B, Hep C)

Evaluation

- Evaluate for FB (tooth fragment), superficial vs deep infxn, N/V exam distally; ensure complete exploration in the position which injury occurred
- Lac near MCP joint during altercation should be considered a human bite, or "fight bite"—bacteria may spread to nearby soft tissue, joints, or deeply along tendon sheaths
- Obtain x-ray to assess for fx, air in joint, retained FB; serology typically unnecessary for uninfected wounds
- Consider surgical c/s for deep wounds, significant infxn, N/V compromise, or complex facial injury

Treatment

- Local wound care: copious irritation; do not close given high likelihood of infxn–uninfected simple facial lacs <24 h may be closed for cosmetic reasons; delayed 1° closure if closure necessary
- Prophylactic abx: amoxicillin/clav 875/125 mg PO BID × 5–10 d
- Alternative Abx: doxycycline or TMP-SMX or pen VK or fluoroquinolone or cefuroxime PLUS clindamycin or metronidazole OR moxifloxacin
- If late/complicated/needs admit: IV ampicillin/sulbactam 3 g q6h

Disposition

- DC w/ scheduled strict f/u in 24–48 h for wound recheck
- Admx for systemic illness, significant cellulitis, failure of outpt abx therapy, or need for surgical intervention

Pearl

- *Eikenella* (most common), *Staph/Strep* species found in mouth, anaerobes

Cat

Evaluation

- Cat bites often penetrate deep; 80% of cat bites become infected!
- Consider x-ray to assess for fracture, air in joint, tooth fragments
- Extend & explore joint injuries inc in the position that injury occurred

Treatment

- Local wound care w/ debridement, copious irrig & dressing
- Prophylactic abx: amoxicillin/clav 875/125 mg BID or doxycycline 100 mg BID
- Allow for open healing by 2° intention for wounds other than simple, noninfected, facial lac <24 h

Disposition
- Scheduled strict f/u in 24 h for wound recheck; may consider delayed 1° closure if no e/o of infx on abx in 48–72 h

Pearls
- *Pasteurella multocida* most common organism
- Consider cat-scratch dz if pt has tender LAD 1 wk after bite/scratch
- Consider rabies prophylaxis (rabies immunoglobulin + vaccine) if unknown cat

Dog

Evaluation
- Consider x-ray to assess for fracture, air in joint, tooth fragments

Treatment
- Amoxicillin/clav 875/125 mg BID or clindamycin 300 QID + ciprofloxacin 500 mg BID
- 1° closure of nonpuncture wounds after copious irrig possible (only 5% become infected) except when on hand/foot

Disposition
- Scheduled strict f/u in 24 h for wound recheck

Pearls
- Polymicrobial infections; *capnocytophaga* commonly reported in dogs
- Consider rabies prophylaxis if unknown dog as above w/ cats

SNAKE BITES

Crotalinae/Pit Vipers (Rattlesnakes, Copperheads, Water Moccasins)

History
- Rattlesnake bites are the most common snake envenomation in the US
- Pain & swelling around fang marks, attempt identification of snake if possible

Findings
- Local (pain, swelling, ecchymosis, compartment synd), systemic (↓ BP, ↑ HR, paresthesias, rhabdomyolysis), coagulopathies (↓ PLTs, ↑ INR, ↓ fibrinogen), & allergic rxns. Pulmonary edema & cardiovascular collapse reported
- Mojave rattlesnake—delayed neurologic sxs (ptosis, muscle weakness, respiratory depression) reported several hours after bite

Evaluation
- C/s PCC/toxicologist; CBC, BMP, coags w/ fibrinogen & split products, CK, T&C, UA for occult blood; x-rays to r/o retained fang; watch compartment pressures
- PLT & fibrinogen most beneficial for prognosticating severity & need for antivenom, repeat q2–6h until stable

Treatment
- Remove rings, constrictive clothing, general wound care, update tetanus
- Aggressive antivenom (Crotalidae immune Fab) tx for systemic effects or coagulopathy; surgical assessment if compartment synd; supportive care; no proven benefit w/ abx or steroids

Grades of Pit Viper Envenomation (Dynamic)

Grade	Signs/Sxs	Vials of Antivenom
Mild	Local pain, edema. No signs of systemic tox. nl labs	None
Moderate	Severe local pain, edema <50 cm around wound. Systemic tox: n/v. Labs abnl (↓ Hct, ↓ PLTs)	4–6
Severe	Generalized petechiae/ecchymosis, compartment sx, bleeding, ↓ BP, AMS, renal dysfxn, markedly abnl coags	Initial dose 8–12

Disposition
- D/C if absence of any findings 8–12 h postbite envenomation in healthy adults, 12–24 h in children/elderly or if concerns for Mojave rattlesnake envenomation
- ICU admx if antivenom given

Pearls
- Avoid oral or mechanical suction of wound, tourniquets, incision, or suction
- 25% of bites are "dry strikes" (no effect); pit vipers identified by 2 fangs

Elapidae/Coral Snake (*Micrurus fulvius*)

History
- Bitten by brightly colored snake (black, red, & yellow bands), primarily occur in southeastern US

Findings
- Neurotoxic effects predominate; minimal local effects: Tremor/sz, ↑ salivation, respiratory paralysis, bulbar palsy (dysarthria, diplopia, dysphagia)
- Sxs onset w/i a few h but may be delayed for up to 12 h!

Evaluation
- C/s PCC/toxicologist; CBC, BMP, coags/DIC eval not usually indicated, consider pulmonary fxn testing

Treatment
- C/s PCC before giving antivenom as higher risk for allergic rxn; if e/o of neurotoxicity or coagulopathy generally advised to give antivenom. Surgical assessment if concern for compartment synd; supportive care (esp respiratory support)

Disposition
- 12–24 h observation; ICU admx if antivenom given or respiratory compromise

Pearl
- Coral snakes have red on yellow banding, nonvenomous snakes have red band on black background: "*Red on yellow: Kill a fellow. Red on black: Venom lack.*"

Scorpion Bites

Scorpion (*Centruroides exilicauda*)

History
- Burning & stinging w/o visible injury at bite site

Findings
- Usually no visible local injury; possible systemic effects include roving eye movements (pathognomonic), opisthotonos, ↑ HR, diaphoresis, fasciculations
- Mydriasis, nystagmus, hypersalivation, dysphagia, restlessness
- Severe envenomation may cause pancreatitis, respiratory failure, coagulopathy, anaphylaxis

Evaluation
- "Tap test": Exquisite tenderness w/ light tapping in *Centruroides* stings; c/s PCC/toxicologist
- CBC, BMP, coags, LFTs, CK, ECG

Treatment
- Most bites are self-limited & resolve in h, provide supportive care
- BZD for muscle spasm/fasciculations, pain control, tetanus, reassurance
- If severe systemic sxs, 1–2 vials *Centruroides* antivenom; avail from AZ PCC

Disposition
- Admx for observation; ICU admx if antivenom given

Pearl
- Only *C. exilicauda* (bark scorpion) found in Western US produces systemic tox

Spider Bites

Brown Recluse (*Loxosceles reclusa*)

History
- Pt may not remember bite; typically presents w/ pain, pruritus, & a "bull's eye" lesion which develops over 12 h

Findings
- Cutaneous loxoscelism: Pain & blistering followed by necrotic ulcer which may develop over 3–4 d & can take wks to heal
- Systemic loxoscelism: Systemic rxn 1–2 d after envenomation; N/V, f/c, muscle/joint aches, sz, rarely renal failure, DIC, hemolytic anemia, rhabdomyolysis

Evaluation
- C/s PCC/toxicologist, surgery/plastics c/s for lesion >2 cm
- CBC, BMP, coagulation profile, UA

Treatment
- Antivenom not available in US: provide wound care, tetanus, supportive care (eg, hydration, abx, tfx, HD), local debridement
- May consider dapsone 50–100 mg BID to prevent necrosis, hyperbaric O_2, steroids (all are controversial)
- Dapsone causes hemolysis, hepatitis; monitor LFTs, check G6PD level

Disposition
- Admx for observation

Pearl
- Located in S. Central & SW (desert) of US; violin-shaped marking on back
- Many self-reported & unwitnessed spider bites are in fact infectious skin conditions, such as MRSA

Black Widow (*Latrodectus mactans*)

History
- Pain, swelling, & target-shaped lesion; may present w/ severe chest, abdomen, or back pain (may mimic acute MI or surgical abdomen), muscle cramps develop w/i 1 h
- Pain may continue intermittently for 3 d, is often a/w muscle weakness & spasm for wks to mos

Findings
- Severe rxns: HTN, local sweating, respiratory failure, abd rigidity, fasciculations, shock, coma, fatalities rarely

Evaluation
- CBC, BMP, CK, coagulation profile, UA, ECG, +/– abd CT (r/o acute abdomen)

Treatment
- Antivenom if severe rxn not responsive to standard care, hemodynamic instability, respiratory distress, or risk of premature delivery in pregnancy: 1–2 vials over 30 mins (after cutaneous test dose)
- Wound care, tetanus, supportive care: BZD, analgesia

Disposition
- Consider admx for observation & symptom control

Pearls
- Identified black widows by red hourglass-shaped marking found on spider's abdomen

Hymenoptera (Bee, Wasp, Stinging Ant)

History
- Immediate pain & swelling at site of bite

Findings
- Local redness, wheals, blisters, edema; severe systemic signs & allergic rxns may occur

Treatment
- No available antidote. Treat anaphylaxis/allergic rxn; local rxn treated w/ analgesia, cleansing, tetanus prophylaxis, ice packs, & elevation
- If present, stinger should be removed immediately by scraping it from the wound

Disposition
- Close wound care f/u; prescribe epinephrine autoinjectors in cases of anaphylaxis

Pearls
- The more rapid onset of sxs, the more severe the rxn; IgE-mediated allergic rxn
- Rapid onset: 50% D in 30 mins, 75% in 4 h; usually see fatal rxn following prior mild rxn
- Delayed rxn similar to serum sickness can present 10–14 d after a sting/bite

Jellyfish Stings

History
- Swimming in seawater w/ jellyfish

Findings
- Painful lines of papular lesions ("tentacle tracks") & urticarial eruptions last min to h
- Systemic rxns rare; vomiting, muscle spasm, paresthesias, weakness, fever, respiratory distress, Irukandji synd: Rare, severe chest/abd/back pain, HTN, GI sx

Evaluation
- CBC, BMP, LFT, CK, coagulation profile, UA, ECG, cardiac enzymes

Treatment
- Analgesia, supportive care
- Tentacles should be removed w/ forceps; nematocysts should be scraped off w/a knife/blade after dusting w/ talcum powder & covering w/ shaving cream
- Analgesia & after nematocyst removal wash w/ hot (40 °C) salt water (helps w/ pain)
- Antivenom available for serious systemic effects (cardiopulmonary arrest, severe pain) from the Commonwealth Serum Laboratory in Melbourne, Australia

Disposition
- D/C if mild & pain controlled, admx for observation o/w

Pearls
- Box jellyfish are severely toxic, can induce respiratory & myocardial arrest in min
- Use seawater/vinegar (not urine!) to wash; freshwater causes nematocysts to fire

OCCUPATIONAL EXPOSURE

Approach
- Institutional guidelines vary regarding occupational exposures of HC workers to bodily fluids
- Refer to CDC/local experts for recs on postexposure prophylaxis (PEP)
- 24 h National Clinicians' Postexposure Prophylaxis Hotline (PEP line): (888) 448-4911

History
- Any percutaneous injury, MM exposure, or exposure of nonintact skin to any blood & other bodily fluids considered potentially infectious
- RFs: High-risk procedures, use of equipment w/o newer safety designs, failure to follow universal precautions

Findings
- Physical examination nl; should be documented for future reference

Evaluation
- Test source pt: consent & obtain HIV (4th gen Ab/Ag), HBsAg, & HCV RNA. If known HIV+ source pt c/s ID for appropriate regimen based on source pt's regimen
- Test HCP: HIV (4th-gen Ab/Ag) & Hep C Ab, obtain HBsAb & anti-HBs if HBV immune status is unknown
- Check B-hCG, CBC, BMP, LFTs, & UA before initiating PEP

Treatment
- Clean wounds w/ soap & water; MM w/ copious irrig
- HIV PEP: Goal to initiate tx w/i 1–2 h and up to 72 h; may stop tx if source pt results HIV neg. Continue tx for 28 d if source pt HIV+

Antiretrovirals for HIV Exposure	
Special Considerations	**Regimen**
General	TDF/FTC (300/200 mg) QD + DTG (50 mg QD) × 4 wks
Pregnant or potential childbearing	TDF/FTC (300/200 mg) QD + RAL (400 mg BID) × 4 wks
Known drug-resistant HIV+ source	TDF/FTC (300/200 mg) QD + DTG (50 mg QD) OR DRV (800 mg QD) × 4 wks
Reduced renal function	TAF (200/25 mg) QD × 4 wks

- HBV PEP: Anti-HBs titer ≥10 mIU/mL is considered immune and no PEP recommended. Start vaccination series if HCP is unvaccinated & Hep B immune globulin (0.06 mL/kg IM) if source pt is HBsAg+. HBIG must be given w/i 1 wk of exposure & provides up to 75% protection for 3–6 mos
- HCV PEP: No PEP for HCP exposed to HCV; management involves early dx & tx if HCV seroconversion occurs. Consider direct acting antiviral tx as soon as HCV seroconversion is documented

Disposition
- F/u w/ ID specialist; fully inform risks & benefits of tx & non-tx

Pearls
- ~80% ↓ rate of HIV transmission w/ immediate initiation (w/i 2 h) of PEP
- Needle-stick seroconversion rates: HIV + source pt: 0.3%; Hep B + source pt: 23–62%; Hep C + source pt: 0–7%

Percutaneous Exposure Risk for HIV Seroconversion	Odds Ratio
Injury resulting in deep wound	OR 15
Injury from large-gauge (<18) hollow-bore needle	OR 14
Injury from device w/ visible source pt's blood	OR 10
Injury from needle placed in pt's artery or vein	OR 5.9
Injury obtained during an emergency procedure	OR 5.6
Exposure from pt w/ terminal AIDS	OR 4.8

Engl J Med 1997;337(21):1485.

BURNS

Approach
- Early airway assessment, determine need for intubation (soot in airway, edema, voice Δ, deep facial burns, ↓ O_2 sat; transfer to burn center if intubated)
- 100% O_2 or O_2 by NRB mask until CO & other inhalation tox assessed
- Evaluate for concomitant trauma (fall, blast injury); maintain c-spine precautions
- Start IVF resuscitation early (almost universally required)
- Keep room warm to ↓ insensate losses

History
- Determine burn mechanism (thermal, electrical, chemical, radiation, or friction) duration of exposure, depth of burn, extent of injury, existing circumference burns, risk of smoke inhalation, potential associated trauma, & existing comorbid states

Findings
- Assess depth & extent of injury

Burn Classifications by Depth			
Degree	**Areas of Involvement**	**Clinical Findings**	**Sensation**
1°: Superficial	Epidermis only	Erythematous, indurated area w/o blisters, blanching	Painful
2°: Superficial partial thickness	Epidermis & superficial dermis	Erythematous or mottled, indurated, blisters, blanching	Painful
2°: Deep partial thickness	Epidermis, deep dermis	Waxy white, blisters, nonblanching	Painful
3°: Full thickness	Epidermis, entire dermis	Pale white, leathery, black, charred, nonblanching	Not painful
4°: Fourth degree	Epidermis, dermis, SQ, muscle, & bone	Visible muscle & fascia	Not painful

Evaluation
- ABC's!
- Check CO level, CN (combustion of synthetics/plastics), CBC, BMP, CK, lactate, ABG, LFTs, coags, tox, T&S, UA, CXR, & advanced imaging if trauma suspected

Treatment
- Airway management: Intubate early if serious inhalational burn is suspected
  - Toxic inhalation (cough, dyspnea, carbonaceous sputum, soot in oropharynx): Intubate or perform fiberoptic airway exam early; delay could cause ↑ airway edema → airway compromise, difficult/impossible intubation
- If >15% TBSA, aggressive IVF resuscitation
  - Parkland formula calculates IVF requirement in 1st 24 h after burn:
    - 4 mL × weight (kg) × TBSA (2nd- & 3rd-degree burns)
    - Give ½ over 1st 8 h, other ½ over next 16 h; use LR to avoid NAGMA w/ NS
- Urinary catheter placement: Target urine output: 0.5–1 mL/kg/h (~30–50 mL/h)
- Early & generous analgesia: Morphine IV q5–10min titrated to pain
- Burn mgmt: Irrigate w/ NS, remove debris, clothing, jewelry, & ruptured blisters (prevent future infection)
  - Apply silver sulfadiazine (antipseudomonal) ointment to denuded areas
  - Bacitracin only on face (silver sulfadiazine may cause discoloration)
  - Immediate escharotomy for full-thickness circumferential burns that compromise distal N/V status or significantly ↓ chest compliance
- Tetanus prophylaxis, no role for steroids or immediate IV abx

Disposition
- Admit 2° burns 10–20% TBSA (or 5–10% if <10 y/o), circumferential or if meet criteria to transfer to burn unit

Criteria for Transfer to Burn Unit
Burns >20% BSA (or >10% if age <10 or >50)
3rd-degree burns >5% BSA or 2nd-degree burns >20% BSA
Burns involving face, eyes, ears, hands, feet, or perineum
Burns a/w significant electrical, chemical, inhalational, or traumatic injury
Burns suspected to be related to abuse
Burns to pts w/ special psychosocial or rehabilitative care needs

Pearls

- Initial injury may be difficult to estimate; burns evolve & must be reevaluated in 24 h
- Smoke contains other potential toxic gasses: consider cyanide tox, methemoglobinemia, & caustic gas injury

Figure 10.1 The rule of nines for estimating total body surface area burned. (Reprinted with permission from Mick NW, Peters JR, Egan D, et al. *Blueprints Emergency Medicine*. Lippincott Williams & Wilkins; 2006.)

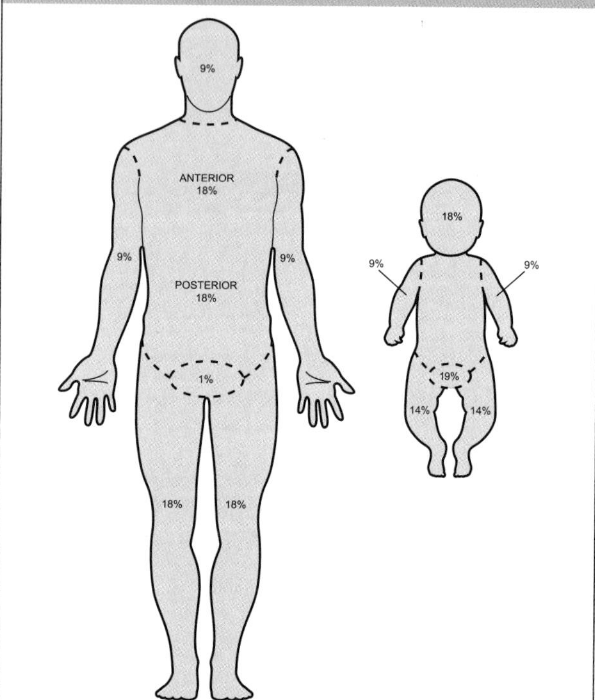

CARBON MONOXIDE POISONING

Approach

- Early airway assessment, determine need for intubation (AMS)
    - 100% O_2 or O_2 by NRB mask until CO assessed
- Call regional poison control center ([800] 222-1222) for advice & locations of local hyperbaric chamber if necessary

History

- Exposure to CO from combustion, faulty heating, closed-space fire, defective automobile exhaust; often multiple people exposed/symptomatic

Findings

- Mild poisoning: Frontal HA, N/V, dizziness/confusion
    - May have subtle psychomotor abnormalities: ataxia, muscle rigidity, tachycardia, retinal hemorrhage, ↓ visual acuity, cyanosis, or pallor
- Severe exposure: Syncope, coma, sz, arrhythmia, ↓ BP, & death
- Bright venous blood or cherry red skin is suggestive however not frequently observed

Evaluation
- Check CO, ABG, BMP, EKG, pregnancy; CN & methemoglobin w/ smoke inhalation
- Pulse oximetry not useful b/c it will detect carboxyhemoglobin (COHgb) as oxyhemoglobin
- ABG alone not useful b/c pO_2, a measure of dissolved O_2, will be nl; check ABG for COHgb via co-oximetry
  - Level is weakly correlated w/ tox but it confirms significant exposure
  - Level of <10–15% may be nl in smokers
- Higher risk for myocardial injury: Check ECG esp if baseline CAD, risk fx, or high CO
- Assess for suicide attempt; may need psychiatry c/s

Treatment
- O_2 via NRB (60% O_2) at least, ideally deliver 100% O_2
- Airway management: If AMS, hypoxemia or shock → intubate
- Cardiac monitoring; admx if dysrhythmia or e/o ischemia on ECG
- Hyperbaric O_2 tx controversial but recommended by Undersea & Hyperbaric Med Society, potential long-term neuro sequelae benefit
- Fetal Hgb has higher affinity for CO than adult Hgb; lower threshold for hyperbaric O_2 in pregnant women

Indications for Hyperbaric O_2 in CO Poisoning
Transient or prolonged unconsciousness (syncope, coma)
CO level >25%
Persistent neurologic disturbances
E/o end organ ischemia (encephalopathy, CP, EKG Δ,'s)
Severe acidosis (pH <7.1)
Pregnancy w/ CO level >20% or signs of fetal distress

Disposition
- Admx based on level & clinical findings; D/C asx pt w/ HbCO <5%

Pearls
- CO is the most common cause of death from acute poisoning & fires; reversibly binds Hb more avidly than O_2 → functional anemia
- May see delayed neurologic sequelae (personality Δ, HA, sz, parkinsonian Δ) 2–40 d after exposure; virtually universally resolve w/i 6 mos
- Half-life of COHgb: 360 mins on RA, 90 mins on 100% NRB, 30 mins hyperbaric

DYSBARISM

Background
- Dysbarism refers to cx from dynamic pressure & gas chgs during scuba diving ascent or decent stages while breathing compressed air

Approach
- Careful hx: Length, depth, # of dives, interval btw dives, comorbid dz, sinus pain during dive, intoxication, onset of sxs, dive relative to decompression limits
- Divers Alert Network, Duke University: (919) 684-8111, 24-h med advice

Decompression Sickness (DCS)

History
- Improper dive & ascent times, depth; sx can develop during or after ascent (1–24 h), longer if air travel

Findings
- Findings spec to mild Type I & more serious Type II DCS

Types of Decompression Sickness	
Type I: "the bends"	• MSK: extremity/joint pain w/o localized tenderness or erythema • Skin: Pruritus, rash, mottling or marbling of skin, violaceous rash • Lymphatics: Venous stasis • Inflate BP cuff to 150 mmHg over affected joint; if relieves pain, confirms dx
Type II: CNS or pulm gas embolism	• Pulm: Pleuritic pain, respiratory distress, nonproductive cough "the chokes," RV failure "air lock," circulatory failure, shock, death • Neuro: Ataxia "the staggers", mimics spinal cord trauma; ext weakness & paresthesias, moves proximally, focal neuro deficit, AMS, SZ

Evaluation
- Cardiac monitor, CBC, CMP, O_2 sat, tox screen, CO level, coags, CXR, CT Brain

Treatment
- Consider hyperbarics: goal of recompression to ↓ mechanical obstruction of air bubbles, ↑ tissue O_2 delivery
- 100% O_2 (NRB mask), place pt in L lateral decub & mild Trendelenburg, hyperbaric O_2, IVF (UOP 1.5 mL/kg/h) for recompression
- Sx tx: Intubation, needle decompression, sz control

Disposition
- Ground transport, or low-flying air transport (cabin pressure <1000 ft)
- Admit to institution w/ hyperbaric O_2 capability

Pearls
- Spectrum of illness: formation of small nitrogen gas bubbles in blood & tissues
- Depends on location & degree of bubble formation
- ↑ freq w/ longer & deeper dives, comorbid illness (COPD, CAD, PFO, asthma)
- Residual paralysis, myocardial necrosis, other ischemic injuries possible; early recognition & tx imperative
- Wait >12–48 h btw diving & flying, no diving for 7 d after DCS I, 28 d after DCS II

MIDDLE EAR BAROTRAUMA

History
- Most common d/o among divers; usually occurs on descent; ↑ pain w/ ↑ water pressure on TM, equilibration via Eustachian tubes, rupture occurs b/w 5 & 17 ft → pain relief; vertigo, N/V, hearing loss

Findings
- Reversible Bell palsy from increased pressure to facial nerve in severe cases

Evaluation
- Concomitant eval for inner ear barotrauma

Treatment
- Nasal vasoconstrictor drops/spray to open fluid from middle ear; antihistamines, analgesia, pinch nose & swallow to displace fluid through Eustachian tube

Disposition
- ENT f/u in 2 wks

Pearl
- No benefit w/ abx; use occlusive earplugs when diving/showering until TM healed
- Atmospheric pressure at sea level = 760 mmHg = 14.7 psi: 1 atm
  - Each descent of 33 ft under water ↑ pressure by 1 atm

Other Dysbarisms	
Inner ear barotraumas	• Occurs during descent; nausea, vertigo, tinnitus, hearing loss • Insufflation in ear canal using otoscope produces nystagmus • Conservative mgmt, 1-wk bed rest, elevated HOB, no Valsalva
Facial barotraumas	• Neg. pressure generated in airspace created by mask over face • If pt doesn't force exhale through nose, get conjunctival edema, petechial hemorrhages over face, subconjunctival hemorrhages
PTX/Pneumomediastinum	• Results from barotrauma, seen on CXR • Pleuritic pain, dyspnea, subcutaneous emphysema/crepitus • Unless hemodynamic compromise or tension, not life threatening
Arterial gas embolism (AGE)	• Most serious complication of pulmonary barotrauma • Sudden onset stroke sxs in 10 mins of surfacing, dyspnea, hemoptysis • Look for PFO, shouldn't dive again, emergent recompression
Nitrogen narcosis	• "Rapture of the deep:" due to ↑ CNS nitrogen concentration • S/S of Etoh/benzo intoxication: euphoria, false sense of well-being, confusion, loss of judgment, disorientation, inappropriate laughter, ↓ motor control, paresthesias • Occurs at 100 ft; can leads to drowning but resolves w/ ascent

ELECTRICAL INJURY

Background

- Current: volume of electrons flowing through an object per sec; in amperes (A)

Approach

- Identify electrical injury class: high voltage (>1000 V) or low voltage (<1000 V); current cannot be directly measured but is directly proportional to voltage
- Identify electrical injury category: classic pattern (entrance & exit wound), electrical arc burn, thermal burn from electrical source, or lightning strike

Types of Current	
Direct current (DC)	Occupational, high voltage: Current flows in 1 direction only; most pts are thrown from this exposure & suffer blunt trauma
Alternating current (AC)	Home, low voltage: 3 × more dangerous than DC of same voltage due to continuous muscle contraction/tetany from current alternating direction of flow; pt "can't let go"
Arc injury	Pt trapped in electrical arc b/w 2 objects; mostly serious b/c of ↑ risk of blunt trauma & temp as high as 2500–5000 °C causing burn

History

- Usually obvious & reported (eg, occupational injury of electrician, home handyman); pt reports minor shock (tingling); related to home appliance use
- Toddler w/ burns to corners of mouth (chewing) or hands (playing w/ socket)
- Injury from an electrical weapon (stun gun/Taser) by security or law enforcement
- Victim of lightning strike

Findings

- Pulm: Respiratory arrest via chest wall paralysis or resp center of brain possible
- Cardiac: Dysrhythmias common; VF more common w/ low-voltage AC, asystole w/ high voltage AC or DC
- Neuro: Autonomic dysfxn, motor & sensory loss; "keraunoparalysis" vasospasm resulting in paralysis, cyanosis, mottling, & pulseless lower extremities
- Renal: Rhabdomyolysis & ATN from tissue necrosis & myoglobin related AKI
- Skin: Wounds may appear minor & entry/exit wounds may be present (examine bottoms of feet for exit); often findings significantly underestimate true extent of internal injuries
- MSK: Long-bone fx, scapular fx, shoulder dislocation, spinal fx from mechanical trauma caused by whole body tetanic contractions or trauma of being thrown back

Evaluation

- ECG, CBC, BMP, cardiac enzymes, CK, UA (myoglobin), coags, consider advanced &/or plain imaging for possible concomitant trauma

Treatment

- Resuscitate, eval for trauma, immobilize c-spine, continuous cardiac monitoring
- High-volume & aggressive IV crystalloid resuscitation (NS, avoid K-containing fluids)
- Avoid Parkland or thermal burn-based IVF resuscitation formulas based on external findings as skin findings belie true extent of internal injury
  - Use physiologic parameters & target urine output: 0.5–1 mL/kg/h
- If rhabdomyolysis (↑ CK, +UA dip), maintain high UOP until urine dip neg
  - Goal serum pH 7.45–7.55
  - Alkaline urine (pH > 6.5) to ↑ excretion of acidic myoglobin by ↑ solubility; D5W + 150 mEq $NaHCO_3$ OR D5 ¼ NS or D5 ½ NS + 100 mEq $NaHCO_3$
  - Diuresis w/ Lasix 20–40 mg IV or mannitol 25 g IV (then 12.5 g/kg/h) prn
- Treat wounds the same as thermal burns (10 d)
- Compartment pressures ± fasciotomy if sx of compartment synd
- Splint injured extremities in best "position of fxn" to minimize contractures

Disposition

- <1000 V, nml ECG, mild cutaneous burns, nl urine dip: observe in ED for 2 h then D/C
- >1000 V, abnml ECG, report of syncope, hx of CAD: admit obs tele
- Hemodynamic instability, ECG Δ's, myoglobinuria, severe injury, partial/full thickness burns: admit ICU; severe burns to burn center

Pearls

- Electrical injuries are often minor, but may be more serious than they 1st appear. If any concern, observe for 6–12 h
- Pediatric oral "bite" burns may develop delayed labial artery bleed at 2–3 wks

HIGH-ALTITUDE ILLNESS

Background
- Caused by acute exposure to hypobaric hypoxia (low PO_2) usually above 8K ft
- Altitude illness is generally considered as a progressive spectrum from acute mountain sickness (AMS) to HACE
- Acclimatization allows body to minimize effects of hypoxia; ↑ RR (↓ $PaCO_2$), ↑ CO, ↑ hematopoiesis & 2,3-DPG production (favors O_2 release to tissues)
- Takes 5–7 d for full effect; inherent acclimatization ability varies by individual

Approach
- HAPE may be fatal w/in h unless treated; early recognition & symptomatic relief is key

History
- Rapid ascent to altitude >8K ft, risk increased by exertion, past h/o altitude illness
- Flu-like sxs, "hangover," HA, fatigue, DOE, sleep disturbance, N/V, dizziness, paresthesia
- Sxs manifest 6–12 h after ascent, subside in 1–2 d or may progress to HAPE, HACE

Findings
- Depends on severity of altitude illness
- AMS/HACE represent a continuum of the same dz process

Summary of High-altitude Illnesses		
Dz	**Signs & Sxs**	**Altitude & Course**
AMS (most common)	Hangover like, HA + GI upset, insomnia, fatigue, lightheaded, Lake Louise Scoring system	8–10K ft; onset 6–12 h, peak 1–2 d, duration 3–5 d
HACE	HA, ataxia, slurred speech, AMS (hallucinations), insomnia, stupor, coma, herniation, death	>12K ft; onset 1–3 d, peak 5–9 d, resolves 3–7 d after descent
HAPE	SOB at rest, fatigue, HA, anorexia, cyanosis, rales, tachypnea, tachycardia, cardiopulm collapse	>14,500 ft; onset 2–4 d, resolution 1–2 d after descent
High-altitude retinal hemorrhage	Usually asx, sometimes central scotoma	>17,500 ft; onset 1-3 d; resolves 1–3 wks

Evaluation
- Clinical Dx; also consider alt etiologies to explain findings
- HAPE: CXR (patchy infiltrates), US (comet tails), pulse oximetry (relative hypoxia)
- HACE: Head CT neg, MRI (white matter Δ showing ↑ edema)

Treatment
- All cases of HAI: Descent! If unable → O_2, symptomatic relief, bed rest; Hyperbaric O_2 chamber used as temporizing measure until descent
- Severe AMS & HACE: Dexamethasone: 8 mg PO/IV/IM × 1, then 4 mg q6h; acetazolamide 250 mg q6h
- HAPE: Nifedipine: 60 mg ER daily (or 30 mg BID) PO; consider sildenafil 50 mg TID (used to ↓ pulm HTN) & inhaled β-agonist (salmeterol; clears alveolar fluid) INH q12h
- Prophylactic meds: start 1 d prior to ascent & continue 2–3 d at max altitude
  - AMS/HACE: Acetazolamide: 125–250 mg PO q12h; alt: Dexamethasone 2 mg q6h or 4 mg BID
  - HAPE: Nifedipine: 60 mg ER Daily (or 30 mg BID) PO; consider: Tadalafil 10 mg q12h, sildenafil 50 mg q8h; Dexamethasone: 8 mg PO × 1, then 4 mg PO q6h
- Avoid in tx: Morphine sulfate, nitrates, diuretics; may be harmful

Disposition
- Admit if hypoxic, dyspnea at rest; prognosis excellent for survivors

Pearls
- Avoid abrupt ascent, spend 1–2 nights at intermediate elevation, descend to sleep
- Severity a/w underlying med conditions (COPD, HTN, SSD, pregnancy)

HYPOTHERMIA

Background
- Multiple classifications of hypothermia based on severity & etiology

Approach
- Careful hx: Determine degree & etiology of hypothermia (environmental exposure vs acute medical cause)
- Environmental hypothermia can occur even in the absence of freezing weather (malnourished pt, elderly)
- Many medical etiologies: Hypothyroidism (myxedema coma), hypoglycemia, hypoadrenalism, sepsis, hypothalamic lesion (eg, 2/2 trauma, tumor, stroke), dermatologic conditions that prevent heat conservation (burns, erythrodermas)
- If unresponsive, check BS/give D50, give naloxone 2 mg

History
- Environmental exposure, drug use, trauma, comorbid illnesses

Findings
- Based on degree of hypothermia

Classifications of Hypothermia		
Temp	**Physiologic Response**	**Clinical Presentation**
Mild (32–35 °C)	Increased: HR, BP, CO, RR, metabolic activity, shivering, cold diuresis	Dizziness, lethargy, confusion, amnesia, apathy, dysarthria, nausea, ataxia, loss of fine-motor skills
Moderate (28–32 °C)	Decreased: HR, BP, CO, RR, metabolic activity, cold diuresis, shivering stops	Delirium (paradoxical undressing), stupor, pupillary dilatation, ↓ reflexes
Severe (<28 °C)	Decreased: HR, BP, CO, RR, metabolic activity, no shivering	Unresponsive, fixed & dilated pupils, rigid, very cold skin, coma, pulm edema; ↑ risk of ventricular fibrillation & asystole

Evaluation
- Obtain core temp (bladder, rectum, esophagus: all may be inaccurate)
- Cardiac monitor, CBC, CMP (↑ K bad sign), tox screen, coags, fibrinogen, lipase (cold-induced pancreatitis), CK, UA (rhabdo), lactate, ABG, CT brain, CXR
- ECG w/ characteristic Osborn waves (J pt elevation), <32 °C/90 °F
- ECG w/ interval prolongation (PR, QRS, QT), AF w/ slow ventricular response

Treatment
- ABC's! Resuscitate, prevent further heat loss, remove wet clothes, start rewarming appropriate to degree of hypothermia, & tx cx
- Maintain horizontal position, avoid movement, limit manipulation to essential tasks. However, this should not prevent CPR or other critical interventions
- Monitor ECG, check for pulse q1min; chest compressions may cause ventricular dysrhythmias, perform only if no pulse
- Cardiac arrest:
  - Initiate ACLS protocol w/ emphasis on aggressive rewarming
  - Do not cease resuscitative efforts until core temp >32–35 °C, may take several h; "*You're not dead until you're warm & dead*"
  - After ROSC: goal temp of 32–34 °C
- Consider alt dx: may give hydrocortisone 100 mg IV or levothyroxine μg IV if slow to respond to rewarming measures

Rewarming Strategies by Severity of Hypothermia		
Temperature	**Rewarming Strategy**	**Dispo**
Mild (32–35 °C)	Passive external rewarming (PER): remove wet clothes, blankets	Likely D/C
Moderate (28–32 °C)	Active external rewarming (AER): warm blankets, radiant heating to core (prevent afterdrop effect)	Admit, cardiac monitoring
Severe (<28 °C)	AER & Active internal rewarming (AIW): Warm IVF (40 °C), thoracic lavage, extracorporeal blood rewarming (ECMO, cardiopulm bypass)	Admit ICU

Disposition
- Based on severity of hypothermia (table above)

Pearls
- Core temp afterdrop phenomena: Rewarming cold & acidemic extremities will lead to recirculation and may cause recirculation a drop in core temp, resulting in deadly arrythmias
- Consider femoral line placement if needed to avoid cardiac stimulation (vs IJ, SC)

FROSTBITE

History
- Cold exposure, numbness of body part → loss of sensation

Findings
- Distal body part most commonly affected (fingers, nose, toes, ears)
- Caused by both immediate cell death from cold & delayed injury from inflammatory response
- Skin initially white, waxy, insensate → erythematous, edematous, painful 48–72 h after rewarming → bleb formation, devitalized tissue demarcation over weeks

Evaluation
- Check core temp to look for systemic hypothermia
- Bone scan (Technetium [Tc]-99 scintigraphy): Identifies tPA candidacy after thawing & used for long-term viability assessment

Frostbite Injury Classification After Rewarming			
Grading	**Skin Findings**	**Bone Scan**	**Prognosis**
Grade 1	Simple erythema	Not indicated	Excellent
Grade 2	Cyanosis to distal phalanx	↓ Radiotracer uptake	Likely tissue amputation
Grade 3	Cyanosis to proximal phalanx	Absent Radiotracer uptake	Likely digit amputation
Grade 4	Cyanosis to tarsal/carpal	Absent Radiotracer uptake	Likely limb amputation

Treatment
- Handle tissue gently, keep extremity elevated, sterile/nonadherent dressing
- Rapid rewarming of frozen extr in gentle warm water bath (40–42 °C), ROM exercise in bath, avoid water temp falling outside of range; 30 mins if superficial/60 mins if deep
- Systemic thrombolysis: tPA indicated in grade 3 & 4 injury on bone scan after rewarming, w/in 24 h, w/o CIs, & in coordination w/ burn center
  - IV tPA protocol: Start 0.15 mg/kg over 15 mins, then 0.15 mg/kg/h × 6 h (max 100 mg); after tPA start enoxaparin 1 mg/kg SQ BID × 14 D
- Wound care: Topical aloe vera q6h; aspirate & debride clear blisters, only aspirate (do not debride) hemorrhagic blisters to avoid desiccation, infection of deeper tissues
- Tetanus prophylaxis, consider ppx abx
- Early surgical intervention not indicated other than escharotomy for circumferential limb lesions (very uncommon)

Disposition
- Refer to burn service; consider admx for 24–48 h to observe for progression

Pearls
- Long-term cx: cold insensitivity, paresthesias, nail loss, joint stiffness
- Avoid refreezing, if unable to maintain warmth to affected part (eg, prehospital) do not rewarm

HYPERTHERMIA

Background
- Spectrum of heat-related illnesses inc heat rash, cramps, syncope, stroke

Approach
- Careful hx: Determine etiology of hyperthermia: External (environmental) or internal (toxic/metabolic) factors, environmental hypothermia can occur even in absence of exertion (malnourished pt, chronically ill, elderly)
- Look for medication related hyperthermia: MH, NMS, SS
- Use rectal thermometer to determine core temperature

External Heat Emergencies

Heat Cramps

History

- Brief, intermittent, severe muscle cramping not a/w elevated ambient temp (misnomer); rather exercise induced muscle cramps. Often in abd or calf muscles

Findings

- Euthermic, clinical signs of dehydration

Evaluation

- BMP (↓ Na, ↓ Cl), urine lytes optional (↓ urinary Na & Cl from sweating)

Treatment

- Oral salt or electrolyte repletion tablets or sports drinks; IV hydration rarely required; relaxation & stretching for acute discomfort

Disposition

- Home after observation for sx relief

Pearl

- Related to electrolyte deficiency; electrolyte enhanced sports drinks may be helpful although may cause diarrhea due to the high sugar content

Heat Edema

History

- Swollen feet/ankles after long periods of sitting/standing due to hydrostatic pressure, vasodilation & orthostatic pooling → vascular leak, interstitial fluid accumulation
- No underlying hepatic, lymphatic, cardiac, or venous dz

Findings

- Euthermic, BLE pitting edema w/o signs of CHF or renal failure

Evaluation

- BMP, UA for proteinuria, CXR for pulm edema, ECG

Treatment

- Elevate lower extremities, provide support hose
- No evidence that diuretics help

Disposition

- Home after reassurance, PCP f/u

Pearl

- Dx of exclusion

Heat Rash (Prickly Heat, Miliaria, Lichen Tropicus)

History

- Sweat gland blockage w/ localized inflammatory response
- Often seen in pts newly arrived to subtropical/tropical areas or during heat waves

Findings

- Euthermic, erythema w/ pruritic vesicles, primarily in intertriginous areas, then becomes anhidrotic
- Occasionally will become superinfected, usually *Staph*

Evaluation

- None

Treatment

- Treat pruritus: Diphenhydramine 25–50 mg PO or hydroxyzine 25 mg PO
- Desquamate skin w/ chlorhexidine antibacterial soap or salicylate-containing topical scrub

Disposition

- Home, PCP f/u

Pearl

- Avoid routine talcum powder application, which may block sweat glands

Heat Syncope

History

- Syncopal event following strenuous activity; misnomer as ambient heat is only indirectly a/w "exercise-induced collapse"
- Exercise → vasodilation → cessation of activity → ↓ central venous return → syncope

Findings

- Euthermic, nl exam

Evaluation

- Gluc, EKG, & eval for other causes of syncope
- Syncope/presyncope sx should resolve w/i 30 mins, if not consider further w/u

Treatment

- PO or IV hydration

Disposition

- Home, PCP f/u

Pearl

- Dx of exclusion, diagnose only in young healthy pts w/ no cardiac dz

Heat Exhaustion

History

- Gradual onset, extreme fatigue in warm/humid weather following strenuous activity, profuse sweating, dizziness, N/V; often pale w/ cool, moist skin
- Inadequate PO intake

Findings

- Mild hyperthermia, may reach 40 °C (104 °F), nl mental status

Evaluation

- BMP for electrolyte imbalance, UA (rhabdomyolysis uncommon)

Treatment

- IV hydration (PO if pt tolerates), replace w/ NS (or alternate w/ ½ NS if ↑ Na)

Disposition

- Observation w/ continued hydration until normothermic w/ good UOP

Pearl

- No value w/ fever-reducing medications

Heat Stroke

History

- Acute onset when compared to heat exhaustion
- Classic: Occurs during heat waves, affects susceptible pts: extremes of age, chronically ill, CF, burns, chronic alcohol use, homeless, psych dz, on diuretics or antichol
- Exertional: Occurs in pts who are overwhelmed by heat overproduction: athletes, military recruits, thyroid storm, pheochromocytoma, sympathomimetic o/d

Findings

- Hyperthermia >41 °C/106 °F, CNS dysfxn: Confusion, disorientation, delirium
- Classic: Anhidrotic, tachypnea
- Exertional: Diaphoretic until "sweat gland fatigue"
- Muscles usually flaccid in HS, if rigid consider NMS, etc

Evaluation

- BMP (electrolyte imbalance, ↓ blood sugar), LFTs (hepatic damage common), coags (DIC possible but uncommon), CK & UA (rhabdo common in exertional heat stroke); consider CT brain & CSF analysis
- DDx for hyperthermia is vast, consider: infxn, CNS, tox, endocrine, onc, etc

Treatment

- Aggressive fluid resuscitation: Cooling procedures → vasoconstriction, can ↑ BP so may need to guide fluid status by UOP, IVC US, CVP, etc
- Rapid cooling indicated, ↓ by 0.2 °C/min → 39 °C/102.2 °F to avoid overshooting
- Ice water immersion: Can ↓ core temp in 10–40 mins
- Evaporation: Spray water mist & use fan, maintains cutaneous vasodilation, avoids heat generation by shivering, 7 × more efficient than ice packing but 2 × as fast
- Adjunctive cooling strategies: Strategic ice packs near large blood vessels (ant neck, axilla, groin), ice water gastric lavage at NS 200 mL/h
- Consider Mannitol 50–100 g IV for suspected cerebral edema
- Treat rhabdo w/ IVF, HD if anuric; reverse coagulopathy

Disposition

- Admit for ongoing tx & cooling

Pearls

- Avoid alcohol sponge baths, dantrolene
- Avoid antipyretics (APAP damages liver, salicylates aggravate bleeding)

- Avoid α-adrenergic drugs (promote vasoconstriction, ↑ hepatic/renal damage, CO same)
- Avoid atropine/anticholinergics that ↓ sweating; use BZD to stop shivering
- Avoid neuroleptics (chlorpromazine): ↓ sz threshold, interfere w/ thermoregulation, etc

Internal Heat Emergencies

Malignant Hyperthermia (MH)

History
- Acute ↑ body temp after administration of inhaled anesthetic or succinylcholine
- Genetic abnlty of skeletal muscle sarcoplasmic reticulum → inappropriate Ca release → severe tetany & spasm (heat); often FH of adverse rxn to anesthesia

Findings
- Acute hyperthermia after anesthetic, hypercapnia (early sign), muscular rigidity, masseter muscle spasm, acidosis, tachycardia, rhabdomyolysis

Evaluation
- Check core temp, electrolytes, CK, blood gas (mix met & res acidosis), coags, EKG

Treatment
- Stop offending agent & supportive care
- Dantrolene 2.5 mg/kg bolus IV ASAP, repeat doses of 1 mg/kg until sxs subside

Disposition
- Usually occurs in OR, admx for supportive care

Pearl
- MH hotline: 1-800-MH-HYPER (1-800-644-9737), ask for "Index Zero"

Neuroleptic Malignant Syndrome (NMS)

History
- Subacute (d/wks) exposure to any dopamine antagonist (antipsychotic, antiemetic)
- W/d from anti-Parkinson's meds (L-dopa or dopamine agonists)
- Dopamine blockade → severe muscle rigidity, dysautonomia, hyperthermia

Findings
- NMS Tetrad: Hyperthermia, muscular rigidity (lead pipe), AMS, & autonomic dysfxn

Evaluation
- CBC, BMP(↑ K), LFTs, CK, UA (myoglobinuria), blood gas (met acidosis), tox screen

Treatment
- Stop offending agent! Mainstay is supportive care & aggressive cooling measures
- Benzos first line tx for rigidity & hyperthermia; consider dantrolene (as for MH) or dopamine antagonists (bromocriptine 2.5 mg PO q8h, amantadine 200 mg PO q12h)
- Treat rhabdomyolysis w/ IVF, alkaline urine (pH > 6.5) to ↑ myoglobin excretion
- Keep Na in IVF close to 154 mEq/L; add $NaHCO_3$

Disposition
- Admx; mortality 10–20%

Pearl
- NMS hotline: 1-888-667-8367

Serotonin Syndrome (SS)

History
- Recent (w/i 24 h) therapeutic use, inadvertent ingestion, or intentional suicide attempt w/ known serotonergic agent (SSRI, MAOI, amphetamine, MDMA, tramadol, etc)

Findings
- Hunter criteria: Serotonergic ingestion w/ either: clonus (ocular or inducible or spontaneous) & agitation/diaphoresis, or hyperreflexia & tremor, or ↑ temp & hypertonia
- Mydriasis, ↑ HR/BP, diaphoresis, flushed skin, V/D, tremors, akathisia, SZ

Evaluation
- CBC, BMP, LFT, CK, UA, coags, tox screen, consider CT brain & CSF analysis
- Clinical dx, must confirm h/o serotonergic agents; consider toxic, metabolic, infectious, oncologic, CNS, or other tox etiology

Treatment
- Stop offending agent, supportive tx, whole body cooling, treat rhabdo w/ IVF
- BZD: May require high doses to eliminate muscle rigidity & hyperthermia

- Dantrolene not recommended: May ↑ central serotonin metabolism & production
- Nonsp serotonin inhib: Cyproheptadine 12 mg PO then 2 mg PO q2h

Disposition

- Admx; ICU for severe cases w/ autonomic instability; obs for mod cases; mild cases may be safely discharged after 6 h ED obs; most resolve w/ no sequelae in 24–36 h after starting tx

Pearl

- Most common cause of death is uncontrolled hyperthermia

Differentiating NMS & Serotonin Syndrome		
	NMS	**SS**
Etiology	• A/w neuroleptic use • Idiosyncratic rxn to therapeutic doses	• A/w serotonergic agents • Manifestation of tox
Timing	• Slow onset (d → wks)	• Rapid onset & progression (24 h)
Sxs	• Bradykinesia, lead-pipe rigidity	• Hyperkinesia, clonus, tremors
Tx	• BZD • +/– Dantrolene/Bromocriptine	• BZD • ± Cyproheptadine

LIGHTNING INJURY

Background

- Acts as direct current → asystole; heart's intrinsic automaticity usually restarts in SR but CNS injury & concussion may cause respiratory arrest w/ secondary cardiac arrest

Approach

- Early & continuous cardiac monitoring for dysrhythmias
- Evaluate for concomitant trauma (fall, injury); maintain c-spine precautions
- Reverse triage in field: Lightning victims that appear dead should get CPR as pts can be pulseless w/ fixed, dilated pupils, & still have good survivability

History

- Usually obvious, reported lightning strike near pt; often witnessed collapse

Findings

- TM rupture, transient vasospasm (cool ext), symp nervous system instability
- Various burn patterns
  - Linear: Caused by steam production during flashover (charge passes over surface of body only) where sweat accumulates
  - Punctate: Multiple cigarette-like burns
  - Feathering: Not actual burns; electron showers make a ferning pattern on skin (Lichtenberg figures)
  - Thermal: Usually from burnt clothing
- Ocular pathology: Corneal lesions, hyphema, vitreous hemorrhage, retinal detachment, cataracts develop long term
- Keraunoparalysis: Transient paralysis that can occur, likely 2/2 vasospasm, LE > UE, usually resolves in h, still will need eval for true spinal cord pathology 2/2 trauma

Evaluation

- ECG, CBC, BMP, CK (rhabdomyolysis), UA (myoglobin), CT brain if unresponsive

Treatment

- Resuscitate, eval for trauma, immobilize c-spine, continuous cardiac monitoring
- High-volume IV crystalloid (NS); same tx as electrical injury (10f)
- Urinary catheter placement: Target urine output 1–1.5 mL/kg/h (200–300 mL/h)
- If rhabdomyolysis (↑ CK, +UA dip), maintain high UOP until urine dip neg
- Treat wounds the same as thermal burns (10 d), tetanus, wound care, etc
- Splint injured extremities in best "position of fxn" to minimize contractures & edema

Disposition

- If asx & nl exam, can be discharged; good prognosis if survive in field
- ECG Δ, myoglobinuria, entry/exit burns, partial/full thickness burns: admit to burn center

Pearl

- Lightning causes ~50–300 Ds in US each year, 25–30% of lightning strike victims die, of those that survive ~75% have permanent disability

DROWNING

Background
- "A process resulting in primary respiratory impairment from submersion or immersion in a liquid medium" (2010 AHA)
  - Submersion: Airway under liquid surface (underwater) leading to direct aspiration
  - Immersion: Airway remains above liquid surface w/ proximity to splashing liquid
- >4000 drowning Ds annually in US; toddlers & teenage boys at greatest risk
- Freshwater vs saltwater vs chlorinated pool water: No difference, theoretical diff only
- 1° insult to lung; water moves across alveolar–capillary membrane, destroys (freshwater) or washes out (salt water) surfactant → hypoxia
- Diving reflex = immersion of face in water <68 °F, blood shunts from periphery → brain & heart → apnea, bradycardia, hypothermia → ↓ metabolic demand prevents/delays severe cerebral hypoxia

Approach
- Careful hx: Possible diving (cervical spine or head) injury vs 1° drowning, intoxicants, comorbidity, submersion time, water temp, initial rescuer response (ACLS)
- Extricate pt, remove wet clothing, ABCs, ACLS, intubation as appropriate
- Maintain cervical spine immobilization if suspicion for head or neck injury (diving, pool accident)
- Consider D50 or naloxone if AMS

History
- Submersion or immersion event

Findings
- Variable presentation (awake, coma, cardiac arrest)
- Wheezes/rales/rhonchi, ecchymosis/crepitus/other signs of trauma on exam

Evaluation
- CBC, BMP, LFTs, tox, CXR may show pulmonary edema or aspiration 2–6 h after event, CT brain & c-spine if concern for trauma

Treatment
- ABCs, intubation or supplemental O_2, CPR, ACLS, Foley placement
- Measure core temp, treat for hypothermia if indicated to temp 30 °C/86 °F
- Ventilator PEEP 5–10 mm H_2O to ↓ intrapulmonary shunting

Disposition
- Admx for continued tx, watch for signs of ARDS/VALI
- May develop pulm Δ even after mild submersion, observe asx pts for at least 8 h

Pearls
- Prophylactic abx & glucocorticoids not indicated; if infx ensues consider water-borne sources (PsA, aeromonas, etc)
- Artificially induced hypothermia does not improve outcome

ANAPHYLAXIS

(*J Allergy Clin Immunol* 2020;145(4):1082; *Ann Allergy Asthma Immunol* 2024;132(2):124)

Approach

- Eval & treat anyone w/ potential anaphylaxis immediately; can deteriorate rapidly w/ resp/cardiac arrest w/i min
  - In a study of fatal anaphylactic rxns, median time to resp/card arrest: 5 mins (2/2 drug), 15 mins (2/2 venom), 30 mins (2/2 food) (*Clin Exp Allergy* 2000;30(8):1144)

Definition

- Anaphylaxis—systemic hypersensitivity rxn that is typically acute onset and potentially life threatening
- Clinical dx and multiple definitions exist, inc National Institute of Allergy and Infectious Diseases (NIAID) 2006 criteria and more recent World Allergy Organization (WAO) 2022 criteria (see *Ann Allergy Asthma Immunol* 2024;132(2):124)
- Typically has multisystem dysfxn: Skin (eg, urticaria), mucosa (eg, swelling of lips/tongue/uvula), GI (eg, cramping abdominal pain, vomiting), respiratory (eg, bronchospasm, wheezing, stridor, hypoxia), circulatory (eg, hypotension, syncope)
- DDx: Anaphylactoid rxn, angioedema, malignancies a/w flushing (eg, carcinoid), scombroid tox, systemic mastocytosis, other causes of shock or respiratory collapse (*J Allergy Clin Immunol* 2005;115:S485)

Anaphylaxis & Anaphylactic-Like Syndromes	
Pathophysiology	**Definition**
Anaphylaxis	IgE-mediated rxn → typically multisystem involvement as above; multiple causes; requires repeat exposure but trigger not always known
Anaphylactoid rxn	Non–IgE-mediated rxn, can appear identical to anaphylaxis, but doesn't require prior exposure (eg, iodine-contrast)
Angioedema (*West J Emerg Med* 2019;20(4):587)	Bradykinin &/or histamine-mediated, subdermal/submucosal non-pitting edema, typically of the face, airway, & GI tract. May be 2/2 ACEI, C1-esterase deficiency, idiopathic

History

- Sudden onset is key; sxs can involve many organ systems—hives, swelling of tongue/throat, bronchospasm, stridor, vomiting, abdominal cramps, presyncope/syncope
- Assess recent exposures: Foods (inc but not limited to nuts, egg, shellfish), meds (abx, NSAIDs, vancomycin, iodine contrast; ACEI for angioedema), enzymes (insulin, trypsin, etc), airborne allergens (pollen, mold), venoms (bees, fire ants, snakes), exercise induced, latex, idiopathic
- Check PMH for atopy, hypersensitivity synds, or hereditary angioedema

Physical Examination

- May have urticaria, facial, or oropharyngeal swelling, stridor, wheezing, ↓ BP

Evaluation & Treatment

- Labs not routinely indicated; consider serum tryptase during acute event esp if idiopathic, recurrent or severe anaphylaxis or if dx uncertain (tryptase elevation spec but insensitive for IgE-mediated rxns)
- Remove allergen
- Epinephrine IM in anterolateral thigh is mainstay of tx for anaphylaxis; 0.01 mg/kg to maximum of 0.5 mg in adults or 0.3 mg in children (use 1 mg/mL solution)
  - When autoinjectors available, recommended to give 0.1 mg if available (or 0.15 mg) to infant 7.5–15 kg w/ anaphylaxis; give 0.15 mg to child 15–25 kg; give 0.3 mg autoinjector if pt >25 kg (can give 0.5 mg dose if pt >50 kg and available)
  - If needed, can repeat dose q5–15min; if incomplete response to IM epi, can start epi gtt
  - Consider adjunctive txs (below) after Epi; note steroids do not have role in treating acute rxn (slow onset of action, do not reverse acute sxs)

Treatment	
Type of rxn	**Tx Approach**
Adjunctive txs for allergic rxn	H1 antihistamine: Diphenhydramine 25–50 mg PO or IV or cetirizine 10 mg PO or IV for urticarial sxs
	H2B: Famotidine 20 mg
	Consider prednisone or methylprednisolone

Anaphylaxis (*J Allergy Clin Immunol* 2020;145(4):1082; *Ann Emerg Med* 2006;47:373)	**Airway compromise:** Consider early intubation, consider fiberoptic/awake
	All txs for allergic rxn (IV)—as above
	IVF bolus
	IM Epinephrine: As above, (Repeat prn, ± infusion, 1st line, do not delay)

- H1 + H2 antihistamines > H1 antihistamine alone for urticaria (*NEJM* 2004;351:2203)
- Epi & cardiac dz: Place on monitor → epi is relatively contraindicated w/ CAD, but still critical intervention if anaphylaxis; mortality of anaphylaxis w/o epi >> mortality from arrhythmia 2/2 epi
- Glucocorticoids may be given as adjunctive tx for delayed sxs, but no clear e/o acute benefit (*Cochrane* 2012;4:CD007596; *Ann Allergy Asthma Immunol* 2024;132(2):124)

Disposition
- Home after short observation period (1–2 h): Pts w/ either local rxns (w/o airway involvement) or delayed-presentation generalized rxn (w/o airway involvement)
  - Provide EpiPen Rx (esp if unknown cause) & allergist f/u
- **Biphasic rxns** (*J Allergy Clin Immunol* 2020;145(4):1082): May occur in 1–20% of cases; occur 1–48 h after initial sxs resolve; higher risk if severe or require >1 dose of epi, wide pulse pressure, unknown trigger, cutaneous sxs, drug trigger in children
  - No evidence that glucocorticoids &/or antihistamines prevent biphasic rxns
  - Must observe at least until sxs resolve; consider prolonged observation if required epi or if high risk for biphasic rxn; no clear data on recommended duration of observation & consider early D/C (*Allergy* 2014;69(6):791)
  - Risk of clinically important biphasic rxn small (<0.5%) (*Annals Emerg Med* 2014;63(6):736)
- Admit to ICU: Severe anaphylactic rxn (multiple epi, epi gtt, airway compromise)

Pearls
- ACEI can cause angioedema at any time, independent of length of use
- PCN allergy: IgE-mediated allergy confers low (~1%) risk of cross-reactivity w/ cephalosporins; however, avoid if rxn is severe (*NEJM* 2006;354:601)

ONCOLOGIC EMERGENCIES

See also Section I (Cardiac tamponade), Section II (Respiratory distress, Hemoptysis), Section V (Altered mental status, Seizure, Brain tumor, CNS infections), Section IX (SIADH, Hypercalcemia), Section XII (Cauda equina syndrome)

NEUTROPENIC FEVER

Overview (*Clin Infect Dis* 2011;52(4):e56; *J Oncol Pract* 2019;15(1):19)
- **Definition:** Fever (single temp >38.3 °C *or* temp >38 °C for 1 h) + Neutropenia (ANC <500 *or* predicted <500 w/i 48 h *or* "functional neutropenia" [eg, AML])
- **Approach:** Early IV access, IVF, & early abx for all pts; some pts will not end up having identifiable infxn, but those who do can deteriorate quickly
- **Etiology:** Infxn found in 40–50% (bacteremia in 10–30%, most commonly GNRs/GPCs); fungal infxn rare unless neutropenia >1 wk; consider also viral, drugs (chemo), VTE, tumor burden

Differential for Fever in Neutropenic pt	
Category	**Source**
Bacterial	HEENT (sinusitis, mucositis, otitis, pharyngitis), Pulm (PNA, TB), GI (colitis, typhlitis, mucositis, hepatobiliary), GU (UTI, pyelo), cardiac (endocarditis), neuro (meningoencephalitis, epidural abscess), skin (cellulitis, line-related infxn, abscess [inc perianal])
Viral	Influenza (in epidemics), RSV, other viral pathogens, HSV, CMV, EBV
Fungal	Candidiasis, aspergillosis (most common life threatening)
Drug related	Many chemo agents can cause immune-mediated febrile rxns

History
- Date of fever onset & last chemo (ANC nadirs 7–10 d after chemo), prior infxns, recent abx, sick contacts, social hx; thorough ROS
- Assess RFs warranting inpt care: MASCC score (see *Disposition*)

Physical Examination

- Examine skin, mouth, lung, abdomen, catheter/surgical sites, perirectal area (No DRE)

Evaluation

- CBC w/ diff, Chem 10, LFTs, coags, UA/urine cx, blood cx (at least 2 + BCx from any catheter port if present), ± CXR, viral testing, & sputum cx if resp sxs
- ±Additional labs: Culture (stool/sputum/peritoneal/CSF), *C. diff* PCR
- Imaging: Consider imaging of chest, abdomen/pelvis, sinuses, brain based on context

Low-Risk Criteria for Neutropenic Fever	
Adults (*J Clin Oncol* 2000;18:3038; *J Clin Oncol* 2018;36(14):1443)	Age <60, minimal sxs, no ↓ BP, solid tumor, no COPD, no fungal infxn, no dehydration, anticipated brief neutropenic periods; MASCC score ≥21; no additional concerning clinical criteria (eg, see Table 1 in *J Clin Oncol* 2018;36(14):1443)

Treatment (*Clin Infect Dis* 2011;52(4):e56; *J Clin Oncol* 2018;36(14):1443)

- Resuscitation w/ IV fluids, vasopressors, empiric abx (delay to abx a/w worse outcomes) (*Antimicrob Agents Chemother* 2014;58:3799)
- Empiric tx depends on risk level (see above): Low risk (PO, outpt) vs high risk (IV, inpt)
  - Low risk: Ciprofloxacin or levofloxacin PLUS amoxicillin/clavulanate (or clindamycin [if PCN allergic])
    - If no RFs, mortality & tx failure w/ oral tx = similar to IV tx (*Cochrane* 2013;10:CD003992)
- High risk: Antipseudomonas (piperacillin-tazobactam, cefepime, meropenem, or imipenem)
  - If PCN-allergic: Ciprofloxacin plus clinda, or aztreonam plus vancomycin
  - If complication: Consider adding AG or quinolone for additional GNR synergy
  - If c/f line-infxn, PNA, hypotension, cellulitis: Add vancomycin
  - If MDRO, consider use of carbapenem (if ESBL), addition of vancomycin (if MRSA), or addition of linezolid or daptomycin (if VRE)
  - Antifungals generally not routinely indicated except if strong hx, shock, or recent HSCT

Disposition

- Admit all high-risk pts; low-risk pts (based on clinical judgement, MASCC and CISNE scores, see Figure 2 in *J Clin Oncol* 2018;36(14):1443)) can consider D/C only if close outpt f/u guaranteed by discussion w/ oncologist
- CISNE score may outperform MASCC Risk Index in identifying low-risk pts who present to ED for eval (*Ann Emerg Med* 2017;69(6):755)

Multinational Association for Supportive Care in Cancer (MASCC) Risk Index			
Criteria	**Pts**	**Predictive Performance of Fever Resolution w/o Serious cx**	
No or mild sxs	5		
No hypotension (SBP >90 mmHg)	5		
No active COPD (O_2, steroids, bronchodilators)	4	**Total Pts**	**PPV (%)**[a]
Solid tumor or no hx of previous fungal infxn	4	≥17	84
No dehydration	3	≥19	86
Mod symptom burden	3	≥20	90
Outpt status	3	≥21	91
Age <60 y	2	≥22	94

[a]PPV of fever resolution w/o med cx. From *J Clin Oncol* 2000;18(16):3038–3051. Table 6.

Clinical Index of Stable Febrile Neutropenia (CISNE)					
Criteria	**Pts**	**Rate of Adverse Outcome by Points**			
ECOG performance status ≥2[a]	2		**Total Points**		
Stress-induced hyperglycemia	2	**Outcome**	**0 (%)**	**1–2**	**≥3 (%)**
Active COPD	1	Cx	1.1	6.2	36.0
Chronic cardiovascular dz	1	Bacteremia	9.1	9.0	15.5
Mucositis NCI grade ≥2[b]	1	Mortality	0.0	0.0	3.1
Monocytes <200/μL	1				

J Clin Oncol 2015;33(5):465. [a]ECOG (Eastern Cooperative Oncology Group) Performance Status: 0 (fully active, able to carry on all predisease performance w/o restriction), 1 (restricted in physically strenuous activity but ambulatory & able to carry out work of a light or sedentary nature), 2 (ambulatory & capable of all self-care but unable to carry out work activities; up & about more than 50% of waking h), 3 (capable of only limited self-care; confined to bed or chair more than 50% of waking h), 4 (completely disabled; cannot carry on any self-care; totally confined to bed or chair). Source: *Am J Clin Oncol* 1982;5:649.

[b]NCI Mucositis Grades: 0 (none), 1 (painless ulcers, erythema, or mild soreness in absence of lesions), 2 (painful erythema, edema, or ulcers but eating/swallowing possible), 3 (painful erythema, edema, or ulcers requiring IV hydration), 4 (severe ulceration or requiring parenteral or enteral nutritional support or prophylactic intubation). *Cancer* 2004;100(9 suppl):1995.

Neutropenic Enterocolitis (Typhlitis)

Overview

- **Definition:** Rare life-threatening dz of neutropenic pts, characterized by mucosal injury, bowel edema & distention, bacterial translocation; cecum ± ileum & other colon
- **Approach:** Early IV abx, IVF, surgical consultation

History

- Abd pain (RLQ or diffuse), diarrhea, fever; ± n/v, abdominal distention, GIB
- Onset may correspond to WBC nadir (7–10 d after chemo)

Physical Examination

- Always assess for rebound tenderness; no DRE given neutropenia

Evaluation

- CBC (typically ANC <500), Chem 10, LFTs, lactate, blood Cx
- CT A/P w/ IV contrast (bowel thick/dilated, pneumatosis), ±Upright abd XR if CT delay (can show intramural gas) or c/f perforation (subdiaphragmatic air)

Treatment

- Supportive: IVF, analgesia, antiemetics, NGT PRN for bowel decompression
- Early abx as for neutropenic fever (see above); add flagyl
- May need surgical intervention if e/o perforation or bowel necrosis

Disposition

- Admit, may need ICU

Tumor Lysis Syndrome

Overview (*NEJM* 2011;364(19):1844; *Oncology* 2011;25(4):378)

- **Definition (Cairo–Bishop):**
  - Laboratory TLS: ≥2 metabolic abnltys (>25% ↑ K, ↑ PO_4, ↓ Ca, ↑ uric acid) present in a 24-h period w/i 3 d before or 7 d after the start of chemo (can also be spontaneous)
- Clinical TLS: Laboratory TLS PLUS renal, neurologic, &/or cardiac dysfxn that is not the result of chemotherapy itself (ie, e/o AKI [GFR ≤60], arrhythmia, szs, death)
- **Etiology:** Rapid destruction neoplastic cells → release of nucleic acids, K, PO_4 → uric acid (from nucleic acids), AKI (2/2 uric acid), ↓ Ca (2/2 PO_4)
- Typically 48–72 h after starting cytotoxic cancer tx, a/w large, rapidly proliferating, tx-responsive tumors (esp acute leukemia, non-Hodgkin lymphoma, Burkitt)
- **Approach:** Obtain ECG immediately (look for signs ↑ K), and put on cardiac monitor, resuscitation w/ IV fluids

History

- Diverse sxs (need high index of suspicion prior to labs): Lethargy, nausea, vomiting, confusion, myalgias, edema, CHF, hematuria, cardiac dysrhythmia, sz, muscle cramps, tetany, syncope, sudden death, sepsis like sxs
- Assess last chemo, but may be presenting sign of malignancy

Evaluation

- Serial Chem 10 (↓ Ca, ↑ PO_4, ↑ BUN/Cr, ↑ K), ↑ uric acid (draw on ice), ↑ LDH (marker of tumor proliferation), UA (urine pH), CBC w/ diff, VBG, Foley (r/o postrenal AKI)
- Close UOP measurement for pts w/ TLS and pts at risk of TLS

Treatment (*NEJM* 2011;364(19):1844)

- Correct electrolyte d/o (↑ K, ↑ PO_4, ↓ Ca), except use Ca tx in hyperK cautiously (may worsen $CaPO_4$ crystals in kidneys & worsen AKI), and similarly treat symptomatic hypocalcemia w/ lowest Ca dose necessary for symptom relief (*see also Section 9*)
- Maintain UOP at least 2 cc/kg/h: IVF ± loop diuretic PRN
- Reduce uric acid: Allopurinol (prevents uric acid formation) *or* rasburicase (more effective; breaks down existing uric acid); give rasburicase in consultation w/ oncology
  - Rasburicase (compared to allopurinol): Lowers mean peak PO_4 & uric acid, less AKI, reduces need for HD; superior in multiple trials
- Avoid $NaHCO_3$ for urine alkalinization: ↓ uric acid crystals, but also ↑ $CaPO_4$ crystals
  - Consider only if no rasburicase available *AND* nl serum PO_4
- HD: If persistent ↑ K, severe acidosis, volume overload, uremia, severe ↑ PO_4 or ↓ Ca

Disposition

- Clinical TLS should be admitted to ICU; pts w/ AKI, laboratory TLS should be admitted at least to tele bed vs ICU

Superior Vena Cava Syndrome

Overview

- **Definition:** Intrinsic/extrinsic SVC obstruction causing upstream high venous pressure
- **Etiology:** Malignancy (eg, lung [non–small-cell lung cancer ~50% cases], mediastinum) in majority of cases; other causes include thrombosis (eg, a/w implantable device), rarely TB & syphilitic aortic aneurysm *(NEJM 2007;356(18):1862)*

History & Physical Examination

- Facial swelling, upper extremity, swelling ± laryngeal edema (cough, hoarseness, stridor), dyspnea, cerebral edema (HA, confusion), or ↓ venous return (hypotension)
- Time course of sxs (usually subacute over weeks)
- Hx of malignancy, smoking hx, cancer screening hx
- Check for upper extremity or facial/oropharyngeal edema, distended neck or chest veins, flushing, cyanosis, JVD, abnml lung sounds, neuro deficits inc Horner synd

Evaluation

- Chem 10, CBC, CXR, CT Chest (w/ IV contrast) ± CT Head (r/o ICH), bedside echo

Treatment *(NEJM 2007;356(18):1862; Crit Care Med 2012;40:2212)*

- Severity of sxs, acuity of worsening, & type of malignancy dictate intervention & urgency
- Elevate head of bed (decrease ICP and edema)
- If 2/2 malignancy: Chemo, radiation, endovascular stenting (stenting can be performed before tissue dx)
  - Glucocorticoids commonly used to reduce swelling, but uncertain benefit
- If 2/2 thrombosis: A/C (if concurrent HA: r/o ICH 1st), remove line if able and 2/2 indwelling catheter
- If cerebral edema or airway obstruction: C/s rad-Onc, interventional radiology from ED; intubate if impending airway obstruction

Disposition

- Admit for expedited w/u (eg, bx of mass) & tx in symptomatic pts

Hyperviscosity Syndrome and Leukostasis

Overview

- Hyperviscosity synd: Clinical sxs & physical findings c/w increased serum viscosity due to pathologic elevation of cellular (WBC –> leukostasis; polycythemia) or acellular (protein) contents in the circulation leading to low flow & prolonged bleeding
  - Most common in Waldenström macroglobulinemia (leading cause; can be presenting symptom), multiple myeloma, acute leukemia (2/2 cellular proteins)
- Leukostasis *(Blood Rev 2012;26:117)*: WBC is sufficiently high to cause vascular congestion leading to end-organ dysfxn, no single threshold of WBC count; CNS and lungs most commonly affected

Manifestations

- Pulmonary: SOB, tachypnea, hypoxemia, crackles/rhonchi on auscultation
- CNS: Confusion, hallucinations, HA, ataxia, coma, ICH, neuro deficits, blurred vision
- Mucosal bleeding
- Other: Retinal hemorrhage, MI, limb ischemia, priapism, renal vein thrombosis, renal infarct

Evaluation

- CBC w/ differential & smear, BMP, LFTs, coags, lactate, consider trop/BNP
- CXR or CT chest, head CT or MRI

Treatment

- Reduction of blood viscosity: IVF, avoid RBC tfx (increase viscosity)
  - Leukopheresis or plasmapheresis, hydroxyurea, or chemotherapy to reduce leukocyte or other cell count (high risk of TLS)

Disposition

- Admit, may require ICU

Immunotherapy Toxicity

Overview *(Ca Cancer J Clin 2020;70(2):86)*

- Immunotherapy manipulates the immune system to reactivate antitumor responses
- Examples: Targeted cytokines, checkpoint inhs, adoptive cell therapy, oncolytic viruses, cancer vaccines

Checkpoint Inhibitors

- Immune checkpoint proteins can be expressed by tumor cells to evade immune response; immune checkpoint inhs bind to these tumor ligands to overcome this pathway and disinhibit T-cell antitumor function
- Examples are anti–CTLA-4, PD-1, & PD-L1 Abs, used to treat cancers inc melanoma, RCC, lung cancer, H+N SCC, gastric cancer, Hodgkin lymphoma, etc
- Adverse effects include inflammatory toxicities (multiple possible manifestations inc dermatologic, pneumonitis, colitis, hepatitis, hypothyroidism, thyroiditis, hypophysitis, arthritis, and more rarely encephalitis, nephritis, uveitis, myocarditis, cytopenias, etc)
- Tx of toxicities involves steroids & immunosupp, close consultation w/ oncology

Adoptive Cellular Therapy

- Chimeric antigen receptor (CAR) T cell therapy: genetically engineered autologous T cells that bind to tumor antigen, used in the tx of B-ALL, DLBCL, multiple myeloma
- Cytokine release synd: Potentially life threatening systemic inflammatory response, p/w fever, constitutional sxs (rash, malaise), may progress to multiorgan failure & circulatory collapse, DDx also includes sepsis, occurs 1–14 d after tx, treat w/ IL-6 receptor antagonist (Tocilizumab) (*NEJM* 2013;368:1509); ranges from grade 1 (fever) to grade 4 (fever PLUS hypotension requiring more than one pressor or hypoxia necessitating PPV)
- Hemophagocytic lymphohistiocytosis/macrophage activation synd: P/w HSM, liver dysfxn, hyperferritinemia, hypofibrinogenemia, coagulopathy, renal dysfxn, pulmonary edema, hemophagocytosis
- Immune cell-associated neurotoxicity synd (ICANS): Usually develop tremor, dysgraphia, expressive aphasia, apraxia, & impaired attention, pts progress to mute & akinetic (awake, mute, unable to follow commands), may progress to subclinical szs & cerebral edema; treat w/ high-dose steroids in close consultation w/ oncology

SICKLE CELL DISEASE

Overview

- **Pathophysiology:** Recessive beta-globin mutation (usually HbSS) → structurally abnl HbS → deoxygenated form polymerizes → RBC sickles → ↓ ability of RBCs to deform → hemolysis & microvascular occlusion → tissue ischemia & reperfusion injury

Acute Presentations of Sickle Cell Disease	
Acute anemia	**Aplastic crisis:** Reduced marrow production (eg, parvo B19) combined w/ short existing RBC half-life **Splenic sequestration:** Sequestration of RBCs in spleen **Hyperhemolytic crisis:** 2/2 hemolysis
Vaso-occlusive crisis (VOC)	Can manifest as pain (migratory, progressive), tissue infarction (stroke, renal necrosis, aseptic necrosis, hepatic), priapism
Acute chest synd	Resembles PNA; fever, dyspnea, hypoxia, CXR infiltrates; in one study 13% required mechanical vent; mortality up to 9%; ~3/4 occur w/ VOC (*N Engl J Med* 2000;342(25):1855); potential triggers include fat embolism, infxn, PE
Acute on chronic pain	May be orthopedic in origin; caused by AVN of joints, bone infarct, chronic osteo or ulcers; pain is persistent in same location w/ flares, located in bones or joints
Infxn	At risk for infxn w/ encapsulated organisms 2/2 functional asplenia, low threshold for labs, UA, CXR, cultures, consideration of LP, arthrocentesis, empiric abx if fever
Other	Stroke (may be symptomatic or "silent"; w/o primary prevention overt stroke in 10% children w/ HbSS dz); priaprism (ischemic) (*JAMA* 2014;312(10):1033)

- **Approach:** Initiate empiric analgesia early, can decompensate quickly; maintain high index of suspicion for infxn, IVF if concern for hypovolemia

History & Physical Examination

- **HX:** Assess location, duration, & severity of pain; similarity to prior crises; CP, or respiratory sxs; infectious sxs
- **PE:** Assess joints and ROM in areas affected; respiratory status; neuro deficits

Evaluation

- CBC w/ diff (compare to baseline), Chem 20 (↑ bili in hemolysis), reticulocyte count (↑ in hemolysis or sequestration; ↓ in aplastic crisis), LDH (elevated), ABG (if hypoxic)
- Imaging as directed by sxs: CXR (if CP or c/f acute chest synd), x-ray/MRI (if c/f osteomyelitis or avascular necrosis), CTA chest (if c/f PE); CTA/MRI (if c/f stroke)

Treatment

Acute Treatment in SCD (*JAMA* 2014;312(10):1033)	
Aplastic crisis	pRBC tfx
Splenic sequestration	Immediate IVF if hypovolemia, c/s hematology and initiate pRBC tfx
VOC	O_2, +/– IVF, rapid analgesia (generally IV opioids for severe pain; NSAIDs if pt has had relief w/ NSAIDs and no CIs; check pain plan w/ outpt hematologist if possible), do not transfuse unless other indication for pRBC
Acute chest synd	O_2, Abx (CTX and azithromycin), pain control, exchange tfx; AC if dx PE; discuss need for pRBC tfx &/or exchange tfx w/ hematology, incentive spirometry use
Acute stroke	O_2, IVF, discuss exchange tfx w/ hematology, consider pRBC tfx if delay to exchange tfx; data on reperfusion therapies (eg, thrombolytics, mechanical thrombectomy) for ischemic stroke in SCD is limited, consider tPA if o/w eligible and engage in shared decision making but admin should not delay simple or exchange tfx; discuss eligibility for thrombectomy w/ neurology (*Blood Adv* 2020;4(8):1554)
Other severe organ injury (eg, hepatic)	O_2, IVF, pRBC tfx, discuss exchange tfx w/ hematology
Sepsis (any cause)	Broad-spectrum abx, esp if indwelling line

Chronic

- Hydroxyurea: ↑ fetal hemoglobin (HbF) leading to decreased polymerization of deoxygenated HbS & ↓ pain crises, frequency & duration of hospitalizations, & risk of acute chest synd (*NEJM* 1995;1332:1317), ↓ mortality (*NEJM* 2003;1289:1645), needs time to work so not practical in ED

Disposition

- Home: If pain controlled, no e/o acute chest synd; close hematology f/u
- Admit: Requiring further IV pain control, any acute complication as detailed above

ABNORMAL BLEEDING

Overview

- Etiology & tx depend on nature of problem (plt count, plt fxn, clotting time, etc)
- Can be congenital or acquired from drugs, associated disease, or iatrogenic causes

Differential Diagnosis for Abnormal Bleeding	
1° Problem	**Potential Causes**
↓ plt count	ITP, HUS/TTP, DIC, HELLP synd (if pregnant), SLE, HIT, splenic sequestration (eg, NHL, myelofibrosis, cirrhosis), bone marrow failure (eg, aplastic anemia, heme malignancy), massive tfx/dilution, chronic systemic dz
↓ plt fxn	vWD, meds (eg, ASA/NSAIDs, clopidogrel, GP IIb/IIA inh), chronic systemic dz (eg, uremia, cirrhosis, leukemia/MDS)
↓ clotting cascade	DIC, meds (eg, warfarin, DOACs), factor deficiency (eg, hemophilia), chronic systemic dz (eg, malnutrition, cirrhosis), massive tfx/dilution

History & Physical Examination

- Bleeding hx (w/ menses, surgery, dental procedures, trauma), easy bruising, meds, family hx bleeding disorders
- Bleeding synds can present in many organ systems, inc several at once:

Hx			
System	**Manifestation**	**System**	**Manifestation**
HEENT	Gingival bleeding, epistaxis	GU	Hematuria, menorrhagia
CNS	ICH, epidural hematoma	MSK	Hematoma, hemarthrosis
Pulm	Hemoptysis	Skin	Petechiae, purpura, ecchymosis
GI	Hematemesis, melena, hematochezia		

- Physical exam may suggest sp bleeding problem:
  - Petechiae: ↓ plt count
  - Purpura: ↓ plt count, ↓ plt fxn, problem w/ blood vessels or connective tissue
  - Ecchymosis: ↓ clotting cascade, problem w/ connective tissue, trauma
  - Deep muscle or joint bleeding: ↓ clotting cascade

Evaluation
- CBC w/ diff, Chem 7, coags; consider LFTs, peripheral blood smear, DIC panel (fibrinogen, D-dimer, LDH, haptoglobin), direct Coombs

IMMUNE THROMBOCYTOPENIA

Overview
- **Definition:** Isolated TCP due to immune Ab-mediated destruction of PLTs (PLT count <100 k/μL); either 1° (idiopathic) or secondary (2/2 virus, meds, autoimmune dz, pregnancy, vaccine)
- Common associated meds: Quinine, antimicrobials (linezolid, rifampin, vancomycin, sulfa), anticonvulsants (phenytoin, valproic acid, carbamazepine), thiazides, histamine antagonists, NSAIDs/tylenol, chemotherapies (*NEJM* 2007;357(6):580)
- Dx of exclusion: R/o TTP/HUS, HIT, hematologic d/o (eg, malignancy, MDS, HIV)

History & Physical Examination
- Acute/subacute petechiae ± e/o bleeding (see above; assess for ICH, GIB, etc); always ask about new meds, recent infectious sxs, pregnancy

Evaluation (*Blood* 2011;117(16):4190)
- CBC w/ diff (↓ plt count, o/w nml), peripheral smear (no schistocytes), coags (nml), T+S
- HIV/HCV recommended on all pts to r/o alt cause, *H. pylori* can be associated as well

Treatment (*Blood* 2011;117(16):4190; *Blood Adv* 2019;3(23):3829)
- Adults: If asx, tx rarely indicated if PLTs >30K & no bleeding, trauma, or surgery
- Children: Manage mild cases expectantly, treat if active bleeding

Tx for ITP		
Adults	No bleeding, Plt >30K	May manage expectantly; close f/u
	No bleeding, Plt <30K	Prednisone (0.5–2 mg/kg/d), OR dexamethasone (40 mg/d for 4 d)
		IVIG (1 g/kg/d) × 1–2 d
		Anti-D Ig (Rh+ pts only) (75 μg/kg/d)
	Bleeding, Plt <50K	Combine tx above, transfuse
Children	No bleeding or minor bleeding, any plt count	Observation, no tx indicated; close f/u
	Non–life-threatening mucosal bleeding	Steroids: Prednisone 2–4 mg/kg/d PO (max 120 mg daily) × 5–7 d
		Anti-D Ig (Rh+ pts only) (75 μg/kg/d)
		IVIG: 0.8–1 g/kg IV × 1 dose
	Major bleeding	Combine tx above, transfuse

- Transfuse PLTs as per guidelines below (*see Transfusion section*)
- Steroids: 1st-line preferred agent, 50–75% response, often by 3 wks
- IVIG: Equivalent but quicker remission compared to steroids; c/s w/ hematology
- Anti-D Ig: As effective as IVIG, but shorter infusion, longer response; c/s w/ hematology
- 2nd-line tx should be discussed w/ consultant: Thrombopoietin receptor agonist (eltrombopag or romiplostim), rituximab, splenectomy, etc
- No role for plasmapheresis in tx of ITP

Disposition
- Home: If no active bleeding, PLTs >20K for adults (no PLT cut-off for children)
- Admit: Any adult pt w/ PLTs <20K &/or any pt w/ active bleeding

HEPARIN-INDUCED THROMBOCYTOPENIA (HIT)

Overview (*Blood Adv* 2018;2(22):3360)
- **Definition:** TCP (PLT <150K) or 30–50% drop in plt count after starting heparin
  - More common w/ unfractionated heparin, but occurs as well w/ LMWH
- **Pathogenesis:** HIT type II due to IgG target complexes of heparin & PF4 → plt activation → ↑ thrombosis
  - Thrombosis (arterial or venous) in 30–50% pts: PE, DVT > limb ischemia, stroke > MI

History & Evaluation
- Can have sxs of TCP (if PLTs very low), thrombosis (even w/ nl plt count), or be incidental discovery; very rarely causes bleeding

- Usual occurrence 5–10 d after starting heparin, more rapid onset if recent heparin exposure
- Anti-PF4 enzyme assays highly sens, poorly spec (good NPV); combine lab testing w/ clinical probability (hi, med, low) based on 4Ts score: Δ plt count (>50%, 30–50%, <30%), plt nadir (>/20K, 10–19K, <10K), timing (5–10 d or ≤1 d if exposure w/i 30 d, >10 d, <4 d without recent exposure), thrombotic cx, & alternative causes (yes, possible, no) (*J Thromb Haemost* 2006;4:759)

Treatment (*Blood Adv* 2018;2(22):3360)
- STOP heparin + any device/flush that contains heparin (even if thrombotic cxs)
- Initiate nonheparin a/c (even if no thrombosis): Argatroban, bivalirudin, DOAC
- Avoid vitamin-K antagonists, as will decrease protein C → ↑ thrombosis
  - Avoid PLT tfxs unless bleeding or high risk of bleeding
- Recurrence w/ future heparin may be low if neg for PF4 Ab >100 d after Dx (*NEJM* 2001; 344:1286)

Disposition
- Admit for monitoring & IV A/C

Hemolytic-Uremic Syndrome (HUS) & Thrombotic Thrombocytopenic Purpura (TTP)

Overview (*NEJM* 2006;354(18):1927; *NEJM* 2014;371(7):654)
- **Definition:** Systemic (TTP) or intrarenal (HUS) microvascular occlusive d/o 2/2 PLT aggregation → migroangiopathic hemolytic anemia (MAHA) + TCP & microvascular thrombosis
- **Pathogenesis:** TTP a/w ADAMTS13 deficiency (normally cleaves vWF, resultant inability to cleave vWF → plt activation → microthrombi); HUS a/w *E. coli* O157:H7, shiga toxin leading to defective complement activation & regulation

History & Physical Examination
- TTP: Acute/subacute, can be subtle & non-sp (classic pentad of MAHA, TCP, fever, neurologic and renal abnormalities is rare); adults > children
  - MAHA: Vague sxs (abd pain, nausea, weakness) 2/2 diffuse microvascular thrombi
  - TCP: E/o bleeding, skin findings (petechial, purpura)
  - Neuro sxs: AMS, stroke, szs, fluctuating deficits, confusion; neuro sxs present only 50%
  - AKI: Can be mild
  - Fever: Uncommon, low-grade when present; no other cause
- HUS: Acute onset, bloody diarrhea & abd pain, f/b TCP & renal failure; children > adults
  - Classic triad: MAHA + TCP + renal failure (anuria/oliguria, HTN)
- Always ask about triggers: HUS (contaminated food), TTP (meds, systemic dz, HSCT)

Evaluation
- CBC w/ diff (↓ Hct, ↓ Plt), Chem 20 (↑ Cr), peripheral smear (schistocytes), coags (nml), ↑ LDH & reticulocytes, ↓ haptoglobin, fibrinogen & D-dimer (nml), UA/preg, direct Coombs (neg), T+S; send testing for ADAMTS 13 deficiency if c/f TTP

Treatment
- C/s hematology, consider renal c/s early
- TTP: Plasma exchange (↑ survival @ 6 mos), FFP (if delay to plasma exchange), steroids (prednisone 1–2 mg/kg/d or methylprednisolone 1 g/d, data on efficacy limited)
- HUS: Supportive; pts commonly need dialysis, pRBCs prn for severe anemia, control of BP (CCB), avoid abx & antimotility agents
- Do not give PLTs → ↑ microvascular thrombosis

Disposition
- Admit, may require ICU

Disseminated Intravascular Coagulation (DIC)

Overview (*J Intensive Care* 2014;2:15)
- **Definition:** Acquired life-threatening consumptive coagulopathy a/w diverse dz
- **Pathogenesis:** Widespread activation of coagulation → thrombosis of small/midsized vessels → organ dysfxn, ↓ PLTs/coagulation factors → bleeding & thromboembolism
- Can have mild bleeding, massive bleeding, thrombosis, progression to multiorgan failure

Causes of DIC	
Cancer	Solid tumors, hematologic malignancy (eg, acute promyelocytic leukemia), metastasis
Infxns	Sepsis, bacteremia, viral infxn
Trauma	Severe trauma, burn, head injury, fat embolism
Obstetrics	Amniotic fluid embolism, abruptio placentae, HELLP synd

History & Physical Examination

- Underlying systemic dz is necessary for dx (see above)
- Chronicity of sxs; signs/sxs of bleeding (hyperfibrinolysis), end-organ damage (hypercoagulation)

Evaluation

- CBC w/ diff (↓ PLTs [usually <100K]), ↑ PT, ↑ PTT, ↑ D-dimer, ↓ fibrinogen, ↑ LDH, ↑ Fibrin degradation products, e/o end-organ damage (↑ lactate, ↑ Cr); consider cultures, imaging, further eval based on sxs/underlying dz
- Different scoring systems used to help in dx of DIC (*Thromb Haemost* 2011;105(1):40)

Treatment (*J Thromb Haemost* 2013;11:761)

- Tx of underlying disorder is mainstay of tx (abx, surgery, chemo, etc)
- Transfuse if bleeding, risk of bleeding, or need for procedure: PLTs (if bleeding + plt <50K, or plt <10–20K w/ risk of bleeding), FFP (if INR >1.5; beware large volume may be required, start w/ 15 mL/kg), cryoprecipitate (if fibrinogen <1.5 g/dL despite FFP), prothrombin complex concentrate (if bleeding & FFP delayed/not possible [eg, volume])
- Heparin/LMWH if thromboembolism predominates (LMWH may be superior to UH)

Disposition

- Admit to ICU

VON WILLEBRAND DISEASE (VWD)

Overview (*Blood* 2017;130(22):2386)

- **Definition:** Most common inherited bleeding d/o caused by ↓ vWF (↓ quantity [type 1] (partial deficiency) is most common, 3 (near complete)] or impaired function [type 2]); vWF carries factor VIII & enables plt adhesion/aggregation; rarely acquired
- **Etiology:** Precursor vWF cleaved by ADAMTS13 (see TTP above) → circulating vWF activated by vascular damage → vWF binds collagen → plt aggregation
  - ↓ vWF leads to ↓ plt aggregation & ↑ factor VIII degradation

History & Physical Examination

- Mucocutaneous bleeding, menorrhagia, bruising, epistaxis, hemarthrosis, hematomas
  - 5–20% of pts w/ menorrhagia will have vWD (sometimes requiring TAH)
- Most pts aware of their hx (60–80% will have bleeding after surgery), often w/ family hx

Evaluation

- CBC w/ diff, T&S, coags (↑ PTT); ↓ vWF Ag, ↓ vWF activity (ristocetin cofactor), ↓ factor VIII activity

Treatment

- Life-threatening bleeds: Important to increase levels of both vWF & factor VIII
- DDAVP: Most useful in type 1 vWD, where sufficient & functional vWF exists in noncirculating form; limited utility in severe bleeds; DDAVP causes endothelial release of vWF & ↑ circulating vWF levels (no chgs in overall vWF); efficacy variable; dose 0.3 μg/kg IV or 1–2 spray IN
- vWF replacement: Most useful in type 2 or 3, where endogenous vWF either dysfxnal or absent; options include cryoprecipitate (requires up to 8–12 bags), plasma-derived vWF/factor VIII concentrate (Humate-P), or recombinant vWF + factor VIII
- Adjunct tx: Antifibrinolytics (eg, TXA, aminocaproic acid); high-quality data lacking

Disposition

- If severe or significant bleeding, admit; if D/C, f/u w/ hematology

HEMOPHILIA A/B

Overview

- Definition: X-linked (usually male) d/o 2/2 ↓ factor VIII (hem A) or factor IX (hem B)

Hemophilia Dz Severity		
Severity	**Factor Concentration (% of nml)**	**Manifestations**
Mild	5–40 IU/dL (5–40%)	Severe bleeding w/ major trauma
Mod	1–5 IU/dL (1–5%)	Severe bleeding w/ minor trauma
Severe	<1 IU/dL (<1%)	Spontaneous IM bleeding

History & Physical Examination
- Bleeding (GI, GU, mucosa), hematoma, hemarthroses (knee, ankle, elbow), bruising
- Gusto Classification of bleeding severity (*Circulation* 2011;123(23):2736):
  - Severe: ICH or bleeding that results in hemodynamic instability
  - Mod: Requires tfx but doesn't lead to hemodynamic instability
  - Mild: Bleeding that does not meet above criteria

Evaluation
- CBC (nml PLTs), nml INR, ↑ PTT (can be nml if mild hemophilia), T&S, bleeding time nml, Imaging PRN based on clinical scenario
- Consider testing inc mixing studies, testing for VWD, measurement of factor levels

Treatment (*Haemophilia* 2013;19(1):e1; *Haemophilia* 2020;26(S6):1)
- Alternative to factor concentrate or tx for minor bleeds:
  - Hemophilia A: DDAVP (0.3 μg/kg IV, 150 μg IN kids/300 μg IN adults) increases factor VIII concentration 3–6 × 2/2 release of vWF; cryoprecipitate also can be used given high concentration of factor VIII & vWF
  - Hemophilia B: Transexamic acid (25–50 mg/kg/dose PO)
- Mod–severe bleeds: Factor VIII/IX concentrate based on extent of deficiency
  - Factor VIII dose: Typically 50 IU/kg or (wt [kg] × 0.5 × desire factor concentration rise)
  - Factor IX dose: Typically 100 IU/kg or (wt [kg] × 1 × desire factor concentration rise)
  - If severe (eg, ICH), give factor even prior to diagnostic testing
  - If pts have developed inhs to factor VIII, consider use of factor VIIa or prothrombin complex (bypass factor VIII in clotting cascade)

TRANSFUSIONS

See Section 18 for transfusions in trauma.

Overview
- **Approach:** Obtain type & screen for any pt who may need tfx

Transfusion Product Sp	
Irradiated	Use for pts w/ cellular immunosupp (eg, neonates, HSCT, congenital immune def); destroys donor T cells (↓ GVHD)
Leuko-reduced	Use for tpx pts or pts requiring multiple tfxs; removes WBCs (↓ CMV, ↓ rejection against donor product, ↓ febrile nonhemolytic rxn)
Washed	Use for pts w/ hx of tfx allergic rxns & IgA deficiency; removes plasma components (↓ allergic rxns); very time intensive
Pheresis	Single donor (vs pooled-donor); refers to PLT tfx

Packed Red Blood Cell Transfusion (*Ann Intern Med* 2012;157:49; *JAMA* 2016;316(19):2025)
- **When to give:** Restrictive strategies ↓ adverse events, mortality (*Cochrane* 2012;(4):CD002042)
  - All pts: Hgb ≤7, Hgb >7 + acute, ongoing, or significant sxs
  - Cardiovascular dz: Hgb ≤8, Hgb >8 + acute, ongoing, or significant sxs
- **What to give:**
  - Emergent tfx: O neg to females w/ childbearing potential, O positive to males
  - In massive tfx (expected >10 U PRBC/d), give FFP, PLTs, Ca as well
- **How much to give:**
  - Neonates: ↑ Hgb by 3 g/dL for 10–15 mL/kg of PRBCs
  - Adult: ↑ Hgb by 1 g/dL or Hct by 3%, for each 1 U PRBCs
- **What to monitor:**
  - Signs/sxs tfx rxn (eg, fever, SOB, hypoxia)
  - Electrolytes: Esp if large volume PRBC (↑ K, ↓ Ca)
  - O_2: Pts w/ CHF may require concurrent diuresis

Platelet Transfusion (*JAMA* 2025;334(7):606–617; *Chest* 2025;168(3):661–676)
- **When to give based on 2025 clinical practice guidelines:**
  - PLT <10K: Regardless of s/s of bleeding or comorbidities
  - PLT <20K: If pt undergoing lumbar puncture or low risk interventional radiology procedure
  - PLT <50K: Serious active bleeding or need for invasive procedure

- PLT <100K: Need for ophthalmologic or neurosurgical procedure
- Dengue-related TCP and no major bleeding–no PLT tfx
- **How much to give:** ↑ PLTs by 5000–10,000 for each 1 U PLTs

Fresh-Frozen Plasma Transfusions (*Transfusion* 2010;50(6):1227)
- **When to give:** Massive tfx (*see Trauma section*); reversal of warfarin (4-factor PCC more effective & less volume); coagulopathy (eg, DIC); TTP/HUS (if delay to plasmapheresis); replacement of factor deficiencies (targeted factor conc preferred)
- **How much to give:** 10–20 mL/kg will ↑ coagulation factors by 20–30% (1U FFP = 200 mL); consider giving concurrent diuretic if e/o or known hx of CHF

Cryoprecipitate Transfusions (*BC Medical J* 2007;49(8):441)
- **When to give:** Fibrinogen level <1 g/L; factor XIII deficiency, hemophilia A, vWD, bleeding related to thrombolytic therapy
- **Contains:** Factor VIII, XIII, fibrinogen, vWF
- **How much to give:** 1 U/5–10 kg body weight, will raise fibrinogen by 0.5 g/L

Anticoagulation Reversal

Approach (*Ann Emerg Med* 2020;76(4):470)
- Hold further doses of anticoagulant
- Supportive care: Gastric lavage or activated charcoal (if o/d w/i 1 h), apply pressure to site of bleeding if possible, transfuse (as indicated), consider TXA
- Agent-spec reversal: If bleeding life threatening or at critical site (eg, ICH, hemoptysis, GIB) or need for emergent procedure/surgery
- Also consider indication for AC (eg, valvular vs nonvalvular A fib; recent stent)

Reversal of Common Anticoagulants (*Ann Emerg Med* 2020;76(4):470)		
Antiplatelet agent	Minor bleed	Weigh risks/benefits of holding antiplatelet
	Severe bleed	Hold antiplatelet agent, consider DDAVP[a] Plt tfx in absence of significant TCP may be harmful for some pts[b]
Heparin	Protamine (1 mg/90–100 U heparin in last 2–3 h; max 50 mg)[c]	
LMWH	Protamine may be partially (60–80%) effective (dosing above)[c]	
Warfarin[d]	INR <4 No bleeding	Decrease or omit single warfarin dose F/U for INR check w/i 48–72 h
	INR 4–10 No bleeding	Omit 1–2 warfarin doses and f/u INR check Vitamin K 1–2.5 mg PO × 1 if risk for bleeding F/U for INR check w/i 24–48 h
	INR >10 No bleeding	Hold warfarin (until F/U INR recheck) Vitamin K 2.5–5 mg PO × 1 F/U for INR check w/i 12–24 h
	INR >1.5–2 Serious bleed	Hold warfarin Vitamin K 5–10 mg IV (risk of anaphylactoid rxn) Prothrombin clotting complex (25–50 IU/kg, max 2500–5000 IU) w/ vitamin K FFP (10–15 mL/kg) only if PCC unavailable
DOAC	Dabigatran	Idarucizumab reverses bleeding w/i min[e] OR if unavailable, recombinant factor VIIa or activated PCC may have effectiveness[h]
	Rivaroxaban	Consider risks/benefits of Andexanet, if available: Dose based on time since last dose[g] OR if unavailable, 4-factor PCC may have effectiveness[f]
	Apixaban	Consider risks/benefits of Andexanet, if available: Dose based on time since last dose[g] OR if unavailable, 4-factor PCC may have effectiveness[f]

[a]*Crit Care Med* 2016;44(12):2251. [b]*Lancet* 2016;387(10038):2605. [c]*American College of Chest Physicians Evidence-Based Clinical Practice Guideline on Antithrombotic and Thrombolytic Therapy*, 8th ed. [d]*Circulation* 2012;125:2944. [e]*NEJM* 373(25):2413. [f]*Thromb Haemost* 2018;118(5):842. [g]*NEJM* 2019;380(14):132. [h]*AAEM Clinical Practice Statement 2017.*

Pearls
- Irreversible antiplatelet agents inhibit life of PLT (7–10 d)
- Vitamin K takes 6 (IV) to 24 (PO) h to reverse warfarin; IV may cause anaphylactoid rxn in rare instances (push slowly over 30 mins)
- 4F-PCC contains factor II, VIII, IX, X, protein C+S, heparin, albumin
- 4F-PCC superior to FFP, may have fewer adverse events (*Lancet* 2015;385(9982):2077)
  - Adverse events: W/ 4F-PCC mostly 2/2 thrombosis; w/ FFP mostly 2/2 volume
  - Risk of thrombosis also w/ other methods of AC reversal inc Andexanet; note the U.S. Food and Drug Administration (FDA) considers risks of Andexanet to outweigh its benefits

TRANSFUSION COMPLICATIONS

Approach

- Always obtain consent before giving a tfx
- If e/o rxn: **Stop tfx**, check bag, label, & send remaining products to blood bank, provide supportive care
  - May be possible to resume tfx in mild allergic rxn only (see below)
- If febrile, obtain CBC, smear, direct Coombs, UA, Gram stain, BCx (pt & product)

Common or Critical Transfusion rxns		
Rxn	**Incidence***	**Note**
Febrile (nonhemolytic)	1:100	Recipient Ab against donor antigens or release of cytokines from blood; dx of exclusion **HX:** Fevers, chills, tachycardia ± transient HTN **TX:** Antipyretics, monitor to r/o infxn (septic tfx) or hemolysis (acute hemolytic rxn) **Pearl:** Consider washed products
Allergic	1:1000	Histamine-mediated; more common w/ PLT tfx **DX:** Pruritus, urticaria ± angioedema, e/o anaphylaxis, SOB/wheezing, hypotension **TX:** H1 antihistamine; bronchodilators; if anaphylaxis then add H2 antihistamine, glucocorticoids, IM epi; can restart tfx if sxs were local only & full resolution (stop if recurs) **Pearls:** If hx of tfx allergic rxn, consider washed products & H1B premed; no role for steroid premed
Anaphylactic	1:10,000	
Febrile (acute hemolytic)	1:10,000	Can be immune or non–immune-mediated; blood product error (eg, ABO incompatibility, incorrect preparation): **DX:** Fever (1st sign) → flank pain, f/c, SOB, AKI, hemoglobinuria, anemia, DIC, shock w/i 24 h **TX:** If fever, monitor for other sxs; IVF/diuretics for UOP **Pearls:** Differs from delayed hemolytic rxn (1:2500 [1:10 in SCD]; 2/2 Abs against non-ABO groups; occurs 1 wk after tfx; dx by Hgb not rising as expected, +Coombs, ↑ Bili, jaundice, f/c; no tx needed); Ab hx should be noted for future tfxs
TACO (tfx-associated circulatory overload)	1:10,000	Excess volume &/or rate of tfx, ↑ risk if hx of CHF, CKD, large volume or rapid rate (eg, hemorrhage) **DX:** SOB, ↓ O_2, ↑ BNP, ↑ CVP, & JVD, peripheral edema, pulm edema w/i 6 h of tfx **TX:** O_2, diuresis, NIPPV prn **Pearl:** If at risk of TACO, administer tfx slowly (eg, over 3–4 h), consider diuresis prior to tfx
TRALI (tfx-related lung injury)	1:100,000	Proposed etiology: Donor Abs bind recipient WBCs → pool in pulm capillaries → ↑ permeability → non-cardiogenic pulmonary edema **DX:** SOB, ↓ O_2, CXR w/ b/l infiltrates; fever/hypothermia, hypotension/HTN; generally w/i 6 h of tfx (can be delayed) **TX:** Supportive (O_2, low tidal-volume vent if requires intubation/mechanical ventilation)
Septic	1:100,000	Infected blood product, most common w/ PLTs **DX:** Fever, rigors, hypotension; +BCx (pt & product) **TX:** Broad-spectrum abx (inc antipseudomonal)
Viral infxn	Variable	HBV (1:2M), HCV (1:2M), HIV (1:2M), CMV (1:3M)

*Incidence estimates are per unit transfused; rounded to nearest factor of 10. *Lancet* 2016;388(10061):2825; *JAMA* 2003;289:959; *NEJM* 1999;340:438; *Blood* 2019;133:1854.

EMERGENCIES IN THE TRANSPLANT PATIENT

Approach to the Solid Organ Transplant Patient *(Am J Emerg Med 2016;34(11):2200)*

- Signs and sxs of disease may be subtle
  - Transplanted organs lack native innervation so pain may be unreliable
  - Immunosupp blunts inflammatory response to infxn
- Categories of cx include infxn, rejection, drug tox, & other organ spec cx
- Hx: Time since tpx, reason for tpx, hx of infxns (pt &/or donor), rejection, & other cx, immunosupp regimen & compliance
- C/s w/ tpx team

Medication Adverse Effects

- Common maintenance regimens include calcineurin inhs (cyclosporine, tacrolimus), antimetabolites (azathioprine, mycophenolate mofetil), rapamycin inhs (sirolimus, everolimus) &/or corticosteroids
  - Drug levels can be obtained for cyclosporine, tacrolimus, sirolimus, which each have narrow therapeutic window
  - Many drug–drug interactions
- Common side effects: Nephrotoxicity, anemia, electrolyte derangements, metabolic synd, GI sxs, adrenal suppression, osteoporosis, neurotoxicity, malignancy

Infectious Complications

- Incidence is 25–80% in 1st y after tpx
- Can be subtle: Immunosupp can diminish classic sxs (eg, fever, localizing sxs), radiographic signs, or lab results; maintain high index of suspicion

Infections in Posttransplant pts	
0–1 mos post-tpx (early)	Nosocomial (bacteremia, VAP, surgical infxn, CAUTI) Preexisting or donor derived (HIV, HCV, TB, fungal)
1–6 mos post-tpx (intermediate)	Immunomodulating viral infxns (CMV, EBV BK virus, HCV/HBV, herpes viruses) Opportunistic infxns (mycobacteria, candidiasis, endemic mycosis, PJP, toxo, cryptococcus, strongyloides)
>6 mos post-tpx (late)	Healthy tpx pts: Mild increase in community acquired infxn (PNA, Influenza, EBV, RSV Legionella, listeria, UTI) Pts w/ chronic viral infxn: Progressive disease (HBV, HCV, CMV, EBV HSV) Pts w/ chronic rejection: Aggressive immunosuppressive tx increases risk of late infxns

Graft Rejection

- Recipient immune-mediated rxn against tpxed organ (esp microcirculation)
- Frequency & sxs of rejection vary by organ tpx type
  - Kidney 20%; liver 64% acute rejection, 23% late rejection; cardiac 30% (acute); lung ~1/3 w/i 1 year
- Essential to involve tpx team if considering dx of rejection
- Biopsy for definitive dx
- Occurs in three phases
  - Hyperacute: Usually in immediate postop period due to preformed Abs, rare w/ donor-recipient matching, results in complement activation & thrombosis
  - Acute: Occurs d–wks after tpx or if immunosupp stopped
  - Chronic: Occurs mos–y after tpx, results in gradual failure over time
- TX: High-dose IV steroids; may require additional tx, c/s tpx team

Signs & Symptoms of Transplant Rejection	
Renal (20%)	Sxs: Often asx; fever, malaise, oliguria, graft pain; HTN, tenderness over graft Mechanism: Interstitial fibrosis & tubular atrophy DX: Labs (↑ BUN/Cr, abnml lytes); urine lytes (r/o other dx); Renal US w/ Doppler w/ ↑ resistive indices, biopsy
Liver (60% w/i 6 weeks; 23% late)	Sxs: Fever, malaise, abd pain, organomegaly, ascites Mechanism: Fibrosis of bile ducts, arteries, & veins DX: Labs (↑ LFTs); RUQUS w/ Doppler (r/o other dx [eg, thrombosis]), biopsy

Cardiac (30% <6 mos)	Sxs: SOB, orthopnea, palpitations, arrhythmias, near-syncope, edema, GI Sxs if R heart predominance (RUQ pain, nausea), generally no CP Mechanism: Arteriosclerosis & chronc allograft vasculopathy DX: Labs (↑ Troponin, BNP), ECG w/ ST/T-wave chgs, BSUS w/ systolic/diastolic dysfxn; CXR w/ edema, biopsy
Lung (30% <1 y)	Sxs: SOB, cough, +/– abnl lung sounds (eg, crackles, wheezing) Mechanism: Inflammation leading to airway obstruction DX: Labs (↑ eos), CXR can be nml, Chest CT generally needed, bronch/biopsy

Organ-Specific Complications

Renal Transplant

- UTI (most common): Always culture; consider strongly dual-abx & admx
- Peri-tpx hematoma (2–3%): Graft pain, ↓ H/H, U/S (may need CT)
- Arterial stenosis (10%): HTN, ↓ UOP, edema; U/S w/ flow limitation; tx w/ stent
- Venous thrombosis (4%): Graft pain/erythema, ↓ UOP, n/v; U/S (may need contrast CT); often results in graft failure & need for graft replacement
- Ureteral obstruction (3–6%): ↓ UOP, edema; U/S w/ hydronephrosis; if no correction w/ Foley, may need percutaneous intervention for urinary drainage
- Urinary leakage (2–5%): ↓ UOP, perineal edema; U/S w/ peritransplant fluid collection; urology c/s
- Lymphocele (5–15%): Abd swelling/pain; U/S w/ hydrocele (CT for definitive dx)

Liver Transplant

- Hepatic artery thrombosis (4–12%): Doppler U/S 90% Sens; mortality 80% w/o tx
- Hepatic artery stenosis (14%): Doppler U/S 70% Sens; may need angiography for dx
- Pseudoaneurysm: Can cause hemobilia, hemoperitoneum, GIB; dx w/ U/S or CT
- Biliary strictures: May be asx 2/2 denervation; U/S (Sens up to 66%), MRCP (Sens 95%); tx stent
- Biliary leaks (2–25%) & bilomas: Tx w/ stenting over leak, drain & abx (if biloma)

Cardiac Transplant

- Allograft vasculopathy (30–70%): Chronic & progressive; rapid atherosclerosis in transplanted organ; may have s/s of ischemia, or be asx 2/2 denervation (inc sudden cardiac arrest), dx w/ cath, cardiac POCUS eval for wall motion abnormalities; tx requires CABG or repeat tpx
- Bradycardia: 2/2 sinus or AVN trauma; refractory to atropine 2/2 loss of vagal innervation, tx w/ epi or isoproterenol, may need PPM
- Tachyarrhythmias: Can be 2/2 rejection, consider cardioversion
  - A fib/flutter: BB > CCB (2/2 med interaction)
  - SVT: Half-dose adenosine 2/2 sens of transplanted heart, vagal maneuvers ineffective 2/2 loss of vagal innervation
  - Ventricular dysrhythmia: Cardioversion & ICD for sustained dysrhythmia

Lung Transplant

- Airway anastomotic stenosis, tracheobronchomalacia (increase in granulation tissue), necrosis; p/w SOB/stridor; CT may help, but bronch is definitive dx; may need stent
- Fistula: Depending on tract, may present w/ PTX, crepitus, hemoptysis, dx w/ CT
- Pulm artery stenosis: Early & late post-tpx; SOB, ↓ O_2, LE edema, ↓ BP; dx w/ CTA chest, may need dilatation & stent
- Pulm vein thrombosis: Early after tpx; SOB, ↓ O_2, LE edema, ↓ BP; dx w/ CTA chest, tx w/ AC, thrombolysis if unstable
- Phrenic nerve injury (3–9% lung tpx; 40% of heart–lung tpxs): SOB; CXR ↑ hemidiaphragm
- Pl lining cxs: PTX, hemothorax, chylothorax, dx w/ CXR &/or CT

Stem Cell and Bone Marrow Transplant (*Curr Oncol* 2019;26(3):187)

- Hematopoietic stem-cell tpx (HSCT): Infusing stem cells (obtained from peripheral blood, bone marrow, or umbilical cord units) after short course of chemotherapy &/or radiotherapy
- Used for the tx of hematologic malignancies (multiple myeloma, lymphoma, AML, ALL, MDS, myeloproliferative neoplasms), nonmalignant conditions (aplastic anemia, bone marrow failure synds, SCD, thalassemia, immune deficiencies)
- Can be autologous (cells collected from recipient) or allogeneic (from another individual)

Complications of Stem Cell Transplant	
Pre-engraftment period (start of conditioning through neutrophil recovery)	• 2/2 tox from chemo &/or radiotherapy regimen • Pancytopenia, GI tox • Infxn (2/2 neutropenia, gram [+] & [–] bacteria, HSV, candida, aspergillus) • Organ dysfxn (2/2 endothelial dysfxn, hepatic sinusoidal obstruction synd, diffuse alveolar hemorrhage, thrombotic microangiopathy)
Early postengraftment period (neutrophil recovery to post-tpx day 100)	• Acute GVHD (only in allogeneic HSCT): 2/2 transplanted immune cells recognizing recipient as foreign, affects skin, GI system, liver; sxs include rash, diarrhea, n/v; treat w/ steroids • Infxn (impaired cellular & humoral immunity, opportunistic organisms, fungal, viral reactivation)
Late postengraftment period (day 100 & later)	• Chronic GVHD: Can affect skin, myositis & fasciitis, salivary & lacrimal glands, lung (obstructive or restrictive), GI; treated w/ steroids & immunomodulators • Relapse of primary disease • Increased risk of cardiovascular dz, metabolic dz, secondary malignancies, reproductive dysfxn, neuropsychiatric disorders

Approach
- Careful hx: Anatomic distribution, unilateral vs b/l, acute vs chronic, a/w erythema or dermatologic findings; hx of trauma
- Assess for paresthesia or neuropathy
- Complete MSK, neuro, & vascular exam

Differential	
Pathophysiology	**Differential**
Cardiovascular/Renal	Heart failure, volume overload, nephrotic/nephritic synd, ascites, PAD, arterial occlusion, venous stasis
Infectious/Inflammatory	Cellulitis/abscess, arthritis, phlebitis, necrotizing fasciitis, myositis, diabetic foot infection
Heme/Onc/Lymph	Acute/chronic DVT, cancer, lymphedema
Neuro	Spinal stenosis, diabetic neuropathy, other neuropathies, complex regional pain synd (CRPS)
Trauma, Environmental	Compartment synd, fracture, dislocation, hematoma

PERIPHERAL VASCULAR DISEASE

Claudication

History
- Ischemic muscle pain reproducible w/ exertion, improves w/ rest
- Pts often place legs in dependent position to improve flow
- 1–2% have chronic critical limb ischemia: pain at rest, nonhealing ulcers, dry gangrene

Findings: May have nl exam at rest w/ or w/o ↓ peripheral pulses; shiny, smooth skin

Evaluation
- Careful neurovascular exam, obtain Doppler if difficult to palpate pulse
- Look for S/S of critical ischemia: Rest pain, paresthesias, ulcers, ↓pulses, coolness
- ABI <0.9 is diagnostic of PAD (1–1.4 nl; 0.5–0.89 abnml; 0.4–0.49 severely reduced)

Management: If concern for critical ischemia or acute dz, c/s vascular surgery

Disposition
- Admit acute dz
- If chronic and stable exam, D/C home w/ PCP (medical mgmt) & vascular surgery f/u, strict return instructions

Acute Extremity Arterial Occlusion

History
- Known PVD and/or RFs (HTN, tobacco, known CAD, AF/AFL, postangiogram, or following other endovascular procedure)
- Abrupt onset of pain w/ reduced/diminished pulses, may have paresthesias
- Later findings: Poikilothermia, pallor, paralysis

Findings
- Cold, mottled extremity, ↓ pulse, motor weakness, +/– bruit
- Tenderness to palpation out of proportion of exam or ↓ sensation

Evaluation
- Bedside Doppler of all pulses, inc unaffected extremities; ABI
- Labs: CBC, BMP, coags, T+S ± lactate
- CT angiogram; differentiate chronic PVD vs other etiology (aneurysm, dissection, embolism) & useful for emergent operative planning
- Evaluate for atheroembolic source; ECG for arrhythmia

Treatment
- Immediate vascular surgery consultation for potential revascularization; if vascular surgery not available, transfer to facility w/ vascular surgery capability
- A/C (eg, heparin IV bolus f/b 18 U/kg/h infusion)

Pearl
- Ischemic tissue death starts by 4 h; may be sooner in pts w/ chronic arterial insufficiency

Measurement of Ankle–Brachial Indices (ABIs)	
1	W/ pt lying supine, measure SBP at ankle & ipsilateral brachial artery Place cuff over biceps to measure brachial SBP & over calf to measure ankle SBP Place Doppler over brachial pulse upper-extremity measurement & over posterior tibial artery or DP pulse for ankle measurement Inflate cuff until Doppler pulse no longer heard, then deflate and record pressure at which Doppler signal reappears

2	ABI = higher pressure b/w PT and DP of that leg divided by higher brachial SBP (b/w both arms) nl ABI = 1–1.4, <0.9 defines presence of PAD ABI <0.9 indicates lower-extremity diminished flow

Trauma

Compartment Syndrome

History

- Can occur in any closed fascial space, most commonly in leg & forearm
- Hx of trauma (fracture esp tibia; crush injury), burns, rhabdomyolysis, tight cast/dressing, hemorrhage (anticoagulants, coagulopathy), postischemic swelling, animal bites

Findings

- Rapid progression; pain out of proportion to exam, tense compartment, pain w/ passive stretch of muscles that run through compartment (see the table below), paresthesias, pallor of the extremity, taut or rigid compartment. LATE: decreased pulse, paralysis

Evaluation

- Measure compartment pressures: Nl <8 mmHg; emergent fasciotomy if delta pressure (DBP – compartment pressure) is <30 mmHg
- Historically, absolute compartment pressure above 30 mmHg was used as a diagnostic threshold. Some protocols still reference absolute pressure cutoffs; however, most modern guidelines recommend using delta pressure (DBP – compartment pressure) b/c it better accounts for perfusion
- Stryker instrument: Enter each compartment perpendicular to the skin
- A-line manometer: Attach 18G needle to A-line manometer; check that the compartment pressure being measured is at the same height as the manometer transducer
- If obtain labs: CBC, BMP, coags, CK, UA (myoglobinuria), T+S

Treatment

- Immediate orthopedic/surgical c/s for potential fasciotomy

Disposition

- Admit to ortho either for OR, or for serial manometry & neurovascular checks if compartment pressures nondiagnostic but evolving compartment synd suspected

Pearls

- Pain out of proportion is the earliest sign and should raise suspicion of compartment synd even if other sxs are absent
- Can occur w/ open fx (eg tibial fx); wound may not relieve muscle compartment pressures

Lower-Extremity Compartments & Associated Muscles	
Deep posterior	Flexor digitorum longus, tibialis posterior, flexor hallucis longus
Superficial posterior	Soleus & gastrocnemius
Lateral	Peroneus longus, peroneus brevis
Anterior	Tibialis anterior, extensor hallucis longus, extensor digitorum longus

LOWER BACK PAIN

Approach

- Careful hx: Location, unilateral vs b/l, acute vs chronic, fever, neuro sxs, incontinence, syncope, hx of trauma or cancer, worse at rest or at night, A/C

Historical "Red Flags" for Back Pain	
For cauda equina	Saddle anesthesia, LE weakness, urinary or fecal incontinence
For fracture	Age >70, any trauma w/ age >50, chronic steroids, osteoporosis, sxs of cancer (eg, weight loss, B sxs)
For malignancy	Elderly, sxs of cancer, worse when supine, >1 mo of sxs
For infection	Fever, IVDU, HIV, ESRD, DM, immunosuppression, hx of TB
For aortic/vascular	Abd pain, "tearing" pain, syncope

- PE w/ thorough neuro exam, straight leg raise, pulses, rectal tone, gait
- Imaging not routinely indicated: consider "red flags" above, neuro exam, point tenderness
- Many require only analgesia & f/u but always consider life- & limb-threatening conditions

Differential	
Pathophysiology	**Differential**
MSK	Acute lumbosacral strain, SI joint dysfxn, piriformis synd, fracture
GI	Abdominal aortic aneurysm/dissection, pancreatitis, cholecystitis, ulcer (±perforation)
Trauma	Vertebral fx (eg, compression fx), retroperitoneal bleed (can be minor/ no trauma but on anticoagulant)
Infectious	SEA, discitis, OM, pyelonephritis/perinephric abscess, herpes zoster
Neuro	Cauda equina synd or cord compression, herniated disc, spinal stenosis, radiculopathy, transverse myelitis
Rheumatologic	Rheumatoid arthritis, ankylosing spondylitis, OA
GU/GYN	Nephrolithiasis, pyelonephritis, prostatitis, endometriosis, PID
Vascular	Spinal epidural hematoma, aortic dissection
Neoplasm	Malignancy (eg, multiple myeloma), bony metastasis

TRAUMA

See Section 18 for further review of spinal trauma.

Acute Lumbosacral Strain

History
- Usually hx of precipitating event: twisting, lifting, new workout. Acute/subacute onset
- Should have no "red flag" sxs

Findings: Paravertebral muscle spasm & tenderness; nl neurovascular exam

Evaluation: No indication for imaging in acute setting

Treatment
- NSAIDs > APAP; if severe, can consider short course opioids or muscle relaxant (eg, cyclobenzaprine 5 mg TID); early activity (no bed rest!)
- Muscle relaxants of questionable value, many side effects (anticholinergic, sedation)

Disposition: D/C home w/ PCP f/u, consider PT referral; strict return instructions

Pearl: Lumbar strain is the #1 cause of LBP in ED but a dx of exclusion; consider "red flags"

Vertebral Compression Fracture

History: Acute-onset LBP usually in elderly pts w/ +/– trauma, osteopenia, smoking, chronic steroids

Findings: Midline spinal tenderness, usually no neuro findings

Evaluation: X-ray of spine first; consider advanced imaging (CT vs MRI)

Treatment
- Usually stable fx; analgesia +/– brace for comfort
- C/s spine for >50% compression, unstable fx, neuro deficits, or multiple fx

Disposition: Admit for intractable pain, any neuro findings, unstable fx, multiple fx

Pearl: Look for neoplastic cause if no other RFs or hx, esp in elderly

NEUROLOGIC

Cauda Equina Syndrome

Definition: Compression of distal lumbosacral nerve roots (many causes; trauma, infxn, disk herniation, neoplasm, spinal stenosis)—*neurosurgical emergency!*

History
- LBP shooting down 1 or both legs & neuro sxs: saddle paresthesias, LE weakness, urinary retention w/ overflow incontinence, loss of bowel control or sexual dysfxn; pts w/ recent trauma or pts w/ cancer w/ possible mets
- Determine time course of sxs

Findings: ↓ rectal tone, urinary retention/incontinence, saddle anesthesia, ↓ reflexes, LE weakness

Evaluation
- MRI is imaging test of choice
- Postvoid residual (nl <50–100 mL)

Management: Emergent NSGY c/s for surgical decompression; emergent XRT for select patient w/ malignancy, consider IV steroids if definitive management is delayed

Lumbar Spinal Stenosis

Definition: Narrowing of lumbar spinal canal from degeneration, facet arthritis, or subluxation

History: 40+ y/o, often b/l low back pain, pseudoclaudication (pain w/ walking), improves w/ sitting & flexion of back (walk hunched over to keep back flexed)

Findings: Nl exam, often nl SLR, pain w/ back extension

Evaluation: Emergent imaging not needed if nl neuro exam; CT, MRI are diagnostic

Treatment: Pain mgmt w/ NSAIDs; PT is mainstay of nonsurgical mgmt; surgery if severe

Disposition: PT referral; close f/u w/ PCP & spine

Herniated Disc

History
- Most common 30–50 y/o, presents w/ acute radiculopathy; hx of waxing/waning back pain shooting down leg (past the knee) ± paresthesias
- Exacerbated by leaning forward, coughing, sneezing, & straining (stretches nerve root)

Findings
- See table below (L4–L5 is most common)
- SLR test correlates w/ nerve root irritation only if reproduced sxs extend below knee; Ipsilateral SLR is *sens*, contralateral SLR is *spec*

Management
- Neuro intact: Analgesia, DC home. MRI (or CT myelogram if MRI not feasible) if no improvement in 4–6 wks

Disposition: Typically D/C if no red flags; o/w may need imaging/spine consultation

Pearl: Sciatica is lumbar disc herniation impinging on sciatic nerve

Lumbar Nerve Root Compression			
Root	**Pain**	**Sensory Loss**	**Weakness**
L4	Hip, anterior thigh	Anteromedial thigh to medial aspect of foot	Weak quadriceps; ↓ knee jerk
L5	Lateral thigh/calf; dorsal foot, big toe	Lateral calf, dorsal foot, big toe	↓ extensor hallucis longus
S1	Posterolateral thigh, calf, heel	Back of thigh & calf; toes, lateral heel	Gastrocnemius; ↓ ankle jerk
S2–S4	Sacrum, perineum	Perineum	Bowel/bladder; sexual dysfxn

Infectious

Spinal Epidural Abscess

History
- Most common sxs: Fever, back pain, and neuro deficit; however, classic triad present in minority of SEA patients
- High-risk population: IVDU, DM, ESRD, immunocompromised, recent instrumentation, spinal trauma

Findings
- Classic sequence: Back pain → root pain/radiculopathy → motor weakness, sensory Δ, bowel/bladder dysfxn → paralysis
- Typically elevated inflammatory markers +/– leukocytosis though neither spec
- Bacteremia and/or osteomyelitis are common; each are RFs for and potential cx D/C of SEA

Evaluation: MRI w/ IV contrast (gadolinium) is imaging of choice

Treatment
- Empiric abx (after obtain BCx): Cover *Staph* (inc MRSA), *Strep*, Gram-neg bacilli. CTX 2 g IV PLUS Vancomycin 20 mg/kg +/– antipseudomonal (cefepime, ceftazidime, or meropenem) for recently hospitalized pts, hx of DM, or device infx
- Spine surgery consultation; do not delay abx for pre-tx specimen to confirm dx!

Disposition: Admit, may require OR w/ spine surgery for decompression & drainage

Pearl: Avoid LP to prevent introduction of organisms into CSF

Neoplastic

Bony Metastasis

History: >50 y/o, 1 mo of sxs, weight loss. Commonly breast, lung, kidney, prostate, thyroid

Findings: Tenderness of spine to palpation; lumbar spine most common location

Evaluation
- Plain film (not sens). CT/MRI (or outpt bone scan) if x-ray not definitive
- MRI & spine/oncology consultation if cord synd or neuro findings

Treatment
- Pain control, oncology f/u
- If cord compression, administer dexamethasone 10 mg IV; immediate spine c/s

Pearls
- May be osteolytic (more prone to pathologic fx), osteoblastic, or mixed
- 1° malignancy (esp multiple myeloma) should also be considered, esp in elderly
- Many bony mets missed on x-rays/CT; review films w/ radiologist specifically

JOINT PAIN

Approach
- Careful hx; anatomic distribution, single vs multiple joints, acute vs chronic, a/w fevers, skin Δ; hx of trauma; A/C use
- Eval for systemic sxs in conjunction w/ chief c/o joint pain
- Arthrocentesis if concern for septic arthritis

Differential	
Pathophysiology	**Differential**
Trauma	Fx, dislocation, hemarthrosis, ligamentous injuries
Infectious	Non-GC septic arthritis, GC septic arthritis, reactive arthritis (associated w/ infxn), tenosynovitis, Lyme dz
Rheumatologic	Gout, pseudogout, rheumatoid arthritis, psoriatic arthritis, OA
Other MSK	OA, Bursitis, tendonitis, osteonecrosis

Etiology of Common Regional Joint Pains		
Region	**Type**	**Findings**
Shoulder	Rotator cuff injury	Inflammation or tear of rotator cuff tendons from direct trauma or overuse Pain in deltoid area of shoulder, worse w/ moving arm overhead or w/ direct pressure (sleeping); weakness "Empty Can Test": Weakness w/ resisted abduction of arm elevated at 90°, forward flexion at 30°, thumbs down Other physical exam maneuvers include drop arm test Tx w/ NSAIDs, avoidance of aggravating movements, PT, subacromial steroid injections if no improvement Note calcific tendonitis near rotator cuff also common cause of shoulder pain; dx on x-ray, initial treatment is similar w/ NSAIDs, PT, possible steroid injections
	Frozen shoulder (adhesive capsulitis)	Gradual ↓ ROM (active & passive) of glenohumeral joint due to joint capsule pathology; +/– preceding injury; can be precipitated by prolonged immobilization Pain at extremes of ROM Tx w/ NSAIDs, PT, 2–4-wk oral corticosteroids
	Acromioclavicular synd	Arthritis or injury to AC ligaments Acute or chronic, possible hx of trauma TTP & swelling of AC joint, pain worse w/ cross-body adduction Acute injury tx w/ sling

Elbow	Lateral epicondylitis (tennis elbow)	Pain along lateral epicondyle at attachment of extensor tendons of wrist ↑ pain w/ resisting wrist flexion Tx w/ rest, activity adjustments, NSAIDs, ±steroid injections
	Medial epicondylitis (golfer's elbow)	Less common than tennis elbow Pain along medial epicondyle at insertion of common flexor tendon Resistance to wrist extension w/ elbow in extension ↑ pain Tx w/ rest, activity adjustments, NSAIDs, ±steroid injections
Hip	Trochanteric bursitis	Common cause of hip pain (lateral aspect) Pain ↑ w/ walking, direct pressure, climbing stairs, ↓ at rest TTP of greater trochanter; resisted abduction of hip ↑ pain Tx w/ NSAIDs, PT, corticosteroid injections
Knee	Patellar tendonitis (jumper's knee)	Pain at inferior aspect of patella following or during repetitive running, jumping, kicking Tx w/ rest, NSAIDs, knee brace, PT, strengthening exercises for quads & hamstrings
Ankle	Achilles tendonitis	Pain, swelling, tenderness, over Achilles tendon from repetitive trauma & microscopic tears from overuse (ballet, distance running, basketball) ↑ pain w/ dorsiflexion Tx w/ rest, heat, NSAIDs, shoe modification, heel lift to ↓ Tendon stretching, PT, stretching exercises

Tenosynovitis

Definition

- Inflammation of tendon & tendon sheath. Can result in chronic pain, disability, ↓ ROM

Types of Tenosynovitis		
Type	**Hx & Findings**	**Management & Disposition**
De Quervain tenosynovitis	Repetitive pinching of thumb & fingers Pain improved w/ rest; no hx of acute trauma Most common in middle-aged women Pain at radial aspect of wrist, worse w/ passive ROM of thumb, ulnar deviation of wrist w/ thumb cupped in closed fist (Finkelstein test)	Rest, NSAIDs Thumb spica Steroid injection Surgery if needed Good prognosis
Stenosing flexor tenosynovitis (trigger finger)	Progressive clicking, and later locking of thumb or finger in flexion f/b sudden release Most common in middle-aged women, diabetics Pain in proximal tendon sheath in distal palm ±Palpable tendon thickening or nodularity May require manipulation to release	NSAIDs Splint 4–6 wks ±Steroid injection Surgical release if injection fails Good prognosis
Infectious flexor tenosynovitis	May develop after puncture wound, lac, bite, cracked skin, high-pressure injury Usually *S. aureus*, *Strep* **Kanavel signs:** 1. Fusiform ("sausage") swelling of finger 2. Flexed position of finger 3. Severe pain w/ passive extension 4. Tenderness along flexor tendon sheath	**Admit** to ortho/hand Abx +/− surgery Splint & elevation Fair prognosis even w/ abx, surgery

Gout

History

- Middle-aged pt w/ abrupt (often recurrent) onset single joint pain, swelling, erythema, warmth; may be precipitated by minor trauma, illness, medication or diet chgs
- RFs: Age, HTN, CKD, DM, obesity. Systemic etiologies: Cancer, hemolysis
- 75% monoarticular, classically affects 1st MTP joint (aka "Podagra")

Findings

- Red, swollen, tender, warm joint (MTP > ankle, knee, fingers, wrist, elbow)
- Inflammation often extends beyond the joint itself, causing swelling and tenderness in the surrounding soft tissues
- Tophi overlying effected joints indicate chronic gouty dz

Evaluation

- Arthrocentesis: If 1st episode (no prior tap), unclear dx, or concern for septic joint
- Joint fluid: Needle-shaped, neg birefringent crystals; always send for culture
- Serum uric acid level is of no value
- X-ray findings in chronic gout include bony erosions, punched out lesions, calcified tophi

Treatment

- Consider side effect profile when selecting treatment option
- NSAIDs (no aspirin). eg, indomethacin or naproxen for duration of attack (~3–10 d)
- OR Colchicine (D 1: 0.6 mg PO TID; D 2: 0.6 mg BID until flare resolution)
- OR steroids (prednisone 30 mg PO daily 7 d)
- Allopurinol for chronic prevention; no role in acute mgmt of gout attack

Disposition

- D/C home w/ pain control unless intractable pain; lifestyle modification education (↓ consumption of EtOH & purine-rich foods)

Pearl

- Gout is a result of monosodium urate crystal deposition

Pseudogout (Acute Calcium Pyrophosphate Crystal Arthritis)

History

- Elderly pt w/ abrupt-onset, single-joint pain, swelling, erythema, warmth; precipitated by minor trauma or illness; medication or diet chgs

Findings

- Red, swollen, tender, warm joint (knee > wrist most common; Podagra rare)

Evaluation

- If unclear dx, concern for septic joint, perform arthrocentesis
- Joint fluid: Rhomboid shaped, positively birefringent crystals
- X-ray findings: Chondrocalcinosis (seen w/ calcium pyrophosphate deposition, does not indicate arthritis), subchondral sclerosis, radiopaque calcifications

Treatment

- Same as gout

Disposition

- D/C home w/ pain control

Pearls

- Calcium pyrophosphate deposition dz can be asx, or acute crystal arthritis
- RFs: ↑ Ca, ↓ Mg, ↓ PO_4, hemochromatosis, parathyroid dz; consider metabolic dz if presentation at age <60 y

---

Bursitis

Definition

- Inflammation of bursa, which are flattened sacs lined w/ synovial membrane that helps facilitate movement; bursitis is usually due to overuse, trauma, or OA, but can be septic

History

- Discrete area of pain, swelling, erythema, warmth over a joint
- Less than half of bursitis is septic; trauma is most important RF for septic bursitis
- Most common in joints that are subject to repetitive stresses (elbow, knee), but can be deep (hip) esp in setting of instrumentation (eg, acupuncture, surgery)

Findings

- Warm, swollen, fluid-filled pocket outside the joint ± erythema
- Tenderness, fever, associated cellulitis suggest septic bursitis
- Should have minimal pain or limitation of joint movement; o/w consider septic arthritis

Evaluation

- If concern for septic bursitis, perform bursa aspiration (WBC >2k is suggestive); obtain bursal fluid culture for definitive dx
- Deep bursae may require aspiration by ortho or IR
- Often clinically difficult to differentiate from septic arthritis; may need arthrocentesis

Treatment

- Rest, ice, elevation, analgesia, ±steroid injection
- If septic bursitis: Abx for *MRSA/Strep* coverage (vancomycin & cefazoline IV; trimethoprim/sulfamethoxazole & cephalexin PO)
- C/s ortho for f/u as these have high outpt failure rate & may need surgical bursal excision or serial aspirations

Disposition

- D/C w/ pain control if no ortho intervention, ±abx
- Admit for fulminant infxn, immunocompromised pt, significant surrounding cellulitis

Pearl

- Prepatellar (carpet layer's knee) & olecranon bursitis (student's elbow) are most commonly infected; usually due to local trauma and *Staph* infxn

---

INFECTIOUS

Septic Arthritis (Nongonococcal)

History

- Acute onset of painful, swollen, warm, tender joint, often w/ fever
- Hallmark is severe pain w/ active or passive ROM
- All joints are at risk but most commonly knee > hip. In peds, hip is most common
- High-risk groups include pts w/ hx IV drug use, immunocompromised

Findings

- Usually single joint involvement; can see multijoint involvement in disseminated GC dz
- Pain w/ minimal passive/active ROM or axial load; warmth, redness, swelling

Evaluation

- X-ray to identify effusion, FB, fracture
- Arthrocentesis to differentiate from inflammatory arthritis or OA: Gram stain & culture, cell count, protein & gluc, crystal analysis, synovial lactate; positive: WBC >50,000 w/ PMN predominance (>75%). However, WBC <50,000 does not exclude septic arthritis, as may be lower esp if abx already administered, if lyme or GC arthritis; prosthetic joint infxn p/w substantially lower WBC
- Labs: Consider ESR, CRP, blood cx to isolate, UA, CXR for infectious w/u

Management

- Ortho c/s for operative washout (if arthrocentesis c/f septic arthritis); hip may need orthopedics or IR for arthrocentesis
- Abx generally after arthrocentesis & blood cultures taken; *S. aureus* is most common
- Gram stain w/ GP cocci: Vancomycin
- Gram stain w/ GN bacilli: 3rd-gen cephalosporin or antipseudomonal cephalosporin
- Neg Gram stain: Immunocompetent adult w/o trauma: vancomycin. Immunocompetent adult w trauma: vancomycin & 3rd-gen cephalosporin. Immunocompromised or IVDU: vancomycin & antipseudomonal cephalosporin
- Supportive care: Hydration, antipyretics, pain control

Disposition: Admit for abx, likely operative washout, ortho observation

Pearls

- Septic hips may not present w/ classic signs; can be subtle presentation
- Presence of crystals in the joint fluid does NOT r/o a septic joint
- Overlying cellulitis is relative CI for arthrocentesis; avoid cellulitic area during tap
- If hardware is present, discuss risk/benefit w/ orthopedics prior to arthrocentesis
- Intra-articular steroid injection for pain relief in septic arthritis is contraindicated

Gonococcal Septic Arthritis

History

- Young, sexually active pt usually w/ single painful, swollen, warm, & tender joint
- May be polyarticular or migratory; smaller joints (elbow, wrist, ankle) commonly involved
- Urethral or vaginal D/C of GC infxn may be present

Findings

- Any clinical manifestations of *Neisseria* GC infxn (cervicitis, malodorous, purulent vaginal D/C in female or dysuria & penile D/C in male)
- Swollen, tender, warm & extremely painful knee and/or small joint(s), usually slightly flexed at rest, more painful w/ ROM; may have tenosynovitis
- A painless diffuse maculopapular rash w/ necrotic/pustular centers may be present
- RUQ abdominal pain may indicate Fitz–Hugh–Curtis synd

Evaluation

- Same as non-GC septic arthritis + cervical (female) & urethral (male) cultures; blood, pharynx & rectal cultures (based on RFs) to ↑ likelihood of definitive dx
- Screen for other sexually transmitted infxns inc chlamydia, HIV, syphillis

Treatment

- Arthrocentesis, ortho c/s, splint joint in physiologic position for comfort
- 3rd-generation cephalosporin (CTX 1 g IV QD), total treatment duration at least 7 d; add doxycycline 100 mg PO BID × 7 d for chlamydia co-infxn
- Supportive care: Hydration, antipyretics, pain control

Disposition: Admit for abx, ortho observation, possible need for operative washout

Pearls

- Gram stain & culture from GC septic arthritis more often neg than non-GC septic joints
- Intra-articular steroid injection for pain relief in septic arthritis is contraindicated

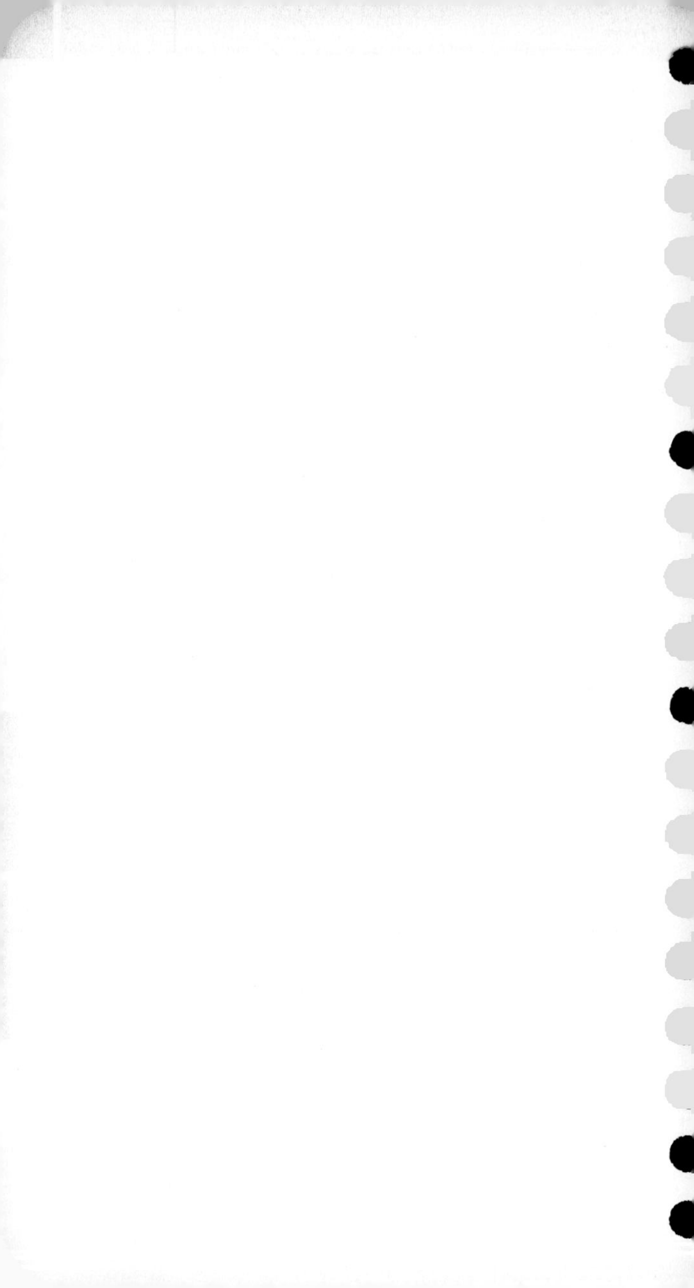

Approach

- Nature of ear pain, associated sxs, duration, fevers, hearing loss; diabetes

Otalgia Differential	
Location	**Differential**
Outer ear	OE, malignant OE, trauma, FB, herpes zoster oticus, perichondritis, allergic angioedema, juvenile spring eruption, frostbite, sunburn, tumor
Middle ear	AOM, OME, bullous myringitis, eustachian tube dysfxn, cholesteatoma
Mastoid air cells	Mastoiditis

Otitis Externa (Swimmer's Ear)

Definition

- Infxn (Acute: PsA, *S. aureus, S. epidermidis;* Chronic: *Aspergillus, Candida*) of the outer ear due to breakdown of natural barriers

History

- Summer, water exposure, cotton swab trauma, hearing aids, pain/itching/drainage

Physical Findings

- Pain w/ movement of tragus/helix, edema/erythema/exudate in canal, red TM, white/gray debris, ±abscess, conductive hearing loss if severe

Treatment

- Remove debris, irrigate w/ 1.5% hydrogen peroxide if TM intact, drain abscess if present
- Mild infxns: Topical acetic acid/hydrocortisone × 7 d; Avoid w/ ruptured TM
- Severe: Topical antipseudomonal abx + steroid × 7 d (eg, Ciprofloxacin + hydrocortisone)
  - Use wick (cotton, gauze, or cellulose) 10–12 mm into canal × 2–3 d to allow med delivery
  - If TM rupture, extension beyond canal or immunocompromised, add oral abx (eg, cipro)
- No swimming + keep ear dry in shower × 1 wk (ear plugs or cotton ball w/ petroleum jelly)

Disposition

- Home: Diabetic/immunocompromised w/ simple OE or any pt w/ severe OE = close f/u

Malignant (Necrotizing) Otitis Externa

Definition: Aggressive infxn (95% PsA) of the outer ear canal to skull base/bony structures, usually in elderly diabetics/immunocompromised

History: Ear pain extending to TMJ (pain w/ chewing), nocturnal pain, swelling, otorrhea

Physical Findings: Toxic, febrile, granulation tissue, severe inflammation, ±CN palsy

Evaluation: ESR/CRP/blood and ear cultures. CT temporal bone to eval for bony erosion which is diagnostic, then MRI to appreciate extent of involvement, underlying osteomyelitis, & intracranial extension

Treatment

- 1st line: IV ciprofloxacin; Increasing rates of resistance
- 2nd line: Ceftazidime, cefepime, meropenem, OR piperacillin/tazobactam
- Consider amphotericin B or voriconazole for aspergillus in HIV/immunocompromised

Disposition: Admx for IV abx ± operative debridement

Pearls

- 10% mortality
- Cx: Cerebral/epidural abscess, osteomyelitis, dural sinus thrombophlebitis, meningitis

Acute Otitis Media

Definition

- Effusion in the middle ear w/ acute inflammation caused by infxn (agents: *S. pneumoniae, H. influenzae, M. catarrhalis,* viral)

History: Unilateral ear pain, fever (25%), winter/spring, common 6 mos–5 y/o, URI

Physical Findings: Bulging TM, loss of light reflex/TM mobility (most sens), effusion, erythema (not sufficient alone to diagnose AOM), purulent drainage

Differential: OME (effusion w/o infxn), bullous myringitis (bullae on TM, same tx), otitis-conjunctivitis (caused by *H. influenzae*)

Treatment
- Many improve w/ no abx w/o cx
- Pain control: APAP/ibuprofen
- Nonsevere acute OM: Amoxicillin to start in 72 h if sxs do not improve
- Severe (<6 mo, b/l, bulging TM, otorrhea, fever >39 °C, systemically ill) = immediate abx
- Pediatric:
  - 1st line: Amoxicillin 90 mg/kg/d (max 1 g PO BID) × 5 d if >2 y/o, × 10 d if <2 y/o
  - Amoxicillin-clavulanate if recent abx, recurrent AOM or concurrent conjunctivitis
- Adult:
  - Amoxicillin-clavulanate 875/125 mg BID × 5–10 d (Higher dose amox recommended for age >65, immunocompromise, recent abx (<30 d)

Disposition: D/c, PCP f/u 2–3 d

Pearls
- Cx (rare): Meningitis, mastoiditis, persistent effusion/cholesteatoma → hearing loss
- If TM perforation, consider ofloxacin otic drops BID × 10 d

Mastoiditis
Definition: Extension of infxn from the middle ear into the mastoid air cells

History: Unilateral ear pain, fever, HA

Physical Findings: Mastoid tenderness, erythema, fluctuance over mastoid, outward bulging pinna

Evaluation: CT to eval extent/destruction of the septa of the air cells, MRI for intracranial cx, ENT c/s

Treatment
- Abx: Vancomycin OR linezolid ± antipseudomonal
- ±Myringotomy/tympanostomy; mastoidectomy (Indications for mastoidectomy include subperiosteal abscess, intracranial extension, not simply 50% air cell involvement)

Disposition: Admx, possible operative debridement

Pearl: Cx include labyrinthitis, meningitis, dural sinus thrombosis, petrositis, osteomyelitis, brain abscess, subperiosteal abscess, hearing loss, facial paralysis

HEARING LOSS

Approach
- Nature, acuity of onset, unilateral/b/l, associated pain/systemic sxs

Hearing Loss Differential

Cause	Differential
Infxns	Mumps, measles, influenza, herpes simplex, herpes zoster, CMV, mononucleosis, syphilis (sudden onset), viral cochleitis, meningitis
Vascular	SCD, Berger dz, leukemia, polycythemia, fat emboli, hypercoagulability, stroke
Metabolic	Diabetes, pregnancy
Conductive	Cerumen impactions, FB, OM, OE, barotrauma, trauma, TM rupture, cholesteatoma, traumatic ossicle disruption, Ménière's
Medications	Aminoglycosides, furosemide, salicylates, antineoplastics
Other	Presbycusis, congenital malformation, noise exposure, acoustic neuroma

Cerumen Impaction/Foreign Body
Definition: Buildup of earwax or FB in the external canal

History: Unilateral hearing loss, placement of FB in ear, drainage, pain

Physical Findings: Visualization or cerumen/FB in ear

Treatment
- Irrigate the external canal w/ room temperature NS (cold/hot NS can cause nystagmus/vertigo/nausea), past FB if possible. Do not irrigate batteries/perforated TM
- For live insects, use liquid lidocaine, isopropyl alcohol, or mineral oil to asphyxiate prior to removal
- For cerumen: Instill colace, mineral oil, carbamide peroxide or H_2O_2 for 15 mins to dissolve, then irrigate
- For FB: Alligator forceps OR cyanoacrylate (glue) to cotton-tipped applicator, hold against object for 60 sec; OR try suction for smooth objects

- Re-examine ear postextraction for TM rupture, canal damage, or residual FB. Consider topical abx if canal damaged

Disposition: D/c

Ruptured Tympanic Membrane

Etiologies include trauma (open hand slap over ear, lightning), FB (cotton swab, pipe cleaner), barotrauma (high altitude, diving), infxn (OM)

History: Pain, hearing loss

Physical Findings: Perforation of TM, ±blood in the canal

Treatment

- Keep ear dry (earplugs during shower, no swimming)
- Abx (eg, ofloxacin otic drops) needed if pre-existing infxn, contaminated water exposure, blood occluding canal, or drainage from associated middle ear trauma
- Operative repair likely if >¼ of TM damaged

Disposition

- Minimal hearing loss: D/c, PCP f/u in 4 wks for audiogram + repeat ear exam; persistent perforation or hearing loss at that time needs ENT referral
- Admit in acute trauma w/ associated facial nerve injury, severe vertigo, or basilar skull fracture. ER c/s to ENT if significant hearing loss for expedited f/u

ODYNOPHAGIA

Approach

- Nature, acuity of onset, duration, associated sxs (cough, fever, drooling, voice Δ, dysphagia, difficulty breathing)

Odynophagia Differential	
Cause	**Differential**
Infxns	Viral (respiratory viruses), herpangina (enterovirus), HSV, HIV, infectious mono (EBV, CMV), bacterial (*S. pyogenes, gonorrhea, N. meningitides, M. pneumoniae, Chlamydia, S. aureus, H. influenzae, C. diphtheriae, Legionella*), fungal (*Candida*), peritonsillar abscess, epiglottitis, retropharyngeal abscess, Ludwig angina, Lemierre synd
Systemic	Kawasaki, SJS, thyroiditis, Behçet synd, PFAPA synd
Trauma	Penetrating, FB, laryngeal fx, caustic ingestion, retropharyngeal hematoma
Tumor	Tongue, larynx, thyroid, leukemia

Group A *Streptococcus Pharyngitis* ("Strep Throat")

Definition: Infxn of the oropharynx caused by Group A Beta Hemolytic Strep

History: Sore throat, odynophagia, myalgias, fever; no cough, coryza, or conjunctivitis

Physical Findings: Erythematous oropharynx, tonsillar exudate, cervical LAD

Evaluation

- Centor criteria: Fever >38 °C, tonsillar exudate, tender LAD, absence of cough
- Rapid strep: Sens 70–90%, spec 95% (send culture if neg given low sens)
- GABHS culture: 90–95% sens
- Consider NAAT for chlamydia/gonorrhea (if oral sex exposure), or Monospot for EBV

Treatment

- There are multiple conflicting guidelines (*NEJM* 2011;364:648). One reasonable approach:
  - If *0–1* Centor criteria met: No testing, no tx
  - If *2–3* Centor criteria met: Rapid strep, treat if positive, confirm w/ culture
  - If *all* Centor criteria met: No testing, yes tx
- Abx: Benzathine PCN 25,000 U/kg max 1.2 million U IM × 1 OR PCN VK, OR amoxicillin. If PCN allergy: Cephalosporin, clindamycin, or azithromycin
- Dexamethasone 0.6 mg/kg max 10 mg × 1 ↓ time to pain relief (*BMJ* 2017;358:j4090)

Disposition: D/c

Pearl: Treat w/ abx to prevent scarlet fever, rheumatic fever, abscess, mastoiditis. Poststrep glomerulonephritis is not prevented w/ abx

Croup (Laryngotracheobronchitis)

Definition

- URI in children (6 mo–6 y, most common <3 y) usually by parainfluenza virus causing inflammation/exudate/edema of subglottic mucosa

History: Barky cough, worse at night, low-grade fever, following 2–3 d of URI sxs

Physical Findings: High-pitched inspiratory stridor, barking cough, hoarse voice, tachycardia, tachypnea

Westley Croup Severity Score (*Am J Dis Child* 1978;132:484)	
Inspiratory stridor	None = 0, w/ agitation = 1, at rest = 2
Retractions	None = 0, mild = 1, mod = 2, severe = 3
Air entry	nl = 0, mildly decreased = 1, severely decreased = 2
Cyanosis	None = 0, w/ agitation = 4, at rest = 5
Level of alertness	nl = 0, altered = 5
Score ≤2 = mild, 3–5 = mod, >6 = severe	

Evaluation: Neck XR typically low clinical value → narrow subglottic trachea ("steeple sign")

Treatment

- Calm child, monitor pulse oximetry
- Supportive care (no clear benefit): Cool mist, steam from shower, cold night air Dexamethasone 0.6 mg/kg, max 16 mg (↓ sxs, ↓ repeat visits) (*Cochrane Syst Rev* 2018;8:CD001955)
- Mod–severe or stridor at rest: Nebulized racemic epinephrine 0.5 mL of 2.25%. If epinephrine given, observe for >3–4 h for rebound stridor
- Severe respiratory distress: Heliox, bag-valve-mask, intubation by skilled provider

Disposition

- Admit if no improvement in ED, hypoxic, persistent stridor at rest, <6 mo old, unable to tolerate PO, requiring multiple doses of epinephrine
- Croup severity score ≤4 can usually be D/C, score ≥8 may require ICU

Pearl: Consider bacterial tracheitis if recent croup w/ acute worsening (toxic, high fever, severe respiratory distress)

Epiglottitis

Definition

- Inflammation of the epiglottis caused by *H. influenzae, Staph, Strep*, other bacteria/viruses
- Can lead to rapidly progressing, life-threatening airway obstruction

History

- Sore throat, muffled "hot potato" voice, odynophagia, respiratory distress, fever
- ↓ Pediatric incidence w/ use of Hib vaccine, now more common in adult diabetics

Physical Findings: Dysphonia, stridor, drooling, sitting in tripod position

Evaluation

- Lateral neck XR (77–88% sens): Epiglottis >8 mm ("thumbprint"), loss of vallecular air space
- Adult: If nl XR → indirect or fiberoptic laryngoscopy (have surgical airway ready)
- Pediatric: Avoid agitation (↑ risk of acute airway obstruction), do NOT attempt to visualize in the ED. OR for DL w/ anesthesia & ENT/surgery (*Curr Infect Dis Resp* 2008;10(3):200)

Treatment: Airway monitoring + Abx (CTX OR ampicillin–sulbactam, add clindamycin or vancomycin if concern for MRSA); no proven benefit w/ steroids or racemic epinephrine

Disposition: ICU admx

Pertussis (Whooping Cough)

Definition: Lower respiratory tract infxn by *B. pertussis* (Gram-neg rod)

Presentation

- Commonly a prolonged course (aka "hundred-day cough")
- Stages: (1) *Catarrhal* (most infectious): 2 wks mild URI sxs; (2) *Paroxysmal:* 2–8-wk intense paroxysmal cough ± posttussive emesis, inspiratory "whoop"; (3) *Convalescent:* Several wks of chronic cough
- ↑ Risk if unvaccinated, but immunity wanes after ~12 y; ↑ morbidity if <6 mo old

Evaluation

- Rapid PCR, nasopharyngeal culture, antipertussis toxin IgG if ≥1 y since last vaccine
- May develop PNA; consider CXR if refractory to abx

Treatment

- Droplet precautions/isolation × 5–7 d, abx (only effective in reducing transmission, not sxs)
- Azithromycin × 5 d or clarithromycin × 7 d, albuterol prn, treat household contacts
- Low threshold for empiric tx in infants, pregnant, healthcare workers

Disposition: Admit <6 mo–1 y/o or ill appearing (*Evid Based Child Health* 2012;7(3):893–956)

Lemierre Syndrome

Definition

- Septic thrombophlebitis of internal jugular vein w/ *F. necrophorum* (anaerobe) or oral strep
- Septic emboli to lung are common (can be confused w/ R-sided endocarditis)

History

- Usually previously healthy young adults w/ high fever, sore throat ± cough
- Typical course is pharyngitis that improves & then f/b severe sepsis

Physical Findings: Unilateral neck swelling, tenderness, induration

Evaluation: Contrast CT of neck +/– chest

Treatment: Abx: Piperacillin–tazobactam, carbapenem OR CTX + metronidazole. Consider adding vancomycin if catheter associated. Anticoagulation is controversial

Disposition: Admit (*Lancet Inf Dis* 2012;12(10):808–815)

SINUSITIS

Definition

- Inflammation of the paranasal sinuses. Usually viral or allergic. Acute <4 wks, chronic >12 wks
- Common bacterial etiologies: *S. pneumoniae,* nontypable *H. influenzae, M. catarrhalis*
- PsA is seen in HIV, CF, or after instrumentation
- Mucormycosis is invasive fungal sinusitis (*Rhizopus*) in diabetics or immunocompromised

Presentation

- Mucopurulent d/c, postnasal drip, cough, sinus pressure, positional HA, ±fever
- Typically progresses over 7–10 d & resolves spontaneously
- Sxs >7 d, worsening course, or worsening after improving, all suggest bacterial dz
- Consider sinusitis w/ positional HA that is worse when bending forward
- Sphenoid sinusitis is a difficult Dx, often presents late; classically worse w/ head tilt
- Nasal purulence alone does not indicate bacterial infxn (*Acta Otolaryngol* 2002;122:192)

Evaluation

- Clinical, no routine imaging. CT sens but not spec, can r/o cx
- Cx include orbital cellulitis, osteomyelitis, cavernous sinus thrombosis, cerebral abscess, meningitis, frontal bone abscess (Pott puffy tumor)

Treatment

- Supportive (analgesics, antipyretics, decongestants, steroids, antihistamines if allergic)
- Intranasal steroids (eg, fluticasone) have small proven benefit for sx control (*Cochrane* 2013)
- Abx *not routinely indicated*
  - Reserve for pts w/ sxs >7 d, worsening sxs, fever, purulent d/c, or high risk for severe infxn or cx
  - Amoxicillin-clavulanate (45 mg/kg/d max 875–125 mg PO BID) × 5–7 d
  - RFs for resistance: high-dose amoxicillin-clavulanate (90 mg/kg/d max 2000 mg BID)
  - Second line: fluoroquinolone, doxycycline, clindamycin + 3rd-gen cephalosporin

Disposition

- Vast majority are managed outpt
- Admit if toxic, severe HA, high fever, immunocompromised, poor f/u

Pearl

- Sphenoid/ethmoid sinusitis is less common than maxillary sinusitis but has significant potential cx (eg, orbital cellulites, cavernous sinus thrombosis)

EPISTAXIS

Definition: Bleeding from the nose. 90% of cases are anterior & involve Kiesselbach plexus on the septum. 10% of cases are posterior & arise from a branch of sphenopalatine artery

History

- Etiologies include URI (most common), trauma, nose picking, env. irritants (dry air), intranasal drug use, neoplasm, FB, polyps, anticoagulation/TCP
- RFs: Cirrhosis, diabetes, anticoagulation, antiplatelet tx, HTN, hematologic disorder

Physical Findings
- Evaluate w/ nasal speculum after having pt blow nose to express clots

Evaluation
- Can usually identify anterior source on exam; posterior bleeds are heavy, brisk, can cause airway compromise. If still bleeding after anterior packing, consider posterior source
- Check hct if extensive/prolonged bleeding, INR if on warfarin

Treatment
- Anterior
  - Start w/ oxymetazoline (Afrin) 3 sprays & hold pressure for 15 mins
  - May also insert cotton pledgets soaked in tranexamic acid, cocaine, lidocaine, epinephrine, or phenylephrine
  - Once vasoconstricted, try to identify a focal bleeding site, then use silver nitrate cautery in ring around bleeding (will not work on active bleeding; caution on septum)
  - If bleeding has stopped, observe for 60 mins; if recurs, insert a lubricated nasal tampon or Vaseline gauze packing (*Otolaryngol Head Neck Surg* 2020;162(1):8–25)
  - If nasal tampon is not successful, pack the contralateral side
- Posterior
  - Bleeding can cause airway compromise & be life threatening
  - Commercial double balloon device OR pass Foley catheter through nose into posterior pharynx, fill balloon, hold gentle traction
- No evidence to support use of antihypertensives in epistaxis control (*NEJM* 2009)

Disposition
- Anterior: D/c w/ 48-h f/u for packing removal, typically w/ prophylactic abx for TSS (unproven) (eg, cephalexin, amoxicillin-clavulanate, or topical mupirocin)
- Posterior: Admit w/ ENT c/s—may need sphenopalatine artery ligation/embolization
- B/l packing: Admit for tele observation; trigeminocardiac reflex, increased risk of bradycardia, and asystole

EYE PAIN & REDNESS

Approach
- Ask about FB exposure, chemicals, trauma, contact lens use, freshwater exposure
- *Always* check visual acuity. Use topical anesthetics (tetracaine, proparacaine) for exam
- Complete eye exam: Visual acuity (corrected), visual fields, external inspection, periorbital soft tissue & bones, extraocular movement, pupils (inc swinging light test for afferent pupillary defect), pressure (tonometry), slit lamp (lids, conjunctiva, sclera, cornea w/ fluorescein, anterior chamber, iris, lens), fundoscopy

Acute Angle-Closure Glaucoma
Definition: Increased IOP due to ↓ aqueous outflow. Generally due to reduced angle of anterior chamber in setting of dilated pupil pushing against trabecular meshwork

History
- Sudden onset of severe unilateral pain, HA, N/V, blurry vision, halos
- May be triggered by dim light, mydriatic drops, stress, sympathomimetics, anticholinergics

Physical Findings
- Unilateral perilimbal eye injection, ↓ VA, "steamy" (cloudy) cornea, nonreactive midsize pupil (5–7 mm), shallow anterior chamber, ↑ IOP >40 mmHg (nl <20), firm globe

Treatment
- *Immediate ophtho c/s; need for urgent laser peripheral iridotomy*
- *Reduce aqueous production:* Timolol 0.5% 1 drop q30min (avoid if CI to systemic βB), apraclonidine 1% 1 drop q30min (α-2 agonist), acetazolamide 500 mg IV (avoid in sulfa-allergic pts). Allow 1 min b/w each med. Repeat dosing until IOP <40 mmHg
- *Facilitate aqueous outflow* (miotics): Pilocarpine 2% 1 drop q15min until pupil constricts
- *Decrease vitreous volume* (osmotics): Mannitol 1–2 mg/kg IV over 30–60 mins

Disposition
- Per ophtho recs: Admit for intractable vomiting or need for systemic agents

Critical Dx		
Etiology	**Features**	**Management**
Caustic injury (chemical)	Hx: Chemical exposure PE: Corneal burns (esp w/ alkali), pain, blepharospasm	*Immediate ophtho c/s* Immediate copious (2–4 L) irrig until pH = 7
Acute angle-closure glaucoma	See discussion above	See discussion above
Retrobulbar hematoma	Hx: Often due to trauma, but also spontaneous in coagulopathy or due to tumor PE: Decreased acuity, diplopia, proptosis, afferent pupillary defect, rock hard to palpation	IOP >20 = orbital compartment synd *Immediate ophtho c/s* Lateral canthotomy if: • Conscious, ↑ IOP, ↓ VA • Unconscious, IOP >40 & proptosis • CI: ruptured globe
Penetrating trauma/scleral penetration	Hx: Blunt (blow to orbit or globe) or penetrating PE: ↓ acuity, afferent papillary defect, classically teardrop-shaped pupil, Seidel sign (aqueous leak on fluorescein)	Apply eye shield *Immediate ophtho c/s* IV abx Tetanus prophylaxis CT scan to assess for FB
Corneal ulcer/keratitis	Hx: Pain, FB sensation, photophobia, tearing, blurry vision. Recent contact lens use, UV light exposure, Bell palsy, or abrasion PE: Fluorescein: Corneal infiltrate (white spots/haze) around sharply demarcated "scooped out" epithelial defect • Herpes: Dendritic • UV keratitis: Many punctate ulcers (snowfall pattern)	*Immediate ophtho c/s* May need to debride or culture prior to abx (caused by bacteria, fungi, acanthamoeba) • Moxifloxacin or fortified cefazolin/tobramycin gtt • Cycloplegics • Acyclovir if suspect HSV
Orbital cellulitis (vs preseptal cellulitis)	Orbital cellulitis: Posterior to orbital septum, drains into cavernous sinus *Both orbital & preseptal:* • May have fever, leukocytosis • Lid swelling, erythema, warmth • Eye tenderness • ±Conjunctivitis, chemosis *Suspect orbital cellulitis if:* • Ill appearance, high fever • Pain w/ extraocular movement • Ophthalmoplegia/diplopia • Visual impairment • Proptosis • Increased IOP	*Immediate ophtho c/s* for orbital cellulitis IOP >20: Ophtho emergency CT orbit to r/o FB, abscess Obtain blood cx Start IV abx (vancomycin + CTX or ampicillin/sulbactam) In diabetics, consider mucormycosis *Admit all orbital cellulitis* If preseptal cellulitis, outpt abx w/ amoxicillin-clavulanate & ophtho recheck in 1 d Cx: vision loss, cavernous sinus thrombosis, CNS involvement, abscess, osteomyelitis
Emergent Diagnoses		
Hyphema	Hx: Pain, ↓ visual acuity, usually after blunt trauma PE: Gross or microscopic blood layering in anterior chamber, ±fixed & dilated pupil	First r/o open globe and orbital compartment synd *Discuss w/ ophtho-"eight ball" hyphema requires urgent f/u* IOP >30: Treat as glaucoma IOP <20: Use cycloplegic to prevent iris motion for pain control Elevate HOB 45 degrees Screen for FH of sickle cell Most can be D/C home w/ 1–2 d recheck, rx eye patch, activity restriction, glucocorticoid eye gtt and HOB elevation Return for ↑ pain or ↓ vision

Corneal abrasion/FB	Hx: Pain worse w/ blinking, photophobia, FB sensation PE: Conjunctival injection. Evert lids to look for FB. Use fluorescein to eval • Rust ring = metallic FB • Seidel test to r/o corneal penetration	If high velocity: XR or CT to r/o ocular penetration If embedded FB, remove w/ 27G needle tip under magnification, or burr Give tetanus prophylaxis Abx (erythromycin), use quinolone if contact use or freshwater exposure DC home w/ *ophtho f/u in 1–2 d* for recheck, rust ring removal if needed. No contacts until resolved
Anterior uveitis/ iritis	Def: Inflammatory process involving anterior chamber, iris, ciliary body, or choroid Hx: Usually due to trauma, autoimmune dz, or infxn (HSV, Lyme). Unilateral painful red eye, "deep" pain, blurred vision, photophobia Physical Findings: Perilimbal injection, photophobia (consensual suggests iritis), ± ↓ visual acuity, slit lamp shows anterior chamber cell & flare	• Traumatic iritis: Cycloplegic for comfort, *ophtho f/u in 1–2 d* • Inflammatory: Cycloplegics, c/s *ophtho* for possible steroids • Infectious: Treat the underlying infxn w/ systemic therapies, and c/s *ophtho* for possible ocular steroids
Other Causes of Red Eye		
Conjunctivitis (allergic, viral > bacterial)	Def: Inflammation of mucus membranes that line sclera/lids. Usually viral Hx: Drainage, irritation, pruritus, crusting, concurrent URI PE: Injection/edema, usually sparing limbus, o/w nl exam Gonorrhea = copious, green exudate	Culture if neonate or concern for *Chlamydia, gonorrhea* Warm soaks, artificial tears Antihistamine if allergic Abx if concern for bacterial: • Erythromycin, Polytrim • Quinolone if contact lens or freshwater exposure D/c home, ophtho f/u in 2 d if not improving C/s *ophtho if gonorrhea suspected*
Lid disorders (blepharitis, chalazion, dacrocystitis, hordeolum/ stye)	*Blepharitis:* Inflamed eyelid margins *Chalazion:* Inflamed meibomian gland (subcutaneous lid nodule) *Dacryocystitis: nasolacrimal duct* infxn. Inflamed lacrimal sac w/ redness, tenderness *Hordeolum (stye):* Abscess in eyelash follicle or lid margin (can be external or internal)	*Blepharitis:* Warm compresses *Chalazion:* Warm compresses, gentle massage *Dacrocystitis:* R/o periorbital or orbital cellulitis. If mild, d/c w/ clindamycin & warm compresses. Admit for IV abx, ophtho c/s if systemically ill *Hordeolum:* Warm compresses

VISION CHANGE & VISION LOSS

Approach

• Complete eye exam: Visual acuity (corrected), visual fields, external inspection, periorbital soft tissue & bones, extraocular movement, pupils (inc swinging light test for afferent pupillary defect), pressure (tonometry), slit lamp (lids, conjunctiva, sclera, cornea w/ fluorescein, anterior chamber, iris, lens), fundoscopy, & full neuro exam

Differential of Vision Δ & Loss	
	Differential
Painful	Trauma, glaucoma, uveitis, corneal ulcer, temporal arteritis, optic neuritis
Painless	Amaurosis fugax/TIA, central retinal artery/vein occlusion (CRAO/CRVO), vitreous hemorrhage, retinal detachment, lens dislocation, hypertensive encephalopathy, pituitary tumors, macular disorders, toxic ingestions (toxic alcohols, heavy metals), sz

Differential of Diplopia	
	Differential
Monocular	Astigmatism, cataracts, lens dislocation, medication induced
Binocular	Entrapment, CN palsy, intracranial mass effect, thyroid dz, microvascular dz

Central Retinal Artery Occlusion

Definition: Retinal artery occlusion, most commonly embolic; represents a CVA equivalent

History

- Sudden painless, monocular vision loss (or visual field cut if branch of retinal artery), may have transient loss prior to complete loss (amaurosis fugax)
- RFs: HTN, DM, CVA, AF, carotid dz, hypercoagulable, vasculitis, endocarditis, SCD

Physical Findings

- Afferent pupillary defect, funduscopic exam shows cherry-red spot at fovea, pale optic disc (late finding)
- May have carotid bruit, irregular HR, murmur; r/o temporal arteritis

Evaluation

- CBC, ESR
- Embolic w/u: Neuroimaging (CT/CTA or MRI/MRA), carotid imaging, echo, EKG

Treatment

- Initiate immediately (>2 h = irreversible vision loss). No proven therapies.
- *Immediate ophthalmologic c/s, also consider neuro consultation*
- Intermittent globe massage (to try to dislodge embolus & move it further downstream) & breathe into bag (increased CO_2 causing vasodilation)
- Reduce IOP as in glaucoma (eg, acetazolamide, mannitol, timolol); vasodilators to improve blood flow (eg, NTG)
- Anterior chamber paracentesis, surgical decompression, anticoagulation, intra-arterial thrombolysis w/ tPA, hyperbaric O_2

Disposition: Admit

Pearl: Cardiac embolus most common in >40 y/o, coagulopathies most common in <30 y/o

Central Retinal Vein Occlusion

Definition: Retinal vein occlusion, usually thrombotic

History

- Sudden painless monocular vision loss (may be gradual onset)
- RFs: CAD, HTN, glaucoma, venous stasis, hypercoagulable, DM, vascular dz, smoking

Physical Findings: Afferent pupillary defect, funduscopic exam w/ retinal hemorrhages/disk edema ("blood & thunder"), cotton wool spots

Management: Immediate ophtho c/s. Outpt hypercoagulability and cardiovascular w/u

Disposition: Home w/ ophtho follow up (may require intravitreal medications)

Temporal Arteritis (Giant Cell Arteritis)

Definition: Granulomatous inflammatory vasculitis of medium/large arteries

See Section on Headaches in Chapter IV: Neurology

Optic Neuritis

Definition

- Inflammation of the optic nerve usually due to focal demyelination
- A/w MS (⅓ pts will be diagnosed w/ MS), but also sarcoidosis, SLE, leukemia, alcoholism, syphilis, idiopathic, postviral

History: Vision loss (minimal → complete over days to wks), ↓ color perception, pain w/ eye movement

Physical Findings

- ↓Visual acuity, afferent pupillary defect, central scotoma, optic disc swelling/pallor

Evaluation: MRI shows inflammation of optic nerve, 20% have other demyelinating lesions; lumbar puncture may be used to test for oligoclonal banding

Treatment: Immediate ophthalmology/neuro c/s; IV methylprednisolone, IVIG, or plasma exchange

Disposition: Admit

Retinal Detachment

History

- Painless, classically "curtain-like" visual field deficit, "coal dust" or "spider webs," floaters, photopsia (scintilla)
- RFs include myopia, trauma, surgical hx (cataract removal), DM, HTN, malignancy (breast CA, melanoma, leukemia), SCD, eclampsia, prematurity

Physical Findings: Visual field cut, "billowing" retina, may see pigmented vitreous or visible line demarcating detachment (usually by indirect ophthalmoscopy)

Evaluation: Bedside ED ocular U/S highly sens for detachment (hyperechoic membrane attached to optic disc, does not cross midline), must differentiate from posterior vitreous detachment (no attachment to optic disc, crosses midline)

Management

- Immediate ophtho c/s if suspected
- If macula still attached, surgical repair indicated w/i 24–48 h
- Most inflammatory retinal detachments are treated medically (NSAIDs, steroids), but sometimes require emergent surgery depending on etiology, size, location

Disposition: Admit if acute

TOOTHACHE

Toothache Differential	
Trauma	Dental fractures, tooth subluxation, tooth avulsion, intrusion/extrusion
Atraumatic	Dental caries, pulpitis, pericoronitis, periapical/periodontal abscess (see Section 4), acute necrotizing ulcerative gingivitis (ANUG), alveolar osteitis

Tooth Numbering	
Upper right 1, 2, 3, 4, 5, 6, 7, 8 (midline)	Upper left (midline) 9, 10, 11, 12, 13, 14, 15, 16
Lower right 32, 31, 30, 29, 28, 27, 26, 25 (midline)	Lower left (midline) 24, 23, 22, 21, 20, 19, 18, 17

Dental Fractures

Definition

- Ellis I: Enamel only (typically painless)
- Ellis II: Enamel + dentin (painful)
- Ellis III: Enamel + dentin + pulp (pain + bleeding)

Evaluation: Consider CXR in trauma pt for aspirated fragments

Management

- Dental blocks & oral analgesia
- Ellis I: Smooth sharp edges if needed, dental f/u in 2–3 d
- Ellis II: Cover w/ calcium hydroxide paste, zinc oxide paste, glass ionomer composites (pulp necrosis 1–7%), dental f/u in 24 h
- Ellis III: Cover w/ calcium hydroxide paste, zinc oxide paste, glass ionomer composites (pulp necrosis 10–30%), dental c/s or urgent referral for pulpotomy/pulpectomy, urgent (<24-h) dental f/u
- Type II & III: PCN V or clindamycin rx recommended, limited evidence (*Dent Traumatol* 2020;36(4):314–330)
- If bleeding → gauze soaked in epinephrine, inject lidocaine w/ epinephrine into pulp

Tooth Subluxation & Avulsion

Definition: Loose teeth or loss of teeth due to trauma

Evaluation: X-ray if mobility suggests alveolar fracture

Management

- Dental blocks & oral analgesia
- Minimal mobility: Soft diet 1–2 wks, dental f/u in 2–3 d
- Grossly mobile: Stabilize w/ periodontal paste or splint, *dental f/u in 24 h*
- Avulsion: Only permanent teeth should be replanted. Transport tooth in Hank solution or milk (preserves up to 8 h). Hold by crown, do not touch root. Clean w/ nl saline rinse, replace tooth to socket w/ stabilization if w/i <60 mins. 1% loss of tooth survival for every minute out. *Immediate dental c/s w/ f/u in 24 h*

Dental Caries

Definition: Bacterial infxn of hard tooth structure (enamel, dentin, & cementum)

Presentation: Tooth pain, poor dentition

Management: Dental block & oral analgesia, dental f/u in 1–2 d

Periapical Abscess

Definition: Bacterial infxn of alveolar space

Presentation: Severe tooth pain, often fluctuant abscess

Management: Dental block. I&D if fluctuant. Abx (PCN V or clindamycin), warm saline rinses, dental f/u in 1–2 d

Acute Necrotizing Ulcerative Gingivitis (ANUG, Trench Mouth)

Definition

- Polymicrobial infxn of gums causing bleeding, deep ulcers, & necrotic gums
- RFs: Poor oral hygiene, local trauma, smoking, immunodeficiencies

Presentation

- Rapid onset diffuse mouth pain, halitosis, fever, gum bleeding
- Gingival erythema/edema, interdental papillae ulceration, gray pseudomembrane

Management: Oral anesthetic solution (viscous lidocaine), dilute hydrogen peroxide rinses QID or chlorhexidine, and abx (amoxicillin-clavulanate, metronidazole OR clindamycin), *dental f/u in 1–2 d*

Pearl: Cx: Vincent angina–spread to pharynx & tonsils

Alveolar Osteitis (Dry Socket)

Definition: Irritation of bone exposed to the oral cavity after premature disintegration of blood clot 3–5 d after tooth extraction

History: Sudden onset, severe pain after dental extraction, foul odor/taste

Management: Dental block, oral analgesia, irrigate socket, pack w/ iodoform gauze soaked in medicated dental paste or eugenol. Abx (PCN, clindamycin). *Dental f/u in 1 d*

THE PEDIATRIC PATIENT

Relevant Differences in Physiology

- Young children = larger surface area-to-mass ratio, more easily lose heat to environment; tx: warm w/ blankets/warmers as soon as possible
- Healthy children compensate to maintain BP –> hypotension, a late finding in shock
- Earliest sign of CV compromise is tachycardia –> Any unexplained tachycardia is a red flag & should be investigated
- Airway anatomy: Larynx is more anterior, epiglottis is more "floppy," occiput & tongue are relatively larger; tx: towel roll, NPA

Vital Signs

Pediatric Vital Signs			
Age	**HR**	**Systolic Hypotension**	**RR**
Neonate (<28 d)	90–205	<60	30–60
Infant (1–12 mos)	90–190	<70	24–40
Toddler (1–2 y/o)	80–140	70 + (age in years × 2)	22–37
Preschool (3–5 y/o)	65–120		20–28
School-age (6–11 y/o)	58–118		18–25
Adolescent (12–15 y/o)	50–100	<90	12–20

PEDIATRIC CRITICAL CARE

Airway

- Pretreatment: Atropine (0.02 mg/kg, max 1 mg) PRN bradycardia; lidocaine (1–1.5 mg/kg) PRN if ↑ ICP
- Sedation: Etomidate (0.3 mg/kg); ketamine (1–2 mg/kg IV)
- Paralysis: Succinylcholine (1–2 mg/kg IV); rocuronium (0.6–1.2 mg/kg)
- ETT size: 3 mm cuffed (newborns); (age/4 + 4) – 0.5 mm cuffed (>1 mos); approx. depth (cm) = ETT size × 3
- Laryngoscope size: 0 (<2.5 kg); 1 (<3 y); 2 (3–12 y); 3 (12 y to adult)

Shock

- Start w/ 20 cc/kg NS, up to 3 boluses (for distributive/hypovolemic)
- Dopamine (2–20 µg/kg/min); epinephrine (0.05–1 µg/kg/min) for cold shock; norepinephrine (0.05–1 µg/kg/min) for warm shock; dobutamine (2–20 µg/kg/min) for cardiogenic shock; in septic shock, favor norepinephrine or epinephrine over dopamine
- Consider hydrocortisone if at risk for adrenal insufficiency
- In trauma, start w/ 20–40 mL//kg NS; then add 10–20 mL/kg PRBCs

INFANTILE COMPLAINTS

Approach

Common Neonatal Presentations	
Pathophysiology	**Complaint**
GI	Poor feeding, reflux/regurgitation, vomiting, diarrhea, constipation, jaundice
Infectious dz	Fever
Other	Crying/colic, BRUE, sudden infant death synd (SIDS)
Respiratory	Stridor, apnea, cyanosis

History

- Events during pregnancy, delivery, gestational age & weight @ birth, alertness, diet, frequency of diaper Δ, crying patterns, color Δ; FH

Findings

- Weight, VS, color; undress baby → full exam

Pearl

- Many signs/sxs are nonspecific: Abnl tone, weak suck, decrease PO intake, jaundice, abnl breathing, peripheral cyanosis, vomiting

Poor Feeding

Approach

- Check for appropriate weight gain (5–7% wt loss during 1st wk nl, then gain 1 oz/d for 1st 3 mos), take a careful hx/physical exam to identify any other abnlty

Treatment

- If weight gain is appropriate & pt has no other concerning findings, attempt feeding trial

Disposition

- Pts w/ appropriate wt gain who have a reassuring eval and tolerate POs in ED may be D/C home w/ parental reassurance & outpt f/u; all other pts require further eval (see w/u for inconsolability below)

Constipation

Approach

- Differentiate functional (no underlying condition) from pathologic constipation

Constipation Differential

Pathophysiology	Differential
Obstruction	Bowel obstruction, anal atresia, meconium ileus, viral illness w/ ileus
Metabolic	Hypothyroid, hypercalcemia, heavy metal poisoning
Neuro	Cerebral palsy, Down synd, spina bifida occulta, neuromusc dz
Other	Dehydration, rectal prolapse, anal fissure, botulism, Hirschsprung dz

History

- Sx time course, Δ in stool consistency, baseline stooling patterns, 1st meconium passage after birth (>24–48 h = abnl), recent illness, V/D, fever, ingestion of honey

Findings

- Abd (distension), rectal exam (patency, stool @ vault), neuro exam (CNs, muscular tone)

Evaluation

- KUB (select cases, not routine use); consider Chem 7, TSH, Ca, heavy metal screen

Treatment

- For functional constipation: Glycerin suppository, disimpaction, increased water b/w feedings, consider bisacodyl, lactulose, enemas (toddlers and older children), high fiber diet in older children
  - In infants avoid fleets enemas (risk of hypocalcemia), mineral oil (risk of aspiration PNA)

Disposition

- Functional constipation → D/C w/ PCP f/u: Pathologic causes warrant further w/u & may require admx

Crying and Colic

Definition

- Colic: Recurrent pattern of inconsolable crying & irritability lasting >3 h/d on >3 d/wk, 3 wks–3 mos of life. Benign GI colic is Dx of exclusion

Approach

- Excessive crying/colic are nonsp complaints that can be the presenting signs of benign GI distress or life-threatening dz

Colic Differential

System	Differential
CNS	Meningitis/encephalitis, ICH
HEENT	FB in eye, corneal abrasion, OM, pharyngitis
Cardiac	CHF, SVT
GI	Gastroenteritis, intussusception, appendicitis, anal fissure, GERD, incarcerated hernia, benign GI colic, constipation, milk allergy
GU	Testicular torsion, UTI
Other	Hair tourniquet (finger, toe, penis), trauma, child abuse, extremity fracture, septic arthritis, drug ingestion, electrolyte disturbance

History
- Timing of crying, trauma, fever, medication ingestion, feeding hx, complete ROS & PMH

Findings
- Observe behavior, thorough physical exam

Evaluation
- UA; consider further testing (eg, abd U/S, x-ray, tox screen) to r/o spec etiologies

Treatment
- Treat the underlying d/o

Disposition
- Home: If etiology is thought to be benign & pt has cry-free period in ED
- Admit: If pt w/o clear etiology identified & no cry-free period in ED

Brief Resolved Unexplained Event (BRUE)

Definition
- Observed episode characterized by all 4 of the following:
  - (1) infant <1 y, (2) asx on presentation, (3) no explanation for the event after conducting hx & physical, (4) h/o sudden brief & now resolved episode
- And at least 1 of the following:
  - (1) Cyanosis or pallor, (2) absent or irregular breathing, (3) marked change in tone, (4) altered level of responsiveness
- Considered high risk if it meets any of the following criteria:
  - (1) Episode duration >1 min, (2), Age <2 mos, (3) h/o prematurity, (4) Prior BRUE, (5) CPR needed by medical provider, (6) Any concerning hx (eg, FH sudden death or SIDS) or exam (eg, abnl neuro or cardiac exam, findings c/f NAT)

BRUE Differential	
Pathophysiology	**Differential**
Cardiac	Arrhythmia, CHD, myocarditis, hemorrhage
GI	GERD
Infectious	UTI, sepsis
Metabolic	Hypoglycemia, inborn error of metabolism
Neuro	Sz, head trauma, hydrocephalus, meningitis/encephalitis
Other	Toxins/drugs, FB, NAT, nl periodic breathing, factitious disorder imposed on another
Respiratory	Respiratory infxn, airway obstruction, breath-holding spell

History
- Obtain 1st-hand account of event when possible—duration, appearance of child (central vs peripheral cyanosis, pallor, etc), preceding sxs, prior episodes, presence of apnea or gagging, muscle tone, sz-like activity, spontaneous or facilitated recovery

Findings
- Thorough physical exam inc evaluating for NAT

Management
- Eval depends if low vs high risk; consider pertussis screen if c/f exposure
- Low risk: Consider observation on pulse oximetry, PO trial, education/reassurance
- High risk: Observation on pulse oximetry, testing based on DDx

Disposition
- Pts w/ low-risk BRUE and reassuring observation/PO trial, D/C w/ f/u & CPR teaching
- Infants w/ high-risk BRUE require admx for observation & further reeval

Pearl
- Definitive etiology of the BRUE is found in only ~50% of pts

---

Sudden Infant Death Syndrome (SIDS)

Definition
- Death of child <12 mos of age that is unexplained after careful investigation, autopsy, exam of the scene, & hx; most common @ 2–5 mos

Approach
- Approach parents of SIDS pts w/ sympathy, as child abuse rare in SIDS

Risk Factors for SIDS	
Infant	Male, preterm or mx birth, low birth weight, recent viral illness, sibling w/ SIDS, prone or side sleeping position, heavy layers, bed sharing, soft bed surface
Maternal	Age <20 y/o, low SES, inadequate prenatal care, illness during pregnancy, smoking during pregnancy and/or postpartum, use of illicit drugs

Prevention

- Remind parents to lay their children on back for every sleep, use firm bed surface, avoid bed sharing, avoid smoking, avoid soft objects near sleeping infant to reduce risk

---

CYANOSIS

Approach

- Differentiate cyanosis that is central (mucous membranes, tongue, trunk—suggesting cardiopulmonary pathology, eg, 2/2 R-to-L shunt) vs peripheral (feet, hands, lips 2/2 peripheral vasoconstriction)

Definition

- Acrocyanosis: Blueness in hands, feet, around mouth seen in newborns, 2/2 peripheral vasoconstriction and variable perfusion of the extremities → nl & resolves w/i 1st few d of life
- Breath-holding spell: Prolonged period w/o attempt to breathe a/w intense crying from pain, anger, fright → benign, but Dx of exclusion

Cyanosis Differential	
Pathophysiology	**Differential**
Hypoventilation	Apnea, breath-holding spell, sz
Respiratory	Upper airway obstruction, lung dz, bronchiolitis/asthma
Cardiovascular	Cyanotic congenital cardiac dz, persistent pulm HTN of newborn
Other	Sepsis, hypothermia, methemoglobinemia, CN^-, acrocyanosis of the newborn

History

- Age of onset, central or peripheral, med ingestion, recent illness, environmental exposures
- Δ w/ crying: Improvement → respiratory etiology (↑ alveolar recruitment); exacerbation → cardiac etiology (↑ CO)

Findings

- Appearance (ill or well), VS, respiratory distress, heart murmur

Evaluation

- Pre- and postductal pulse oximetry, obtain CXR, ECG, echo if suspicion for cyanotic CHD
- Hyperoxia test: Compare ABG on RA on 100% O_2 for 10 mins, PO_2 of >150 suggestive of pulmonary rather than CHD etiology
- Improvement in O_2 sat w/ O_2, lack of murmur, nl ECG → suggests pulmonary process
- No Δ in O_2 sat w/ O_2, murmur, abnl ECG → c/f cardiac cause → obtain echo

Treatment

- O_2, identify then tx underlying condition
- Consider PGE_1 for pts <2 wks of age in circulatory failure c/f ductal-dependent CHD (note risk of apnea w/ PGE_1 administration)

Disposition

- Admit any pt who is ill appearing, low O_2 sat or PaO_2
- C/s cardiology for any pt w/ suspected congenital cardiac dz

PEDIATRIC JAUNDICE

Definition

- Yellowish discoloration of skin/tissue/body fluids from ↑ bilirubin production or ↓ excretion

Approach

- Bilirubin: Formed from degradation of hemoglobin → bound to albumin in blood (unconjugated/indirect) → conjugated in liver by glucuronyl transferase (conjugated/direct) → excreted in bile

History

- diff depends on age (neonates ≤4 wks), gestational age, breast-feeding status
- Time of onset of sx: Yellowing of skin, dark urine

Physical Findings

- Scleral icterus, jaundice, cephalocaudal progression

Labs

- Total and direct bilirubin, LFTs, CBC (hemolysis/anemia → Coombs test, smear, ABO/Rh type), reticulocyte count, serum haptoglobin
- Neonates → unconjugated can be physiologic, treat to prevent kernicterus; conjugated always pathologic

Differential Dx of Unconjugated Hyperbilirubinemia in Children	
Hemolytic disorders	ABO or Rh(D) incompatibility
	G6PD deficiency
	Sickle cell anemias
	Thalassemias
	Hereditary spherocytosis
	HUS
Enterohepatic recirculation	Hirschsprung dz, pyloric stenosis, GI obstructions
Other	Cephalohematoma, birth trauma, hypothyroidism, Down synd, polycythemia, Gilbert synd, Crigler–Najjar synd (deficiencies in glucuronyl transferase)

Benign Neonatal Hyperbilirubinemia

Definition

- Elevated unconjugated bilirubin in the 1st wk of life, 60% newborns will be jaundiced (peaks 2–5 d), due to low activity of glucuronyl transferase, increased production, & increased enterohepatic circulation

Evaluation

- Total and direct bilirubin, CBC (hemolysis/anemia → Coombs test, smear, ABO/Rh type)

Management

- Ensure below threshold for phototherapy, even if asx (see **bilitool.org**); phototherapy thresholds depend on gestational age and RFs for neurotoxicity (*Pediatrics* 2022;150(3):e2022058859)

Pearls

- Consider pathologic jaundice: Onset before 24 h of life; if persists beyond 1st wk of life; ↑ bilirubin >5 mg/dL/d; if symptomatic
- Cxs of severe hyperbilirubinemia: Kernicterus (bilirubin deposition in basal ganglia → neurodevelopmental deficits)
  - Neurotox RFs: Prematurity, albumin <3, hemolytic dz, sepsis
- Sepsis can rarely present as jaundice

Breast-Feeding Jaundice

Definition

- ↑ unconjugated bilirubinemia in breast-fed infants, generally related to inadequate milk intake, early onset after birth (peaks d 3–5)
- Insufficient breast milk intake –> ↓ stooling –> ↑ enterohepatic circulation

Evaluation

- Total/fractionated bilirubin, CBC

Management

- Breast-feeding support; see **bilitool.org** for phototherapy thresholds

Breast Milk Jaundice

Definition
- Unconjugated hyperbilirubinemia after 1st wk of life, can persist for up to 3 mos
- Sufficient intake and nl weight gain
- Thought that substances in breast milk prevent conjugation & excretion of bilirubin

Evaluation
- Total/fractionated bilirubin, CBC

Management
- Determine if above phototherapy threshold (**bilitool.org**); if Tbili <12 mg/dL continue breastfeeding and monitor; if Tbili >12 mg/dL consider alternative etiologies

ABO and Rh Incompatibility/Hemolytic Disease

Definition
- Hemolytic dz caused by maternal antibodies against fetal A or B type proteins or maternal Rh antibodies (sensitized from previous pregnancy) against Rh-positive fetus (Rh incompatibility)

History
- Jaundice w/i 1st 24 h of life, dark urine, lethargy

Physical Findings
- Severe jaundice, scleral icterus, ill appearing

Evaluation
- Total/fractionated bilirubin, CBC (hemolysis/anemia → Coombs test, smear, ABO/Rh type)

Management
- Phototherapy (see **bilitool.org**), exchange tfx
- Admit

Conjugated Hyperbilirubinemia

Definition
- Pathologic increase in direct bilirubin leading to jaundice (conjugated bilirubin >20% of total, or >2 mg/dL)

History
- Yellowing of skin, dark urine, acholic stools, lethargy, ± genetic synd/metabolic synds/sepsis

Physical Findings
- Severe jaundice, scleral icterus; if ill appearing, consider infxn

Evaluation
- Total/fractionated bilirubin, CBC, BCx, blood smear, LFTs, blood type, KUB if signs of obstruction, U/S: Biliary obstruction, UA, Ucx

Management
- Hydration, tx based on cause (see below)
- Admit

Differential Dx of Conjugated Hyperbilirubinemia in Children	
Biliary obstruction	Biliary atresia
	Choledochal cyst
	Primary sclerosing cholangitis
	Gallstone (usually pigmented stone from hemolysis in sickle cell/ thalassemia)
Infxns	TORCH infxn (toxoplasmosis, rubella, CMV, & herpes virus)
	Bacterial sepsis
	UTI
	Viral hepatitis

Metabolic	Cystic fibrosis
	Galactosemia
	a1-antitrypsin deficiency
	Wilson dz
Drugs	Aspirin
	APAP
	Iron
	Sulfa
Miscellaneous	Reye synd
	Neonatal lupus
	Neonatal hepatitis, autoimmune hepatitis

PEDIATRIC FEVER

Approach

- Fever (38 °C or 100.4 °F) mgmt is different in pediatric population compared to adults
- ABCs, check O_2 saturation, rectal temperature is most accurate (oral temp next best)
- Need for abx & hospitalization depends on age, exposures, vaccination status, suspected/identified source, severity of infxn
- Introduction of *H. influenzae* & pneumococcal vaccines have changed the incidence & etiology of febrile illness in pediatric populations

Fever Differential	
Pathophysiology	**Differential**
Pulmonary	Bronchiolitis, croup, pertussis, pharyngitis, PNA, viral URI
GI	Appendicitis, gastroenteritis, rotavirus
GU	UTI, pyelonephritis
Noninfectious	SCD, Kawasaki dz, MIS-C, rheumatologic & oncologic etiologies
Misc infxns	Cellulitis, HIV, sepsis, varicella, epiglottitis, measles, meningitis, mumps, OM, omphalitis, roseola, rubella, scarlet fever, osteomyelitis, HSV, enterovirus, bacterial conjunctivitis, nonsp viral synds

Febrile Neonate 0–21 d Old

- Difficult to localize source of infxn; any fever high-risk 2/2 immature immune sz; risk of occult bacterial infxn; standardized w/u to dx serious bacterial illnesses (*Pediatrics* 2021;148(2):e2021052228)
- Exposures (travel, ill family members) & immunizations useful to note

History

- Fever >38 °C or 100.4 °F, rectal considered standard; fussy, irritable, poor feeding
- Assess frequency & # of wet diapers, capillary refill, fontanelles, tears to estimate dehydration
- Ask about any rashes (viral exanthems, meningococcus)

Evaluation

- Sepsis w/u required: see table below

Treatment

- Less than 1 mo: IV ampicillin + either gentamicin or ceftazidime or cefotaxime
- Consider adding acyclovir 20 mg/kg IV q8h if concern for potential herpes infxn & vancomycin IV if critically ill or maternal RFs to resistant infxn
- Treat other identified bacterial source appropriately

Disposition

- If 0–21 d or <90 d & ill appearing, admit & follow cx even if all labs nl

Febrile Child 22–28 d Old

Evaluation

- For select well appearing, full-term infants w/ no obvious source of infxn can consider deferring LP; see table below (*Pediatrics* 2021;148(2):e2021052228)

Treatment

- If well appearing and no known source, should give IV abx if results suggest UTI or bacterial meningitis; consider IV abx particularly if inflammatory markers ↑

Disposition

- Limited subset may be appropriate for D/C home after dose IV abx w/ f/u in 24 h

---

Febrile Child 1–24 mos

History

- Vulnerable immune system
- Exposures (travel, ill family members) & immunizations helpful

Findings

- Irritable, poor feeding; elicit hydration status via # of wet diapers, tears, fontanelle, capillary refill
- Ask about any rashes (viral exanthems, meningococcus)

Evaluation

- Guidelines differ for 29–60 d vs 2–24 mos; (see table below; *Pediatrics* 2021;148(2):e2021052228)

Treatment

- If well appearing 29–60 d old, no known source, consider IV abx if inflammatory markers ↑
- If ill appearing w/ fever, 1 dose ceftriaxone (50 mg/kg IV & 24-h admx for cx)
- Treat identified bacterial source appropriately

Disposition

- If well appearing w/ neg w/u & fully immunized, D/C home w/ close f/u
- If well appearing w/neg w/u & incomplete immunization:
  - WBC >15k (ANC >9000), give empiric abx (ceftriaxone IV or IM) & 24 h f/u or admit if f/u uncertain
  - WBC <15k (ANC <9000), D/C w/o abx, but close f/u in 24–48 h

Pearl

- Prevalence of occult bacteremia if well-appearing, otw healthy 3–36 mos is <1%

Eval of Pediatric Fever by Age (see *Pediatrics* 2021;148(2):e2021052228)

Age	Temp	Appearance	Eval
0–21 d	>38 °C	Any	Straight cath UA & Ucx CBC w/ diff, BCx, procalcitonin, CRP CXR if ↑ RR, respiratory sxs CSF culture, cell count, Gram stain, gluc, protein, ± HSV if ↑ risk; ± enterovirus PCR Stool culture if diarrhea is present
22–28 d	>38 °C	Well	CBC w/ diff, BCx, procalcitonin, CRP If pos UA –> cath UCx If inflammatory markers nl –> consider LP If inflammatory markers ↑ –> LP required
29–60 d	>38 °C	Well	CBC w/ diff, BCx, procalcitonin, CRP If pos UA –> cath UCx If inflammatory markers nl, no need for LP If inflammatory markers ↑ –> consider LP
2–24 mos	>39 °C	Well	UTICalc (see https://uticalc.pitt.edu/) to determine need for UA & Ucx CXR if ↑ RR, respiratory sxs CBC w/ diff, BCx if c/f occult bacteremia
		Ill	UA & Ucx CBC w/ diff, BCx, procalcitonin, CRP If neg, LP CXR if ↑ RR, respiratory sxs

CONGENITAL HEART DISEASE

Approach

- Consider Dx in pts w/ sudden-onset cyanosis, hypoxemia, and/or shock, typically in the 1st 1–2 wks of life, though some pts present wks to years later
- Differentiate cyanotic vs noncyanotic, & ductal vs nonductal dependent CHD
- Pre- and postductal pulse oximetry, obtain CXR, ECG, echo if suspicious for CHD
- Hyperoxia test: Compare ABG on RA & on 100% O_2 for 10 mins, PO_2 of >150 suggestive of pulmonary rather than CHD etiology
- Give PGE1 to any pt w/ suspected ductal-dependent lesion & circulatory compromise

Definition

- Cyanotic lesions: Congenital cardiac dz w/ R-to-L shunt
- Ductal-dependent lesions: Congenital cardiac dz in which fetal life depends on a PDA, either from impaired systemic or pulmonary blood flow

Congenital Heart Dz Differential	
Type of Lesion	**Differential**
Cyanotic	Tetralogy of Fallot, [a]transposition of the great vessels, truncus arteriosus, [a]pulmonary atresia, [a]critical PS, [a]tricuspid atresia/Ebstein anomaly, total anomalous pulmonary venous return, [a]hypoplastic L heart, [a]interrupted aortic arch
Noncyanotic	PDA, ASD, VSD, AS, [a]critical aortic coarctation, PS

[a]Ductal dependent.

History

- Cyanosis, fussy baby, poor feeding

Findings

- ↓ O_2 sat, cyanosis, ↓ BP, cardiac murmur, hepatomegaly, check 4-extremity BPs

Evaluation

- ABG, response to O_2, CXR, ECG, echo

Treatment

- O_2, consider PGE_1 (alprostadil): 0.05–0.1 μg/kg/min (max 0.4 μg/kg/min) if c/f ductal-dependent lesion, side effects: bradycardia, hyperthermia, hypotension, & apnea
- Inotropic support w/ dobutamine, dopamine or epinephrine & intubation PRN

Disposition

- Cardiology c/s, ±cardiac surgery c/s, admit

Pearls

- Pts w/ ductal-dependent lesions p/w circulatory failure, usually during 1–2 wks of life
- Acyanotic lesions may p/w CHF

Tetralogy of Fallot

Approach

- Recognize/tx "Tet" spells w/ knee to chest positioning

Definition

- 4 defects: PA stenosis, VSD, RV hypertrophy, & deviation of aortic origin to the R (overriding); degree of severity dictated by degree of RV outflow tract obstruction

History

- Presentation usually w/i 1st few y of life, though rarely into adulthood
- Cyanosis (often during feeds), ↓ PO intake, agitation, ↑ RR; ↑ sxs w/ exercise, szs, CVA
- **"Tet" spell:** Infundibulum spasm → ↑ RV outflow obstruction → cyanosis, respiratory distress

Findings

- ↓ O_2 sat, systolic ejection murmur, cyanosis, squatting pt (to ↓ R-to-L shunting)

Evaluation

- See above, ECG (RAD, RVH, RAE, RBBB), CXR (boot-shaped heart), CBC, VBG

Treatment

- See above, 100% O_2, calm child, bring knees to chest; consider morphine & IV fluid bolus, correct hypoglycemia, consider propranolol, phenylephrine, intubation

Disposition
- Cardiology, cardiac surgery c/s, admit

Pearl
- Onset determined by slowly ↑ infundibulum hypertrophy → ↑ RV outflow tract obstruction → ↑ RV hypertrophy → ↑ R-to-L shunt; thus, presentations at later age have poorer long-term outcomes

PEDIATRIC RESPIRATORY

PNEUMONIA

History
- Fever, cough; quality of sputum usually cannot be ascertained (children often swallow secretions); recent URI, malaise, lethargy, n/v, SOB, nasal flaring & grunting
- Older children: Cough, SOB, abd pain, neck stiffness
- Infants/neonates: Difficulty feeding, tachypnea, restlessness, or lethargy
- RFs: Lack of immunizations/incomplete immunizations, travel, daycare

Bacterial (10–40%)
- Abrupt, follows URI, appearing ill, usually <5 y

Atypical
- Fever, malaise, & myalgia, HA, photophobia, sore throat, & gradually worsening nonproductive cough

Viral
- Nontoxic, associated upper airway sxs (runny nose, nasal congestion)

Physical Examination
- Fever, tachypnea (most sens), O_2 saturation; full pulmonary exam (rales, rhonchi, decreased breath sounds)

Evaluation
- **Labs:** CBC (elevated WBC), Chem 7 (severe dehydration), BCx (if seriously ill); consider viral panel (inc RSV)
- **Imaging:** CXR

Treatment
- Supportive: IVF (if dehydrated), O_2 monitoring & therapy
- Viral: Supportive
- Abx (duration is generally 5–7 d), add vancomycin if critically ill
  - *Neonate*—generally ampicillin + gentamicin inpt
  - *1–3 mos*—3rd-gen cephalosporin + macrolide inpt
  - *3 mos–5 y*—3rd-gen cephalosporin + macrolide (inpt) or high-dose amoxicillin (outpt)
  - *5–18 y*—3rd-gen cephalosporin + macrolide (inpt) or macrolide alone (outpt) vs amoxicillin (outpt) if c/f typical bacterial PNA
  - If c/f atypical PNA – azithromycin preferred

Disposition
- Home: Immunizations up to date, HD stable, on room air, >3 mos
- Admit: Tachypnea (>70 breaths in <12 mos & >50 breaths in older children), retractions in infants, respiratory distress, nasal flaring, cyanosis or hypoxemia (O_2 <92%), intermittent apnea, grunting, poor POs, signs of dehydration, social concerns, inadequate f/u, sepsis, immunosuppressed, comorbidities, cx, virulent pathogens

ASTHMA AND BRONCHIOLITIS

History

Asthma
- Cough (usually early), dyspnea & wheezing (generally worse at night). Consider frequency, severity, duration, home txs, required past txs, baseline peak flow, number of ED visits, hospitalizations, ICU admx, intubations
- Triggers: Exercise, infxn, cold air, allergens, any respiratory irritant

Bronchiolitis (usually <2 y of age)
- Fever, cough, wheezing, variable degree of respiratory distress; viral exposure (RSV most common, but also parainfluenza, adenovirus, influenza, rhinovirus, human

metapneumovirus, COVID-19). Often prior 1–3-d hx of nasal congestion & mild cough
- RFs for severity: Prematurity, low birth weight, <12 wks old, pulmonary or cardiac dz, airway defect, congenital dz, immunodeficiency, neurologic dz

Physical

Asthma

- Tachypnea, tachycardia, inspiratory/expiratory wheezes, decreased or no air movement, accessory muscle use, anxious/agitated; consider using asthma severity score (eg, Pediatric Asthma Severity Score)

Bronchiolitis

- Same as asthma; may hear crackles & have signs of other infxns such as OM

Evaluation

- **Pulse oximetry:** Continuous, unless very mild sxs
- **Labs:** Usually not necessary, clinical dx; consider viral testing if admx
- **Imaging:** CXR only if concomitant PNA suspected or if c/f FB aspiration
- **Peak flow** (asthma): In children >6 y (compare to predicted based on height)

Treatment

- Supportive: ABCs, O_2 therapy (O_2 sat >90%)

Asthma

- Mild/mod:
  - **Albuterol:** 0.15 mg/kg (max 5 mg) q20–30min × 3 doses (short-acting beta-agonist)
  - **Ipratropium bromide:** 250 μg/dose (<20 kg) OR 500 μg/dose (>20 kg) q20–30min × 3 doses may decrease need for hospitalization
  - **Steroids:** Dexamethasone 0.6 mg/kg PO (max 16 mg) preferred OR methylprednisolone 1–2 mg/kg IV (max 60 mg)
- Severe (add):
  - **Albuterol:** As above but may be used continuously
  - **Magnesium:** 25–75 mg/kg IV (max 2 g) once over 20 mins (optimal dose unknown)
  - **Heliox:** 80% helium/20% O_2. Use only if O_2 saturation can be maintained above 90%
  - **Terbutaline or epinephrine:** Terbutaline 0.01 mg/kg SC (max 0.4 mg) q20min × 2 doses and/or epinephrine 0.01 mg/kg SC (max 0.4 mg) q20min × 3 doses
- Ventilation:
  - **Noninvasive** (BiPAP): May reduce respiratory fatigue & improve oxygenation/ventilation
  - **Intubation:** For impending respiratory failure; use large ETT; consider permissive hypercapnia (increased expiratory time & low VTs to prevent barotraumas). Consider ketamine for induction (bronchodilating properties)

Bronchiolitis

- Supportive tx is mainstay inc humidified O_2, suctioning, oral hydration
- Consider HFNC if mod/severe respiratory distress
- Trial of albuterol if suspected reactive airway dz, continue only if response
- Nebulized hypertonic saline not routinely used; not a/w decreased hospital LOS after controlling for heterogeneity (*JAMA Pediatr* 2016;170(6):577)

Disposition

Asthma

- Reassess in 2 h (more frequent if sxs more severe) after nebulizers, steroids, O_2 therapy
- Home: Improved peak flow (to >70% predicted), significant improvement in RR/O_2 saturation; D/C w/ inhaled beta-agonist, consider repeat dexamethasone dose @ 24–48 h (vs steroid burst; see *Adult Asthma Table* for further home management) w/ close f/u
- Admx:
  - Floor: Persistent wheezing w/ nasal flaring, ↑ RR, hypoxia, & unable to tolerate POs
  - ICU: If pt maintains severe wheezing/poor air movement w/ peak flow <50% & worsening tachypnea or possible impending respiratory fatigue, PCO_2 >42 mmHg, need for PPV or intubation, requiring continuous nebs, heliox, or terbutaline

Bronchiolitis

- Home: Age >2 mos, no hx of intubation, RR <45, no/mild retractions, O_2 sat >92%, tolerating PO
- Admx: Age <6 wks, apnea, hypoxia, persistent respiratory distress, significant comorbidities or immunosuppression, dehydration

Bronchopulmonary Dysplasia

Definition

- Chronic lung dz in preterm neonates w/ hx of ICU, malnutrition, exposure to high O_2 concentrations, mechanical ventilation, inflammation, infxn (sepsis, postnatal infxns) & PPV → impaired alveolar/pulmonary vascular development

Dz Severity	
Severity of BPD	**O_2 Supplement >36-wk Postmenstrual Age**
Mild	None
Mod	<30% O_2
Severe	>30% O_2 &/or pos pressure

History

- Preterm birth, hx of ICU stay w/ supplemental O_2, mechanical ventilation, recent respiratory infxn, poor feeding, need for O_2 support at 28 d

Physical Examination

- Abnl VS, nasal flaring, retractions, grunting, wheezes, rales, decreased breath sounds

Evaluation

- CXR—hyperinflation, cystic areas, scarring; RSV testing to guide dispo

Treatment

- Supportive; O_2, consider inhaled & systemic corticosteroids, abx (see *Pediatric Pneumonia*), bronchodilators (see *Pediatric Asthma*), furosemide (1 mg/kg q6–12h, titrate to effect)

Disposition

- Admx: If increased respiratory distress, hypoxia, hypercarbia, new pulmonary infiltrates, inability to maintain oral hydration, RSV infxn

Upper Airway Emergencies

Definition

- Actual or impending obstruction of the upper airway

Approach to the Patient

History and Exam

- Agitation or fidgeting, cyanosis, AMS, choking, SOB, increased work of breathing, panic, unconscious, unusual breathing noises, voice change
- ROS **(fever, drooling)**, PMH/MEDS **(see differential chart)**

Diagnostics

- CXR and/or neck x-ray, esp if abnl O_2 sat & temp

Treatment

- O_2, calm the child, head tilt, chin lift, "position of comfort" (upright while leaning forward)
- Largely will depend on hemodynamic stability & degree of airway obstruction

Upper Airway Obstruction Differential	
Pathophysiology	**Differential**
Structural	Tracheomalacia, laryngomalacia, tumors, macroglossia
Infectious	Peritonsillar abscess, epiglottitis, retropharyngeal abscess, bacterial tracheitis, croup
Other	Allergic rxn, chemical burns, FB aspiration, trauma

Foreign Body/Upper Airway Obstruction (See Adult Respiratory Section)

Croup (Laryngotracheobronchitis)

Definition

- Viral infxn primarily of the larynx & trachea (parainfluenza common), ages 6 mos–6 y

History

- Hoarseness, barking cough & inspiratory stridor w/ variable degree of respiratory distress; preceded by nonsp respiratory sxs (rhinorrhea, sore throat, cough); fever is usually low grade

Physical Examination
- Inspiratory stridor, retractions, decreased air entry; assess for stridor at rest

Evaluation
- Labs: None
- Imaging: Not routinely indicated; obtain if c/f alternative dx (eg, FB aspiration)
- CXR: PA view may show steeple sign, (subglottic narrowing), lateral view may reveal a distended hypopharynx (ballooning) during inspiration

Treatment
- Supportive: Humidified air, O_2, keep child as comfortable as possible
- Steroids: Dexamethasone (0.6 mg/kg × 1, max of 16 mg)
- Racemic epinephrine (2.25% solution) neb: 0.05–0.1 mL/kg (max 0.5 mL) diluted in 3 mL NS (may repeat q20–30min), for children w/ stridor at rest, requires 2–3-h observation for "rebound stridor"

Disposition
- Home: If maintaining O_2 saturation; advise symptomatic tx w/ Tylenol & humidified air
- Admit: If hypoxia, depressed sensorium, mod to severe respiratory distress, persistent sxs s/p txs above, stridor at rest, poor oral intake/dehydration

Epiglottitis

Definition
- Pharyngeal infxn classically due to *H. influenzae;* incidence in children has declined since introduction of *H. influenzae* vaccine, most common organisms now include *S. pyogenes, S. aureus, S. pneumoniae*

History
- Fever is usually 1st sx w/ abrupt onset sore throat, stridor, labored breathing, drooling muffled/hoarse voice, age 2–7 y, lack of cough

Physical Examination
- Toxic, irritable, anxious, sitting in tripod or sniffing position (chin hyperextended & leaning forward), drooling, retractions, adenopathy; may visualize edematous epiglottis on oral exam (do not attempt oral exam if c/f impending airway obstruction)

Evaluation
- **Labs:** Postpone IV & labs until airway secured; CBC, BCx, Chem 7
- **Imaging:** Lateral neck x-ray not required if high or low suspicion; findings: swollen epiglottis (ie, thumbprint sign), thickened aryepiglottic folds, obliteration of the vallecula, & dilation of the hypopharynx

Treatment
- Supportive: O_2 therapy, keep child as comfortable as possible; place child & caregiver in a quiet & controlled environment for complete eval/tx
- Airway: Preferable secured in OR under controlled environments, but if not available, consider ketamine sedation & fiberoptic vs VL intubation (single attempt) w/ cricothyrotomy kit at bedside for emergent surgical airway; tracheostomy
- Abx: Ceftriaxone or cefepime PLUS Vancomycin
- c/s: ENT or anesthesia for STAT OR airway

Disposition
- Admit: All to the ICU

Pearls
- Avoid procedures which may cause distress to the pt & further compromise airway
- Give child or parent Yankauer suction to maintain secretions & alleviate associated anxiety

Bacterial Tracheitis

Definition
- Infxn of subglottic region causing edema, pseudomembrane formation; polymicrobial (*S. aureus, S. pneumoniae, H. influenzae, Pseudomonas, Moraxella*), average age 3 y

History
- Preceding URI infxn w/ rapid deterioration, high fevers, age 3 mos–5 y

Physical Examination
- Stridor, retractions, tachypnea, barking cough, wheezing, high fevers, toxic appearing

Evaluation
- Labs: None
- Imaging: X-ray shows subglottic & tracheal narrowing, irregular tracheal margins, PNA

Treatment
- Supportive: O_2, frequent suctioning; assess need for intubation, use one size smaller ETT
- Broad-spectrum abx: 3rd-gen cephalosporin or ampicillin-sulbactam PLUS vancomycin

Disposition
- ICU

PEDIATRIC ABDOMINAL PAIN

Approach
- Nature of pain: Duration, location, constant/intermittent, relation to eating, associated sxs
- PMH: Previous abd surgeries, prematurity
- Exam: Always perform genital exam in males to r/o testicular torsion
- Labs: CBC, CRP, BMP, UA, LFTs, lipase if in the upper abdomen

Abd Pain Differential		
Location	**Infancy**	**Childhood/Adolescence**
Mechanical	Malrotation w/ midgut volvulus, intussusception, hernia, Meckel diverticulum, Hirschsprung	Constipation, hernia, Meckel diverticulum, bowel obstruction
Inflammatory/ infectious	NEC	Gastroenteritis, appendicitis, HSP, pancreatitis, gastritis, biliary tract dz, colitis
GU	UTI	UTI, renal colic, pregnancy/ectopic, PID, testicular/ovarian torsion
Other	Colic, trauma, NAT	DKA, trauma, sickle cell, toxic ingestions, PNA, strep pharyngitis

APPENDICITIS

History
- Diffuse/periumbilical pain → localizing to RLQ, anorexia, n/v, irritability (may be the only sx in age <2), fever

Physical Findings
- RLQ tenderness, rebound/guarding, pain w/ coughing/hopping/percussion, Rovsing sign (RLQ pain w/ palpation in LLQ), psoas sign (RLQ pain w/ hip extension), obturator sign (RLQ pain w/ leg flexion + internal hip rotation)

Evaluation
- Labs: CBC w/ diff, CRP, UA (sterile pyuria/mild hematuria), hCG (if female)
- Consider use of score (eg, Pediatric Appendicitis Score) to inform risk of appendicitis
- Imaging: U/S (90% sens: much lower if perforated/large habitus/operator dependent) -> CT scan (95% sens/spec) if U/S equivocal & high suspicion

Treatment
- Surgical c/s for operative mgmt; start abx (ceftriaxone 50 mg/kg IV [max 2 g] + metronidazole 10 mg/kg)

Pearls
- 90% of children <2 y/o have perforation at presentation (thinner-walled/looser omentum → ↑ perforation)
- Young children may not have anorexia

INTUSSUSCEPTION

Definition
- Invagination of part of bowel into another, most commonly ileocolic (most frequent cause of SBO in <6 y/o)

History
- Age 3 mos–3 y (peak 5–9 mos), M > F, vomiting, intermittent fussiness/crying/ inconsolability w/ drawing legs to chest, cramping abd pain, lethargy (esp in infants)

Physical Findings

- Not tender b/w episodes, abd tenderness, RUQ sausage-like mass, heme + stool, "currant jelly" stool (late finding in <1/3 of pts)

Evaluation

- Upright plain abd film to r/o free air, crescent sign; U/S (95% sens/spec): Target sign, bull's eye, doughnut, pseudokidney sign

Treatment

- Pneumatic/hydrostatic enema (diagnostic and therapeutic; 90% successful; main risk is perforation); surgical c/s for operative mgmt if enema fails

Disposition

- PO challenge and observation; consider D/C w/ strict return precautions vs admit

Pearls

- <3 y/o likely idiopathic
- Enema is contraindicated if peritoneal signs or c/f perforation
- If >3 y/o, consider abnl lead point (eg, tumor, Meckel, polyp)

Malrotation with Midgut Volvulus

Definition

- Malrotation & weak fixation of the duodenum & colon during embryologic development → twisting of the mesentery causing duodenal obstruction/SMA compression → necrosis

History

- Neonate (1/3 in 1st mo life, most in 1st y, some older) acute abd pain, bilious vomiting, ±distension, irritability/lethargy, FTT

Physical Findings

- Ill appearing/dehydration, heme + stool/grossly bloody, abd tenderness, often peritonitis

Evaluation

- Infant ill appearing, bilious emesis, and/or peritonitic –> high suspicion –> surgery c/s
- Upright plain films: "Double bubble" (dilated stomach & duodenum, can also occur in duodenal atresia), pneumatosis, SBO; U/S: "Whirlpool sign"; upper GI series (diagnostic): "Corkscrew sign," coiled spring appearance of jejunum

Treatment

- Immediate surgical c/s for operative mgmt, NGT, NPO, abx, fluids

Disposition

- Admx

Incarcerated/Strangulated Hernia

Definition

- Defects in the abd wall that allow protrusion of abd contents through the inguinal canal

History

- More commonly male, abd/groin/testicular pain, inguinal fullness w/ prolonged standing/ coughing, vomiting, irritability in infants

Physical Findings

- Intestine/BS in scrotal sac; unable to reduce (incarcerated); dusky skin (if strangulated)

Evaluation

- Scrotal/abd U/S if physical exam is unclear, x-ray can be used to r/o free air

Treatment

- Reduction: Place in Trendelenburg → gentle pressure ± ice analgesic/BZD; >12-h concern for perforation/ischemia → surgical mgmt

Disposition

- Admx if operative mgmt required

Meckel Diverticulum

Definition

- Omphalomesenteric duct remnant w/ 60% containing heterotopic gastric (80%) or pancreatic tissue

History

- Any age (sxs usually begin <2 y/o), ±LLQ pain, melanotic stool (acid secretion → ulceration/erosion of mucosa; usually painless), vomiting, SBO, intussusception

Physical Findings

- LLQ mass, heme + stool/brisk bleeding, abd distension

Evaluation

- Technetium scan (Meckel scan): Identifies heterotopic gastric tissue (90% sens)

Treatment

- Type & cross/transfuse for brisk bleeding, surgical c/s for Meckel diverticulectomy

Meckel's Rule of 2s
2% of the population
2× more common in males than females
~2% of those w/ Meckel are symptomatic
2 inches long
2 ft proximal to ileocecal valve
Presents in the 1st 2 y of life
2 main types of epithelium: gastric & pancreatic

Necrotizing Enterocolitis (NEC)

Definition

- Inflammatory condition of intestinal wall, bacterial overgrowth w/ translocation, spectrum from mucosal injury to necrosis

History

- Preterm neonate (90%), age <1 mo (usually 1st d of life), bilious vomiting, abd distension, bloody stool, new feeding intolerance

Physical Findings

- Ill appearing, hypotension, lethargic, abd tenderness, heme + stools, diarrhea

Evaluation

- Abd x-ray: Pneumatosis intestinalis (75%), portal venous air, ileus

Treatment

- NPO, hydration/tfx, NGT, broad-spectrum abx (eg, ampicillin plus gentamicin plus metronidazole), surgical c/s

Disposition

- Admit

Pearls

- Bell stages: I. Vomiting, ileus, II. Intestinal dilation/pneumatosis on x-ray, III. Shock/perforation
- Cxs: DIC, strictures, obstruction, fistulas, bowel resection/short gut synd

Hirschsprung Disease

Definition

- Absence of ganglion cells in the myenteric plexus of the colon → constant contraction & proximal dilation → constipation, obstruction (4:1 male predominance)

History

- Chronic constipation, delayed 1st meconium, FTT, abd distension, vomiting

Physical Findings

- Sx in 1st d to wks of life, palpable stool in abdomen, tight sphincter, fecal mass in LLQ, no stool in rectal vault, "squirt" sign—explosive release of stool when finger is withdrawn from rectum

Evaluation

- Abd x-ray: Dilated colon/fecal impaction/air fluid levels; Barium enema or anal manometry; Dx → biopsy (aganglionosis)

Treatment

- Outpt surgical eval

Disposition

- D/C unless cx (eg, perforation, enterocolitis)

PEDIATRIC NAUSEA AND VOMITING

Approach

- Common sxs of many dz processes (eg, intra-abd causes, metabolic derangements, toxic ingestions, neurologic causes)

History

- Relation to eating, bilious (require eval for obstruction) vs nonbilious, ability to tolerate POs, urine output, presence of bloody stools, HA, AMS

Labs

- Consider CBC, BMP, LFTs, lipase, serum gluc (↑ risk of hypoglycemia), UA

Treatment

- Treat underlying cause, antiemetics in pts >6 mos, hydration (PO or IV)

Nausea & Vomiting Differential		
Location	**Infancy**	**Childhood/Adolescence**
Mechanical	GERD, malrotation w/ midgut volvulus, intussusception, pyloric stenosis	Constipation, hernia, Meckel diverticulum, bowel obstruction
Inflammatory/ infectious	NEC, gastroenteritis, sepsis, meningitis, PNA, OM	Gastroenteritis, OM, appendicitis, pancreatitis, HSP, biliary dz
GU	UTI	UTI, renal colic, pregnancy/ ectopic, PID, testicular/ ovarian torsion
CNS (persistent vomiting w/o systemic/GI sxs)	Hydrocephalus, intracranial injury/ tumor	Hydrocephalus, intracranial injury/tumor, migraine
Metabolic	DKA, urea cycle defects, fatty acid oxidation disorders, amino acidopathies, organic acidurias	DKA, urea cycle defects, fatty acid oxidation disorders, RTA, adrenal insufficiency
Other	Toxic ingestions, trauma, Reye synd	Trauma, toxic ingestions

Pyloric Stenosis

Definition

- Hypertrophy of the pylorus, 5:1 male-to-female ratio

History

- 2–5 wks of age (rare after 3 mos), nl feeding after birth → nonbilious (± blood streaked) projectile vomiting after feeding, weight loss, hungry, lethargy

Physical Findings

- RUQ olive-size mass, dehydration (loose skin, sunken eyes, dry mucous membranes)

Evaluation

- BMP (hyperchloremic hypokalemia metabolic alkalosis)
- U/S study of choice: + pylorus >3 mm thick, >16 mm long, 95% sens; upper GI series: "String sign," abd x-ray: Dilated stomach

Treatment

- Hydration, electrolyte repletion, surgical c/s for pyloromyotomy

Disposition

- Admit

Gastroesophageal Reflux Disease

Definition
- Loose esophageal sphincter → retrograde passage of food into esophagus

History
- <2 y/o, nonbilious vomiting/spitting during/after eating, irritability, type of formula (cow vs soy; to help differentiate from milk protein intolerance)

Physical Findings
- Sandifer synd: Startled/jerky movements after eating, often confused for sz

Evaluation
- Outpt w/u: 24 pH probe (most sens), nuclear milk scan, barium swallow, heme + stools (if esophagitis present), bloody diarrhea can indicate formula allergy

Treatment
- Small feeding volumes w/ burp breaks, keep semiupright for 30–40 mins after eating, thicken feeds by adding cereal
- Most do not require acid-reducing agents, but consider PPI trial if GERD (vs GER)

Disposition
- Home

Gastroenteritis

Definition
- Vomiting & diarrhea caused by infectious source

History
- Vomiting & diarrhea, abd discomfort, sick contacts, travel

Physical Findings
- Lethargy, dehydration (skin turgor, cap refill, mucous membranes, tears, VS)

Evaluation
- BMP (if severely dehydrated), stool culture/ova/parasites (protracted/bloody diarrhea)

Treatment
- Electrolyte correction, hydration (PO preferred, IV PRN), most self-resolve, avoid antimotility agents (↑ pain/cramping/prolonged sxs)
- Ondansetron PRN if >6 mos; consider abx for certain infxns (see table below); consider zinc if developing country

Disposition
- Home or admit (eg, if severe dehydration, bicarb <16 mEq/L, inability to tolerate POs)

Etiology-sp Sxs & tx of Gastroenteritis			
Agents	**Classic Hx & Findings**	**ED Intervention**	**Clinical Pearls**
Viral			
Rotavirus	Watery diarrhea, in fall (Southwest)/winter (Northeast) mos; common among children attending daycare or preschool	Hydration	Very infectious; routine vaccination to prevent infxn
Adenovirus	Watery diarrhea w/ concurrent respiratory illness, conjunctivitis; usually in spring or early summer	Hydration	
Norwalk virus (Norovirus)	Watery diarrhea w/ fever, HA, & myalgia	Hydration	Major cause of diarrhea outbreaks
Bacterial			
C. jejuni	Watery or bloody diarrhea w/ fever & crampy abd pain	Hydration & azithromycin, erythromycin, or ciprofloxacin	Contracted through contaminated food or water; can cause GBS

Shigella	Diarrhea possibly w/ blood/mucus/pus a/w fever, HA, & abd pain	Hydration; fluoroquinolone, Bactrim (TMP/SMX), ampicillin, or azithromycin	Contracted through contaminated food or water; increasing abx resistance
Salmonella	Watery or bloody diarrhea w/ fever	Hydration; if high-risk invasive dz ciprofloxacin, azithromycin, ampicillin, or Bactrim (TMP/SMX)	Abx can induce a carrier state Treat only if risk of invasive dz (eg, <3 mos, SCD, immunosuppression)
E. coli	Watery diarrhea (ETEC) vs bloody diarrhea (EHEC)	Hydration; generally avoid abx	Tx w/ abx may trigger HUS in pts w/ *E. coli* 0157 (controversial)
V. cholerae	Profuse watery diarrhea, "rice water" stools	Hydration; tetracyclines or azithromycin	
V. parahaemolyticus	Watery, sometimes bloody diarrhea in pt who ingested inadequately cooked seafood	Hydration; doxycycline, fluoroquinolones	Risk of sepsis in pts w/ liver dz
Y. enterocolitica	Diarrhea possibly w/ blood/mucus/pus a/w fever, vomiting, & RLQ pain	Hydration	Can mimic appendicitis
C. difficile	Diarrhea a/w recent abx use	Hydration; Metronidazole PO or vancomycin PO	Toxic megacolon very rare in children, but possible
S. aureus	Foodborne toxin mediated w/ abrupt, dramatic onset of sxs w/i 2–6 h of ingestion	Hydration, supportive care	
Parasitic			
G. lamblia	Watery diarrhea & excessive, particularly malodorous, flatulence; exposure to daycare or mountain streams	Hydration & supportive care; metronidazole PO	
C. parvum	Diarrhea often a/w water exposure	Hydration; if immunocompetent, consider nitazoxanide (for those ≥1 y/o)	Choline resistant; pts should not swim for 2 wks after sxs resolve

PEDIATRIC GU/RENAL

Urinary Tract Infection

History

- Adolescents: Dysuria, urgency, frequency, hematuria; fever; flank pain, abd pain
- Young children: Fever (2–23 mos can use UTICalc [see https://uticalc.pitt.edu/] to guide likelihood of UTI), enuresis, foul-smelling urine, abd pain, n/v
- Infants: Fever, irritability, poor feeding, vomiting, jaundice, FTT

Physical Examination

- Fever, suprapubic tenderness, bladder fullness; CVA tenderness; consider assessing for vaginitis

Evaluation
- **Labs:** UA/Ucx (may require straight cath for clean specimen); Chem 7 (dehydration), CBC/BCx (if considering sepsis)
- Renal U/S in young child b/w 2 mos & 2 y w/ 1st UTI
- VCUG for recurrent infxns, poor urinary stream, palpable kidneys, unusual organism, HTN, bacteremia or sepsis that fails to respond to abx, unusual presentation, or hydronephrosis/scarring seen on renal U/S

Treatment
- Supportive: Oral rehydration if child able to tolerate o/w establish IV for hydration
- Abx (usually *E. coli*):
  - IV: Cefazolin or ceftriaxone or gentamicin
  - PO: Cephalexin or cefdinir or augmentin

Disposition
- Home: Stable, tolerating POs, nontoxic appearing; PCP f/u in 2–3 d
- Admit: <2 mos old, toxic appearing, vomiting/unable to tolerate POs, signs of urinary obstruction, suspected sepsis, underlying comorbidities, ↑ Cr

---

Fluid and Electrolyte Abnormalities

Definition, History, Physical Examination, Evaluation
- See *Abnormal Electrolytes (Section IX)* for etiologies

Treatment
- Supportive: Continuous cardiac monitoring, obtain EKG, O_2 sat monitoring
- Electrolyte monitoring: Chem 7, Ca (& ionized Ca), Mg, phosphorus
- Electrolyte correction:
  - Hyponatremia: See *Adult Metabolic section*; determine volume status; children should not be corrected >10 mEq/L/d in hypovolemia; acute onset <48-h hyponatremia can be corrected more quickly over 24 h; 3% NS 3–5 mL/kg for severe neuro sx (ie, szs); tx underlying cause
  - Hypernatremia: See *Adult Metabolic section* for Na correction (goal Na reduction rate of 0.5 mEq/L/h); consider vasopressin/DDAVP for DI
  - Hypokalemia: Correct alkalosis, hypomagnesemia
    - IV: 0.5–1 mEq/kg/h IV (max 40 mEq/dose) over 1–2 h. Goal ↑ potassium by 0.3–0.5 mEq/L (require ECG monitoring)
    - PO: 1–4 mEq/kg/d PO in divided doses (max 20 mEq/dose)
- Hyperkalemia:
  - Calcium gluconate: 100 mg/kg/dose IV, up to adult dose
  - Calcium chloride (code situation): 10–20 mg/kg/dose IV, up to adult dose over 2–5 mins
  - Gluc + insulin: 1 g/kg IV of $D_{25}W$ (max 25 g) + 0.1 U/kg/dose IV (max 10 U) regular insulin
  - Sodium bicarbonate: 1–2 mEq/kg/dose IV (max 50 mEq) over 5–10 mins
  - Albuterol: 2.5–10 mg nebulized (dose based on weight)
  - Furosemide: 1–2 mg/kg IV/PO
  - Kayexalate: 1 g/kg PO (max 30 g)
  - Dialysis
- Hypocalcemia:
  - Symptomatic: Calcium gluconate: 100 mg/kg IV slowly over 5–10 mins to control szs; use calcium chloride (dose as in hyperkalemia) in code situation
  - Asx: Calcium carbonate: children: 20–65 mg/kg/d PO divided QID
- Hypercalcemia:
  - NS: (Weight-based bolus + 1.5 times maintenance); furosemide
  - C/s endocrine, consider bisphosphonates, calcitonin
  - Dialysis: In extreme hypercalcemia & renal failure
- Hypomagnesemia:
  - PO: Magnesium gluconate 10–20 mg/kg/dose TID/QID
  - IV: Magnesium sulfate 25–50 mg/kg IV over 2–4 h (max 2 g)
- Hypermagnesemia:
  - NS infusion, furosemide 1 mg/kg/dose q6–12h; titrate to effect
  - Calcium gluconate/calcium chloride (same dose as hyperkalemia)
  - Dialysis: Severe renal failure, cardiac or neuromuscular dysfxn

Disposition
- Home: Mild, asx electrolyte abnlty may be D/C home w/ PCP f/u in 1–2 d for repeat labs
- Admit: All pts w/ symptomatic electrolyte abnlty should be admitted & monitored; consider ICU-level care for unstable pts or those w/ severe cardiac or neurologic disturbances

PEDIATRIC ENDOCRINOLOGY

Pediatric Diabetic Ketoacidosis

History
- Fatigue & malaise, n/v, abd pain, polydipsia, polyuria, polyphagia, weight loss, dehydration, AMS/HA (may be signs of cerebral edema), fever/sxs of infxn (cough, URI sxs, dysuria, rash); toddlers may not p/w classic sxs
- RFs: Infxn/illness, poor compliance w/ insulin, growth, inadequate caregiver

Physical Examination
- AMS, tachycardia, tachypnea, Kussmaul respirations, normo- or hypotensive, delayed capillary refill, mottled, lethargy/weakness, fever, n/v, acetone on breath

Evaluation
- Labs: FSG, Chem 10 (elevated anion gap acidosis, pseudohyponatremia, total body K generally depleted despite lab value, ↓ phosphorus, ↓ Mg), urine/serum ketones, beta-hydroxybutyrate, HgbA1C, UA, CBC w/ diff, lactate, lipase, LFTs, urine hCG, VBG; ABG if hemodynamically unstable or comatose; blood & Ucxs if febrile
  - Corrected Na = measured Na + (1.6 × [measured gluc – 100]/100)
  - Definition: Gluc >200 + venous pH <7.3 or bicarb <18 + ketonemia or ketonuria
- ECG: T wave Δ (hyper/hypokalemia)
- Imaging: If concern for focal infxn or precipitant that warrants imaging

Treatment
- Supportive: Continuous cardiac monitoring, O_2 sat monitoring, 2 large-bore IVs, evaluate & treat sources of infxn
- Electrolyte monitoring: Gluc fingerstick q1h (goal = 150); Chem 7, Ca, Mg, phosphorus, beta-hydroxybutyrate, and VBG q2h

Acute Tx (see *Pediatr Diabetes* 2022;23(7):835–856)	
Medication	**Dose/Frequency**
IV hydration	NS bolus 10–20 cc/kg over 20–30 mins (before electrolytes result) + maintenance (assume fluid deficit 5–10% BW maintenance fluids should have Na in 0.45–0.9% range) "Two-bag system" often used, rate 1.5 maintenance Add dextrose once serum gluc <250 mg/dL
Insulin	0.1 U/kg/h w/o insulin bolus (consider 0.05 U/kg/h if pH >7.15) *Persistent anion gap:* Continue drip *Anion gap resolved:* Δ to SC insulin (overlap IV w/ SC by 2–3 h)
Electrolyte repletion	Potassium: if K <3.5 give K before starting insulin (promotes K entry into cells); Add 20–30 mEq/L IVF (K: 3.5–5) OR 40 mEq/L IVF (K <3.5). Replete when K <5.5 HCO_3: ↑ risk of cerebral edema; avoid use Phosphate: Replete if <2, monitor for hypocalcemia
Mannitol or hypertonic saline (signs of cerebral edema)	*Mannitol:* 0.5–1 g/kg IV over 10–15 mins (may repeat in 30 mins if no improvement) *Hypertonic saline:* 2.5–5 cc/kg over 10–15 mins × 1

Disposition
- Admit: All pts; hemodynamically unstable, pts w/ cerebral edema/AMS, or newly diagnosed diabetes pts should go to the ICU; some settings may require ICU for insulin infusion

Pearl
- Children at greater risk of developing cerebral edema (watch for HA, vomiting, AMS), which has 25% mortality rate; avoid insulin bolus & large-volume isotonic fluid boluses

Pediatric Hypoglycemia

Definition

- Gluc <50 in children; gluc <40 w/ age 3–24 h; gluc <50 in infants >24 h of age

Hypoglycemia Differential	
Pathophysiology	**Differential**
Congenital	Glycogen storage disorders, disorders of gluconeogenesis, disorders of fatty acid metabolism
Autoimmune/ endocrine/ neoplasm	Hypothyroidism, insulinoma, hypopituitarism, adrenal insufficiency, glucagon deficiency, GH deficiency
GI	Liver pathology, Reye synd
Other/meds	Oral hypoglycemics, pentamidine, alcohol ingestion, salicylates, sepsis, other critical illness

Approach to the Patient

History

- Irritability, sweating, jitteriness, feeding problems, lethargy, cyanosis, tachypnea, and/or hypothermia. May be a/w sepsis, congenital heart dz, ventricular hemorrhage, tox, & respiratory distress synd, PMH/meds (see chart)

Physical Examination

- Hypotonia, lethargy, cyanotic, hypothermic, apneic, tachycardic, pallor, vomiting, tremulousness, sz

Evaluation

- Labs: FSG, Chem 7, LFTs, serum insulin, UA (ketones), C-peptide (low in exogenous insulin, high in insulinoma or sulfonylureas); growth hormone, cortisol, glucagon levels; tox screen if indicated

Treatment

- Gluc replacement
  - PO: Gluc paste, fruit juice (preferred), or formula/breast milk for infants
  - IV infants: IV bolus: 10% dextrose: 2 mL/kg then recheck in 15 mins
  - IV children: IV bolus: 10% dextrose at 5 mL/kg then recheck in 15 mins
  - IM: Glucagon 0.03 mg/kg/dose SC q20min PRN up to × 3 (not to exceed 1 mg/dose)

Disposition

- Home: If obvious cause treated, sx reversed, tolerated high-carbohydrate meal
- Admit: No obvious cause, toxic ingestion w/ oral hypoglycemic, long-acting insulin, persistent sxs

PEDIATRIC NEUROLOGY

Pediatric Seizure

Approach

- ABCs, check O_2 saturation, temperature, determine if still seizing
- Immediate bedside gluc fingerstick, consider administering empiric gluc
- If actively seizing, quickly administer suppression medications
- Hx: Description of events before & after sz and sz episode, fever, associated sxs (HA, photophobia, vomiting, visual Δ, ocular pain), focal neurologic sxs, prior sz
- Assess for head or neck trauma, meningismus, skin findings (petechiae, café-au-lait spots, port-wine stain, ash leaf spots), ↑ ICP (bulging fontanelle)
- Thorough neurologic exam; Todd's paralysis: Transient paralysis after a sz
- CBC, CMP, tox screen, anticonvulsant levels, UA, CXR, other infectious w/u
- Consider CT or quick brain MRI if persistent AMS, neurologic deficit, or trauma
- Consider LP after head imaging if persistently AMS, fever, & c/f CNS infxn
- EEG o/p unless concern for nonconvulsant status epilepticus
- Status epilepticus is continuous sz activity lasting >5 mins or recurrent sz w/o return to baseline MS
- Can result in cerebral hypoxia, lactic & respiratory acidosis, hypercarbia
- Dispo: Dependent on etiology and exam/results of eval

Sz Differential	
Pathophysiology	**Differential**
Neurologic	Status epilepticus, febrile sz, degenerative CNS dz (neurofibromatosis, tuberous sclerosis, Sturge–Weber synd), epilepsy, cerebral palsy
Head injury	IPH, SAH, SDH, epidural
Infxn	Meningitis, encephalitis, brain abscess, toxoplasmosis, tetanus, neurocysticercosis
Metabolic	Hypoglycemia, hyperglycemia, hyponatremia, hypernatremia, hypocalcemia, hypomagnesemia, alkalosis, pyridoxine deficiency
Toxic	Lead, PCP, amphetamine, cocaine, aspirin, CO, organophosphates, theophylline, lidocaine, lindane, drug w/d
Neoplasm	Brain tumor
Pediatric	Reye synd, CMV congenital syphilis, maternal rubella, PKU
Vascular	Embolism, infarction, HTN encephalopathy, malformations
Other	Psychogenic nonepileptic szs (PNES), hyperventilation, breath-hold spells, missed anticonvulsant dose/insufficient dose, inborn errors of metabolism, syncope

Primary Seizures

History

- Presence/absence of aura, abrupt onset & termination of sz activity, stereotyped purposeless behavior, fecal or urinary incontinence, postictal confusion or lethargy
- Characteristics depend on type of sz; may have LOC

Evaluation

- As above

Treatment

- Acute vs chronic meds, airway mgmt often w/ only nasal trumpet, supplemental O_2
- **Abortive tx**
  - 1st line: BZD (can repeat × 1 after 3–5 mins)
    - IV: lorazepam 0.1 mg/kg up to 4 mg; IM or IN: midazolam 0.2 mg/kg up to 10 mg; PR: diazepam 0.2–0.5 mg/kg (based on age) round to nearest 2.5 mg up to 20 mg
  - 2nd line >28 d: Levetiracetam 60 mg/kg (max 4.5g) OR fosphenytoin 20 mg PE/kg (max 1.5 g) OR valproic acid 40 mg/kg (avoid if liver dz); if persistent sz given alternative 2nd-line agent
  - 2nd line <28 d: Phenobarbital (20 mg/kg IV load), watch for hypotension & bradypnea
  - 3rd line: Midazolam 0.1–0.2 mg/g IV bolus –> 0.1 mg/kg/h drip OR pentobarbital 5 mg/kg bolus –> 1 mg/kg/h drip
  - 4th line: Propofol & intubation
- If refractory szs, give pyridoxine 100 mg IV; consider thiamine 100 mg IV in adolescents
- **Long-term Anticonvulsant Medications**
  - If known sz disorder & subtherapeutic levels, load w/ chronic med
  - Long-term anticonvulsants not routinely indicated for 1st unprovoked sz

Pearls

- Keep diff broad even if known sz d/o, esp if tx med levels
- If meningitis suspected, give abx preemptively while awaiting confirmation
- Pseudoseizure (PNES) is dx of exclusion
- Consider neuro c/s if starting new long-term med in 1st-time sz (will need close f/u)

Epilepsy

History

- Typical sz recurrence, may be a/w lip biting, incontinence of bowel or bladder f/b lethargy/combativeness & confusion (postictal period); may or may not have LOC

Evaluation

- As above

Management

- Acute vs chronic meds, airway mgmt often w/ only nasal trumpet, supplemental O_2
- Dispo depends on the precipitant, change from baseline
- Neuro f/u for medication adjustment if indicated

Pearls

- Keep diff broad even if known sz d/o, esp if tx med levels
- Systemic illness, such as URI or fever, can lower sz threshold

Cerebral Palsy

History

- Nonprogressive lesion sustained during brain development → motor, speech, & learning disabilities, high risk (50%) for szs. Prematurity is the biggest RF

Findings

- Depends on type of cerebral palsy:
  - Quadriplegia: Hypotonic trunk & spastic extremities
  - Diplegia: Spastic lower extremities, ↑ DTRs, clonus, & "scissoring"
  - Hemiplegia: Unilateral spasticity, usually UE > LE
  - Athetoid/Dyskinetic: Writhing, involuntary movements of extremities
  - Ataxic: Unsteady, uncoordinated movements
  - Hypotonic: Low muscle tone

Evaluation

- Head CT or quick brain MRI if new-onset sz or recent trauma
- Outpt EEG if new onset sz or Δ in sz pattern or frequency

Treatment

- Standard sz tx

Disposition

- Neuro f/u for medication adjustment if indicated

Pearls

- Pts w/ cerebral palsy often have breakthrough sz & low sz thresholds, look for underlying illness (URI, PNA, UTI, etc) or other precipitant; adjust outpt meds w/ primary neurologist
- Pts w/ cerebral palsy may also commonly present to the ED w/ aspiration, PNA, feeding difficulties, G-tube malfxn, UTIs

Pediatric Sz Types	
Sz Type	**Findings**
Generalized absence	Staring spell w/ loss of motor/speech activity, w/ brief LOC
Generalized tonic–clonic	Contracted posture f/b rhythmic jerking movements of extremities in pts w/ impaired consciousness
Atonic	Sudden loss of muscle tone
Myoclonic	Repetitive, rhythmic muscular contractions
Focal aware	Unilateral tonic–clonic movements, nl consciousness
Focal w/ impaired awareness	Unilateral tonic–clonic movements w/ impaired consciousness, both cerebral hemispheres involved
Somatosensory	Focal; numbness, tingling, paresthesias, or visual Δ
Autonomic	Focal; Δ in HR, pupil size, sweating, aphasia
Infantile spasms	<1 y/o; spasms of neck, trunk, extremities; often in clusters

Febrile Seizures (*Pediatrics* 2011;127(2):389–94)

History

- Sz a/w T ≥38 °C (100.4 °F) in child b/w 6 mos & 5 y of age
- No hx of prior afebrile sz; no evidence CNS infxn or other clear precipitant

Findings

- Simple febrile sz: Generalized sz activity, lasts <15 mins, no recurrence in 24 h, not focal
- Complex febrile sz: Last >15 mins OR >1 sz in 24-h period OR focal component

Evaluation

- If actively seizing, treat w/ abortive medication esp if >5 mins
- Evaluate for source of fever; full neurologic exam when at baseline
- Antipyretic, observation until pt back to baseline, parental reassurance
- Routine blood tests, EEG, and neuroimaging not required for simple febrile sz
- Consider neuro c/s for complex febrile sz

Disposition

- 1st febrile sz, nonfocal exam, reassuring ED w/u can be D/C w/ f/u

Pearls

- Consider meningitis/encephalitis, esp in unvaccinated children; perform LP if concern
- Febrile sz not a/w brain damage; low-risk epilepsy ~2%,
- Incidence of another febrile sz is ~35%
- >2 febrile sz/y or >3 total febrile sz should be evaluated for other etiologies

Pediatric Meningitis

History
- HA, fever, neck stiffness, lethargy, AMS, n/v, rash, irritability, sz, vaccination status, recent abx use

Findings
- Meningismus (stiff neck) occurs <15% of the time in children <18 mos old, bulging fontanelle, petechial rash, irritability/lethargy, hemodynamic instability, fever, sz

Evaluation
- If bacterial etiology suspected, abx should be given immediately, then LP (see Section 5)

Treatment
- Abx
  - <1 mo: Ampicillin + gentamicin OR cefepime +/– vancomycin if c/f MRSA
  - >1 mo: Vancomycin plus ceftriaxone 1st line
- Consider adding IV acyclovir if c/f HSV encephalitis (20 mg/kg q8h for <3 mos; 10–15 mg/kg q8h for 3 mos–12 y, 10 mg/kg q8h for ≥12 y)

Clinical Pearl
- Ampicillin necessary to cover *Listeria* in infants

PEDIATRIC LIMP

Approach
- Examine abdomen, genitalia, spine, hips, long bones, knees, ankle, feet; observe gait
- Careful hx from pt & caregiver: Acute vs chronic, fevers, skin Δ; trauma
- Obtain x-rays, although pain is often referred (classically, knee pain referred from hip)
- Consider systemic sxs in conjunction w/ chief c/o joint pain

Limp Differential	
Pathophysiology	**Differential**
Trauma	Fracture, dislocation, sprains, hemarthrosis, back pain
Hematologic	Sickle cell anemia, hemophilia
Neuromuscular	Peripheral neuropathy, muscular dystrophy, myositis
Infectious	Septic arthritis, transient synovitis, osteomyelitis, gonococcal arthritis, discitis, epidural abscess, lyme
Rheumatologic	Juvenile rheumatoid arthritis, gout, pseudogout, lupus, rheumatic fever, reactive arthritis
GI/GU	Psoas abscess, testicular torsion, orchitis, appendicitis
Musculoskeletal	Legg–Calvé–Perthes dz, SCFE, Osgood–Schlatter dz
Neoplastic	Leukemia, Ewing sarcoma, osteosarcoma, osteochondroma

Infectious

Septic Arthritis of the Hip

History
- Most commonly in children <3 y/o, but can occur at any age
- Limp or refuse to walk, hx of fever & irritability (sxs may be more subtle in infants)

Findings
- Often febrile & toxic appearing
- Flexed, externally rotated, abducted hip; antalgic gait (if walking)
- Significant pain w/ ROM but not necessarily warm, swollen, or erythematous

Evaluation
- ↑WBC, ↑ CRP, ↑ ESR arthrocentesis shows ↑WBC, +Gram stain & +culture
- Consider lyme testing
- X-rays & U/S may show effusion

Treatment
- Orthopedic consultation for drainage & washout in the OR
- Abx: IV Vancomycin & ceftriaxone
- Pain control

Disposition
- Admit for surgical wash-out

Pearl
- Most cases pediatric septic arthritis in lower extremities: Hip > knee > ankle
- Kocher criteria described to help predict probability septic arthritis of Hip; 4 factors: Temp >38.5 °C, WBC >12, ESR >40, refusal to bear weight
- CRP >20 is also predictive

Predicted Probability of Septic Arthritis of Hip (%)	
No. of Factors	**Kocher Criteria**
0	<0.2
1	3
2	40
3	93.1
4	99.6

Results above from initial study of children with hip pain (*J Bone Joint Surg Am* 1999;81(12):1662–1670).

Transient (Toxic) Synovitis

History
- 3–6 y/o, M:F 2:1, acute or chronic unilateral hip, thigh, or knee pain
- May have low-grade fever, possibly recent URI

Findings
- Nontoxic appearing
- Limited hip ROM 2/2 pain; mild restriction of passive ROM to internal rotation & extension; most sens to log roll
- Antalgic gait, painful to palpation

Evaluation
- X-ray of hip nl; may show effusion
- WBC & ESR nl or slightly ↑; afebrile children w/ nl labs can generally avoid arthrocentesis
- U/S can diagnose effusion, but cannot differentiate type

Treatment
- Pain control w/ NSAIDs, heat & massage

Disposition
- Orthopedic f/u, consider crutches to keep weight off hip until pain resolves

Pearls
- Most common cause of acute hip pain in children from 3- to 10 y; arthralgia & arthritis secondary to transient inflammation of the synovium of the hip
- Recurrence rate <20%, most develop w/i 6 mos, no ↑ risk for juvenile chronic arthritis, few may develop Legg–Calvé–Perthes dz

---

Musculoskeletal

Legg–Calvé–Perthes Disease (Idiopathic Avascular Necrosis of Femoral Head)

History
- Most commonly in 5–7 y/o w/ limp & pain in groin, thigh, or knee; worse w/ ↑ activity
- No fever or irritability, no hx of trauma; more common in males > females

Findings
- Nontoxic appearing, antalgic gait
- ↓ Hip ROM secondary to pain w/ possible thigh atrophy, ↑ w/ internal rotation & abduction

Evaluation
- WBC & ESR nl
- X-rays often nl initially; frog-leg views helpful
  - Widening of cartilage space
  - Subchondral fx of femoral head; linear lucency in femoral head epiphysis
  - Femoral head opacification & flattening known as coxa plana

Treatment
- Goal is to avoid severe degenerative arthritis, maintain ROM, relieve weight bearing
- Orthopedic eval; bone scan & MRI more diagnostic than x-rays

Disposition
- Orthopedic f/u, crutches to keep weight off hip until pain resolves

Pearls

- Idiopathic osteonecrosis of capital epiphysis of femoral head; 15–20% cases are b/l
- Caused by interruption of blood supply to capital femoral head → bone infarction
- Better prognosis at younger onset; proportional to degree of radiologic involvement
- A/w Stickler synd: Rare condition, most common cause pediatric retinal detachment; consider screening w/ Cambridge "LCP-Plus" score (*Arch Dis Child* 2023;108(10):789–791)

Slipped Capital Femoral Epiphysis (SCFE)

History

- 12–15-y/o boy or 10–13-y/o girl, c/o limp & groin, thigh, or knee pain; obesity is key RF
- If sxs >3 wks, considered chronic
- If unable to bear weight, considered unstable (higher cx rate)

Findings

- Affected leg externally rotated, shortened w/ pain when flexing hip; antalgic gait

Evaluation

- nl temp, WBC, ESR
- X-ray: Femoral head is displaced posteriorly & inferiorly in relation to femoral neck w/i confines of acetabulum ("scoop of ice cream slipping off cone"); AP & frog-leg views best (avoid frog-leg if c/f unstable)

Treatment

- Orthopedic c/s for operative internal fixation; nonweight bearing; goal to prevent AVN of femoral head

Disposition

- Admx for orthopedic surgery

Pearls

- Obesity is the RF; genetics play role; bilaterality more common in younger pts who also tend to have metabolic/endocrine disorders
- If traumatic hip injury w/ obvious external rotation & shortening of the leg, do not force ROM as this can worsen epiphyseal displacement

Osgood–Schlatter Disease

Definition

- Microtrauma to the tibial tubercle tuberosity apophysis occurring due to overuse

History

- Preteen/adolescent w/ knee pain, more common in males; worse w/ activity, better w/ rest

Findings

- Edema & pain of tibial tubercle; enlarged & indurated tibial tuberosity
- Tender over anterior knee, esp over thickened patellar tendon
- Pain reproduced by extending knee against resistance, stressing quads or squatting w/ knee in full flexion, running, jumping, kneeling, squatting, stairs

Evaluation

- Clinical dx. X-ray may show swelling over tuberosity & patellar tendon; no effusion

Treatment

- Guided by severity: Range from decreasing activity in mild cases to rest in severe cases
- NSAIDs for pain control, ice, ±crutches

Disposition

- D/C home w/ pain control

Pearls

- One of the most common causes of knee pain in adolescent; benign & self-limited
- B/l in ~25% of cases; 50% give hx of precipitating trauma

PEDIATRIC EXANTHEMS

Refer to Section 8 "Dermatology" for additional relevant content

ERYSIPELAS

Definition

- Infxn caused most commonly by *Strep pyogenes*

History
- Any age but > in children <3 y

Physical Findings
- Red, hot, tender area of skin, sharp demarcation, acute onset ±fevers

Treatment
- Penicillin G 60,000–100,000 units/kg/dose q6h

Viral Exanthem

Definition
- Diffuse rash caused by nonpolio enteroviruses (coxsackievirus, echovirus, enterovirus) & respiratory viruses (eg, adenovirus, parainfluenza virus, influenza, RSV)

History
- Any age, recent viral illness

Physical Findings
- Diffuse blanchable erythematous macules on trunk & extremities

Treatment
- Supportive

Disposition
- Home

Hand-Foot-and-Mouth Disease

Definition
- Caused by coxsackievirus B

History
- Summer/fall, 1–4 y/o

Physical Findings
- Ulcerative oral lesions on soft palate, macular → pustular → crusted lesions on palms/soles, resolves in 5–6 d

Treatment
- Supportive

Disposition
- Home

Impetigo

Definition
- Secondary infxn in pts w/ underlying dermatoses caused by *S. aureus* & *Strep pyogenes*

History
- Warm humid summer mo, any age

Physical Findings
- Papule/vesicle → golden crusted lesions commonly around mouth & on cheeks

Treatment
- Topical abx (2% mupirocin 1st line), or oral dicloxacillin, 1st-gen cephalosporins

Disposition
- Home

Kawasaki Disease

Definition
- Systemic vasculitis of microvessels of unknown etiology, often self-limited

History
- Febrile illness, peak onset 18–24 mos, usually in children <5 y of age

Physical Findings (*Circulation* 2017;135(17):e927–e999)
- To make dx classic Kawasaki dz, need unexplained fever × 5 d + 4 of the following:
  - Edema and erythema of hands/feet and/or periungual desquamation

- B/l bulbar conjunctival injection
- Polymorphous rash-may be maculopapular, resemble erythema multiforme, or erythroderma
- Cervical LAD
- Mucous membrane Δ of oropharynx (ie, strawberry tongue, cracked lips, erythema of pharyngeal mucosa)

- If do not have all of these features may have incomplete Kawasaki dz; consider if prolonged fever w/o etiology, esp in infants, and some of features above

Evaluation
- Typical lab findings: CBC w/ diff (↑ WBC, ↑ PLT), ↑ LFTs, ↑ ESR, ↑ CRP, sterile pyuria on UA
- Also obtain ECG, echocardiography (for coronary artery aneurysm, other cardiac cx)

Treatment
- High-dose ASA 100 mg/kg/d divided QID (consider avoiding if also influenza+)
- IVIG 2 g/kg (reduces risk of coronary artery aneurysms)
- Can consider adding steroids for pts at high risk of IVIG resistance; however lack reliable predictor of high-risk pts in North America

Disposition
- Admit

Complications
- #1 cause of acquired heart dz in children
- Cxs: Coronary artery aneurysm, CHF, MI, dysrhythmias, valvular insufficiency, gallbladder hydrops, uveitis

---

SERUM SICKNESS

Definition
- Immune-complex–mediated type III hypersensitivity rxn

History
- Any age but > in children <3 y, fever, arthralgias, rash, possible etiologies include blood products, antitoxins (eg, spider or snake envenomations), meds

Physical Findings
- Fever, rash (urticarial, serpiginous)

Treatment
- Supportive as dz is self-limited, resolves in 2–3 wks, discontinue offending agent
- Short course of corticosteroids can be used for severe arthralgias

Disposition
- Home

IGA VASCULITIS (HENOCH–SCHÖNLEIN PURPURA)

Definition
- Small-vessel vasculitis, predominantly in children age 2–11 y/o but can also affect adults

History
- Commonly p/w rash, develops into purpura; fever, arthralgia, abd pain, bloody stools, hematuria; preceding respiratory infxn (eg, Group A beta-hemolytic *Strep*)

Physical Findings
- Palpable purpura in dependent regions and/or petechiae, fever, joint swelling, guaiac pos, scrotal edema

Diagnosis
- Clinical; other findings may include: CBC (↑ WBC, ↑ PLT, anemia), ↑ ESR, antistreptolysin antibodies (+ in 50%), UA (hematuria, proteinuria, pyuria), abd U/S (intussusception), scrotal U/S

Treatment
- Majority is self-limiting w/ resolution in a few wks; supportive, NSAIDs, treat underlying infxn
- Corticosteroids does not prevent recurrences, which occurs in ~1/3, but can be used for severe arthritis, renal involvement, GI, scrotal, or CNS cx

Disposition

- Home unless cx: HTN, oliguria, obstruction, intussusception, GIB

Complications

- Intussusception (most common GI cx), renal failure, bowel obstruction, perforation, hypertensive encephalopathy, acute scrotal pain (mimics torsion), pancreatitis, CNS cx (sz, neuro deficits)

NONACCIDENTAL TRAUMA

History

- Historical factors that raise concern: Injuries not consistent w/ stated mechanism, mechanism not consistent w/ developmental stage, inconsistent histories, unexplained delay in care, presentation at mx care sites w/ traumatic injuries
- RFs: Age <5 (<1 y highest risk), prematurity, chronic medical conditions, disability, young parent, poor social support

Physical Findings

- High-risk bruises, high-risk fractures, burns (esp forced immersion burns in stocking & glove pattern or patterned contact burns in shape of object), head trauma, retinal hemorrhages, traumatic retinoschisis should raise concern
- High-risk bruises: Nonambulatory child; see **TEN-4-FACESp** decision rule (below)
- High-risk fractures: Rib fractures (esp posterior), mx fractures (esp different stages healing), metaphyseal (corner) fracture, femur or humeral fracture <18 mos, unusual fracture w/o severe witnessed mechanism (ie, scapula, sternum, vertebrae), nonambulatory child

Evaluation

- Thoroughly document pertinent hx & physical; consider uploading photos to medical record following institutional protocols
- **TEN-4-FACESp** – validated clinical decision rule to help screen children <4 y w/ bruising; acronym stands for findings c/f NAT: bruising to **T**orso, **E**ars, **N**eck, **F**renulum, **A**ngle of the jaw, **C**heeks, **E**yelids or **S**ubconjunctivae, or bruising anywhere in children ≤**4** mos, or any patterned bruising (*JAMA Netw Open* 2021;4(4):e215832)
- Recommended w/u based on age and clinical eval
- Labs: CBC, coags; if abd trauma – LFTs, lipase, UA; if fx – PTH, Ca, Phos, Vit D
- Skeletal survey (routine if ≤2 y), CT head (if c/f head trauma, +/– MRI), consider additional imaging based on eval

Management

- Physicians, along w/ other members of health care team, are mandated reporters in US
- If any concern, report to child protective services (w/ help of child abuse team &/or ED social worker, if available)
- Consider if other children from the same household/school/location may be at risk
- Admx for suspected NAT

THE PSYCHIATRIC PATIENT

Definitions (*Emerg Med Clin North Am* 2020;38(2):419–435)

- *Focused medical assessment:* The process of excluding a medical cause of the pt's presentation and evaluating for illness or injury requiring acute care, preferred to the ambiguous term *medical clearance*
- Risk assessment: The dynamic consideration of a pt's psychological and social well-being to determine likelihood of harm to self or others

Approach

- Triage based on risk to self or others
- Psychiatric presentations requiring prioritization: suicidal ideation, homicidal ideation, acute psychosis, mania, agitation, or combativeness
- Determine capacity of pt to consent to or refuse care
  - Legal considerations and rules for involuntary psychiatric eval vary by state
- Consider whether psychiatric sxs are due to underlying organic medical illness. High risk for organic medical illness: >65 yo, >45 yo w/ new-onset psychiatric sxs, cognitive deficits, decreased alertness or delirium, focal neuro findings, substance abuse/w/d, abnl vital signs, ROS or exam w/ head trauma

"Organic" Disorders That Mimic Psychiatric Disease	
Pathophysiology	**Differential**
Neurologic	Brain tumor, head trauma, ICH, encephalopathy, epilepsy, dementia, hydrocephalus, CVA, migraine, vasculitides
Other	Porphyria, Autoimmune encephalitis
Infxns	Meningitis, encephalitis, UTI, PNA
Medications	Polypharmacy, benzodiazepines, anticholinergics, SSRIs, opioids, digoxin, furosemide, warfarin, hydrochlorothiazide
Toxicologic	EtOH, substance abuse, ODs, w/d
Metabolic/endocrine	Hypo/hyperglycemia, hypoxia, thyroid dysfxn, parathyroid dz, electrolyte abnlty, hyper/hypocortisolism

- Perform risk assessment for self-harm, neglect, or violence
- Offer antipsychotic/anxiolytic medications early to decrease need for restraints and resulting injury

History

- Find quiet & secluded area given potential of history to invoke shame, fear, or guilt
- Ask open-ended questions about thoughts and feelings, prior suicidal/homicidal ideation, prior suicide attempts, prior psych history inc hospitalizations, prior/current psych medications, drug/alcohol use, current living situation, access to firearms
- Mnemonic for classic depressive sxs (SIG E CAPS): **S**leep, **I**nterest, **G**uilt, **E**nergy level decreased, **C**oncentration, **A**ppetite, **P**sychomotor activity, **S**uicidal ideation
- Mnemonic for pts w/ increased suicide risk (SAD PERSONS): male **S**ex, **A**ge (<19 or >45), **D**epression, **P**revious attempt, **E**tOH abuse, **R**ational thinking loss, **S**ocial support lacking, **O**rganized plan, **N**o spouse, **S**ickness
- Whenever possible, obtain collateral from partners, family members, friends, & outpt providers

Physical Examination

- Critical eval of abnl vital signs (ie, tachycardia & hyperthermia suggest SS, NMS, or infxn)
- Head-to-toe physical exam inc thorough neurologic exam looking for e/o organic illness
- Mental status exam noting appearance, speech, eye contact, motor activity, affect, mood, perceptions, thoughts, insight, & judgment

Clinical Features of High-Risk Psychiatric Presentations	
Diagnosis	**Clinical Features**
Suicidal ideation	Thoughts of self-harm, can be active (w/ plan) or passive (w/o plan), often a/w mood disorders such as major depressive disorder & bipolar disorder
Homicidal ideation	Thoughts of hurting others, often a/w psychosis
Psychosis	Loss of contact w/ reality, a/w delusions & hallucinations, often seen in schizophrenia spectrum disorders
Mania	Abnormally elevated or expansive mood, affect, and energy, often w/ flight of ideas & pressured speech, a/w bipolar disorder

Agitation	Excessive verbal or motor arousal, often characterized by verbal or physical escalation
Catatonia	Inability to move normally, can be retarded (psychomotor depression, mutism, rigidity) or excited (psychomotor agitation, purposeless movements)

Evaluation

- Obtain ECG for baseline QTc given majority of psychotropic medications prolong the QT interval
- Routine laboratory testing is not indicated except if concerned for organic medical illness
- Despite this, CBC, BMP, LFTs, urine toxicology (& pregnancy testing in women of childbearing age) are often requested by receiving psychiatric facilities
- Neuroimaging, CSF analysis, & EEG are only indicated if concerned for organic cause
- All pts w/ concerning psychiatric sxs should be eval by a psychiatrist

Treatment

- There are 5 major classes of psychotropic medications: antianxiety agents, antidepressants, antipsychotics, mood stabilizers, & stimulants
- ED clinicians need to have detailed understanding of nonpharmacologic (seclusion, verbal de-escalation, physical restraints) & pharmacologic restraint strategies
- Always attempt to use least restrictive strategy for the shortest time possible, given physical & pharmacologic restraints come w/ significant risk

Pharmacologic Restraint Strategies[a]

Age	Moderate Agitation	Severe Agitation
<18	Lorazepam: 0.05–1 mg/kg Olanzapine 0.1 mg/kg Clonidine: <35 kg: 0.05 mg PO, >35 kg 0.1 mg PO	Olanzapine: <25 kg: 1.25 mg IM, 25–70 kg: 2.5 mg IM, >70 kg: 5 mg IM Midazolam 0.1–0.2 mg/kg IM
18–65	Lorazepam 2–4 mg PO Psychosis: Olanzapine 5–10 mg PO	Droperidol 2.5–5 mg + Midazolam 2.5–5 mg IM/IV Ketamine 1–2 mg/kg IV (avoid in psychosis)
>65	Quetiapine 25–50 mg PO	Non-PD/LBD: Olanzapine 2.5–5 mg IM PD/LBD: Lorazepam 1 mg IM

[a]There is significant geographic and site-to-site heterogeneity in pharmacologic agitation mgmt strategies. Check for site specific protocols.

- If antipsychotic or anxiolytic w/ prior benefit during similar episode, give this medication
- Long-term tx plan will be guided by a trained mental health clinician
- Most psychiatric illnesses require a comprehensive tx approach inc medications, therapy, & social interventions

Disposition

- Mental health clinicians will perform a dynamic risk assessment to determine the most appropriate disposition
- Pts at high risk of harm to self or others will need admission to an inpt psychiatric facility
- Those w/o high-risk features will typically be offered partial hospitalization programs or outpt services

Pearls

- Always have a high index of suspicion for organic medical illness causing pt's psychiatric sxs
- Given high prevalence of comorbid drug use in this population, always consider that current sxs could be exacerbated by intoxication or w/d & treat accordingly
- Engage pt's partners, family members, friends, & outpt providers for collateral whenever possible
- Be proactive about addressing developing agitation, inc w/ verbal de-escalation, to ensure pt & staff safety and minimize restraint use

GENERAL APPROACH TO THE INTOXICATED PATIENT

Approach

- Have a systemic & consistent approach in eval & mgmt of poisoned pts
- (1) ABCs, resuscitate/stabilize → (2) decontaminate (GI tract, skin, eyes)/enhance elimination (charcoal, dialysis) → (3) treat w/ antidote, if available & indicated
- Consider empiric naloxone, dextrose, thiamine in pts w/ depressed MS. Use flumazenil w/ caution as it may precipitate sz
- Call Poison Control Center: 1-(800)-222-1222

Common Toxidromes	
Drug Class	**Toxidrome**
Anticholinergics	↑ BP, ↑ HR, ↑ RR, ↑ Temp, mydriasis, **dry skin, dry MM, urinary retention, ↓ bowel sounds,** AMS, sz, coma
Sympathomimetics	↑ BP, ↑ HR, ↑ RR, ↑ Temp, dysrhythmia, mydriasis, **diaphoresis,** agitation, ↑ reflexia, sz, coma
Serotonin tox	↑ BP, ↑ RR, ↑ HR, ↑ Temp, mydriasis, **myoclonus**, tremor, ↑ reflexia, diaphoresis, trismus, ocular clonus
Cholinergics	↓ BP, ↓ HR, miosis, ↓ peristalsis, ↑ **salivation, diarrhea, lacrimation, emesis, bronchoconstriction**, AMS, sz
Opioids	↓ BP, ↓ HR, ↓ RR, **miosis,** AMS, pulm edema
Sedative-hypnotics	↓ BP, ↓ HR, ↓ RR, ↓ Temp, AMS, slurred speech, ataxia
Hallucinogenic	↑ BP, ↑ RR, ↑ HR, ↑ Temp, mydriasis, **nystagmus**

History

- Always consider Drug, Dose, & Pt: timing, quantity of ingestion/exposure, access to household chemicals/other meds, coingestions, enteric-coated/extended-release substances

Physical Examination

- VS, mental status, & pupil exam most useful in aiding in classification of excited vs depressed toxidrome

Evaluation

- ECG, FSG, CBC, BMP, LFTs, UA, ABG, lactate, hCG, osmolar/anion gap, x-ray (radiopaque substances)
- Drug levels
  - Exposures for which drug level is useful: APAP, salicylates, theophylline, lithium, Dig, EtOH, carboxyhemoglobin, methemoglobin, iron, methanol, ethylene glycol, lead, mercury, arsenic, organophosphate, anticonvulsants

Treatment

GI Decontamination			
Tx	**Indications**	**Dose**	**Relative CIs**
Activated charcoal	Given ideally w/i 1 h from ingestion	50 g (adults) 25 g (children) Give w/ antiemetics	AMS, ↑ risk of aspiration, late presentation, need for endoscopic eval, poorly absorbed toxins (Fe, Li, EtOH, bowel perforation or obstruction)
Multidose activated charcoal	Significant ingestion of ER meds; aids in ↓ enterohepatic recirculation & ↑ "gut dialysis"	12.5 g/h (50 g q4h or 25 g q2h)	Bowel obstruction or ileus
Whole bowel irrigation	Drugs not absorbed by charcoal, bags of illicit drugs, significant ingestion of ER meds	PEG via NGT 2 L/h (children 500 mL/h) until clear rectal effluent	Low-risk ingestion, risk of aspiration, toxin absorbed by charcoal, ileus or obstruction, obtundation, GI bleed, & persistent vomiting

Dermal Decontamination

- Irrigation w/ copious volumes of H_2O (unless metallic Na, K, or P)

Ocular Decontamination

- Irrigation w/ copious volumes of H_2O until neutral pH (unless dry lime, phenol, or elemental Na or K)

Enhanced Elimination

- Urinary alkalinization w/ $NaHCO_3$ (eg, salicylates, phenobarbital, formic acid)
- HD (eg, ethylene glycol, methanol, lithium, salicylates, severe acidosis)

Common Toxicology Antidotes	
Antidotes	**Toxicologic Agent**
100% FiO_2 +/– hyperbarics	CO/CN
4-factor PCC	Anti-Xa inhs
Antivenom	Snake, black widow spider, brown recluse spider, scorpion envenomation
Botulinum antitoxin	*Clostridium botulinum*
Calcium	CCB, ↑ K, ↑ Mg, ↓ Ca, hydrofluoric acid (HF)
Edetate calcium disodium	Lead
Cyproheptadine, BZD	Serotonin synd
Cyanide kit (amyl nitrite, sodium nitrite, thiosulfate); Cyanocobalamin	Cyanide, smoke inhalation
Dantrolene	Malignant hyperthermia (volatile anesthetics, succinylcholine)
Deferoxamine	Iron
Dig antibody fragments	Digoxin
Dimercaprol	Arsenic, lead, mercury
EtOH	Ethylene glycol, methanol
Flumazenil	Benzos
Fomepizole	Ethylene glycol, methanol
Glucagon	βB, CCB
Hyperinsulinemia–euglycemia therapy	βB, CCB
Intralipid	Local anesthetic tox, βB, CCB
Methylene blue	Methemoglobinemia
N-acetylcysteine	APAP
Naloxone	Opioids
Octreotide	Sulfonylureas
Physostigmine	Anticholinergics
Penicillamine	Copper
Pralidoxime	Organophosphates
Protamine	Heparin
Prussian blue	Thallium, radiation exposure
Pyridoxine	INH
Sodium bicarbonate	TCAs, aspirin
Succimer	Arsenic, lead, mercury
Vitamin K, 4-factor PCC, FFP	Coumadin

Disposition

- Admit for any significant ingestion/exposure; consider transfer for complex presentations & inadequate hospital resources

Pearl

- Hospital tox screens vary → know your hospital's screen to guide your practice

ANTICHOLINERGIC INGESTION

Definition

- Antagonists @ central & peripheral **muscarinic** cholinergic receptor → inhibit parasymp system

Medications w/ Significant Anticholinergic Activity	
Class	**Medication**
Belladonna alkaloids	Atropine, scopolamine, ipratropium
Antiparkinsonian agents	Benztropine
Antihistamines	Diphenhydramine (Benadryl), meclizine (Antivert), promethazine (Phenergan), hydroxyzine (Atarax), dimenhydrinate (Dramamine)
Antispasmodics	Oxybutynin (Ditropan), tolterodine (Detrol), dicyclomine (Bentyl)
Cyclics	Cyclobenzaprine (Flexeril)
Psychopharmacologics	TCA, phenothiazines

History
- AMS w/ medication exposure, ingestion hx, teas, supplements, or polypharmacy

Differential
- Sympathomimetic OD, EtOH/benzo w/d, thyroid storm, sepsis, meningitis, hypoglycemia

Findings
- ↑ HR, ↑ temp, dilated pupils, dry MM/skin, ↓ bowel sounds, urinary retention, myotonic activity, choreoathetosis, picking behavior, confusion/delirium, sz; "blind as a bat, dry as a bone, hot as a hare, mad as a hatter, red as a beet, bloated as a toad"

Evaluation
- ECG **(↑ QRS, QT_c → TCAs, neuroleptics);** BMP, FSG, CK (rhabdo), ABG/VBG, UDS

Treatment
- **Supportive:** IV hydration, external cooling—treat hyperthermia!
- **Decontamination/elimination:** activated charcoal (1 dose, w/i 1 h); HD not effective
- **BZD** (IV): for agitation, szs
- **Physostigmine** (0.5–2 mg IV); severe tox; reverses anticholinergic effects via AChE inhibition
  - NOT for routine use: ↑ risk of intractable szs, AV block, asystole
  - Half-life of physostigmine often shorter than toxidrome!
  - Transdermal rivastigmine potential alternative

Disposition
- Admit; ICU for pts w/ cardiac instability or szs

Pearl
- Rarely fatal unless significant hyperthermia is present

PSYCHOPHARMACOLOGIC INGESTION

Selective Serotonin Reuptake Inhibitors & Serotonin Syndrome

Approach
- Spectrum for serotonin intoxication ranges from mild lethargy to serotonin synd
- Consider serotonin synd for anyone on meds w/ serotonin activity, esp ≥2 agents
- Greatest risk w/i min to h after starting new med or increasing dose of old med

Definition
- SSRI: Selective serotonin reuptake inhs; SRIs: serotonin reuptake inhs (also exhibit activity on epinephrine, norepinephrine, dopamine)

Common Drugs That Inhibit Serotonin Reuptake	
SSRIs	**SRIs**
Fluoxetine, paroxetine, sertraline, citalopram, escitalopram, & fluvoxamine	Venlafaxine, duloxetine, mirtazapine, & bupropion

Drugs w/ Serotonin Activity		
Antidepressants	**Illicit Drugs**	**Other**
SSRIs, SRIs, MAOIs, lithium	Amphetamines, cocaine, LSD, MDMA	Buspirone, levodopa, carbidopa, triptans, tramadol, dextromethorphan, trazodone, mirtazapine, linezolid, methylene blue, fentanyl

Differential for Serotonin Intoxication	
Pathophysiology	**Differential**
Toxic ingestion	Sympathomimetics, MAOIs, lithium, salicylates, anticholinergics, NMS
Chemical w/d	EtOH, sedative-hypnotics
Infxn	CNS, SIRS
Other	Thyrotoxicosis, tetanus, malignant hyperthermia, heat stroke

History
- Most cases present <24 h; obtain detailed hx of prescription rx, OTC meds, illicit drugs

Findings

Hunter Toxicity Criteria Decision Rules (sen/spec: 84%/97%)
Ingestion of serotonergic agent w/ any ONE of the following findings: • Spontaneous clonus • Inducible clonus + agitation or diaphoresis • Ocular clonus + agitation or diaphoresis • Tremor + hyperreflexia • Hypertonia + hyperthermia >38 °C + ocular clonus + inducible clonus

QJM 2003;96(9):635.

Evaluation

- VS, CBC, BMP, LFTs, CK (rhabdo), coagulation studies (DIC), ECG (↑ QRS, ↑ QT_c, torsades), pulse ox, Tele

Treatment

Acute Overdose

- Activated charcoal, admit for monitoring

Serotonin Syndrome

- Supportive: IV fluids, electrolyte correction, external cooling (may require sedation/paralysis for muscle rigidity, which leads to hyperthermia & death)
- Benzos (IV): for agitation, rigidity, szs
- (Controversial) Consider cyproheptadine (12 mg initially then 2 mg PO q2h)

Pearls

Characteristics of Serotonin Syndrome vs Neuroleptic Malignant Syndrome		
Signs & Sxs	**Serotonin Syndrome**	**NMS**
Onset	Sudden	Often over d to wk
Resolution	w/i 24 h	Over ~1 wk
Hyperthermia	Common	VERY common
AMS	Common	VERY common
Autonomic dysfxn	Common	VERY common
Muscle rigidity	Common	VERY common
↑ Total CK	Uncommon	VERY common
Metabolic acidosis	Uncommon	VERY common
↑ Reflexes	VERY common	Uncommon
Myoclonus	VERY common	Uncommon

NEUROLEPTICS, NEUROLEPTIC MALIGNANT SYNDROME

Definition

- Characterized by D_2 antagonism ± **serotonin receptor antagonism**

Common Neuroleptics		
Typical Neuroleptics	**Atypical Neuroleptics**	**Antiemetics**
Chlorpromazine, haloperidol	Aripiprazole, clozapine, olanzapine, quetiapine, risperidone, ziprasidone	Promethazine, prochlorperazine, droperidol

History

- Slurred speech, sedation, anticholinergic toxidrome, extrapyramidal sxs (dystonia, akathisia, parkinsonism, tardive dyskinesia)
- **NMS:** ↑ HR, rigidity, AMS, szs, autonomic instability, metabolic acidosis, rhabdomyolysis
- Parkinsonism hyperreflexia synd: NMS-like synd in pts w/ parkinsonism withdrawing from DA agonists or L-dopa

Evaluation

- CBC, BMP, LFTs, CK (rhabdo), ECG (↑ QT_c, torsades, dysrhythmia), UA (myoglobin)

Treatment

- Dystonia/akathisia: diphenhydramine, benztropine, BZD
- **NMS:** stop offending agent; supportive care w/ cooling measures, IV fluids & benzos; consider: (use remains controversial) dantrolene, bromocriptine, or amantadine

Lithium

Clinical Effects			
System	**Side Effects**	**Acute Overdose**	**Chronic Toxicity**
GI	n/v, diarrhea, abd pain	n/v, diarrhea	n/v
Neurologic	Tremor, weakness	Tremor, rigidity, clonus, ↑ reflexes, lethargy, sz, coma	Tremor, rigidity, pseudotumor cerebri, tinnitus, ataxia, blurred vision, sz, coma
CV	Sinus node dysfxn	↓ BP	↓ BP, ↓ T-wave, ↓ ST seg, sinus node dysfxn, ↑ QTc
Renal	Polyuria	—	Nephrogenic DI (↑ Na), interstitial nephritis, renal acidosis
Endocrine	Goiter, ↓ thyroid, ↑ parathyroid	—	Goiter, ↑ or ↓ thyroid, ↑ Ca

History
- Acute tox: ingestion of >1 mEq/kg (40 mg/kg); GI sxs initially; neurologic findings may develop later
- Chronic tox: commonly seen w/ acute dehydration (Li nearly entirely renally excreted); presents w/ neurologic sxs; may be c/b nephrogenic DI
- Synd of irreversible lithium-effectuated neurotox (SILENT): rare & long-term cognitive & cerebellar dysfxn caused by Li tox

Evaluation
- VS, ECG, CBC, BMP, Ca, Mg, P, TSH, free T4, UA
- Lithium level: not useful in acute ingestion (development of neurologic sx is better reflection of tox); in chronic tox, level >1.5 mEq is significant
- Assess for causes of decreased lithium clearance (eg, dehydration, renal failure)

Treatment
- IV fluids: decreases tox & promotes Li excretion, NS bolus then ½ NS (if ↑ [NA] serum)
- GI decontamination: AC ineffective; whole bowel irrigation may be useful for sustained release preparations if no contraindications
- Sodium polystyrene sulfonate (Kayexalate) has been proposed, but poor evidence and high potential for cxs
- Benzos for szs (avoid phenytoin, which ↓ Li renal excretion)
- HD: for pts w/ severe neurologic sxs, dysrhythmias, clinical deterioration, Li level >5 mEq/L, Li level >4 mEq/L w/ AKI, unlikely to improve in w/i 36 h w/ optimal mgmt

Disposition
- Admit all pts w/ sustained-release ingestions, Li level >1.5 mEq, or new neurologic signs; lesser ingestions can be treated & observed 4–6 h → re√ level ± psychiatry eval

Pearl
- Li has very narrow therapeutic window; consider Li tox in pts w/ AKI or ↓ UOP

Tricyclic Antidepressants

Approach
- Ingestion >10–20 mg/kg potentially life threatening; toxic synds of anticholinergic effects, cardiotox, & szs predominate

Physiologic Mechanism of Toxicity	
Receptor	**Clinical Manifestations**
Histamine antagonist	Sedation, coma
ACh (muscarinic) antagonist	↑ HR, ↑ BP, mydriasis, dry skin, ileus, urinary retention, delirium, hallucinations
α1-adrenergic antagonist	Sedation, orthostatic ↓ BP (vasodilation), miosis (can counteract muscarinic mydriasis)
Amine reuptake inhibition	↑ HR, myoclonus, ↑ reflexes
Na channel inhibition	↑ PR/QRS intervals, RAD, ↓ cardiac contractility, heart block
K channel antagonist	↑ QT interval → torsades de pointes
GABA-A antagonist	Szs

Severity of TCA Toxicity	
Degree of Toxicity	**Clinical Manifestations**
Mild to mod	Drowsiness, confusion, slurred speech, ataxia, dry MM, ST, urinary retention, myoclonus, ↑ reflexes
Severe	SVT, ↑ QRS, ↑ PR, ↑ QT, VT, ↓ BP, sz, coma

Evaluation
- ECG (prolonged PR, QRS, QT; prominent R′ in aVR), CBC, BMP, LFTs, Ca/Mg/P, CK, UA, tox screen, pulse ox, Tele

Treatment
- Supportive: Maintain oxygenation/ventilation, hemodynamics, temp control, IV fluids
- GI decontamination/elimination: AC ± gastric lavage (in significant ingestions)
- SZs: Benzos, $NaHCO_3$
- Cardiotox (QRS >100, new RAD, ↓ BP, &/or ventricular dysrhythmia): $NaHCO_3$ 1–2 mEq/kg boluses titrate to pH 7.50–7.55; then continuous IV (150 mEq of $NaHCO_3$ in 1 L D_5W)
- For persistent cardiotox or ventricular dysrhythmias refractory to $NaHCO_3$ consider lidocaine IV, avoid procainamide or other type Ia or Ic antiarrhythmics
- Lipid emulsion: per ACMT position statement 1.5 mL/kg bolus over 2–3 m –> 0.25 mL/kg for 3 m –> 0.025 mL/kg if improving
- HD not effective

Disposition
- Admit all pts w/ e/o cardiotox or sz; D/C pts w/o sxs at 6 h after ingestion

Pearl
- Antimuscarinic effects are absent in many cases of TCA overdose

ALCOHOLS

Definition
- Ingestions of toxic alcohols: EtOH, methanol, ethylene glycol, & isopropyl alcohol

Approach
- Hx: Type of alcohol ingested, time of ingestion, coingestants
- PE: monitor for airway protection, occult trauma (head injury)
- FSG (may be all that's needed), consider BAL (declines ~20 mg/dL/h), BMP (anion gap, calc osms, LFTs, PT/INR, lactate, serum/urine tox, serum osm, consider CT brain (trauma)
- Osmol calc = 2 × Na + BUN/2.8 + gluc/18 + EtOH/4.6
- Osmol gap = Osmol measured – osmol calc
- Tx: alcohol dehydrogenase inhs, ±thiamine/folate, charcoal not effective

Alcohol Ingestion Differential		
Alcohol	**Toxic Metabolites**	**Anion Gap Acidosis**
EtOH	Acetaldehyde → acetate	No (unless alcoholic ketoacidosis)
Methanol	Formaldehyde → formate	Yes
Ethylene glycol	Glycolaldehyde → glycolate, oxalate	Yes
Isopropyl alcohol	Acetone	No (metabolites not highly toxic organic acids)

Ethanol

History
- EtOH ingestion, found down, lethargy, n/v, ±associated trauma, ±aspiration, gastritis

Physical Findings
- CNS, respiratory depression, slurred speech, ataxia, nystagmus

Evaluation
- FSG (hypoglycemia common in chronic alcohol use), ±BAL (if ingestion uncertain), ±CBC/BMP/LFTs/lipase, ±ECG (if pulse irregular), ±magnesium level

Treatment
- Maintain airway, serial exams, ±IVF/thiamine/folate (given but may not be necessary)

Disposition
- Ambulating w/o ataxia + speaking clearly → D/C

Pearls
- R/o head trauma, CNS infxn, Wernicke encephalopathy, alcoholic ketoacidosis, hypoglycemia, alcohol w/d/DTs, coingestions, SI/HI
- Known EtOH ingestion/intoxication in pt w/ hx of same does not require lab & can be observed until clinically sober
- Clinical sobriety rather than BAL is endpoint for DC, as serum EtOH may remain elevated in chronic alcohol use, and continued observation can result in alcohol w/d

Methanol

Definition
- Ingestion of methanol (peak levels 30–60 mins, 24–30 h ½ life, hepatic metabolism)

History
- Drinking: Paint solvents/antifreeze/windshield-washing fluid/canned fuels/gasoline additives, shellac/copy machine fluid/home heating fuels

Physical Findings
- CNS depression, vomiting, papilledema/hyperemia, visual Δ/loss, gastritis

Evaluation
- ↑ Methanol level, ↑ Osmol gap, ↑ anion gap (profound), BMP, ABG

Treatment
- Fomepizole or EtOH if significant ingestion w/ serum methanol >20 mg/dL, osmol gap >10 mOsm/L, or met acidosis (pH <7.3, bicarb <20 mEq/L)
- Fomepizole: Loading dose (15 mg/kg in 100 mL D_5W over 30 mins) → maintenance (10 mg/kg q12h × 4 doses → 15 mg/kg q12 to methanol concentration <20/dL)
- Consider folic acid or leucovorin to aid in additional clearance
- Dialysis: Vision deficit+ detectible methanol level or >50 mL/dL, osmol gap >10, ingestion >1 mg/kg, severe acidosis, renal failure; very effective & reduces ½ life to 3–6 h

Disposition
- Admit

Ethylene Glycol

Definition
- Ingestion of ethylene glycol (peak levels 30–180 mins, 3–7 h ½ life, 70% hepatic metabolism); metabolites may lead to met acidosis, kidney failure, & death

History
- Drinking: Antifreeze (1° ingredient), coolants, paint, polishes, detergents, fire extinguishers

Physical Findings
- 4 phases: <12 h → ↓ CNS (such as EtOH), gastritis; 12–24 h → ↑ HR/RR/BP/SOB; >12 h → ATN (oxalate crystal deposition); >2 d–2 wks → delayed neurogenic sequela

Evaluation
- Ethylene glycol level (>50 mg/dL serious ingestion), ↑ osmol gap (calculate to quickly estimate ethylene glycol level), ↑ AG, calcium oxalate crystals in urine, beta-hydroxybutyrate (used to distinguish from alcoholic ketoacidosis)

Treatment
- Based presumptive Dx if lvls delayed, maintain airway; supportive care
- Fomepizole: initiate if ethylene glycol lvl > 20 mg/dL &/or osmol gap >10 mOsm/L w/o other alcohol coingestion; loading dose (15 mg/kg in 100 mL D_5W over 30 mins) → maintenance (10 mg/kg q12h × 4 doses → 15 mg/kg q12h to ethylene glycol concentration <20/dL)
- Cofactors: enhance metabolism to nontoxic metabolites; folate/thiamine 100 mg IV q6h/pyridoxine 50 mg IV q6h until resolution of acidemia
- Consider gastric aspirate if ingestion w/in 30–60 mins
- HD: severe acidosis (pH <7.25) + osmol gap >10, renal failure (Cr >1.2 mg/dL), ethylene glycol level >50 mg/dL, deterioration despite supportive care

Disposition
- Admit

Clinical Pearl
- Urine/gastric contents fluoresce w/ Wood lamp due to antifreeze additives (early)

Isopropyl Alcohol

Definition
- Ingestion of isopropyl alcohol (peak levels 30–180 mins, 3–7 h ½ life, 80% hepatic metabolism, lethal dose 2–4 mL/kg)

History
- Drinking: rubbing alcohol, paint thinner, solvents, skin/hair products, nail polish remover

Physical Findings
- Profound ↓ CNS (2–4 × EtOH), fruity odor on breath, respiratory depression, ↓ BP (vasodilation & cardiac depression), gastritis, coma, death; isopropyl alcohol lvl >150 mg/dL presents often w/ coma

Evaluation
- BMP, UA, FSG, isopropyl lvl, nl/mild AG, ↑ osmol gap, ABG, false ↑ Cr (from acetone)

Treatment
- Primarily supportive (rarely lethal); Tx hypoglycemia, ↓ BP, & coma
- Fomepizole & EtOH tx NOT indicated; toxic organic acid metabolites not generated
- Gastric aspiration not effective >30 mins post ingestion
- Dialysis: refractory hypotension, lvls >500 mg/dL

Disposition
- Admit if severe tox, may D/C 2 h after resolution of sxs if no coingestions or SI

Alcohol Withdrawal

Definition
- Abrupt cessation or significant reduction in alcohol intake (begins 6–24 h/peaks 48–72 h after last drink)

History
- Heavy alcohol use w/ cessation, insomnia, anxiety/restlessness, tremors, anorexia, n/v, diaphoresis, visual/tactile/auditory hallucinations, sz, prior hx of severe w/d, presence of concurrent illness

Physical Findings

Alcohol Withdrawal Syndromes		
Syndromes	**Exam Findings**	**Timing**
Mild w/d sxs	Anxiety, tremors, diaphoresis, GI upset w/o AMS	6–36 h
W/d szs	Often tonic–clonic; status epilepticus uncommon	6–48 h
Alcoholic hallucinosis	Auditory, tactile, or visual w/o AMS	12–48 h
DTs	Significant autonomic instability; ↑ BR ↑ HR, ↑ Temp, diaphoresis, agitation, AMS	2–4 d (37% mortality if untreated)

Evaluation
- FSG, CBC, BMP, LFTs/coags (if liver dysfxn suspected), BAL
- Exclude other potential dx (meningitis, trauma, sepsis, toxic ingestion)

Treatment
- Supportive care: goal of reducing sxs & preventing cxs; provide sedation, IVF, correct electrolytes, +/– thiamine/folate; close monitoring & frequently reassessment
- Consider sx-triggered dosing approach via validated scoring system (eg, CIWA, MINDS, SEWS)
- Phenobarbital or BZDs 1st line (diazepam, lorazepam, chlordiazepoxide)

Disposition
- Admit if requiring significant IV medication/DTs ± ICU

Clinical Pearls
- Rarely fatal (increased w/ aspiration due to sz) when treated appropriately
- May require very large doses of IV BZD to control/treat

DRUGS OF ABUSE

Focused Differential		
Class	**Drugs**	**Effects**
Sedative-hypnotics	BZD, barbiturates, gamma-hydroxybutyrate (GHB), opioids	Sedation, ataxia, slurred speech, apnea, hypotension, hypothermia, dysrhythmias

Stimulants/ sympathomimetics	Cocaine, amphetamine, methamphetamine, MDMA, caffeine, ephedrine, dextromethorphan, LSD, bath salts	HTN, tachycardia, agitation, vasospasm/ischemia (CVA/ACS), AMS, anxiety, mania, psychosis, szs, rhabdomyolysis, muscle rigidity, hyperthermia

BENZODIAZEPINES

Definition
- GABA agonists (↑ *frequency* of GABAs Cl^- ion channel opening)

History
- Usu suicidal gesture or abuse, hypnotic/sleep agents (zaleplon, zolpidem, eszopiclone) have similar effects as BZD in overdose

Physical Findings
- CNS, respiratory depression, slurred speech, lethargy, ataxia, hyporeflexia, midpoint/small pupils, ↓ Temp, ↓ BP

Evaluation
- FSG, consider ABG, serum/urine tox, serum drug lvls rarely useful, $EtCO_2$ monitor, Tele, pulse ox if severe tox

Treatment
- Supportive care: Maintain airway protection, tx ↓ Temp, ↓ BP, & coma if necessary
- Antidote: Flumazenil 0.1–0.2 mg, repeat up to 3 mg → caution may precipitate szs!—indications are rare, use only to reverse when known benzo is over administered as part of procedural sedation & must be reversed for life-threatening sxs, monitor for resedation after 1–2 h, may require repeat dose
- Decontamination: Activated charcoal if ingestion occurred w/i 30 mins

Disposition
- Home (rarely require admx) if resolution of sxs after monitoring & if no SI

Pearls
- Monitor for w/d, which is similar in presentation (agitation, szs) & tx to EtOH w/d
- Isolated benzo OD rarely life threatening although usu presents as polysubstance OD

GAMMA-HYDROXYBUTYRATE (GHB)

Definition
- Analog of GABA; GABA(B) & GHB receptor agonist

Physical Findings
- Initial euphoria, AMS/obtundation, ↓ BP, ↓ HR, ↓ Temp, respiratory depression, apnea myoclonus, aspiration, rarely pulmonary edema & SZ

Evaluation
- FSG, ±Serum/urine tox screen (rapidly metabolized → GHB levels not readily available)

Treatment
- Supportive, maintain airway, recovery w/i 2–4 h, resolution w/i 8 hv

Disposition
- Home

OPIOIDS

Definition
- Opioid receptor agonist

History
- Witnessed or reported use of opioids (heroin, methadone, morphine, hydromorphone, fentanyl, oxycodone)

Physical Findings
- ↓ CNS, ↓ RR/BP, apnea, ±miosis, track marks, aspiration, noncardiogenic pulmonary edema (often seen after opiate antagonist naloxone), SZ, QT prolongation/torsade de pointes (methadone)

Evaluation
- Gluc, serum/urine tox screen (for coingestants), $EtCO_2$ monitor, Tele, pulse ox

Treatment

- Antidote: Naloxone – cardiopulmonary arrest: 2 mg IV; apneic pt: 0.2–1 mg IV; bradypneic pt: initiate 0.04 mg IV q2–3min titrate to adequate ventilation (not mental status); doses >5–10 mg require reconsidering dx
- Naloxone infusion: alternative to repeat dosing; initiate at 2/3 (total dose required to restore ventilation) q1h IV; stop if w/d sets it, restart if tox returns.
- Activated charcoal (recent ingestion); whole bowel irrigation (long-acting opioid)

Disposition

- May require ICU admx for long-acting opioid tox (methadone) on naloxone drip
- Connect w/ outpt opiate use disorder tx, offer buprenorphine Rx
- D/C home w/ RX naloxone IN 1 mg each nostril × 1, co-RX for friends/family

Pearls

- Mortality rates after ED nonfatal opioid OD: 1 y (5.5%); 1 mo (1.1%); 2 d (0.25%)

Opioid Withdrawal

Definition

- Cessation or rapid reduction of opioid use in a dependent individual

History

- Chronic opioid use, hyperalgesia, anxiety, n/v, abd pain, diarrhea, myalgias

Physical Findings

- Normal mental status, yawning, rhinorrhea, lacrimation, myalgias, arthralgias, mydriasis, piloerection, ↑ HR, ↑ BP

Treatment

- Opioid agonist tx: methadone 10 mg IM or 20 mg PO or buprenorphine 4–8 mg SL may repeat up to 24 mg if sxs persist in 30–60 mins
- Adjunctive tx: clonidine 0.1 mg PO for w/d sxs; promethazine 25 mg IM/IV for n/v; loperamide 4 mg PO for diarrhea; diazepam 1–10 mg PO for anxiety/cramping

Disposition

- Home or detox

Pearl

- Not life threatening, do not require Admx, may be precipitated by administration of naloxone & caution should be used before treating w/ additional opioids

---

Cocaine

Definition

- Snorting, injecting, smoking, ingesting (body packing vs stuffing) cocaine (peak 5–15 mins, duration 1–4 h, releases norepinephrine/blocks reuptake)

History

- Cocaine use, anxiety, CP, focal weakness (CVA/ICH), sz, psychosis

Physical Findings

- ↑ HR, ↑ BP, ↑ Temp, diaphoresis, euphoria, agitation, delirium, nasal septal perforation, mydriasis, coma, sz, respiratory arrest

Evaluation

- Serum/urine tox screen, troponin (if CP present), ECG (↑ QRS, ischemia), Cr (renal failure), CK (rhabdomyolysis), CT brain (if ICH/stroke suspected), Abd plain film or CT (packers/stuffers)

Treatment

- Supportive care, BZD for anxiety/agitation/CP, treat hyperthermia (ice packs, cooling blankets, cooling mist), sodium bicarbonate for ↑ QRS, lidocaine for wide-complex tachy
- Activated charcoal (recent ingestion), whole bowel irrigation +/– surgical removal (packers/stuffers)

Disposition

- Varies depending on severity; ED obs & DC vs admit depending on degree of tox

Pearl

- Cocaine washout synd: After cocaine binging, MS (lethargy, obtundation), lasts up to 24 h
- Cocaine adulterated w/ the antiparasitic drug levamisole may present w/ leukocytoclastic vasculitis & agranulocytosis

METHAMPHETAMINE ("METH")

Definition
- CNS stimulant, releases catecholamine, inhibits reuptake of catecholamines, & MAOI

History
- Ingestion, snorting, smoking, injection, rectal insertion of methamphetamines & derivatives (LSD, bath salts), ADHD, & narcolepsy medications

Physical Findings
- ↑ HR, ↑ BP, ↑ Temp, diaphoresis, agitation, poor dentition ("meth mouth"), poor hygiene, compulsive scratching lesions ("meth mites"), tremors, psychosis, sz, coma

Evaluation
- Serum/urine tox screen, ECG, consider CT brain (ICH), UA, CK (rhabdomyolysis), BMP, troponin (CP), Tele

Treatment
- Supportive care, BZD for anxiety/agitation/CP, cool hyperthermic pts (ice packs, cooling blankets, cooling mist)
- Activated charcoal (recent ingestion), whole bowel irrigation (packers/stuffers)

METHYLENEDIOXYMETHAMPHETAMINE (MDMA, "ECSTASY"), LYSERGIC ACID DIETHYLAMIDE (LSD)

Definition
- Exact mechanism of hallucinations not known; likely serotonin & dopamine agonism

History
- Ingestion of MDMA, LSD, other hallucinogens

Physical Findings
- ↑ HR, ↑ BP, ↑ Temp, anxiety, mydriasis, hallucinations, sz, tremor, hyperreflexia, diaphoresis, bruxism

Evaluation
- Serum/urine tox screen, BMP (↓ Na due to excessive water ingestion), ECG, consider CT brain (ICH), INR, UA, CK (rhabdomyolysis), troponin (CP), Tele

Treatment
- Supportive care, BZD & haloperidol for agitation, cool hyperthermic pts (ice packs, cooling blankets, cooling mist)
- ±Activated charcoal (recent ingestion)

ANALGESIC OVERDOSE

ACETAMINOPHEN (APAP) POISONING

History
- Witnessed or reported ingestion of any APAP-containing meds (many Rx & OTC drugs)
- Often coingestions w/ other substances

Findings
- 4 stages of APAP poisoning
  - I. Asx (0–24 h)
  - II. GI upset, n/v, abd pain (24–72 h)
  - III. Jaundice, fulminant liver failure, encephalopathy (3–5 d)
  - IV. Recovery (1 wk after) if survives phase III or multisystem organ failure

Evaluation
- APAP level 4 h after ingestion, serum/urine tox for coingestants, baseline LFTs & coags, BMP for calculation of anion gap, preop labs if potential for need for transplant, ECG

Treatment
- Antidote: *N*-acetylcysteine (NAC) is glutathione substitute initiate w/ 8–10 h; do not w/hold even if delay is >24 h
- Acute single ingestion: >200 mg/kg pediatric or 6–7 g adult initiate NAC tx if APAP lvl above nomogram line or near line in at-risk pt (alcoholic, poor nutrition, taking INH) (Figure 16.1)

Figure 16.1 Relation between plasma APAP level and hepatotoxicity correlated with time after ingestion. (Derived from Helms RA, Quan DJ. *Textbook of Therapeutics: Drug and Disease Management*. Lippincott Williams & Wilkins; 2006.)

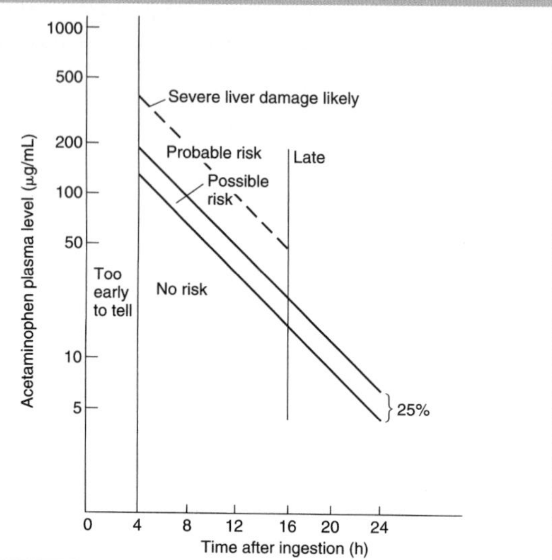

- Chronic ingestion: Report of several doses over 24 h w/ >200 mg/kg × 1 d, 150 mg/kg/d × 2 d, 100 mg/kg/d × 3 d; ↑ LFT/INR; or detectable APAP lvl initiate NAC tx
- NAC dose: NAC 140 mg/kg per NGT × 1, then 70 mg/kg PNGT or 150 mg/kg IV × 1, then 50 mg/kg IV q4h × 5 doses
- NAC duration: Continue × 20 h or until APAP lvl undetectable or LFT/INR clears
- Activated charcoal (recent ingestion), HD (APAP >1000 mg/L + coma/hypotension)

Disposition

- Admx to hospital vs ICU based on clinical picture; transfer to transplant facility
- Consider Psych eval if c/f self-harm attempt

Pearls

- Maximal safe APAP dose 15 mg/kg (up to 1000 mg) QID, max daily dose 3–4 g/24 h
- APAP metabolism produces NAPQI (toxic metabolite) → direct hepatocyte damage
- When coupled to glutathione, NAPQI made inert & is excreted in urine; APAP tox results from overwhelmed/depleted glutathione stores
- Many unintentional APAP OD from confusion b/w pediatric vs infant APAP preparations
- Infant: 80 mg/0.8 mL = 100 mg/mL; children: 160 mg/5 mL (5 mL = 1 tsp) = 32 mg/mL

Salicylate Poisoning (ASA)

History

- Witnessed or reported ingestion of ASA or ASA-containing meds
- Often coingestions w/ other substances, occasionally inadvertent (elderly)
- Suspect ASA poisoning in any pt who reports tinnitus

Findings

- Acute ingestion: 1st 8–12 h: ↑ Temp, ↑ RR (respiratory alkalosis + metabolic acidosis), ↑ HR, ↓ BP, diaphoresis, dysrhythmias, n/v, epigastric pain, AMS; >24 h: Coma, cerebral edema, sz, noncardiogenic pulmonary edema, DIC
- Chronic ingestion: often confused elderly pt taking long-term therapeutic doses; nonspecific findings: AMS, met acidosis, hypovolemia; maintain ↑ index of suspicion!

Evaluation

- Urine/serum tox screen for ASA level & coingestants, BMP(anion gap), CBC, coags, ABG, CXR (pulm edema), ECG
- Acute ingestion: Severe w/ 300–500 mg/kg ingestion or ASA lvl >90–100 mg/dL
- Chronic ingestion: 100 mg/kg/d × 2 d or ASA lvl >60 mg/dL w/ e/o of AMS or acidosis
- In acute ingestion check ASA lvl q4h to ensure that lvls are not rising due to "bezoar" formation or enteric-coated formulation w/ delayed metabolism

Dose-Dependent Severity of Single ASA Ingestion	
Amount Ingested (mg/kg)	**Effect**
<150	None → mild tox
150–300	Mild → mod tox
301–500	Severe tox
>500	Potentially lethal tox

Treatment

- Airway protection if pt tires: hyperventilate & maintain respiratory alkalosis on vent
- Dextrose for hypoglycemia; pts may have ↓↓ CSF gluc but nl serum gluc
- Tx: No antidote but $NaHCO_3$ corrects acidosis & ↑ urine pH to ↑ ASA excretion
- $NaHCO_3$ dosing: 3 amps $NaHCO_3$ to 1 L D_5W or 2 amps $NaHCO_3$ to 1 L ½ NS, bolus over 30 mins; titrate to maintain serum pH >7.45, & urine pH >7.55 & UOP goal 1.5 mL/kg/h; add 20–40 mEq K to replete K exchanged into cells for H^+ ions (hypokalemia prevents effective alkaline diuresis)
- Charcoal (recent acute ingestion), consider whole bowel irrigation for sig ingestion
- HD: Acute pt w/ ASA lvl >90–100 mg/dL & severe acidosis; chronic pt w/ ASA lvl >60 mg/dL w/ acidosis, AMS, or AKI

Disposition

- Admx to floor vs ICU (if symptomatic), observe for at least 6 h (asx, nonenteric-coated, smaller ingestions), screen for SI/psych eval if indicated

Pearls

- ASA uncouples oxidative phosphorylation, causes a 1° metabolic acidosis & 1° (centrally mediated) respiratory alkalosis
- Methyl salicylate (found in BenGay, Icy Hot muscle balm, oil of wintergreen food flavoring) produces ASA tox in very small amounts (1 tsp of oil of wintergreen contains 7 g of ASA)

CARDIAC MEDICATION OVERDOSE

Beta-Blocker (βB) Overdose

History

- Witnessed or reported overingestion of βB (as little as 2–3 × therapeutic dose)
- Children who have been at homes of older relatives taking prescribed medications (in pediatrics "one pill can kill")

Findings

- Symptomatic ↓ HR, ↓ BP, AMS, weakness, bronchospasm
- Lipid-soluble βB (propranolol) – sz/coma; sotalol – ↑ QTc, torsades de pointes
- May have n/v, hypoglycemia, hyperkalemia, heart block, cardiogenic shock, resp arrest

Evaluation

- Specific lvls often unavailable, BMP (gluc, BUN/Cr), ECG (↓ HR, conduction blocks, QRS/QT Δ's), troponin, coingestion screen, blood gas, POCUS to evaluate contractility

Treatment

- Continuous Tele, 2 large-bore IVs, place transcutaneous pacer pads on pt
- Place a cordis in the R IJ or L subclavian vein if transvenous pacing indicated
- Symptomatic ↓ HR & ↓ BP: Glucagon 5–10 mg IV bolus f/b 1–5 mg/h infusion; Atropine 0.01–0.03 mg/kg IV; Isoproterenol 4 mcg/min titrate to effect
- Refractory ↓ HR & ↓ BP: Epinephrine IV 1–4 mcg/min; Consider hyperinsulinemia–euglycemia therapy &/or IV lipid emulsion (benefit in animals & case reports); cardiac pacing
- Bronchospasm: Nebulized bronchodilators
- Wide-complex conduction defects: Sodium bicarbonate 1–2 mEq/kg IV
- Polymorphic VT: Magnesium, isoproterenol, or overdrive pacing

- Activated charcoal (recent OD); whole bowel irrigation (massive OD)
- HD only useful for βB w/ low volume of distribution (acebutolol, atenolol, nadolol, timolol, sotalol) or e/o of renal failure

Disposition

- Admx to floor vs ICU (if symptomatic)
- Clinically significant βB OD develop sxs w/i 6 h; if remain asx, can be D/C unless ingested sustained release formulation (24-h observation)

Calcium Channel Blocker (CCB) Overdose

History

- Witnessed or reported overingestion of CCB
- Children who have been at homes of older relatives taking prescribed medications (in pediatrics "one pill can kill")

Findings

- Symptomatic ↓ HR & ↓ BP (cardiogenic & vasodilatory shock), n/v, weakness, met acidosis (shock state), hyperglycemia (pancreatic suppression), AMS, sz

Evaluation

- Drug lvls not common, BMP, Troponin, blood gas, ECG (↓ HR, ventricular escape rhythm, 2nd- or 3rd-degree AV block; usu nl QRS complex (vs βB OD), serum/urine tox, POCUS to evaluate contractility

Treatment

- Continuous Tele, 2 large-bore IVs, place transcutaneous pacer pads on pt
- Place a cordis in the R IJ or L subclavian vein if transvenous pacing indicated
- Supportive tx: Maintain airway, volume resuscitation & pressors for ↓ BP & ↓ inotropy
- Symptomatic ↓ HR & ↓ BP: Calcium gluconate 3 g slow IV push or calcium chloride 1 g IV q5–10min PRN (central line or secure peripheral line); hyperinsulinemia/euglycemia tx: insulin bolus 1 U/kg + 50 mL $D_{50}W$ IV (w/ additional boluses PRN) goal of serum gluc 100–200 mg/dL (check gluc q10min then q30min; monitor/replete K^+)
- Refractory ↓ HR & ↓ BP: Vasopressors: Cardiogenic shock (epinephrine, dobutamine, isoproterenol, milrinone) vs vasodilatory shock (norepinephrine, vasopressin, phenylephrine); glucagon 0.05 mg/kg bolus repeat in 10 mins (obs for n/v); consider intravenous lipid emulsion 1.5 mL/kg lean body weight bolus IV of 20% lipid emulsion may repeat × 2 for total 3 doses (few pos case reports in verapamil & diltiazem poisonings)
- Activated charcoal (recent OD); whole bowel irrigation (massive OD)
- HD not useful for CCB OD due to extensive protein binding

Disposition

- Admx to floor vs ICU (if symptomatic)
- CCB should be monitored for 6 h or 24 h for sustained release formulations

Digoxin Overdose

History

- Usu in pts on chronic Dig, occasional acute intentional OD occurs (SI attempt)
- Serious tox w/ ingestion as little as 3 mg in adults or 1 mg in pediatrics
- Recent ↓ renal fxn, dehydration, electrolyte abn, illness, recent addition of new med

Findings

- Acute OD: Weakness, n/v, ↑ K, bradyarrhythmia (2°/3° AV block, SA block), tachyarrhythmia (PAT, junctional tach, bidirectional VT, VF)
- Chronic OD: Weakness, fatigue, palpitations, syncope, AMS, n/v, diarrhea, HA, paresthesias, Yellow-green vision (classic but not always present), ECG Δ's (accelerated junctional tach, PAT, AF w/ slowed ventricular response, VT, bidirectional tachy)

Evaluation

- ECG may show a number of cardiac dysrhythmias (see above)
- Dig level, cardiac enzymes, BMP (↑ K in acute OD, nl or ↓ K, ↓ Mg in chronic OD)

Treatment

- Continuous Tele, trend Dig & serum K levels w/ ECG & clinical picture
- Correct electrolyte abnl
- Acute OD:
  - Hyperkalemia: ↑ K is bad prognostic sign; treat immediately w/ calcium (1st drug of choice; "stone heart" phenomena based on weak evidence), gluc/insulin & bicarb

- Bradycardia: Atropine 0.5–2 mg IV, transvenous pacemaker only after failure or unavailable dioxin antibodies (may trigger arrhythmias)
- Antidote: Dig spec Ab (DigiFab): Initiate if dig lvl >6, K >5, high-deg AV block, ventricular arrhythmias, AMS, hemodynamic compromise, massive OD
- Each vial of Dig spec Ab binds 0.5 mg of Dig
- # of Dig spec Ab = (serum Dig [ng/mL] × TBW [kg])/100
- For unknown amount/level, empirically treat w/ 10 vials, repeat once PRN for acute ingestion, 6 vials for chronic ingestion
- VT: Phenytoin & lidocaine safe to control tachydysrhythmias
- Activated charcoal (recent OD); consider repeat activated charcoal if e/o of severe AKI
- HD ineffective due to large Vd

- Chronic OD:
  - Stop Dig
  - Verify need for Dig spec Ab, check Cr, electrolytes

Disposition
- Admx to floor vs ICU (if hemodynamic instability, refractory dysrhythmia)
- If asx, no cardiac dysrhythmias, nl K & dig level, can D/C after 6 h

Pearl
- Many drug interactions (BZD, βB, CCB, diuretics, succinylcholine, some abx)

CAUSTIC INGESTIONS

Background
- Cause tissue injury by acidic or alkaline chemical rxn
- pH <2 is considered strong acid, pH >12 considered strong base
- Severity of tissue injury determined by duration of contact, pH, concentration, type of substance (liquid vs solid)

Approach
- Careful hx: Spec agent, amount, duration, pH, & timing of ingestion, coingestants
- Often accidental in pediatrics & SI in adults; assess mental state as well as physical
- Rapid physical exam: Look for respiratory compromise, stridor, hoarseness, oropharyngeal burns, drooling, subcutaneous air, acute peritonitis (signs of perforation), hematemesis
- Do NOT induce emesis; reexposure could worsen injury
- Do NOT attempt to neutralize ingestions due to possible exothermic rxn

Acid/Alkaline Ingestions

History
- Alkaline: Ingestion of ammonia, cleaning agents: drain, oven, swimming pool, dishwasher detergents, bleach, cement, hair relaxers
- Acid: Ingestion of battery liquid, toilet bowl cleaners, rust or metal cleaning products, drain cleaners, cement cleaning products

Findings
- Alkaline: Liquefactive necrosis—severe injury starts rapidly after ingestion, w/i min of contact, tissues that 1st contact alkali are most severely injured (oropharynx, hypopharynx, esophagus). Tissue edema occurs immediately, may persist for 48 h, progress → airway obstruction. Over 2–4 wks get scar tissue thickening → strictures (depends on depth of burn)
- Acid: Coagulation necrosis → desiccation → eschar formation; stomach most commonly affected; small bowel exposure possible. Eschar sloughs in 3–4 d, then granulation tissue development. Perforation after 3–4 d as eschar sloughs; gastric outlet obstruction if scar tissue contracts over 2–4 wks. Pyloric sphincter spasm may delay gastric emptying & ↑ contact time to 90 mins
- In HF ingestion, ↓ Ca may lead to arrhythmias, sudden cardiac arrest
- Both may cause esophageal perforation

Evaluation
- pH of product & of saliva, CBC, BMP, blood gas, baseline LFTs, UA, preop labs, tox screen; cardiac monitoring, ECG; x-rays (perforation), consider CT for extraluminal air
- Endoscopy if symptomatic, small child, AMS but not if e/o perforation or airway edema

Treatment
- Asx or benign ingestion: No e/o of oral burn, small volume ingestion, accidental → EGD unnecessary; may DC after 6-h ED obs
- Symptomatic or significant ingestion: E/o of burns, large-volume ingestion, SI attempt → Maintain airway, fluid resuscitate, analgesia; broad spect ABX & surgical c/s w/ e/o of perforation; GI c/s for EGD if no e/o of perforation
- Avoid induced emesis, administering neutralizing agents, or corticosteroids

Disposition
- Admit to ICU if symptomatic

CELLULAR ASPHYXIATES

Cyanide Poisoning

Etiology
- By-product of nitroprusside, acrylonitrile (nail polish, plastics, some tattoo ink), cyanogenic glycosides (apricot pits, cassava), cyanide gas (structural fires)
- Mechanism: Binds to cytochrome oxidase, blocks aerobic utilization of O_2, leading to cellular asphyxia

History
- Difficulty breathing, confusion, HA, n/v, AMS, syncope, sz, cardiovascular collapse
- Sxs develop immediately after inhalational exposure, delayed sxs after exposure to nitroprusside, cyanide salts, acrylonitrile, cyanogenic glycosides

Physical Examination
- O_2 saturation often nl; dyspnea/tachypnea, confusion, tachycardia; agonal respirations & cardiovascular collapse a/w severe poisoning
- "Bitter almond" smell (unreliable), bright red venous blood due to high venous O_2 content

Evaluation
- BMP, ↑↑ lactate, ABG (metabolic acidosis), VBG (assess venous/arterial O_2 gradient), cyanide level, carboxyhemoglobin (if smoke inhalation)

Treatment
- Supportive: Maintain airway, O_2 therapy, IV fluids
- Cyanide antidote: 2 FDA approved in US
- Hydroxocobalamin: Adult: 5 g (child: 70 mg/kg) IV over 15 mins may repeat × 1
- Nithiodote: Sodium nitrite 300 mg/10 mL IV at 5 mL/min (induces methemoglobinemia) f/b sodium thiosulfate 12.5 g IV; amyl nitrate no longer FDA approved for CN tox
- Consider activated charcoal (presenting <2 h); no role in HD or hyperbarics

Disposition
- Admit: All pts; consider ICU for pts w/ szs, coma, acidosis, hypotension

Carbon Monoxide Poisoning and Methemoglobinemia

Etiology
Carbon Monoxide
- Smoke inhalation, methylene chloride exposure
- Mechanism: reduces O_2-carrying capacity, shifts O_2 dissociation curve to L

Methemoglobinemia
- Nitrites, dapsone, sulfa drugs, lidocaine/benzocaine, antimalarials, water contamination
- Mechanism: disequilibrium of methemoglobin to hemoglobin; overwhelmed methemoglobin reductase

History
Carbon Monoxide
- Mild: mild HA, DOE; mod: HA, n/v, dizziness, poor concentration; severe: CP, syncope, coma, LOC, & persistent AMS

Methemoglobinemia
- SOB, HA, lightheadedness, fatigue, nausea, tachycardia, CP, syncope

Physical Examination
Carbon Monoxide
- Lethargy, szs, tachycardia, tachypnea, rales, confusion, red skin, or cyanosis

Methemoglobinemia

- "Chocolate" cyanosis, tachycardia; coma, sz, D a/w severe exposure

Evaluation

- ABG & pulse ox: May be falsely reassuring

Labs

- CO
  - CO oximeter, CO level (mild: 10–20%, mod: 20–40%, severe: >40%); mod/severe: ABG (metabolic acidosis), BMP, CBC, cardiac enzymes, UA, CPK, lactate, consider CN level
  - ECG: arrhythmias, signs of MI
- Methemoglobinemia
  - CO oximeter, methemoglobin level; severe exposure: ABG, hemolysis labs (LDH, peripheral smear, haptoglobin, reticulocyte count), type & crossmatch
  - Bedside test: drop of blood on white filter paper will turn chocolate brown (compared to regular venous blood)

Treatment

Carbon Monoxide

- O_2 t½: 200 mins on RA; 74 mins on 100% NRB; 12–20 mins on hyperbaric tx
- Indications for hyperbaric O_2: respiratory failure, LOC, CO level >25%, pregnancy, infants, severe acidosis, neuro deficits, CV dysfxn, exposure >24 h, age >36 y

Methemoglobinemia (symptomatic exposures, level >20%)

- Methylene blue (reducing agent): 1–2 mg/kg of 1% solution IV qh × 2 doses
- Exchange transfusion/hyperbaric O_2: Severe sxs not responsive to methylene blue or if methylene blue is contraindicated (eg, G6PD deficiency)

Disposition

- Admit if CO level >25%, methemoglobin level >20%, dapsone tox, LOC, pts w/ underlying cardiac/neurologic/respiratory dz

Pearls

- Do NOT use methylene blue in pts w/ G6PD deficiency (hemolytic anemia)
- Large amounts of methylene blue may paradoxically elevate methemoglobin levels

---

Hypoglycemics

History

- Oral ingestion of sulfonylureas, meglitinides (eg, repaglinide), or SC/IV insulin (oral insulin is not toxic)
- Agitation, coma, convulsions, confusion, blurry vision, n/v, rapid heartbeat, sweating, tingling of tongue & lips, tremor, dizziness, poor feeding; children may show sxs w/i 5 mins of ingestion
- RF: Extremes of age, polypharmacy, renal or hepatic dz, suicide attempt

Physical Examination

- AMS, generalized weakness, diaphoresis, tachycardia, tachypnea, transient neurologic deficit, pallor, sz, cyanosis, coma, hypothermia

Evaluation

- **Labs:** FSG q1h, BMP, tox screen (if SI or ingestion unknown), C-peptide (present w/ endogenous insulin secretion)

Treatment

- Supportive: ABCs, activated charcoal if recent ingestion
- Dextrose:
  - Oral: Gluc paste, juice
  - IV: 0.5–1 g/kg IV $D_{50}W$ (adults), $D_{25}W$ (children), $D_{10}W$ (neonates) × 1 dose; persistent hypoglycemia: 0.5 g/kg/h $D_{10}W$ (titrate to gluc >100)
- Glucagon: 1 mg/dose IV/IM/SC (if <20 kg, 0.5 mg/dose)
- Octreotide for sulfonylurea or meglitinide overdose

Disposition

- Home: Pts w/ unintentional isolated insulin overdose may be treated & released after effect of insulin wears off depending on rapid vs long acting
- Admit: Pts w/ sulfonylurea overdose must be monitored for at least 8 h

OTHER INGESTIONS

Etiology, Hx, & Sxs of Other Ingestions		
Overdose	**Etiology**	**Sxs of Acute Toxicity**
Insecticides	**Organophosphate** "nerve gas" (Sarin, Tabun, Soman) inhibit AChE & pseudocholinesterase (PChe) in plasma	SLUDGE: Salivation, lacrimation, urinary incontinence, defecation, GI distress, emesis Other: Respiratory depression primary cause of death; AVOID succinylcholine
	Carbamates (used to treat myasthenia gravis)	Similar to organophosphates but shorter acting & may not have neuro sxs (less crossover to BBB)
	Chlorinated hydrocarbons (DDT, chlordane, lindane)	Tremors, paresthesias, szs, AMS, muscle twitching, hyperthermia, arrhythmias, rhabdomyolysis, chemical pneumonitis
Iron	Any iron supplement, tox >20 mg/kg	<12 h: GI (emesis/diarrhea/abd pain; Severe: Bloody emesis/diarrhea, large fluid losses) 6–24 h: Latent phase w/o sxs 24–72 h: Hepatorenal failure 2–6 wks: Chronic GI strictures
Phenytoin/ fosphenytoin		Lethargy, dysarthria, ataxia, dizziness, confusion, horizontal nystagmus, n/v
Hydrocarbons/ volatiles	Baby oil, mineral oil, furniture polish, paint thinner, petroleum jelly, solvents, gasoline, lamp oil kerosene, lighter fluid	Hydrocarbon odor, glue sniffer's rash, chemical pneumonitis, aspiration, confusion, depression, szs, dysrhythmias, n/v, liver failure, burns, cerebellar dysfxn
Herbicides	Paraquat, diquat, Roundup (glyphosate), Glufosinate, Atrazine, Mecoprop, Acetochlor, Dicamba, Pentachlorophenols, Chlorophenoxy, Nitrophenolic, Metolachlor	Dermatologic irritant, mediastinitis, peritonitis, n/v/d, liver failure, CV shock, coma, sz, muscle weakness, renal failure/tubular necrosis/ myoglobinuria, rhabdomyolysis, pulmonary edema, pulmonary fibrosis (paraquat), ICH (diquat)
Heavy metals	Arsenic, bismuth, cadmium, chromium, cobalt, copper, lead, manganese, mercury, nickel, selenium, silver, thallium, zinc	Varies based on poisoning; in general n/v, GI distress, renal failure/ATN, pneumonitis, encephalopathy, abd pain; zinc smells like fish
Rodenticides	Red squill, strychnine, yellow phosphorus, warfarin type/ brodifacoum	Red squill: Cardiac glycoside-like sxs Strychnine: Sz-like appearance w/ extensor posturing, rhabdomyolysis Yellow phosphorus: Garlic odor, oral burns, vomiting, phosphorescent smelling feces, GIB, electrolyte abnl, sz, arrhythmias, renal/hepatic failure Warfarin type/brodifacoum: Long-acting anticoagulation, bleeding risk
Household products	Acids (toilet bowel cleaners), bases (bleach, ammonia), detergents, all-purpose cleaners (glass cleaner, pine oil, turpentine), chlorine, cosmetics	Bases/acids: GI irritation Bases: Pneumonitis, pneumomediastinum Perfume/mouthwash: Depends on alcohol level Pine oil/turpentine: Hemorrhagic pulmonary edema Detergents: GI irritants/corrosives, pulmonary edema Glass cleaner: Ocular, o/w well tolerated

Eval & Tx of Other Ingestions		
Overdose	**Labs/Imaging**	**Tx**
Organophosphates	BMP, ECG, plasma cholinesterase level, lactate, CK, LFTs, CXR	Decontamination; atropine (2–5 mg) IV q5min (endpoint = dried secretions); 2-PAM 1–2 g IV over 30–60 mins, 500–1000 mg/h (will not work on skeletal muscle); BZD (PRN szs/agitation)
Carbamates	Same as organophosphates	Supportive, decontamination, atropine (dose same as organophosphates)
Chlorinated hydrocarbons	Electrolytes (metabolic acidosis, ATN), ECG (arrhythmias), CK (rhabdomyolysis)	Supportive, decontamination, activated charcoal, cholestyramine (do not use in bowel obstruction), BZD (PRN sz/agitation), βB
Iron	Fe level q4h; check BMP, LFTs, lactate, CBC, coags if symptomatic; x-ray/CT KUB may show radiopaque tablets	Decontamination & whole bowel irrigation; supportive/IVF; deferoxamine 15 mg/kg/h (max 1 g/h) over 6 h (for severe sxs, may induce hypotension)
Phenytoin/ fosphenytoin	Check phenytoin or fosphenytoin level; calculate free phenytoin level, albumin level, ECG, BMP	Supportive, activated charcoal, treat hypotension w/ fluids/pressors
Hydrocarbons & other Volatiles	BMP (renal tubular acidosis, hypokalemia), ECG, LFTs (elevated); CXR (infiltrate, bronchovascular markings)	Remove all exposed clothing; supportive care—if intubated, PEEP beneficial
Herbicides	BMP (tubular necrosis, hypernatremia), lipase, CK, urine myoglobin, ECG (dysrhythmias), LFTs, CXR	Irrigate all areas of exposure, IVF, electrolyte replacement, BZD (sz, agitation); activated charcoal Paraquat/Diquat/Glufosinate: Hemoperfusion Chlorophenoxy: Alkaline diuresis via 1–2 amps bicarb + KCl (urine output: 4–6 cc/kg/h) Pentachlorophenols/nitrophenolic: Aggressive cooling, treat hyperkalemia/rhabdomyolysis
Heavy metals	Send off individual levels, BMP (electrolyte abnl, renal failure), CBC (Hct), CXR (pneumonitis)	BAL: Copper, arsenic, lead, mercury NAC: Chromium, cobalt D-Penicillamine: Copper EDTA: Cobalt, lead MDAC/Prussian Blue: Thallium Selenium: Silver Succimer: Lead, copper, arsenic
Rodenticides	CXR, BMP, LFTs, ECG, CXR, CK, Urine hCG, PT/PTT, may check individual levels	Decontaminate, activated charcoal, whole bowel irrigation, supportive, renal failure may require HD
Household material	BMP (hypernatremia w/ bleach), CXR (aspiration PNA)	Supportive: IVF, intubation if necessary; copious irrigation of skin, eye Ingestion: Water, milk to reduce irritation; Pine oil/turpentine: GI decontamination, endoscopy

AIRWAY MANAGEMENT

Approach

- Assess need for intubation

Indications for Intubation
Inability to protect or maintain airway
Inability to ventilate or oxygenate
Impending clinical course

- Anticipated need for airway mgmt in pts at risk for deterioration
- Assess difficulty of intubation early
- In pts w/ acute respiratory failure, BVM ventilation or NIPPV can be a bridge, but not a substitute, to intubation
- **Choose appropriate intubation algorithm**

Airway Algorithms	
Clinical Presentation	**Algorithm**
Standard	RSI
Difficult preoxygenation/agitation	Delayed sequence intubation
Anticipated difficult airway	Awake intubation*
Failed airway: Can't intubate	BVM + oral airway, EGD
Failed airway: Can't intubate, can't ventilate	Cricothyrotomy
Crash airway (near D)	BVM, intubation by any means

- **Choose appropriate intubation tool**
  - VL: 1st choice; higher 1st pass success rate vs DL
  - DL: Most commonly used (Mac or Miller blade)
  - Awake intubation (when difficult laryngoscopy is anticipated or severely deranged physiology prohibits sedation/paralysis): Inhalation and dense topical application of local anesthetic, evaluate airway, intubate via VL or fiber optic, sedate when airway established → *requires cooperative pt, noncrash airway, redundant setup for RSI
  - Mac 3 may improve laryngoscopy and intubation success compared to Mac 4

Pearls

- Have rescue devices at the ready: EGD, cricothyrotomy kit
  - Consider glycopyrrolate 0.2 mg IV w/ ketamine to minimize secretions
- Good BVM technique saves lives
- When unsure or when difficulty predicted, use airway algorithm most experienced intubator is most comfortable and familiar w/—typically RSI

RAPID SEQUENCE INTUBATION

- **Approach to laryngoscopy with direct or video laryngoscope**
  - Optimize positioning (see below)
  - Hold laryngoscope in L hand
  - Hold suction in R hand from the beginning of the attempt; if airway grossly contaminated (ongoing emesis, blood), place additional suction catheter in hypopharynx and leave in place throughout laryngoscopy for continuous suctioning
  - Scissor open mouth w/ R hand
  - Insert blade into midline mouth; if physical obstruction (small mouth opening, VL wire connection, large chest) can insert blade into corner of mouth w/ handle 90° off midline → rotate into midline, gently depress tongue and advance incrementally to identify uvula → epiglottis → vallecula → arytenoids → vocal cords → lift anteriorly (toward ceiling) at 45° angle from horizontal (do not rock blade) → place ETT

The "7 Ps"
Preparation, **P**reoxygenation, **P**retreatment, **P**ositioning, **P**aralysis w/ induction, **P**lacement w/ proof, **P**ostintubation mgmt

- Preparation
  - Monitor O_2 sat, BP, cardiac rhythm, ≥1 IV, O_2 sat probe on opposite arm from BP cuff
  - BVM, **suction**, waveform $EtCO_2$ detector, oral airway, Bougie

- Intubation equipment (eg, laryngoscope): Blade, backup blade, check video monitor/light
- ETT: 7.5–8 (male), 7–7.5 (female); check cuff, load stylet/10-cc syringe; pediatrics tube size = 4+ (age in y/4) → or use Broselow tape
- RSI medications/doses
- Assess for difficult BVM, difficult intubation, & difficult cricothyrotomy → prepare appropriately

Assessing Difficult BVM → MOANS	
Measure	**Comment**
M—mask seal	Beard, lower facial trauma
O—obesity, obstruction	Includes angioedema, Ludwig angina, trauma, etc
A—age	Age >55 y
N—no teeth	Difficulty obtaining seal
S—stiff	Stiff lungs (asthma/COPD, PNA, ARDS, etc)

Assessing Difficult Airway → LEMON	
Measure	**Comment**
L—look externally	Overall gestalt of difficulty
E—evaluate 3-3-2	Can fit 3 fingers into open mouth, 3 fingers b/w tip of chin & chin/neck jxn, 2 fingers b/w chin/neck jxn & thyroid notch
M—Mallampati class	From I (soft palate, uvula, pillars seen) to IV (only hard palate seen)
O—obesity/obstruction	Look for muffled voice, difficulty handling secretions, stridor, sense of dyspnea
N—neck mobility	Eg, C-spine immobilization, ankylosing spondylitis, RA

Assessing Difficult Cricothyrotomy → SHORT	
Measure	**Comment**
S—surgery	Eg, Halo device, recent thyroid surgery
H—hematoma	Anything distorting neck anatomy (includes infection, abscess)
O—obesity	Also consider short neck, SC emphysema
R—radiation	Distorts anatomy
T—tumor	Distorts anatomy, ↑ bleeding

- Preoxygenation: BVM or BiPAP (provide ~100% FiO_2, PEEP) × 3 mins
- Consider passive/apneic oxygenation: Place NC on high flow throughout intubation, prolongs time to desaturation
- Pretreatment: Consider giving 3 min prior to intubation—lidocaine 1.5 mg/kg IV (↓ ICP, in pts w/ ↑ ICP, ↓ bronchospasm in pts w/ reactive airway dz); fentanyl 3 μg/kg IV (↓ ICP in pts w/ ↑ ICP, ↓ HTN response in pts w/ cardiac ischemia, aortic dissection, head bleed)
- Paralysis w/ induction: Always induce prior to paralysis
- Induction: Etomidate (0.3 mg/kg IV), ketamine (1–3 mg/kg IV), midazolam (0.3 mg/kg IV)
- Paralysis: Succinylcholine (1.5 mg/kg IV, if no CI), rocuronium (1.2–1.5 mg/kg IV)
  - Succinylcholine CIs: Large burns, paralysis, crush injury (w/ in 3 d–6 mos), abd sepsis (>3 d), elevated ICP or IOP, hx of MH, neurologic d/o (muscular dystrophy, MS, amyotrophic lateral sclerosis)
  - Rocuronium has no CIs but longer half-life often leads to delayed sedation
- Positioning: Sniffing position, align tragus of the ear w/ the sternal notch, pad beneath occiput and shoulder blades, extend atlanto-occipital joint. If in C-spine immobilization, open collar and hold manual stabilization
- Placement w/ proof: Insert ETT via direct visualization of vocal cords, inflate cuff
- Confirm placement: Waveform $EtCO_2$ detector, auscultate lungs (assess for R-side intubation)
- Secure ETT
- Postintubation mgmt: oral gastric tube, CXR, sedation (benzos, propofol, ketamine), analgesia (fentanyl, ketamine), initiate mechanical ventilation

Pearls

- Consider delayed sequence intubation in agitated pt requiring additional resuscitation, procedures, or preoxygenation prior to intubation via ketamine 1 mg/kg followed by additional interventions before proceeding w/ intubation

CRICOTHYROTOMY

Purpose
- Failed airway (can't intubate/can't oxygenate or ventilate); severe facial trauma, trismus, upper airway obstruction

Equipment
- Scalpel (#10 blade), Bougie, 6.0–6.5 ETT (or tracheostomy tube if available)

Positioning
- Pt supine, hyperextend neck if no CI

Procedure
- Sterile technique if time allows; see *Rapid Sequence Intubation* section above for preparation & postintubation management
- **Open technique**
  - Hold larynx w/ nondominant hand
  - Rest dominant forearm on the pt's sternum to maintain anatomical midline anchor
  - Make generous **vertical incision** w/ dominant hand from thyroid cartilage to cricoid membrane (2–3 cm), through skin & soft tissue. Extend superiorly or inferiorly as needed to ensure adequate exposure to cricothyroid membrane
  - Palpate cricothyroid membrane through incision using nondominant index finger, **not** visualization
  - Make **stab incision** through cricothyroid membrane → extend horizontally until resistance felt → twist scalpel 180° and extend horizontally until resistance felt at opposite side
  - Place finger into incision → place bougie beneath fingertip into airway and advance until hold up at carina → slide ETT over bougie just until balloon is in airway → remove bougie
  - Inflate cuff, confirm placement w/ waveform $EtCO_2$ and b/l breath sounds, and secure tube w/ suture or tube tie

Complications
- Bleeding, misplaced tube, vocal cord damage
- Contraindicated in children <10 y/o, consider needle cricothyrotomy in peds

Pearl
- The hardest part of performing cricothyrotomy is deciding to do it → therefore, always consider this procedure in your airway algorithm—the vast majority of difficult airways are unanticipated
- When using ETT, placement often too deep and into R mainstem. Carefully auscultate breath sounds and retract as needed. Can then trim ETT to reduce extra length
- Consider larger initial vertical midline incision (eg, submentum to suprasternal notch) if no landmarks (obese, anterior neck swelling)

PRIMARY SURVEY

Definition

- Initial survey of the trauma pt for rapid identification of life-threatening injuries

Approach

- Eval in ABCDE order: airway, breathing/ventilation, circulation, disability, exposure/environmental control

1° Survey	
Airway maintenance w/ C-spine immobilization	Talking → airway patent → frequent reassessment Unable to talk → eval for FB/facial fractures/tracheal/laryngeal injury/other obstruction → if obstruction not reversible w/ chin lift/jaw thrust or GCS <8 → intubation w/ C-spine immobilization Severe facial/neck trauma. Be prepared for surgical airway (see Section 17: Airway Management for further details of airway mgmt)
Breathing/ventilation	Eval chest wall excursion/b/l breath sounds/chest wall (flail chest, crepitance, open chest wound, tracheal injury, pulm contusion) → identify/repair injuries that impair ventilation; tension PTX (needle decompression/finger or tube thoracostomy); massive hemothorax (tube thoracostomy → >1500 cc blood out or >200 cc/h or unstable HD → OR), open PTX (occlusive dressing + tube thoracostomy)
Circulation	Hypotension/altered MS/confusion/mottled skin/thready pulse/diminished pulse = hemorrhage/hypovolemia until proven o/w → place multiple large-bore IVs/control external hemorrhage → resuscitate w/ 1 L NS only if hypotensive & blood products unavailable → persistent hypotension; transfuse PRBC (males O^+, females O^-), consider massive tfx protocol (1 PRBC:1 FFP:1 PLTs) if persistent tfx requirements, consider permissive hypotension (SBP 70–100 mmHg) & restrictive use of fluids FAST exam to evaluate for intra-abd hemorrhage → + FAST + persistent hypotension = OR
Disability	Rapid neurologic assessment; AVPU (**A**lert, responds to **V**erbal stimuli, responds to **P**ainful stimuli, **U**nresponsive), GCS
Exposure/environmental	Remove clothes, avoid hypothermia (massive tfxs/environmental exposures), which can lead to coagulopathies (use warmed blankets/IVF)

Glasgow Coma Scale
Eye opening
4—Open eyes spontaneously
3—Open eyes to command
2—Open eyes to pain
1—No eye opening
BEST motor response
6—Obeys commands
5—Localizes pain
4—Withdraws to pain
3—Decorticate posturing (abnl flexion)
2—Decerebrate posturing (abnl extension)
1—None (flaccid)
Verbal response
5—Oriented, fluent speech
4—Confused conversation
3—Inappropriate words
2—Incomprehensible words
1—No speech

Best possible score, 15; worst possible score, 3.

HEAD TRAUMA

Background

- Leading cause of traumatic death in pts <25
- 80% mild (GCS 14–15), 10% mod (GCS 9–13), 10% severe (GCS <9) injuries
- CPP = MAP – ICP
- Target ICP ≤22 mmHg & SBP ≥100
- 1° brain injury: mechanical, irreversible damage caused by mechanical cell damage
- 2° brain injury: alteration in cerebral blood flow → cerebral ischemia, membrane disruption, cerebral edema, free radical generation

Approach

- Hx: Associated sxs (photophobia, vomiting, visual Δ, ocular pain), focal neurologic sxs
- Assess for head or neck trauma, medications, substance abuse
- Check fingerstick blood sugar to r/o hypoglycemia as cause for AMS
- Warning signs for neuroimaging: severe HA, vomiting, worsening over d, aggravated by exertion or Valsalva, neck stiffness, AMS, abnl neuro exam, peri- or retroorbital pain

Skull Fractures

History

- Direct blow to the head, pt c/o pain

Findings

- Skull depression
- Basilar skull fx: Periorbital ecchymosis (raccoon eyes), retroauricular hematoma (Battle sign), otorrhea & rhinorrhea (CSF leak), 7th nerve palsy, hemotympanum

Evaluation

- Noncontrast head CT. CBC, Chem, coags, type & screen, tox screen; plain films not indicated
- CTA to eval for vascular injury if basilar skull fx present

Treatment & Disposition

- Airway mgmt; mgmt guided by underlying brain injury
- Linear skull fx: If closed fx, w/ no other IC injury, may be observed 4–6 h & D/C
- Depressed skull fx: Admit to NSGY, surgical elevation if depressed skull fx > thickness of skull, update tetanus, give prophylactic abx (eg, cefazolin) & consider anticonvulsants
- Basilar skull fx: Admit to NSGY

Pearl

- GCS more indicative of underlying brain injury or hemorrhage

Scalp Laceration

History

- Direct blow to the head, direct bleeding from scalp

Findings

- Often blood has clotted upon ED arrival; has potential for large blood loss
- Blood loss may not be evident in ED, eval for blood loss in field

Evaluation

- Noncontrast head CT if indicated. CBC, Chem, coags, type & screen, tox screen if significant blood loss
- Thoroughly evaluate & explore skull for depressions & large lacerations

Treatment

- Irrigation: Wounds often contaminated despite rich blood supply, direct venous drainage into the venous sinuses can cause significant CNS infxns
- Hemostasis: Use pressure, lidocaine w/ epinephrine, figure-of-8 stitch, Raney clip
- Closure: Staples or modified hair apposition technique can be used if galea not involved
  - If galea involved, repair galea w/ absorbable sutures & close dermis w/ interrupted or vertical mattress sutures using 3-0 Nylon or Prolene
  - Continued bleeding of galea → subgaleal hematoma that often becomes infected

Disposition

- If no other injuries, can D/C. O/w admx & observation

Pearl

- Abx not indicated for properly managed head wound unless gross contamination

Head Injury Classifications			
	Mild	**Moderate**	**Severe**
GCS	14–15	9–13	<9
Hx	Transient LOC, amnestic to event	LOC, amnestic to event	Pt unable to provide hx

Sxs	Mild HA, nausea	Confused or somnolent, often unable to follow commands	Obtunded, cannot follow simple commands
Head CT	Only if indicated (head CT rules); usually neg	All pts	All pts
Eval	Evaluate C-spine, no other testing needed	CBC, gluc, Chem, tox, coags, UA, hCG	CBC, gluc, Chem, tox, coags, UA, hCG
Tx	Observation w/ neuro checks, D/C w/ careful return instructions	24-h admx even if head CT neg, repeat CT if ↓ GCS, AMS	Intubation, NSGY eval, IVF, tight BP control (SBP >100 & <180), treat ↑ ICP (mannitol, hypertonic NS), sz tx

Canadian Head CT Rule[a]
Indications for CT Scan
GCS <15 at 2-h postinjury
Suspected open or depressed skull fx
Age >64
Retrograde amnesia to event for >30 mins
Any sign of basilar skull fx
2 or more episodes of vomiting
Dangerous mechanism

[a]Must have initial GCS 13–15. Exclusion: age <16, seizure, pregnancy, unstable vitals, neuro deficit or anticoagulated. Derived from *Lancet* 2001;357(9266):1391.

Postconcussive Syndrome

History

- Head injury, ±LOC (brief); HA, memory problems, insomnia, dizziness, etc, may last wks

Findings

- Nl neurologic exam, wide spectrum of mild neuro complaints

Evaluation

- Noncontrast CT shows no bleed, but clinically insignificant SAH may have occurred

Treatment

- Symptomatic HA control
- Avoidance of contact sports w/ stepwise return to full activity while monitoring sxs

Disposition

- D/C w/ careful head injury instructions

Pearls

- Thought to be secondary to stretching of white matter fibers at time of injury
- 2nd head injury more dangerous than 1st, "second impact syndrome"

Intracerebral/Intraparenchymal Hemorrhage

History

- Depends on size & location; traumatic, HTN, or hemorrhagic conversion of ischemic CVA

Findings

- Pts commonly c/o HA, n/v

Evaluation

- Noncontrast head CT; CBC, Chem, coags, type & screen

Treatment

- Airway mgmt
- Emergent neurosurgical eval, although most pts are managed nonoperatively; ICP monitor if significant bleed present
- Mannitol or hypertonic saline for ↑ ICP, PPx anticonvulsant medication for traumatic IPH, reserve for clinical or electrographic szs in spontaneous IPH
- Reverse coagulopathy emergently w/ appropriate agent (Vit K vs FFP vs PCC vs factor concentrate) depending on underlying cause of coagulopathy

Disposition

- Most require admx, often based on 6-h repeat head CT

Pearl

- Frontal lobe hematoma may cause disinhibition & personality Δ

Subarachnoid Hemorrhage

History

- Pt c/o "worst HA of life"; acute onset & rapid progression, meningismus, vomiting, photophobia; can often pinpoint exact moment of onset
- Spontaneous (ruptured cerebral aneurysm [~75%], AVM [~10%]) or traumatic

Findings

- HA, n/v, sz, syncope, acute distress
- Acute AMS is indicative of large bleed, usually requires emergent intervention

Evaluation

- Noncontrast CT scan of head, ancillary studies (CBC, BMP, coags, T&S)
- Head CT 95–99% sens for acute SAH w/i 6 h of sx onset
- If CT noncon neg & onset >6 h but high concern for SAH, proceed to CTA vs LP after shared decision making considering risks/benefits of each
- Neg CT + CTA can exclude SAH w/ 99% posttest probability (*Acad Emerg Med* 2010;17(4):444)
- Approx. 3% of population will have asx aneurysm found on CTA
- Large # RBC in CSF on LP highly suggestive of SAH
- RBCs are hemolyzed in CSF, may not be present in large numbers after 12 h or may not be present at all after 2 wks
- Xanthochromia highly suggestive of bleed b/w 12 h & 2 wks (yellow discoloration due to RBC breakdown)
- Check fingerstick blood sugar to r/o hypoglycemia as cause for AMS

Treatment

- Airway mgmt if comatose or not protecting airway, neurosurgical consultation
- ICP & BP monitoring if bleed is significant; a-line, elevate head of bed to 30°
- SPB b/w 90 & 140 mmHg, HR b/w 50 & 90 bpm, nicardipine or labetalol PRN
- Mannitol or hypertonic saline for significant bleed w/ increased ICP
- Nimodipine to decrease vasospasm 60 mg PO q4h × 21 d
- Sz prophylaxis (levetiracetam)

Disposition

- To neurologic ICU

Pearls

- Outcome directly related to amount of intracranial blood
- 30–50% have "sentinel HA" d to wks prior to SAH
- 3rd nerve palsy (pupillary dilation, "down and out" position, ptosis) → PCOM aneurysm

Clinical Findings of SAH	
Findings	**Frequency**
HA	95–100%
Meningismus	Frequent
Transient LOC/syncope	50%
Retinal subhyaloid hemorrhage	6–30%

Hunt–Hess Scale for SAH		
Grade		**Survival (%)**
I.	Asx or mild HA	70
II.	Mod-to-severe HA, nuchal rigidity, no neuro deficits or other CN palsy	60
III.	Confusion, drowsiness, mild focal signs	50
IV.	Stupor or hemiparesis	40
V.	Coma, moribund appearance, posturing	10

Subdural Hematoma

History

- Often caused by acceleration/deceleration tearing injury of bridging veins
- Can be acute (<48 h), subacute (2 d–3 wks), or chronic (>3 wks)

Findings

- Varied. Range from HA w/ nausea to comatose & flaccid

Evaluation

- Noncontrast head CT shows crescent-shaped mass. Check CBC, Chem, Coags, type & screen

Treatment

- Airway mgmt, emergent neurosurgical eval
- If e/o ↑ ICP or midline shift, mannitol or hypertonic saline & anticonvulsant
- Reverse coagulopathy emergently w/ appropriate agent (Vit K, PCC, FFP, factor conc.)

Disposition
- Most require admx, often based on 6-h repeat head CT

Pearls
- More common than epidural hematoma
- Comatose & flaccid pts w/ SDH have an extremely poor prognosis, should discuss w/ family

Epidural Hematoma

History
- Brief LOC followed by "lucid interval," then rapidly progressive deterioration
- Head injury usually in area of temporal bone, causes damage to middle meningeal artery

Findings
- Ipsilateral pupil deviation, occasionally contralateral hemiparesis, n/v, sz, hyperreflexia, +Babinski

Evaluation
- Noncontrast CT often shows lenticular biconcave mass, possible fx of temporal bone
- CBC, Chem, coag panel, type & screen

Treatment
- Airway mgmt, emergent neurosurgical consultation
- Mannitol or hypertonic saline & anticonvulsant if e/o ↑ ICP, midline shift
- Reverse coagulopathy emergently w/ appropriate agent (Vit K, PCC, FFP, factor conc.)

Disposition
- Most require admx, often based on 6-h repeat head CT

Pearl
- Bleeding b/w the dura mater & skull

Indications for Sz Prophylaxis
Depressed skull fractures
Paralyzed & intubated, severe head injury
Sz at the time of injury or during ED presentation
Penetrating brain injury
GCS ≤8
Acute SDH, EDH, or ICH
Hx of szs prior to injury

Diffuse Axonal Injury

History
- Result of tremendous shearing forces seen in high-speed MVCs

Findings
- Pts often present in coma; document best neuro response: May have prognostic value

Evaluation
- Noncontrast CT often nl, must r/o bleed
- CBC, Chem, coag panel, type & screen, tox; look for other etiology for coma
- MRI (nonemergent) will show Δ & can guide prognosis

Treatment
- Emergent neurosurgical consultation for ICP monitor to avoid 2° injury from edema
- Mannitol or hypertonic saline & anticonvulsants

Disposition
- Admit

Pearl
- Prognosis determined by clinical course & difficult to predict

MAXILLOFACIAL INJURY

Definition

Injuries to the soft tissue or bones of the face (50% caused by MVCs)

Approach

Inspection
- Deformities, enophthalmos (orbital blowout fracture), jaw malocclusion, dentition step-offs, nasal septal/auricular hematomas, rhinorrhea (CSF leak), trigeminal/facial nerve deficits, abnl EOM, diplopia, gross visual acuity

Palpation

- Facial prominences for tenderness/bony defects/crepitance/false motion, FB

Radiology

- CT face for most injuries, CTA in injuries at high risk for vascular trauma

Soft Tissue Injury

History

- MVC/bites/assault

Evaluation

- CT only if bony injury/FB suspected

Treatment

- Irrigate/eval for FB/1° closure w/i 24 h, abx (cefazolin, ampicillin/sulbactam, amoxicillin/clavulanate) for contaminated wounds (eg, bites), tetanus vaccine update, plastic surgery repair for nerve damage/extensive repair

Disposition

- Home

Nasal Septal/Auricular Hematomas

History

- Direct trauma to the nose (a/w nasal bone fractures)/ear (classically in wrestlers)

Physical Findings

- Swelling/purple discoloration to the nose or ear. Nasal septum may appear grape-like

Treatment

- Septal: Apply topical anesthetic, incise/evacuate w/ elliptical incision, pack b/l nares, abx (amoxicillin/clavulanate); failure to drain → cartilage necrosis → saddle nose deformity or septal abscess
- Auricular: Anesthetize area w/ auricular block, needle aspiration (small hematomas) or incise along skin folds, evacuate, apply compression dressing, abx (levofloxacin for adults, amoxicillin/clavulanate for pediatric); failure to drain/compress → cauliflower ear/infxn

Disposition

- Home, ENT f/u in 24 h

Nasal Fractures

History

- Direct trauma to the nose

Physical Findings

- Swelling/deformity/ecchymosis to nose. Note patency of nares, any gross deviation, & appearance of septum

Evaluation

- Clinical dx. CT only if significant deformity/persistent epistaxis/rhinorrhea/telecanthus

Disposition

- Isolated nasal fractures → Most home w/ ice × 24 h, plastic/ENT f/u in 5–7 d for reduction, consider reduction in ED if displaced. Pediatric pts have ↑ risk for growth dysplasia

Pearl

- Septal hematoma requires immediate I&D to prevent necrosis

Zygomatic Fracture

Definition

- Fractures of the zygomatic arch or fracture at the zygomaticotemporal suture/zygomaticofrontal suture/infraorbital foramen (tripod fracture)

History

- Direct trauma to face

Physical Findings

- Shallow depression over temporal region, lateral canthal ptosis, trismus, edema, diplopia/vertical dystopia/infraorbital nerve anesthesia (tripod fracture)

Evaluation

- Maxillofacial CT

Treatment

- ENT/OMFS/plastics consult

Disposition
- Home, ENT/OMFS/plastics f/u for delayed ORIF, sinus precautions

Mandibular Fractures
Definition
- Fracture of the mandible (>50% involve multiple fracture sites of the mandible)

History
- Direct trauma to mandible (assaults usually = body/angle fractures, MVC usually = symphysis/condylar fractures)

Physical Findings
- Malocclusion, trismus, sublingual hematoma, associated dental & lingual injury

Evaluation
- Maxillofacial CT preferred (100% sens), esp. if concern for condylar fractures or additional facial trauma. Panorex can be used (86% sens) for isolated mandibular body/symphysis fractures, can miss condylar fracture
- CTA if high-energy mechanism (risk for BCVI)

Treatment
- OMFS or plastic surgery consult: Temporary immobilization (wiring of jaw) or delayed ORIF, abx (PCN, clindamycin) if communicating w/ oral cavity (aka open fx)

Disposition
- Home

Pearls
- Pts w/ temporary wiring must be D/C w/ wire cutters
- Tongue blade test has 89% sens, 95% spec for mandibular fx
- CXR to evaluate for aspirated teeth if unaccounted for missing teeth

Maxillary Fractures
Definition
- Fracture of the maxilla, rare in isolation, a/w significant mechanism, greatest risk of airway compromise, traditionally classified by Le Fort system

History
- Significant mechanism trauma to the face (eg, MVC w/ impact on dashboard/pavement)

Physical Findings
- Midface swelling/mobility, malocclusion of mandible, CSF rhinorrhea

Evaluation
- Maxillofacial CT
- CTA in Le Fort II & III (risk for BCVI)

Treatment
- Airway mgmt (eval for difficult airway, Le Fort II/III highest risk), hemorrhage control (nasal packing/nasal Foley/elevation of head), prophylactic abx (ceftriaxone) for CSF leak to prevent meningitis (controversial), ENT/OMFS consult

Disposition
- Admit

Le Fort Classification	
Le Fort I	Involves only maxilla at level of nasal fossa; free-floating jaw
Le Fort II	Involves maxilla, nasal bones, & medial aspects of the orbits & is described as pyramidal dysfxn
Le Fort III	Involves the maxilla, zygoma, nasal bones, & ethmoids. Extends through the maxillary sinuses & infraorbital rims bilaterally across the bridge of the nose. Is described as craniofacial dysjunction

EYE INJURY

Orbital Fracture
Definition
- Fracture to the wall of the orbit (floor/medial wall most common)

History
- Blunt trauma to eye by object larger than the orbital rim

Physical Findings
- Periorbital swelling/crepitance, tenderness/irregularities to bony orbit, vertical diplopia/limited ROM w/ upward gaze (inferior rectus/inferior oblique entrapment), diplopia/limited ROM w/ lateral gaze (medius rectus entrapment), hypoesthesia of lower lid/cheek (infraorbital nerve entrapment), enophthalmos, ptosis

Evaluation
- Orbital CT (opacification of maxillary sinus or teardrop sign = orbital floor fracture)

Treatment
- Abx (cover sinus flora, eg, amoxicillin/clavulanate), ophthalmology consult if any EOM entrapment or visual acuity Δ (rarely require surgery unless diplopia/entrapment), "sinus precautions" (no nose blowing/sneezing, no sucking on straws/smoking)

Disposition
- Home

Pearls
- Consider associated ocular injury, such as retrobulbar hematoma or malignant orbital emphysema, which can both cause ocular compartment synd
- Pts are at ↑ risk zygomatic tripod fractures/Le Fort II & III fractures

Globe Rupture

Definition
- Full-thickness defect in the cornea/sclera

History
- Blunt (most common at muscle insertion sites/corneoscleral junction) or penetrating (more common) trauma, decreased vision, pain

Physical Findings
- ↓ visual acuity, teardrop-shaped pupil, hyphema, +Seidel test (bright stream of aqueous humor after fluorescein) for corneal perforations, intraocular content extrusion, flattening of anterior chamber, oculocardiac reflex can cause bradycardia, 360° bullous subconjunctival hemorrhage can be seen in posterior rupture

Evaluation
- Orbital CT w/ thin cuts (for foreign body). Obvious globe rupture is contraindication to US

Treatment
- Ophthalmology consult (for surgical repair w/i 1st 24 h), tetanus, abx to prevent endophthalmitis (vanc + ceftazidime/fluoroquinolone), avoid pressure on eye/topical agents/Valsalva (antiemetics, pain control), protective shield

Disposition
- Admit

Pearl
- If concern for globe rupture do not perform IOP measurement

Chemical Burns

Definition
- Burns to sclera/conjunctiva/cornea/lid caused by alkali (oven cleaner, dish soap, detergents, cement, bleach), which cause liquefactive necrosis (deeper injury & ↑ risk of glaucoma) or acid (toilet bowl cleaner, rust remover), which causes coagulative necrosis (superficial injury, corneal ulcers)

History
- Chemical exposure, severe pain, FB sensation, photophobia

Physical Findings
- ↓ visual acuity, conjunctival injection, blepharospasm, corneal edema, lens opacification, limbal blanching

Evaluation
- pH testing of effluent in fornices

Treatment
- Topical anesthetics, irrigation (>2 L NS), use Morgan lens/manual retraction to keep eye open, check pH every 30 mins until pH 7.3–7.7 & 10 mins later, ↑ IOP treat like glaucoma, cycloplegics (cyclopentolate, tropicamide) if ciliary spasm, antibiotic ointment, ophthalmology consult for corneal haziness/perforation/conjunctival blanching

Disposition
- Admit for increased IOP/intractable pain, minor burns: f/u in 24 h

Pearls

- Hydrofluoric acid exposure: Administer 1% calcium gluconate drops during irrigation
- If no pH paper available, can use urine dipstick, for nl pH compare to unaffected eye
- Water irrigation is contraindicated in dry lime & elemental metal exposures

Retrobulbar Hematoma

Definition

- Bleeding in the space surrounding the globe

History

- Blunt trauma, recent eye surgery, pain, vomiting, ↓ visual acuity

Physical Findings

- Afferent papillary defect, ↓ visual acuity, restricted EOM, ↑ IOP (rock hard to palpation), proptosis, periorbital ecchymosis, subconjunctival hemorrhage

Evaluation

- Orbital CT (do not delay treatment to obtain diagnostic imaging)

Treatment

- Immediate ophthalmology consult, decompress w/ lateral canthotomy (for IOP >40 mmHg, consider for >30 mmHg w/ severe visual deficit), elevated head of bed, analgesics, antiemetics, correct coagulopathy
- Serial IOP measurement as hematoma can expand

Disposition

- Admit

Retinal Detachment

Definition

- Separation of retina from underlying retinal pigment epithelium & choroid
- Three types: rhegmatogenous (from hole or tear in retina), tractional (vitreous contracts & pulls on retina, often in severe diabetic retinopathy), exudative (fluid accumulates behind retina, 2/2 inflammatory/infectious condition such as sarcoidosis or syphilis)

History

- Floaters/flashing lights, "mosca volante"—solitary large floater, ↑ IOP, visual loss (macula involvement)

Physical Findings

- Visual field deficit (curtain being pulled down). Dilated retinal exam demonstrates retinal tears/detachment

Evaluation

- POCUS w/ undulating, hyperechoic membrane that is tethered at optic disc

Treatment

- NPO, bed rest, restrict EOM, immediate ophthalmology consult for surgical repair

Disposition

- Admit

Hyphema

Definition

- Accumulation of blood in the anterior chamber caused by rupture iris root vessel (trauma) or sickle cell/DM/anticoagulation
- Grading: Microhyphema (cell & flare on slit lamp), Grade I (<33% anterior chamber filled), Grade II (33–50%), Grade III (>50%), & grade IV (100%). Grade III & above has 50% chance of recovery of 20/50 vision or better

History

- Blunt or penetrating trauma to the globe, dull eye pain, photophobia

Physical Findings

- Microhyphemas: Visualized w/ slit lamp, larger hyphemas: Visualized w/ tangential pen light, total hyphema (high a/w globe rupture): ↑ IOP

Evaluation

- CBC, PT, PTT, INR if w/ bleeding dyscrasia or on anticoagulation
- If any FH of hemoglobinopathy pt should be screened

Treatment

- Immediate ophthalmology consult for >10%/↑ IOP, treat ↑ IOP (timolol, acetazolamide), metal eye shield, cycloplegics (cyclopentolate, tropicamide) if ciliary spasm
- HOB >45% (upright allows blood to settle in anterior chamber/avoid retinal staining)
- Topical anesthesia if no globe rupture, PO/IV analgesia
- Topical steroids may help prevent rebleeding & synechiae

- Limit reading & activity × 1 wk
- Goals: to avoid intraocular HTN (which causes optic nerve atrophy) & rebleeds

Disposition

- Admit for >50%, ↑ IOP, coagulopathy or sick cell
- Urgent ophthalmology f/u

Pearls

- Sickle cell: Avoid acetazolamide/pilocarpine/hyperosmotic, ↑ risk of rapid ↑ IOP → optic nerve injury
- Avoid ASA/NSAIDs 2/2 ↑ rebleed risk
- 10% rebleed (usually more severe) in 2–5 d

Vitreous Hemorrhage

Definition

- Blood in the vitreous humor

History

- Blunt trauma, floaters, blurry vision, vision loss, sickle cell/DM

Physical Findings

- Loss of light reflex, poorly visualized fundus

Evaluation

- POCUS for associated retinal detachment; consider noncontrast CTH if a/w trauma

Treatment

- Immediate ophthalmology consult, HOB >45%, bed rest

Disposition

- Admit if retinal tear/unknown cause

Pearl

- Avoid ASA/NSAIDs b/c ↑ risk rebleed
- Consider nonaccidental trauma if seen in pediatric pt

Subconjunctival Hemorrhage

Definition

- Hemorrhage b/w the conjunctiva & sclera caused by trauma, Valsalva (coughing/straining/vomiting), HTN, coagulopathy

History

- Painless red eye

Physical Findings

- Blood b/w the conjunctiva & sclera

Treatment

- BP control, avoid Valsalva, avoid ASA/NSAIDs, artificial tears for comfort

Disposition

- Home, ophthalmology f/u in 1 wk; typically resolves in 2 wks

Pearl

- Hemorrhagic chemosis and 360° hemorrhage ↑ risk globe rupture

NECK TRAUMA

Definition

- Injuries to the soft tissue, neurovascular or aerodigestive structures of the neck

Approach

- Evaluate 3 main categories of neck injury: vascular, pharyngoesophageal, laryngotracheal (do not place NGT if esophageal/laryngeal injury suspected)

Inspection

- Look for hard signs: airway compromise, subcutaneous emphysema/bubbling, bruit, expanding/pulsatile hematoma, active bleeding/shock, neurologic deficit, hemoptysis, hematemesis

Penetrating Trauma Zones

- Anterior & posterior triangles: Anterior triangle contains most significant structures; it is bordered by anterior SCM, midline, & mandible. Posterior triangle is posterior to SCM, anterior to trapezius, & superior to clavicle
- Three zones: Zone I: sternal notch to cricoid cartilage (highest mortality), Zone II: b/w cricoid & angle of mandible, Zone III: above angle of mandible

Recommended Imaging for Penetrating Neck Injury	
Injury	**Imaging**
Vascular	Unstable → OR for exploration/angiography/embolization Zones I & III → CTA/angiography (high incidence of vascular injury) Zone II → CTA or exploration in OR
Pharyngoesophageal	CTA, Water-soluble contrast swallow study, endoscopy
Laryngotracheal	Unstable → bronchoscopy in OR Stable → CT scan (sens for detecting glottic/cartilaginous injury)

Penetrating Neck Trauma

Definition
- Injury to the neck from GSW, stabbings, projectile objects (shrapnel/glass)

Physical Findings
- Laryngotracheal injuries may have stridor, respiratory distress, hemoptysis, subcutaneous air, dysphonia
- Esophageal injuries may have dysphagia, hematemesis, subcutaneous air
- Vascular injuries may have neuro deficits, expanding/pulsatile hematoma/bleeding, bruit/thrill, hypotension

Evaluation
- CXR (PTX/hemothorax), lateral neck x-ray in trauma bay, CT, CTA
- Trauma labs: CBC, BMP, type & cross, PTT/PT, ABG

Treatment
- Airway mgmt (may be difficult airway), surgical consultation if platysma violation, abx (if ↑ risk contamination from aerodigestive perforation)
- Treat as trauma resuscitation (ABCs, tfx, etc)

Disposition
- Admit if surgical intervention/observation needed

Pearl
- Arrest due to penetrating neck trauma is indication for ED thoracotomy
- Neck exploration decisions based on zone of entry is moving toward approach based on sxs and CT/CTA

Strangulation

Definition
- Neck trauma due to manual strangulation or hanging attempts (3,500 D/y)
- Mechanism of death most commonly due to cerebral anoxia

History
- Strangulation, LOC, voice Δ, attempt to obtain "height of drop" from EMS
- Screen for intimate partner violence, suicidal ideation, & concerns for pt/child safety

Physical Findings
- Dysphonia/dyspnea, dysphagia, stridor, petechial hemorrhages (Tardieu spots), scleral hemorrhage, ligature/finger marks, neuro deficits/coma

Treatment
- Airway mgmt (may be difficult airway), surgical consultation (if needed), consider CTA, abx (if ↑ risk contamination from aerodigestive perforation) (*Ann Emerg Med* 2020;75(3):329–338)

Disposition
- Admit if injuries identified
- Involve forensic, social work, & behavioral health experts as needed for safe disposition

Pearls
- ↑ incidence of ARDS & long-term neuropsychiatric sequelae (selective vulnerability of hippocampus to anoxic injury) in significant strangulation/hanging injury
- Self-inflicted hanging is rarely a/w C-spine injury, see Hangman fracture
- Carotid baroreceptor reflex can trigger bradycardic arrest

Blunt Cerebrovascular Injury

Definition
- BCVI is defined as blunt injury (most often intimal tear) to carotid or vertebral arteries, affecting 1–3% of blunt trauma pts; feared complication is stroke
- Mechanisms incl. motor vehicle crashes, falls, assaults, suicide attempts

History
- Typically seen in pts w/ severe head, face, spine, chest, or abd injuries
- Majority w/ no neurologic manifestations at presentation

Physical Findings

- Findings suggestive of BCVI: Hemorrhage from the neck/mouth/nose/ear, expanding cervical hematoma, bruit, focal neuro deficits (eg, hemiparesis, Horner synd, vertebrobasilar insufficiency)

Indications for CTA Neck	
High-energy mechanism	C-spine fracture, ligament injury, or subluxation
Le Fort II or III or mandible fracture	Basilar skull or occipital condyle fracture
Near hanging w/ anoxic brain injury	Clothesline-type injury or painful/edematous seatbelt abrasion to neck
Scalp degloving	Severe TBI w/ GCS <6
TBI w/ thoracic injuries	Upper rib fractures
Blunt cardiac rupture	Thoracic vascular injury

Derived from: *J Trauma Acute Care Surg* 2020;88(6):875.

Treatment

- Antithrombotic therapy w/ heparin or antiplatelets (eg, aspirin 325 mg), operative repair, or endovascular treatments considered for higher-grade injuries

Disposition

- Most pts will have polytrauma & require admx, isolated low-grade BCVI pt may be discharged w/ close f/u

Pearls

- Must weigh risks & benefits of stroke prevention w/ bleeding risks based on pt's other traumatic injuries
- CTA typically repeated in 7–10 d to screen for resolution of BCVI & determine need for ongoing therapy

CERVICAL SPINE TRAUMA

Definition

- Injury to the bony/ligamentous structure of the cervical spine (C2 24%, C6 20%, C7 19%)

Approach

- Maintain C-spine immobilization until cleared clinically w/o imaging (see table) or radiographically

Palpation

- Midline cervical tenderness, step-offs, neurologic deficits

Radiology

- C-spine CT: 98% sens (gold standard) → obtain MRI if CT demonstrates pathology or neurologic deficits; consider MRI for obtunded/persistent midline tenderness; MRI 97% sens for ligamentous injury
  - Major trauma society guidelines support c-spine clearance in obtunded or intoxicated pt after neg CT and no neurologic deficits
- XR C-spine (52% sens) & flexion–extension XR no longer recommended due to poor sens

Cervical Spine Clearance	
NEXUS Low-Risk Criteria	**Canadian Cervical Spine Rule**
No posterior midline tenderness No focal neurologic deficits Nl alertness No intoxication No painful distracting injury (long bone fracture, visceral injury, large laceration, degloving, burns, injury causing functional impairment)	Inclusion: Age ≥16, GCS 15 NlVS (RR 10–24, SBP >90 mmHg), Injury w/i 48 h, blunt trauma Exclusion: Paralysis/paresthesia, known vertebral dz, repeat visit for same injury, pregnant, previous C-spine surgery 1. Any high-risk factor that mandates imaging? >65 y/o, dangerous mechanism (MVC rollover/ejection/>60 mph, fall from ≥3 ft, bicycle accident, axial load to head) or paresthesias to extremities. If YES, image. If NO, go to q2 2. Any low-risk factor that allows safe assessment of range of motion? Presence of ≥1 low-risk finding (simple rear-end MVC, sitting position in ED, ambulatory after trauma, delayed onset neck pain, no midline tenderness). If YES, go to q3. If NO, image 3. Able to rotate neck 45% L & R? If NO, image
90.7% sens, 36.8% spec for significant C-spine injury	99.4% sens, 45.1% spec for significant C-spine injury

C1 Burst Fracture (Jefferson Fracture)

Definition

- Unstable burst fracture of atlas (C1) causing widening of lateral masses (33% a/w C2 fracture)

History

- Axial load

Physical Findings

- C1 tenderness, neurologic deficit rare (wide canal at C1)

Evaluation

- CT/CTA to eval for associated vertebral artery injury, MRI for ligamentous injury. Disruption of transverse ligament determines instability

Treatment

- C-spine immobilization, spine consult for operative mgmt

Disposition

- Admit

Bilateral Facet Dislocation

Definition

- Anterolisthesis of articular masses of superior vertebra relative to articular surfaces of vertebra below, disrupting all ligamentous structures

History

- Flexion–extension injury, often result of buckling force

Physical Findings

- Often manifests w/ complete spinal cord injury w/ quadriplegia

Evaluation

- CT scan, MRI for ligamentous injury

Treatment

- C-spine immobilization, spine consult

Disposition

- Admit

Odontoid Fracture (C2 Dens)

Definition

- Fracture through the dens w/ variable stability (see table)

History

- Flexion–extension injury

Physical Findings

- C2 tenderness

Evaluation

- CT scan, MRI for ligamentous injury to transverse ligament

Treatment

- C-spine immobilization, spine consult

Disposition

- Likely admit

Dens Fracture Classification	
Classification	**Findings**
Type I	Avulsion fracture through upper part of odontoid process. Stable & does not require surgical intervention. C-collar
Type II	Fracture at the junction of the odontoid process w/ the vertebral body Potentially unstable fracture Nondisplaced: Halo often used to treat, high frequency of nonunion Displaced/angulated: Surgery often performed
Type III	Fracture at base of odontoid that extends down into body of atlas Immobilize w/ halo or collar, does not usually require surgery

C2 Hangman Fracture

Definition

- Unstable fracture of b/l C2 pedicles (↑ risk of C2 anterior subluxation/C2–C3 disk rupture → high mortality)

History
- Hyperextension
- Named due to judicial hangings in which knot is in front of pt & "height of drop" is at least as long as victim

Physical Findings
- C2 tenderness, high-impact trauma, neurologic deficits

Evaluation
- CT/CTA, MRI for ligamentous injury

Treatment
- C-spine immobilization, spine consult for operative mgmt

Disposition
- Admit

Tear Drop Fracture

Definition
- Unstable avulsion of cervical vertebral body at insertion of anterior ligament in extension injury (C2 common) or posterior ligament in flexion injury (C5–C6)

History
- Flexion (MVC, diving in pool) or extension (elderly fall on chin)

Physical Findings
- C-spine tenderness, anterior cord synd (flexion), central cord synd (extension)

Evaluation
- CT/CTA, MRI for ligamentous injury

Treatment
- C-spine immobilization, spine consult

Disposition
- Admit

Pearls
- Atlanto-occipital dislocations & atlanto-axial dislocations are another unstable cervical fracture pattern, but are often immediately fatal
- The mnemonic "Jefferson Bit Off A Hangman's Thumb" can be used to remember the major cervical spine fracture patterns

THORACIC/LUMBAR/SACRAL SPINE TRAUMA

Definition
- Injury to the bony/ligamentous structure of the spine below the level of the neck

Approach
- Maintain logroll precautions
- Examine: Spinal tenderness, step-offs, neurologic deficits, rectal tone
- Thoracolumbar Injury Classification and Severity Scale (TLICS) used for tx decisions

Anterior Wedge/Compression Fracture

Definition
- Compression fracture of the vertebral body (wedge → only anterosuperior vertebral body endplate)
- May be unstable if >50% height loss of vertebral body, significant kyphosis, rotational deformity, or multiple levels involved → Image posterior ligamentous complex

History
- Flexion w/ axial load

Physical Findings
- Focal tenderness, most often no neurologic deficits

Evaluation
- CT scan, MRI if concerns for associated ligamentous instability

Treatment
- Spine consult → Pain control, brace/orthosis, or surgical mgmt based on TLICS

Disposition
- D/C if stable pattern & pain controlled

Burst Fracture

Definition

- Compression fracture of anterior & posterior vertebral body (may be complicated by retropulsed bony fragments → cord injury). Neurologic deficits in 42–58% of pts

History

- Axial load/vertical compression w/ flexion

Physical Findings

- Focal tenderness, ±neurologic deficit

Evaluation

- CT scan, MRI to evaluate posterior ligament complex

Treatment

- Spine consult w/ bracing/orthosis vs surgical fixation based on TLICS

Disposition

- Likely admit

Chance Fracture

Definition

- Compression fracture through the vertebra w/ distraction to posterior elements, can include fractures to body/pedicles/laminae

History

- Back pain after head-on MVC when wearing only a lap belt from flexion–distraction injury

Physical Findings

- Focal tenderness, seatbelt sign, rare neurologic deficit

Evaluation

- CT scan. 50% a/w bowel injury

Treatment

- Spine consult w/ bracing/orthosis (bony injury) vs surgery (ligament injury/neuro deficit)

Disposition

- Admit

Sacral Fracture

Definition

- Fractures of the sacrum (may be a/w pelvic fractures if above S4)
- Denis classification: Zone 1—lateral to neural foramina, 6% sciatic or L5 nerve root deficit; Zone 2—through neural foramina, 28% unilateral L5/S1/S2 lesions; Zone 3—medial to foramina, into spinal canal, 76% w/ bowel/bladder/sexual dysfxn

History

- Buttock/perirectal/posterior thigh pain after direct trauma to sacrum

Physical Findings

- Focal tenderness, neurologic deficits (above S4), careful eval for cauda equina

Evaluation

- CT scan

Treatment

- Spine consult

Disposition

- D/C if isolated & stable

Anterior Cord Syndrome

Definition

- Injury to the anterior cord from blunt or ischemic injury

History

- Flexion/axial load (major trauma), minor trauma (arthritis/spinal stenosis/OA/spinal cord pathology), or infarction/ischemia of anterior spinal artery (aortic dissection/surgery)

Physical Findings

- B/I loss of motor/pain/temperature sensation, dorsal column intact (proprioception/vibratory sense) (see *Sensory & Motor deficit tables*)

Evaluation

- MRI

Treatment

- Spine consult

Disposition

- Admit

Central Cord Syndrome

Definition

- Trauma to central cord → injury of corticospinal motor tracts of UE > tracts of LE (buckling of ligamentum flavum)

History

- Hyperextension of neck, hx of elderly, arthritis, OA, spinal stenosis, syringomyelia

Physical Findings

- Loss of motor fxn in UE > LE, variable sensory loss (See *Sensory & Motor deficit tables*), loss of pain & temperature if nontraumatic

Evaluation

- MRI

Treatment

- Spine consult

Disposition

- Admit

Brown–Séquard Syndrome (Lateral Cord Syndrome)

Definition

- Hemicord transection from penetrating trauma or functional loss from demyelinating lesion

History

- Penetrating trauma (knife or bullet injury) or multiple sclerosis

Physical Findings

- Ipsilateral motor/proprioception/vibration loss, contralateral pain/temperature sensation loss, deficits occur 2 levels below lesion

Evaluation

- MRI

Treatment

- Spine consult

Disposition

- Admit

Deficit by Level of Spinal Injury			
Sensory-deficit Landmarks		**Motor-deficit Landmarks**	
C2	Occiput	C5	Elbow flexion
C4	Clavicular region	C7	Elbow extension
C6	Thumb	C8	Finger flexion
C8	Little finger	T1	Finger abduction
T4	Nipple line	L2	Hip flexion
T10	Umbilicus	L3	Knee extension
L1	Inguinal region	L4	Ankle dorsiflexion
L3	Knee	S1	Ankle plantar flexion
S1	Heel		
S5	Perineal area		

Spinal Shock

Definition

- Loss of vascular tone caused by cord trauma lasting 24–48 h, rarely can last several wk

History

- Spinal cord trauma

Physical Findings

- Hypotension, bradycardia, flaccid paralysis, hyporeflexia

Treatment

- Phenylephrine (neosynephrine peripheral alpha agonist) for BP support

Disposition

- Admit

Pearls

- There is NO evidence to support the administration of steroids in spinal trauma
- SCIWORA (spinal cord injury w/o radiologic abnl): In pediatric pts, if focal tenderness/ neurologic deficits → treat as cord injury regardless of imaging

THORACIC TRAUMA

Definition

- Injuries to the thorax & its structures caused by penetrating or blunt trauma (25% all trauma Ds; immediate: heart/great vessel injury, early: Airway obstruction/tamponade/tension PTX, Late: PNA/PE)

Approach

- Evaluate anatomical categories although many injuries do not occur in isolation: Cardiovascular, pulmonary, skeletal, esophageal, diaphragmatic

Inspection

- External trauma: Open wounds (do not probe wounds: Clot dislodgement → hemorrhage), exit/entrance wounds, flail segments (may require external fixation or PPV), seat belt marks, impaled objects (stabilization → removal in OR)

Palpation

- Crepitus (PTX), unequal pulses (vascular trauma, mediastinal hematoma), wounds below nipple line/tip of scapula ↑ risk abd trauma (25% have both intra-abd + thoracic trauma)

Radiology

- See table

Thoracotomy

- Signs of life (SOL): pupillary response, spontaneous ventilation, extremity movement, pulse, BP, or cardiac electrical activity (*J Trauma Acute Care Surg* 2015;79(1):159–173)
- Penetrating thoracic arrest: Strong recommendation to perform if w/ SOL; consider if CPR <15 mins w/o SOL
- Blunt traumatic arrest: Perform for SOL, or in profound refractory shock. Do not perform if CPR >10 mins & no SOL
- Penetrating extra-thoracic trauma: Consider if CPR <5–15 mins w/ or w/o SOL
- Survival rate s/p thoracotomy in pt w/ blunt trauma <2%, survival rate for arrest from penetrating 15%, cardiac stab wound up to 35% (*J Trauma Acute Care Surg* 2012;73(6):1359)

Thoracic Trauma Treatment Guidelines	
Thoracic Trauma	**General Guidelines**
Blunt trauma	If e/o thoracic trauma exists: CXR, chest CT
Penetrating trauma—traverses mediastinum	Agonal: Thoracotomy Unstable: Place b/l chest tubes Stable: CXR, chest CTA, esophagoscopy, bronchoscopy
Penetrating trauma—does not traverse mediastinum	CXR &/or chest CT for intrathoracic or extrathoracic injury

Traumatic Aortic Rupture

Definition

- Traumatic rupture of the aorta (descending aorta → fixed to thorax) caused by deceleration injury (fall from height, high-speed MVC, T-boned MVC)

History

- Retrosternal/intrascapular pain (80% die immediately)

Physical Findings

- Exam has poor sens for detecting injury, must have high index of suspicion w/ high mechanism
- Hypotension, asymmetric pulses/BP

Evaluation

- CXR (>8 cm widening of mediastinum, esophageal/trachea deviation, loss of aortic knob/aortopulmonary window, L apical cap, fractures of 1st rib/2nd rib/sternum, widening of paravertebral strip), CTA, TEE

Treatment

- Impulse control (esmolol/nitroprusside): HR <100, systolic <100 mmHg, surgical consult

Disposition

- Admit

Pearls

- 90% who survive have contained hematoma near ligamentum arteriosum
- Nl CXR does not rule out aortic injury

Pneumothorax

Definition

- Air in the pleural space (Simple: w/o shift/communicating w/ outside air; Tension: Injury acts as 1-way valve/increased intrapleural pressures; Open: wall deficit/collapse on inspiration/expansion on expiration/ineffective ventilation)

History

- Blunt (simple) or penetrating (tension/open) trauma

Physical Findings

- Decreased BS, hyperresonance; Tension: Tracheal deviation/neck vein distension/hypotension; Open: Chest wound w/ "sucking"

Evaluation

- US to evaluate for lung slide, CXR (treat tension PTX prior to imaging), chest CT

Treatment

- 100% O_2
- Tension: Needle decompression (large-bore needle/IV catheter → 2nd intercostal space, midclavicular line), finger thoracostomy → chest tube to 4th–5th intercostal space mid/anterior axillary line
- Open: Sterile occlusive dressing, → chest tube
- Simple: <10% → serial CXR, mod/large → chest tube directed anteriorly/serial CXR
- Occult: No tx other than O_2
- Prophylactic abx controversial in tube thoracostomy in setting of trauma (*Trauma Surg Acute Care Open* 2019;4:e000356; *Am J Surg* 2021;222(5):1017–1022).

Disposition

- Admit

Pearl

- Chest tube must be placed if mechanical ventilation required

Hemothorax

Definition

- Blood in the pleural space, most common from lung lacerations

History

- Blunt/penetrating trauma

Physical Findings

- Pain, decreased BS, dullness to percussion

Evaluation

- CXR: Costophrenic angle blunting (upright)/diffuse haziness (supine), US, chest CT

Treatment

- Large-bore chest tube directed inferiorly, surgical consult → OR if >1.5 L bloody output initially (>20 mL/kg)/ >200 cc/h (>3 mL/kg/h) or if unstable (↑ likelihood of injury to intercostal/internal mammary/hilar vessels)
- Prophylactic abx controversial in tube thoracostomy in setting of trauma

Pearls

- ~300 cc needed to see hemothorax on CXR
- Retained hemothorax is a/w empyema & pneumonia

Disposition

- Admit

Flail Chest

Definition

- Fracture >3 or more ribs in 2 or more places → discontinuous segment of chest wall → paradoxical movement w/ respiration (5% of thoracic trauma)

History

- Blunt trauma, SOB

Physical Findings

- Respiratory distress, tenderness, crepitus, paradoxical movement of chest wall

Evaluation

- CXR, CT chest

Treatment

- External stabilization (pillow), CPAP (1st line if poor oxygenation/ventilation in awake/cooperative pt → lower mortality/PNA rates vs intubation), ±chest tube placement, pain control (rib block catheter/epidural is best), intubate only if necessary (obtunded, airway obstruction, respiratory distress)

Disposition
- Admit

Pearl
- 35–50% mortality → related to underlying injuries & cx (pulmonary contusions, PNA)

Pulmonary Contusion

Definition
- Injury to lung parenchyma → hemorrhage/edema → V/Q mismatch

History
- Blunt trauma, SOB

Physical Findings
- Respiratory distress, tenderness, tachycardia, hemoptysis, hypoxia ↑ 1–2 d, resolve by 7 d

Evaluation
- CXR: May be nl initially or show b/l alveolar infiltrates

Treatment
- Pain control, pulmonary toilet, O_2 support. Restrict IVF w/ goal of euvolemia. Intubate if needed. Complications include pneumonia & ARDS

Disposition
- Admit

Cardiac Tamponade

Definition
- Hemopericardium → constriction of the heart → decreased CO, most commonly due to penetrating injury (rarely blunt trauma)

History
- Penetrating trauma

Physical Findings
- Beck triad (hypotension/JVD/muffled heart sounds), tachycardia, pulsus paradoxus

Evaluation
- Bedside/formal US: Pericardial effusion/diastolic collapse of RA (early) or RV (more specific), ECG: Low voltage/electrical alternans, CXR: Usually unremarkable

Treatment
- Aggressive IVF (preload dependent)
- Hypotension + pericardial effusion → OR/pericardiocentesis (blood usually clotted, if fresh may be in RV)
- Arrest → thoracotomy

Disposition
- Admit

Pearl
- JVD is rare in trauma pts given hypovolemia

Blunt Cardiac Injury

Definition
- Injury to the myocardium/coronary vessels/valves/septum

History
- Blunt trauma to chest (eg, impact against steering wheel)

Physical Findings
- Chest pain, tachycardia, ±hypotension

Evaluation
ECG: New BBB, dysrhythmias, ST Δ/conduction abnl/RV Dysfxn; cardiac enzymes: nl ECG & neg troponin has NPV 100% (*J Trauma Acute Care Surg* 2012;73(5):S301–S306).

Treatment
- IV fluid resuscitation (RV damage → preload dependence), see table

Disposition
- Admit to Tele

Pearl
- New ECG Δ consider 1° cardiac event → trauma

Cardiac Contusion Evaluation	
Asx, no ECG Δ, no dysrhythmias	Can be D/C home
ECG Δ or dysrhythmia in HD stable pt	24 h of cardiac monitoring
ECG Δ or dysrhythmia in HD unstable pt	Echo ± cardiology consult
Life-threatening dysrhythmias	ACLS guidelines

Esophageal Injury

Definition

- Injury to the esophagus most commonly from penetrating trauma; possible w/ significant epigastric blunt trauma, often will have other severe injuries w/ blunt mechanism

History

- Dysphagia, neck pain, neck swelling, hypersalivation, retrosternal fullness, hematemesis

Physical Findings

- Respiratory distress, neck/chest crepitus, hematemesis, subcutaneous emphysema

Evaluation

- CXR: mediastinal/deep cervical air
- Neck films: eophageal + laryngeal injury → air column in the esophagus
- Flexible esophagoscopy (endoscopy) is 96% sensitive—preferred in stable pt
- CT esophagram w/ water soluble contrast if uncertain (*Radiographics* 2021;41(2):447–461)

Treatment

- Surgical consult, broad-spectrum abx (eg, piperacillin/tazobactam), ±antifungal, PPI
- NPO. Only insert NGT under direct visualization (either during endoscopy or in OR)

Disposition

- Admit

Tracheobronchial Tear

Definition

- Tear to trachea/bronchus, most commonly due to penetrating trauma

History

- Penetrating trauma or severe deceleration injury, often die at scene

Physical Findings

- Crepitus, mediastinal crunch w/ heartbeat (Hamman sign), large persistent air leak or recurrent PTX after chest tube placement (if cervical injury may not have air leak)

Evaluation

- CXR: PTX/pneumomediastinum/"fallen lung sign," chest CT, bronchoscopy (gold standard, may miss injuries >2 cm above carina)

Treatment

- Fiberoptic intubation (in major bronchial lesions → consider double lumen ETT), chest tube placement (may require >1 chest tube)

Disposition

- Admit

Pearl

- May p/w difficulty passing ETT/difficulty w/ ventilation after ETT intubation

ABDOMINAL TRAUMA

Definition

- Trauma to the abdomen & its structures

Approach

Evaluate Main Areas

- Thoracoabdominal region: Nipple line → costal margin. Anterior abdomen: costal margin → inguinal ligaments/pubic symphysis → anterior axillary line; Flank: b/w anterior & posterior axillary lines from 6th rib → iliac crest; Back: inf scapular tips → iliac crest; Gluteal region: Iliac crest → gluteal fold

Inspection

- Entrance/exit wounds (check b/w buttock/thigh/axilla/neck), seat belt sign (↑ risk mesenteric tear/avulsion, bowel perforation, aorta/iliac thrombosis, chance fracture of L1/L2), do not remove objects, cover eviscerated organs in saline-soaked gauze

Palpation

- Peritoneal signs (operative mgmt), rectal exam (high-riding prostate/blood/tone)

Labs

- CBC (Hct may be nl initially in setting of hemorrhage), blood gas, lactate, LFTs, lipase, UA

Radiology

- FAST (90–100% sens for hemoperitoneum, not spec, requires >250 cc fluid), CXR (abd free air), pelvic x-ray (loss of psoas shadow → retroperitoneal injury, location of bullets), CT (definitive test, low sens for early pancreatic/diaphragmatic/bowel injury)

Diagnostic Peritoneal Lavage

- Rarely used given FAST/CT scans, pos study → >10 cc gross blood or enteric contents, blunt trauma >100,000 RBCs, penetrating trauma >5000–10,000 RBC

Approach to Abd Trauma			
Abd Trauma	**Examples**	**Most Common Injuries**	**General Guidelines**
Blunt trauma	Motor vehicle crash, falls, assaults	Spleen, liver, intestine, kidney	Unstable → FAST → OR Stable → FAST, CT (IV contrast only) → OR or serial abd exams
Penetrating trauma—anterior abdomen	GSW, SW	Small bowel, colon, liver, & vascular structures (GSW); liver, small bowel, diaphragm	GSW to anterior abdomen → OR Unstable w/ non-GSW trauma → OR Stable w/ non-GSW trauma → local wound exploration, CT
Penetrating trauma—flank & back	GSW, SW		Unstable → OR Stable GSW → triple contrast (IV, PO, PR) Stable non-GSWs → local wound exploration, CT, serial exams

Notes:
(1) 1° objective is to identify need for surgical exploration.
(2) Peritoneal irritation often seen w/ hollow viscus injury, but not w/ hemoperitoneum.
(3) If fascia penetration is found, f/u w/ DPL, CT, or ex lap. If not, pt can be D/C after wound care.
(4) Intra-abd organ injury occurs in 20% of non-GSW flank injuries & 5–10% of non-GSW back injuries.

Liver Laceration

Definition

- Laceration to liver (most commonly injured organ)

History

- Blunt or penetrating trauma

Physical Findings

- ±RUQ tenderness

Evaluation

- LFTs, Hct, FAST, CT scan

Liver Laceration Grading	
Grade	
Grade I	Subcapsular hematoma <10% surface area; parenchymal lac <1-cm depth
Grade II	Subcapsular hematoma 10–50% surface area; intraparenchymal hematoma <10-cm diameter. Lac 1–3-cm depth & ≤10 cm in length
Grade III	Subcapsular hematoma >50% surface area; ruptured subcapsular or parenchymal hematoma. Intraparenchymal hematoma >10 cm. Lac >3 cm in depth. Any injury in the presence of a liver vascular injury or active bleeding contained w/i liver parenchyma
Grade IV	Parenchymal disruption involving 25–75% of a hepatic lobe. Active bleeding extending beyond the liver parenchyma into the peritoneum
Grade V	Parenchymal disruption of >75% of hepatic lobe. Juxtahepatic venous injury to include retrohepatic vena cava & central major hepatic veins

Treatment

- Surgical consultation for operative vs conservative mgmt (HD stable, serial exams/Hct), IR for embolization

Disposition

- Admit ICU vs floor

Splenic Laceration

Definition

- Laceration to spleen (most commonly injured organ in blunt trauma)

History

- Blunt or penetrating trauma, L shoulder pain (Kehr sign)/chest/flank/upper quadrant pain

Physical Findings
- LUQ pain

Evaluation
- FAST, CT scan: grading of laceration (I–V)

Treatment
- Surgical consultation for operative vs conservative mgmt (HD stable, serial exams/Hct), IR for embolization

Disposition
- Admit ICU vs floor

Splenic Laceration Grading	
Grade	
Grade I	Subcapsular hematoma <10% surface area, capsular tear <1-cm depth
Grade II	Subcapsular hematoma 10–50%, intraparenchymal hematoma <5-cm diameter, parenchymal laceration 1–3 cm not involving vessels
Grade III	Subcapsular hematoma >50% or expanding, ruptured subcapsular/intraparenchymal hematoma, intraparenchymal hematoma >5 cm, splenic laceration >3 cm/involving trabecular vessels
Grade IV	Laceration of segmental or hilar vessels → devascularization of >25%
Grade V	Shattered spleen, hilar vascular injury → complete devascularization

Small Bowel Injury

Definition
- Injury to small bowel (GSW > stab wound > blunt trauma)

History
- Blunt or penetrating trauma, classically handlebar injury

Physical Findings
- Seat belt sign (MVC), peritoneal signs (may be delayed)

Evaluation
- Unstable → FAST/DPL. Stable → CT scan (low sens, fluid collection/bowel-wall thickening/stranding/free air), CXR (rarely shows free air), lumbar XR (Chance fracture)

Treatment
- Surgical consultation for operative mgmt (perforation or devascularization), abx (ceftriaxone/metronidazole)

Disposition
- Admit

Colorectal Injury

Definition
- Injury to colon or rectum (transverse colon most common)

History
- Penetrating trauma (GSW), very rarely seen in blunt trauma (<1%)

Physical Findings
- Hypoactive bowels, peritoneal signs, gross rectal blood

Evaluation
- Triple contrast CT scan (gastrografin, barium is irritating), KUB (air lining psoas)
- Imaging w/ poor sens, definitive eval is w/ exploratory laparotomy

Treatment
- Surgical consultation for operative mgmt (perforation or devascularization), abx (ceftriaxone/metronidazole)

Disposition
- Admit

Duodenal Injury

Definition
- Injury to duodenum (80% a/w other injury)

History
- Penetrating trauma, n/v (obstructing hematoma)

Physical Findings
- Epigastric tenderness, heme pos stool, bloody NGT aspirate

Evaluation
- Upright CXR (free air), CT (duodenal wall hematoma), Upper GI ("coiled spring sign")

Treatment
- Surgical consultation for operative mgmt (perforation or devascularization), abx (ceftriaxone/metronidazole), NGT placement

Disposition
- Admit

Pearl
- 2nd portion most commonly injured (contains bile/pancreatic duct openings)

Gastric Injury

Definition
- Injury to stomach, uncommon

History
- Penetrating trauma

Physical Findings
- Epigastric tenderness, heme pos stool, bloody NGT aspirate

Evaluation
- Upright CXR (free air)

Treatment
- Surgical consultation for operative mgmt, abx (ceftriaxone/metronidazole)

Disposition
- Admit

Pancreatic Injury

Definition
- Injury to pancreas (rare, 3–5% of abd trauma)

History
- Penetrating trauma (40%), epigastric blunt trauma (60%, steering wheel, bicycle handles)

Physical Findings
- Minimal epigastric tenderness (retroperitoneal structure)

Evaluation
- CT scan (low sens early), lipase (may be nl), ERCP for ductal injury

Treatment
- Surgical consultation, low-grade blunt injuries may be managed nonoperatively w/ NGT

Disposition
- Admit

Pearl
- A/w other injuries 90% of the time

Vascular Trauma

Definition
- Injury to abd vasculature (10% of stab wounds, 25% of GSW)

History
- Penetrating trauma; also in blunt trauma (eg, venous plexus or iliac injury in pelvic fx)

Physical Findings
- Distension, expanding hematoma, Grey Turner sign (flank ecchymosis)/Cullen sign (periumbilical ecchymosis) → retroperitoneal hemorrhage

Evaluation
- FAST, CT angiography (if stable), wound exploration

Treatment
- Surgical consultation, unstable → OR; consider REBOA for temporization

Disposition
- Admit

Pearl
- Avoid LE venous access

Diaphragmatic Tear

Definition
- Tear to diaphragm from blunt trauma, ↑ lateral impact (large, L-sided 2–3 × more likely than R, posterolaterally located) or penetrating trauma (small but enlarges w/ time)

History
- Penetrating/blunt trauma, delayed presentation; pain, ±obstruction

Physical Findings
- Bowel sounds over chest

Evaluation
- CXR (50% sens): hemothorax/PTX (penetrating), abnl diaphragmatic shadow (blunt), US, CT scan, careful NGT placement (may be seen in hemithorax)
- Diagnostic laparoscopy is gold standard

Treatment
- Respiratory distress → NGT placement for decompression, surgery consult for operative repair. CXR may be misinterpreted as hemothorax, avoid chest tube placement

Disposition
- Admit

Pearl
- Intrapericardial diaphragmatic rupture/bowel herniation → tamponade

GENITOURINARY TRAUMA

Definition
- Trauma to the structures of the genitourinary tract, uncommon to be life-threat unless significant renal/vascular injury

Approach

Inspection
- Blood at meatus (urethra trauma), blood in vagina, perineal lacerations (do not probe → hemorrhage), scrotal ecchymosis/lacerations, flank bruising

Palpation
- Rectal exam (high-riding prostate/boggy → membranous urethral injury, blood → rectal laceration), testicular disruption

Labs
- UA (microscopic hematuria → no eval; gross blood → serious GU trauma)

Radiology
- RUG: Male w/ blood at meatus (to prevent full urethral tear/false passage w/ Foley), inject 50 cc contrast into urethra → pelvic XR for extravasation
- Cystogram: Instill 400–500 cc contrast into bladder via Foley → AP film or CT scan → repeat image after contrast is washed out (posterior bladder tears)
- CT pyelogram: Complete eval of kidneys

Renal Laceration or Contusion

Definition
- AAST renal injury grading scale
- Minor: Grades I to III—Subcapsular hematoma (Grade I) w/ laceration (Grade II or III)
- Major: Extends to collecting system/vascular injury (Grade IV); involves avulsion of hilum (also called pedicle) which devascularizes kidney, or shattered kidney (V)

History
- Penetrating or high-energy blunt trauma

Physical Findings
- Flank wound, gross hematuria, ±hypotension

Evaluation
- CBC, BMP, UA, Coags, other trauma labs as needed, CT scan w/ delayed phase

Treatment
- Surgery & Urology consult
- Microscopic hematuria only → avoid strenuous exercise/repeat UA in 2 d + until clear
- Subcapsular hematoma or minor lacerations → 24-h obs/serial Hct/serial UA/bed rest
- Ongoing gross hematuria & tfx requirements → angioembolization
- Renal pedicle vascular injury → repair (20% salvage rate) vs nephrectomy

Disposition
- Admit: Major/subcapsular hematoma
- Home: Microscopic hematuria

(*Ther Adv Urol* 2018;10(10):295–303)

Renal Pelvis Rupture

Definition
- Rupture of the renal pelvis

History
- High-velocity deceleration, penetrating trauma

Physical Findings
- Flank ecchymosis, hypotension

Evaluation
- UA, CBC, Coags, BMP, CT scan: extravasation of urine in perirenal space

Treatment
- Urology consult for operative repair

Disposition
- Admit

Pearl
- ↑ risk of infxn in delayed repair

Ureteral Injuries

Definition
- Injury to ureter (very rare), majority are iatrogenic from gyn/uro procedures

History
- Hyperextension, penetrating trauma, forced flexion of L-spine → rupture below UPJ, delayed necrosis from microvascular injury after GSW (rare)

Evaluation
- UA, Hct, CT scan: extravasation of urine, IVP (limited sens)

Treatment
- Urology consult for operative ureteroureterostomy

Disposition
- Admit

Intraperitoneal Bladder Rupture

Definition
- Laceration at dome of bladder w/ intraperitoneal communication

History
- MVC, blunt trauma (burst injury), a/w pelvic fractures

Physical Findings
- Lower abd tenderness, ↓ UOP, hematuria

Evaluation
- UA, Hct, CT cystogram/cystogram: Extravasation of urine

Treatment
- Urology consult for urgent operative repair

Disposition
- Admit

Extraperitoneal Bladder Rupture

Definition
- Rupture of the bladder w/ extraperitoneal spillage

History
- MVC, blunt trauma, a/w pelvic fractures

Physical Findings
- Lower abd tenderness, ↓ UOP, hematuria

Evaluation
- UA, Hct, CT cystogram/cystogram w/ washout: Extravasation of urine

Treatment
- Urology consult (usually nonoperative unless extends to bladder neck), Foley 10–14 d

Disposition
- Admit

Male Urethral Injuries

Definition
- Injury to posterior (prostatomembranous) urethra (a/w pelvic fractures, esp b/l or both ipsilateral pubic rami fx & posterior disruption injuries) & anterior (bulbous/penile) urethra (a/w direct trauma to penis/penile fracture/saddle injuries/falls/GSW)

History
- Blunt or penetrating trauma

Physical Findings
- Blood at meatus, gross hematuria, inability to void

Evaluation
- UA, Hct, RUG (prior to Foley)

Treatment
- Suprapubic bladder decompression if needed, urology consult for 1° repair/fluoroscopic catheter placement/suprapubic cystotomy

Disposition
- Admit

Female Urethral Injuries

Definition
- Injury to female urethra associated most commonly w/ pelvic fractures (rarely saddle injuries, falls, GSW, instrumentation)

History
- Blunt or penetrating trauma, much less common than in males

Physical Findings
- Vaginal bleeding, inability to place Foley, labial edema

Evaluation
- RUG not useful, passage of Foley precludes complete tear

Treatment
- Suprapubic bladder decompression if needed, urology consult for surgical repair

Disposition
- Admit

Testicular Contusion/Rupture

Definition
- Blunt trauma to the testicle leading to contusion or rupture (disruption of tunica albuginea)

History
- Blunt trauma, pain, swelling

Physical Findings
- Ecchymosis, edema, tenderness, inability to palpate testicle due to dislocation

Evaluation
- Testicular US (mod sens/spec for rupture)

Treatment
- Urology consult for surgical repair/clot evacuation (early intervention → ↓ morbidity)

Disposition
- Admit

Penile Fracture

Definition
- Blunt injury to the erect penis when penis is forcefully bent leading to rupture of the tunica albuginea/rupture of corpora cavernosa

History
- "Cracking sound" usually during sexual activity → severe pain

Physical Findings
- Swelling, discoloration (vascular engorgement), ecchymosis, blood at meatus (10–20% a/w urethral injury)

Evaluation
- RUG for urethral injury (concomitant injury in 15–20%)

Treatment
- Urology consult for surgical urethral repair/clot evacuation

Disposition
- Admit

Penile Amputation/Laceration

Definition
- Complete or partial amputation/laceration of the penis

History
- Penetrating trauma, zipper injury

Evaluation
- RUG or testicular US if associated injuries suspected

Treatment
- Amputation: Urology consult (best results if reimplanted in 18 h)
- Simple laceration: Repair w/ absorbable suture
- Zipper injury: Remove zipper w/ mineral oil/wire cutters at zipper median bar to break apart
- Consider penile dorsal nerve block for analgesia if attempting bedside procedures

Disposition
- D/C unless reimplantation required

Female Genital Injuries

Definition
- Injury to ovary, uterus, fallopian tube, vagina (difficult to Dx usually found when evaluating for other injury), a/w pelvic fractures

History
- Blunt or penetrating trauma, vaginal bleeding

Physical Findings
- Blood in vaginal vault, lower abd tenderness

Evaluation
- CT scan, pelvic US (in gravid pt, ↑ risk)

Treatment
- Open vaginal lacerations → abx (ampicillin, gentamicin, Flagyl), Gynecology consult
- Simple vaginal lacerations: Repair w/ absorbable suture

Disposition
- Admit if needed

HIP/PELVIC TRAUMA

Definition
- Trauma to hip or pelvis

Approach

Pelvis Anatomy
- Sacrum, coccyx, & R/L innominate bones (ileum, ischium, pubis) fuse at acetabulum

Inspection
- Perineal edema/lacerations/ecchymosis, blood at urethral meatus, deformities (limb length discrepancy, internal/external rotation), open lacerations

Palpation
- Pulses, pelvic stability (limit manipulation if unstable → clot dislodgement), neurologic exam (strength, sensation, DTRs), rectal exam (blood, high-riding prostate, tone), pelvic exam in females

Radiology
- AP pelvis (can miss sacral fractures/SI joint disruptions → inlet/outlet views), CT scan (superior for acetabular fractures/associated injuries), hip x-ray

Pelvic Fractures

Definition
- Fractures of the pelvis usually caused by significant mechanism (↑ a/w other injuries)

History
- Blunt trauma, lateral/AP compression, vertical shear (fall)

Physical Findings
- External contusion/abrasion/ecchymosis, caution w/ manual compression/distraction of pelvis (may dislodge clot → hemorrhage), evaluate for open pelvic fx as these have 40–50% mortality, hypotension (42–50% mortality), blood at meatus, perineal trauma, neurologic abnl (cauda equina synd, plexopathies, radiculopathies)

Evaluation
- FAST, AP pelvis, CT scan, evaluate carefully for intra-abd trauma as >15% w/ pelvic fx will have intra-abd injury

Treatment
- Unstable: Temporizing measures (wrapped sheet/external binders/external clamps), massive tfx protocol, immediate orthopedic & trauma surgery consult (reduction/external fixation & pelvic packing), IR for hemorrhage control
- Stable: Orthopedic consult

Disposition
- Admit

Pearls
- Type A (inferior pubic rami/avulsion) & type B2 (bucket handle) → most common
- Type B3 (open book) & C (70% have major associated injuries) → most life threatening

Pelvic Fracture Classification (Tile Classification System)	
Type	
Type A: Stable pelvic ring fracture	A1: Avulsion of innominate bone → sudden muscle contraction, Iliac wing (Duverney) fracture → direct lateral to medical trauma A2: Stable or minimally displaced fracture of pelvic ring (ramus/ischium) → elderly fall A3: Transverse fracture of sacrum/coccyx → fall in sitting position
Type B: Partially stable pelvic ring injuries (rotationally unstable/vertically stable)	B1: Unilateral open book (disruption symphysis pubis + SI joint hinge rotation) → AP compression B2: Bucket handle fractures → lateral compression B3: B/I open book fracture → severe AP compression
Type C: Unstable pelvic ring fractures	Distracting vertical sacral fractures/other vertical shear fractures → vertical shear injuries

Vascular Pelvic Injuries

Definition
- Injury to vascular structures of pelvis a/w pelvic fractures (most commonly AP trauma or vertical shear)

History
- Blunt trauma, lateral/AP compression, vertical shear (fall)

Physical Findings
- Unstable pelvis, hypotension resistant to resuscitation

Evaluation
- FAST, AP pelvis, CT scan (if stable), pelvic angiography, consider DPL if FAST neg but HD unstable

Treatment
- Massive tfx protocol, stabilization of pelvis w/ pelvic binder, orthopedic & trauma surgery consult (external fixation & pelvic packing to control hemorrhage), IR embolization for continued hypotension (less effective for venous bleed → high collateralization)

Disposition
- Admit

Acetabular Fractures

Definition
- Fractures to the acetabulum (MVC → knee striking dashboard or lateral intrusion), fall in elderly

History
- Blunt trauma, pain w/ movement of hip

Physical Findings
- Pain w/ movement of hip/compression of sole of foot or greater trochanter

Evaluation
- AP pelvis, lateral hip films (±Judet views), CT scan (if plain films unrevealing)
- 3 types (although some fit in multiple categories)
- Wall: anterior, posterior, posterior wall/column, transverse/posterior wall
- Column: anterior, posterior, both, posterior wall/column, anterior/transverse
- Transverse: transverse, T, transverse/posterior wall, anterior column/transverse

Treatment
- Orthopedic consult for operative mgmt

Disposition
- Admit

Hip Fractures

Definition
- Fractures of the hip (femoral head/neck/trochanter)

History
- Elderly → fall from standing, young → significant mechanism trauma (MVC)

Physical Findings
- External rotation, shortening of leg

Evaluation
- AP pelvis, lateral hip films, CT (if unable to bear weight + neg plain films)

Treatment
- Orthopedic consult for operative mgmt (femoral neck fractures → ↑ risk avascular necrosis of femoral head, surgical repair in <6 h)
- Fascia iliaca or PENG block for pain control

Disposition
- Admit

Pearl
- Hip fracture in elderly → 25% 1-y mortality

Hip Fractures	
Type	
Intracapsular	Femoral head: Rare in isolation, a/w posterior dislocations Femoral neck: ↑ risk avascular necrosis of femoral head, most common in elderly women
Extracapsular	Intertrochanteric: Markedly externally rotated/shortened, elderly fall Subtrochanteric: ↑ risk bleeding into thigh, elderly fall/MVC

Hip Dislocations

Definition
- Dislocation of femoral head from acetabulum (90% posterior)

History
- Elderly fall w/ hx of hip total hip replacement, MVC (knee hitting dashboard, a/w other injuries), athlete running & lands w/ hip flexed/internally rotated & adducted

Physical Findings
- Flexed/adducted/internally rotated hip (posterior)

Evaluation
- AP pelvis, lateral hip films—look for disruption of Shenton line, eval for femoral neck fx
- Obtain CT following reduction to eval for loose bodies, femoral head fx, acetabular fx

Treatment
- Orthopedic consult if fracture or prosthetic hip; reduction under conscious sedation (in <6 h, ↑ risk avascular necrosis of femoral head)

Disposition
- Admit if needed

EXTREMITY INJURY

Definition
- Injuries to the extremities (vascular/bony/soft tissue/nerve)

Approach

History
- Last tetanus (booster if >5 y), hand dominance, time of injury, mechanism (crush/penetrating), neurologic deficit (loss of sensation/motor), environmental exposures (burn/cold), preinjury functional status, occupation or major hobbies

Inspection
- Color (discoloration/ecchymosis/perfusion), soft tissue defects (control hemorrhage during 1° survey), deformities (angulations/shortening), swelling

Palpation
- Pulses, all joints/bones (tenderness), FB, crepitance, strength, sensation, DTRs, range all joints, joint effusions

Radiology
- Plain films guided by PE

Consults
- Orthopedic &/or vascular for open fractures/amputations/vascular injuries/compartment synd, hand surgery for significant hand injuries

Extremity Vascular Injury

Definition
- Injury to the vasculature of the extremities

History
- Blunt trauma (fracture/dislocation → tearing of vessels) or penetrating trauma

Physical Findings
- Obvious vascular compromise → pulseless/pallor/pain/paresthesia/cold, indicators of vascular injury → swelling/pain/↓ cap refill/mottled skin/↓ pulses

Evaluation
- Plain films (blunt trauma), CTA, or angiography (if stable), ankle/brachial index or ankle/ankle index: Abnl if <0.9

Treatment
- Vascular surgery consult for immediate surgical repair (↓ salvage rate if >6 h)

Disposition
- Admit if needed

Extremity Orthopedic Injuries

Definition
- Bony fractures or joint dislocations of the extremities

History
- Blunt trauma or penetrating

Physical Findings
- Deformities, pain, swelling, crepitance, neurologic deficits, diminished pulses

Evaluation
- Plain films, image joint above & below for significant fracture, CT in certain injuries (tibial plateau) or if suspicion for occult fx (eg, unable to bear weight)

Treatment
- Open fractures: Immediate orthopedic consult for operative washout/fixation (<6 h), abx (cefazolin 1–2 g)
- Closed UE fractures + intact neuro exam: splint, outpt f/u (see table)
- Closed LE fractures + intact neuro exam: splint, outpt f/u if able to use crutches (see table)
- Dislocations: ED reduction, pt f/u

Disposition
- Admit if needed

Principles of Immobilization & Referral

Fracture Sites	Splint/Immobilization Technique	Referral Guidelines
Femoral fractures	Temporary traction splints	Emergent ED consult
Knee injuries (w/ no e/o dislocation & no neurovascular compromise)	Knee immobilizer/long leg cast w/ leg flexed 10°	Orthopedic f/u w/i 1 wk
Tibia fractures (not tibial plateau)	Lower-leg posterior splint	Orthopedic f/u in 1–2 d
Ankle fractures	Short-leg walking cast or boot	If fracture fragments well aligned, orthopedic f/u in 1 wk. If angulation or distraction, needs next-d f/u
Hand fractures	Thumb & index finger—radial gutter splint Middle, ring, & little fingers—ulnar gutter splint	If fracture fragments well aligned & fracture is closed, f/u w/ hand surgeon w/i 1 wk

Wrist fractures	Wrist splint/immobilizer unless scaphoid fracture, then thumb spica cast	Orthopedic f/u in 7–10 d unless scaphoid displacement—then f/u in 1 2 d
Distal radius/ulna fractures	Short arm cast	Orthopedic f/u in 1–2 d unless closed reduction results in good anatomic alignment—then f/u in 7–10 d
Humerus fractures	Sling, coaptation splint rarely used	Orthopedic f/u in 7–10 d, sooner if articular surface or tuberosity
Shoulder dislocations	Sling, early ROM to prevent frozen shoulder	Orthopedic f/u in 7–10 d

Pearls
- 5th metacarpal fractures or "Boxer fractures" have a high rate of infxn secondary to breaks in skin from opponent's tooth. Always r/o FB w/ plain radiographs & f/u in 1–2 d in ED or in hand clinic
- Suspicion for scaphoid Fx (snuffbox tenderness, pain w/ thumb axial loading) w/o radiologic e/o fracture requires splinting & orthopedic f/u & repeated x-rays w/i 7 d

Extremity Soft Tissue Injury

Definition
- Injury to the soft tissue of the extremities

History
- Blunt trauma or penetrating (polytrauma, industrial accidents)

Physical Findings
- Soft tissue defects, FBs

Evaluation
- Plain films for FB/underlying fractures, US, CPK (if extensive injury)

Treatment
- Irrigate, explore for FB (↑ risk wound infxn → poor cosmetic outcome), plastic surgery consult (extensive injuries), hand consult for palmar injuries as exploration w/ potential for iatrogenic injury, abx (grossly contaminated wounds)

Disposition
- Admit if extensive, e/o rhabdomyolysis/compartment synd

Extremity Nerve Injury

Definition
- Injury to the nerves of the extremities (a/w fractures/dislocations/lacerations/vascular ischemia/compartment synd)

History
- Blunt trauma or penetrating

Physical Findings
- See table

Evaluation
- Plain films for fracture/dislocation

Treatment
- Reduce fracture/dislocation (↓ pressure on nerve), fasciotomy (compartment synd), orthopedic/plastic surgery consult

Disposition
- Admit if needed

Extremity Nerve Injuries			
Nerve	**Motor**	**Sensation**	**Injury**
Ulnar	Index finger abduction	Tip of little finger	Elbow injury
Median (distal)	Thenar opposition	Tip of index finger	Wrist dislocation
Median (anterior interosseous)	Index tip flexion		Supracondylar fx of humerus in children
Musculocutaneous	Elbow flexion	Lateral forearm	Anterior shoulder dislocation

Radial	Thumb, finger metacarpal extension	1st dorsal web space	Distal humeral shaft, anterior shoulder dislocation
Axillary	Deltoid	Lateral shoulder	Proximal humerus fx, anterior shoulder dislocation
Femoral	Knee extension	Anterior knee	Pubic rami fx
Obturator	Hip adduction	Medial thigh	Obturator ring fx
Posterior tibial	Toe dorsiflexion	Sole of foot	Knee dislocation
Superficial peroneal	Ankle eversion	Lateral dorsum of foot	Fibular neck fx, knee dislocation
Deep peroneal	Ankle/toe dorsiflexion	Dorsal 1st to 2nd web space of foot	Fibular neck fx, compartment synd
Sciatic	Plantar & dorsiflexion	Foot	Posterior hip dislocation
Superior gluteal	Hip abduction		Acetabular fx
Inferior gluteal	Gluteus maximus hip extension		Acetabular fx

Compartment Syndrome

Definition

- A condition in which perfusion pressures < tissue pressures in closed space (fascial compartments) → ↓ circulation/tissue fxn (↑ risk injuries: tibial/forearm fractures, crush injuries, burns, immobilized injuries in tight dressing/cast)

History

- Blunt trauma or penetrating, pain > expected/worse w/ passive muscle stretching

Physical Findings

- Tenderness, tense swelling, classically: pain, pallor, paresthesias, paralysis, pulselessness (late finding). Pain w/ passive stretching is early sign, but not always reliable

Evaluation

- Compartment pressures (measure w/ Stryker or 18 gauge IV + arterial line transducer) >30 mmHg or <20–30 mmHg difference b/w DBP & compartment pressure (if hypotensive necrosis occurs at ↓ pressures), CK

Treatment

- Remove restrictive dressings/casts, elevate extremity, correct BP, surgery consult for fasciotomy (do not delay fasciotomy for surgical availability)

Disposition

- Admit

Crush Syndrome/Rhabdomyolysis

Definition

- Crush injury → release in cellular contents of muscle cells → CK levels >5,000 U/L

History

- Crush injury

Physical Findings

- May have minimal external injury, dark brown/orange urine

Evaluation

- CK levels >5000 U/L, ↑ Cr (15–47% a/w AKI), ↑ potassium, UA (+myoglobin), observe closely for reperfusion synd, esp if in field

Treatment

- IV fluids for UOP >1 mL/g/h; treat hyperkalemia; traditionally alkalization of urine (sodium bicarbonate, 1 amp/1 L NS → urine pH >7 → prevents tubular precipitation of myoglobin) → no difference than NS in prevention of renal failure

Disposition

- Admit

Partial/Complete Amputation

Definition

- Amputation of extremity

History

- Blunt or penetrating trauma (polytrauma, industrial accident)

Physical Findings

- Document motor/neurologic/vascular fxn in remaining limb

Evaluation

- Plain films of stump + amputated fragment, ±angiography (if not going directly to OR)

Treatment

- Limit mobility, hemostasis w/ direct pressure, immediate surgery consult for replantation, abx (cefazolin 1–2 g IV), tetanus update, pack stump w/ sterile NS-soaked gauze, wrap amputated part in cold NS-soaked gauze/place on ice (do not place in direct contact w/ ice or NS)

Disposition

- Admit

Pearl

- Replantation depends on age, vocation, injury severity

WOUND MANAGEMENT

Approach

History

- Time of event (>12 h → irrigate/heal by secondary intention or delayed 1° closure, face/significant soft tissue defect → 1° closure in <24 h), location (suture selection/ time until removal), mechanism (↑ risk FB/contamination), tetanus (booster if >5 y)

Inspection

- FB, wound approximation

Palpation

- Pulses, strength, sensation distal to injury

Laceration

Definition

- Cut or tear to skin & soft tissues

History

- Penetrating or blunt trauma

Physical Findings

- Skin defect, ↓ pulses/sensation/motor (neurovascular injury)

Evaluation

- Plain films only if FB/fracture suspected

Treatment

- Hemostasis: Direct pressure, lidocaine w/ epinephrine if needed, hemostatic agents (eg, thrombin, Surgicel), proximal tourniquet
- Analgesia: Use regional blocks if possible (↓ wound distortion/amt of analgesic needed)

Commonly Used Local Anesthetics

Agent	Trade Name	Class	Concentrations (%)	Maximum Safe Dose	Onset	Duration
Lidocaine (+epinephrine)	Xylocaine	Amide	0.5–2	4 mg/kg (7 mg/kg)	~5 mins	1–2 h 1–4 h
Bupivacaine (+epinephrine)	Marcaine	Amide	0.25–0.5	2 mg/kg (3 mg/kg)	~5 mins	4–8 h 4–8 h
Procaine (+epinephrine)	Novocaine	Ester	0.5–1	7 mg/kg (9 mg/kg)	~5 mins	15–45 mins 30–90 mins

- Irrigation: >500-cc NS (no benefit over tap water), 8 psi of pressure (18 g IV catheter or Zerowet splash shield in 30–60-cc syringe), caution on delicate tissues (eye lids)
- Exploration (through a full ROM): FB, tendons (including in position of injury), fascial planes

Suture Choice		
Body Part	**Suture Size**	**Remove Sutures on Day**
Scalp	Staples or 4-0	7
Face	5-0, 6-0	4–5
Chest	3-0, 4-0	7–10
Back	3-0, 4-0	10–14
Forearm	4-0, 5-0	10–14
Finger/hand	5-0	7–10
LE	4-0, 5-0	10–12

- Use fast-absorbing gut (absorbable suture) for laceration repairs of the face
- Abx: Human & animal bites to hands, face, & genitals prone to infxn; o/w not routinely required

Disposition
- Home

Pearls
- Scarring: Take up to 1 y to fully develop, apply sunscreen/keep covered, apply Vit E
- Hand flexor tendon lacerations: Emergent 1° repair by hand surgeon, splint (wrist 30° flexion, MP joint 70° flexion, DIP/PIP 10° flexion)
- Hand extensor tendon lacerations: Zone IV & VI repair 1° in ED, splint, hand surgery f/u

Foreign Body

Definition
- Retained FB in wound (most common hand/foot) → ↑ risk delayed infxn/granuloma/formation/local compression of structures/embolization/allergic rxns (reactive FBs: wood, organic matter, clothing, skin fragments)

History
- Know FB, ↑ risk wounds: Stepping on glass/punching windows/MVC w/ glass exposure/fall on gravel/pain at IVD site/persistent wound infxns/failure to heal (41% wounds caused by glass)

Physical Findings
- Visible/palpable FB

Evaluation
- Explore wound (adequate anesthesia/hemostasis/probe w/ instrument), plain films for radiopaque FBs (glass, metal, bone, teeth, graphite, gravel), US (submerge part in basin of water for improved resolution to identify superficial FB location)

Treatment
- Not all FB require removal (deep, small, inert, asx, away from vital structures), removal (significant pain, functional impairment, reactive, contamination, near vital structures, cosmetic concerns): May require wound extension, irrigation, fine tip forceps

Disposition
- D/C

Pearl
- Plantar wounds through the sole of a shoe are a/w *P. aeruginosa* infxns and should receive prophylactic Abx coverage

Fingertip Wounds

Definition
- Amputations/laceration/crush to fingertip (skin/volar pulp/distal phalanx/nail/nail bed)

History
- Cutting/crushing injury

Physical Findings
- Amputation, nail bed lacerations, subungual hematoma

Evaluation
- Finger plain film (FB, fracture)

Treatment
- Amputation: Distal to DIP joint → wound care/secondary intention (may need to trim back bone/should always be covered by soft tissue)/abx, significant bone/soft tissue loss → emergent hand surgery consult

- Subungual hematoma: large → nail trephination, small → no intervention
- Nail bed laceration: 1° repair → remove nail, repair w/ 6-0 absorbable suture, replace nail into nail fold (suture or secure w/ tape) to splint nail bed/maintain nail fold (nail growth → 70–160 d)

Disposition
- D/C

ABUSE

Approach

History
- Delays in seeking care, hx inconsistent w/ injury, multiple past injuries, injuries in various stages of healing

Team Approach
- Social work, child protective services, trained sexual assault nurses, pt advocate

Documentation
- Record factual events/injuries, avoid judgments, informed consent for forensic collection/release of information, mandatory reporting for child/elder abuse

Child Abuse

History
- Story inconsistent w/ injuries/child's developmental age, inconsistent stories by caretakers

Physical Findings
- Child neglect: Flattening/alopecia of occiput (supine for long periods of time), decreased SC tissue/prominent ribs/loose skin over buttocks (FTT)
- Child abuse: Bruises/fracture varying stages, bruises in areas not prone to trauma (lower back, buttock, thighs, cheeks, ear pinna), geometric-shaped bruising (belts, cords), scald burns w/o splash marks or in "dip" pattern, multiple deep contact burns, unexplained extremity swelling (long bone spiral fracture, metaphyseal chip fractures, femur fractures in <3 y), posterior rib fractures, MS Δ (shaken baby), suspicious oral/facial trauma (torn frenulum, dental trauma present in 50% of abuse)
- Child sexual assault: Penile/vaginal D/C (STDs), UTI, genital/rectal trauma (inner thigh bruising, rectal tears, loss rectal tone), often no physical findings if delay in presentation

Evaluation
- Skeletal series (children <5 Y), head CT (suspected intracranial injury), dilated eye exam (retinal detachment/hemorrhage → shaken baby), CBC, Coags, LFTs/lipase (abd injury), tox screen, growth measurements, vaginal/rectal/oral swabs

Treatment
- Social work/child protective services, treat injuries as appropriate

Disposition
- D/C per child protective services

Pearls
- Child abuse affects 2–3% children. Physical abuse is a/w low SES
- ↑ risk in children w/ mental/physical disabilities/chronic medical problems
- Consider Munchausen synd by proxy in cases w/ extensive/neg prior w/u
- Most important to suspect abuse & allow trained specialists to opine if abuse occurred

Sexual Assault

History
- Time, date, number/description of assailants, threats made, weapons used, type of assault, drugs used, LOC, post assault activity (Δ of clothing, urination, showering, tampon use), last time of voluntary intercourse

Physical Findings
- Document: Appearance of clothes, scratches, bruising, lacerations (can use toluidine dye to identify vaginal lacerations)

Evaluation
- Imaging as needed, have pt advocate present, pregnancy test, ± STD testing, full rape kit if <72 h (modify as appropriate), vaginal/rectal secretions for acid phosphatase/glycoprotein p30, tox screen
- Many areas will have SANE services available & pt may need transfer for SANE exam, must medically clear pt 1st

Treatment

- Pregnancy prophylaxis (levonorgestrel 0.75 q12h × 2 doses if <72 h since assault; ulipristal if b/w 72–120 h or overweight), STD prophylaxis (Gonorrhea: Ceftriaxone 500 mg IM × 1, Chlamydia: doxycycline 100 mg PO BID × 7 d, Trichomonas: metronidazole 500 mg PO BID × 7 d; Hep B: 1st of 2 vaccines, HBIG; HIV prophylaxis w/i 72 h)

Disposition

- D/C w/ f/u counseling

Pearl

- 1/5 women are sexually assaulted in lifetime, only 7% reported

Intimate Partner Violence

History

- Story inconsistent w/ injuries, frequent ED visits, vague medical complaints, chronic pain (>abd pain), overbearing/controlling partner, injury during pregnancy

Physical Findings

- Injuries face/head/neck/areas covered by clothes (most common)

Evaluation

- Imaging as needed

Treatment

- Photographs as appropriate, determine safety of home/immediate risk (escalating violence, treats, firearms), devise safety plan (avoid sedative/arguments in small rooms/access to firearms, teach children to call 911), social work consult

Disposition

- D/C to shelter if unsafe home

Pearls

- ↑ risk during pregnancy/attempts to leave partner
- Ask about children who may be at risk for abuse
- Universal screening for all pts should be done in the ED

Elder Abuse

Definition

- Includes physical abuse, sexual abuse, emotional/psychological abuse, neglect, financial abuse/exploitation, & abandonment
- Self-neglect is failure of an older adult to provide for their own care & protection

History

- Delayed presentation, hx of med noncompliance/missed appointments, often lives w/ abuser, have dementia, are dependent on abuser for ADLs
- RFs for abusive caretaker: Mental illness, substance abuse, hx of family violence/financial stress/stress of being caretaker

Physical Findings

- Poor hygiene, malnutrition, decubitus ulcers, "urine rash," unexplained injuries to face/head/torso/back/buttocks/limb contractures (restraints)/arms (grabbing)

Evaluation

- Imaging as needed, CBC, BMP, CK (rhabdomyolysis)

Treatment

- Photographs as appropriate, arrange for support services to relieve stress on caretaker (VNA, meals-on-wheels), arrange for home safety eval

Disposition

- Admit if unsafe to go home

Pearls

- May be as high as 5–10% in elderly
- Decreased reporting for fear of institutionalization

CRITICAL CARE AFTER CARDIAC ARREST

Approach

- Repeat ABCDs w/ focused interventions, priority on immediate life threats and stabilization

Post-ROSC ABCDs	
Airway	Intubate if obtunded or resp failure, confirm ET tube placement w/ waveform capnography and b/l breath sounds
Breathing	Lung-protective ventilation (6–8 cc/kg), target normoxia (92–98%) w/ PEEP and FiO_2, target normocapnia ($EtCO_2$ 35–45 mmHg) w/ RR
Circulation	Place arterial line, target MAP 65–80 mmHg, treat dysrhythmia, obtain ECG, perform POCUS RUSH exam
Disability	Evaluate for command following, pupils, motor response, POC gluc, Sz activity

History

- **Witnesses:** Antecedent sxs/injury/ingestion, any initiation of bystander CPR
- **EMS:** Initial rhythm, duration of no-flow (no CPR) and low-flow (CPR) states, interventions

Initial Workup

Post-ROSC Diagnostics	
Labs	CBC w/ diff, BMP, LFTs, VBG/ABG, PT/INR, PTT, iCal, Mg, Phos, Troponin, Lactate, UA +/– BCx, hCG, toxicology studies
Imaging	CXR, CT head, +/– CTA chest, CT abd/pelvis w/ contrast if unclear etiology of arrest
Other	ECG (repeat 15 post-ROSC as may have transient STEMI pattern), TTE, +/– EEG

Evaluation & Management (*Circulation* 2024;149:e168)

- **Neuro:**
  - Cerebral edema common, consider MAP goal 80 mmHg to optimize CPP if suspicion for elevated ICP, prolonged down time, other RFs for cerebral edema
  - Sz common post-ROSC but also may have clinical myoclonus w/o electrographic Sz that does not need Tx, so initiate cEEG for comatose pts
  - Avoid early neuroprognostication in the immediate post-ROSC period
  - Prioritize short-acting agents (ie, propofol, avoid benzos) if sedation needed
  - Monitor core temperature and avoid hyperthermia (maintain <37.8 °C)
- **Cardiac:**
  - Severe myocardial dysfxon likely, if refractory hypoperfusion consult or transfer for mechanical circulatory support (eg, IABP, percutaneous VAD, ECMO)
  - Early coronary angiography can salvage ischemic myocardial tissue, consult cardiology if concerning Hx or ECG even in the absence of STEMI
- **Pulmonary:**
  - Default is lung protective ventilation, but may need higher TV w/ lower RR if clinical context (Hx, vent dynamics) suggests obstructive pulmonary pathology as etiology of arrest
  - Traumatic cxs from chest compressions common (PTX, hemoperitoneum)
- **Heme:**
  - Transfuse for Hgb <7 g/dL
- **GI:**
  - Place enteral tube for gastric decompression and early initiation of feeding
- **GU:**
  - Place Foley (temp sensing if available)
  - If feasible, prioritize LIJ for CVC access to preserve RIJ for HD catheter
  - Reserve sodium bicarb for severe acidosis (pH 7.2, bicarb <20)
- **Endocrine:**
  - Give steroids for refractory shock (eg, hydrocortisone 100 mg IV)
  - Avoid hyperglycemia, target gluc 140–180 mg/dL
- **ID:**
  - Select Abx as indicated based on hx
  - Reasonable to give empirically for refractory shock or if initiating temperature control interventions

PEDIATRIC ADVANCED LIFE SUPPORT (PALS)

Drugs Dosages Used in PALS for Cardiac Arrest and Symptomatic Arrhythmias				
Medication	**Route**	**NI Dose**	**Incremental Dose**	**Maximum**
Adenosine (SVT)	Rapid IV/IO f/b flush	0.1 mg/kg (up to 6 mg)	0.2 mg/kg	6 mg 1st dose 12 mg 2nd dose
Amiodarone (pVT/VF)	Rapid IV/IO	5 mg/kg		15 mg/kg/d (300 mg max)
Atropine (Bradycardia)	IV/IO/ET	0.02 mg/kg	0.04 mg/kg	0.5 mg single dose
Calcium chloride	IV/IO	20 mg/kg		
Calcium gluconate	IV/IO	60–100 mg/kg		
Dobutamine	IV/IO	2–20 μg/kg/min		Titrate to effect
Epinephrine (cardiac arrest)	IV/IO: 0.01 mg/kg (1:10,000)		q3–5min during CPR	1 mg
Gluc (10% or 20% or 50%)	IV/IO	0.5–1 g/kg		2–4 mL/kg 25%
Lidocaine	IV/IO/ET	1 mg/kg		100 mg
Mg sulfate (Torsade's)	IV/IO	25–50 mg/kg		2 g
Naloxone (Narcotic effect)		If <5 y or <20 kg: 0,1 mg/kg If >5 y or >20 kg: 2 mg		Titrate to effect
Procainamide (Tachycardia)	IV/IO	15/mg		
$NaHCO_3$	IV/IO	1 mEq/kg per dose		

Cardioversion in PALS		
Reason	**NI Dose**	**Incremental Dose**
Tachycardia	0.5–1 J/kg	2 J/kg if ineffective
VF/pulseless VT	2–4 J/kg	10 J/kg max or adult dose

MECHANICAL VENTILATION

Indications for Ventilation		
Type of Ventilation		**Indications**
Noninvasive (NIV)	CPAP	Cardiogenic pulmonary edema (ACPE)
	BiPAP	COPD w/ $PaCO_2$ >45 mmHg or pH <7.35
Invasive		Airway protection, ↑ gas exchange, alleviate respiratory distress, assist in pulmonary healing, & allow for NM blockade

Noninvasive Ventilation	
CPAP	**BiPAP**
Mechanism in ACPE → ↓ Preload, ↓ afterload & prevent atelectasis	Mechanism in COPD → CPAP + pressure support → ↓ WOB & improves alveolar ventilation
Benefits in ACPE → ↓ intubation, ↓ mortality, & ↑ hemodynamics & gas exchange	Benefits in COPD → ↓ intubation, ↓ mortality (NNT 12)
Indications w/ possible NIV benefit: Acute hypoxic nonhypercapnic resp failure, acute asthma exacerbation, postextubation/operative or trauma-induced respiratory failure	
CIs: Need for intubation (absolute); AMS, aspiration risk, vomiting, UGIB/epistaxis, facial injury, lethargy precluding compliance, hemodynamic instability, prolonged need for ventilation, & airway obstruction (relative)	

Invasive Ventilation		
Invasive Ventilation Targets	**Description**	**Comments**
Volume targeted	Set tidal volume for assisted breaths; ventilator determines pressure to achieve TV	Standard setting
Pressure targeted	Set inspiratory pressure for assisted breaths	Useful for pts uncomfortable on volume modes
Invasive Ventilation Modes	**Description**	**Comments**
Assist control (ACV)	Preset TV or inspiratory pressure delivered either on ventilator trigger or pt inspiration	Default ventilator mode during resuscitation
Synchronized intermittent mandatory ventilation (SIMV)	Set RR, TV, or pressure; pt can breathe spontaneously, unassisted, b/w assisted breaths	No utility in the resuscitation setting
Pressure support ventilation (PSV)	All breaths triggered by pt and supported by ventilator at set inspiratory pressure	Useful for weaning pts from ventilator

Other Ventilator Settings & Measurements	
Standard, lung-protective settings	ACV, TV 6–8 mL/kg (IBW), RR 12–20, PEEP 5–10 cm H_2O, 100% FiO_2 (wean promptly to maintain SpO_2 92–98%), Pplat <30
PEEP	Positive pressure present during exhalation → maintains patent alveoli → ↓ shunting & ↑ oxygenation (cardiac effects dictate CO & oxygenation); 5 cm H_2O = "physiologic" PEEP Preload: Decreased via ↑ intrathoracic pressure → ↓ venous return Afterload: Decreased via ↓ transmural cardiac pressure
Auto-PEEP	Presence of flow at end expiration due to "breath stacking": ↓ time for exhalation → incomplete expiration → lungs "trap" air → leading to potential compromise of respiratory mechanics & hemodynamics (↓ preload)
I:E ratio	Proportion of time ventilator delivers breath vs allows expiration. ↓ inspiratory time → ↑ expiratory time → improves ventilation & minimizes auto-PEEP in obstructive dz (asthma, COPD)
Pplat	Plateau pressure, measured at end expiration; determined by respiratory system compliance ↑ Pplat w/ obesity, pulmonary edema, ARDS → auto-PEEP, asynchronous breathing
PIP	Peak pressure measured during inspiration affected by airway resistance plus lung/chest wall compliance If ↑ PIP & nl Pplat → cause = airway resistance (bronchospasm, secretions, etc)

Making Changes to the Ventilator	
Improve oxygenation	↑ PEEP, ↑ FiO_2
Improve ventilation	↑ TV, ↑ RR
Reduce auto-PEEP	↓ RR, ↑ expiratory time, ↑ inspiratory flow rate
Permissive hypercapnia	Low TV (4–6 mL/kg) to reduce baro/volutrauma in ALI/ARDS

ANALGESIA & CONSCIOUS SEDATION

Opioids				
Medication	**Nl Dose**	**Incremental Dose**	**Onset of Action**	**Duration**
Morphine	0.1 mg/kg	½ nl dose	5–10 mins	3–4 h
Hydromorphone	0.5–2 mg	½ nl dose	3–5 mins	2–4 h
Fentanyl	0.5–1 µg/kg (25–100 µg)	25 µg	1–2 mins	10 mins–1 h

Benzodiazepines				
Medication	**NI Dose**	**Incremental Dose**	**Onset of Action**	**Duration**
Diazepam	5–10 mg	2.5 mg	1–5 mins	30 mins–2 h
Midazolam	1–5 mg	0.5–1 mg	1–2 mins	15–60 mins
Lorazepam	1–2 mg	0.5–1 mg	1–3 mins	2–6 h

Conscious Sedation Medications				
Medication	**NI Dose**	**Incremental Dose**	**Onset of Action**	**Duration**
Ketamine[a]	1–2 mg/kg IV	1 mg/kg	1–2 mins	10–30 mins
Propofol	1–3 mg/kg IV	0.5 mg/kg	<1 min	8–10 mins
Etomidate	0.2–0.5 mg/kg IV	0.05 mg/kg	<1 min	5–8 mins
Nitrous oxide	30–50%	Constant inhalation	1–2 mins	5 mins

[a]Consider administration w/ glycopyrrolate (0.01 mg/kg) or atropine (0.01 mg/kg) as an antisialagogue.

Reversal Agents				
Medication	**NI Dose**	**Incremental Dose**	**Onset of Action**	**Duration**
Naloxone (opioids)	0.4–2 mg	0.04 mg	1–2 mins	30 mins–1 h
Flumazenil (benzo)	1 mg	0.2 mg	1–2 mins	30 mins–1.5 h

CRITICAL CARE MEDICATIONS

Critical Care Medications		
Drug	**Class**	**Dose**
	Pressors, Inotropes	
Phenylephrine	α_1	50–200 µg/min
Norepinephrine	$\alpha_1 > \beta_1$	0.05–0.5 µg/kg/min, max ~5 µg/kg/min
Vasopressin	V_1	0.04 U/min
Dopamine	D β, D α, β, D	0.5–2 µg/kg/min 2–10 µg/kg/min >10 µg/kg/min, max 50 µg/kg/min
Dobutamine	$\beta_1 > \beta_2$	2–20 µg/kg/min
Epinephrine	$\alpha_1, \alpha_2, \beta_1, \beta_2$	0.05–0.5 µg/kg/min, max ~5 µg/kg/min
	Vasodilators	
Nitroglycerin	NO	5–1000 µg/min
Nitroprusside	NO	0.1–10 µg/kg/min
Enalapril	ACEI	0.625–2.5 mg over 5 mins then 0.625–5 mg q6h
Hydralazine	Vasodilator	5–20 mg q20–30min
Labetalol	$\alpha_1, \beta_1, \beta_2$ blockers	5–20 mg over 2 mins then 20–80 mg q10min or 10–120 mg/h
Nicardipine	NO	2.5–15 mg/h
	Antiarrhythmics	
Amiodarone	Class III	150 mg over 10 mins, then 1 mg/min × 6 h, then 0.5 mg/min × 18 h
Lidocaine	Class IB (Na channel)	1–1.5 mg/kg (100 mg) then 1–4 mg/min
Procainamide	Class IA (Na channel)	17 mg/kg (1 g) over 60 mins, then 1–4 mg/min
Ibutilide	Class III (K channel)	1 mg over 10 mins, may repeat × 1
Propranolol	βB	0.5–1 mg q5min then 1–10 mg/h
Esmolol	β_1 blocker > β_2 blocker	500 µg/kg (20–40 mg) over 1 min, then 25–300 µg/kg/min (2–20 mg/min)
Verapamil	CCB	2.5–5 mg over 1–2 mins, repeat 5–10 mg in 15–30 mins PRN, 5–20 mg/h
Diltiazem	CCB	0.25 mg/kg (20 mg) over 2 mins, reload 0.35 mg/kg (25 mg) × 1 PRN, then 5–15 mg/h
Adenosine	Purinergic	6 mg rapid push, if no response 12 mg rapid push, repeat × 1 PRN

Sedation		
Morphine	Opioid	1–unlimited mg/h
Etomidate	Anesthetic	0.2–0.5 mg/kg
Propofol	Anesthetic	1–3 mg/kg (50–200 mg) then 0.3–5 mg/kg/h (20–400 mg/h)
Diazepam	Benzo	1–5 mg q1–2h
Midazolam	Benzo	0.5–2 mg q5min PRN or 0.5–4 mg then 1–10 mg/h
Ketamine	Anesthetic	1–2 mg/kg (60–150 mg)
Haloperidol	Antipsychotic	2–5 mg q20–30min
Paralysis		
Succinylcholine	Depolarizing	0.6–1.1 mg/kg (70–100 mg)
Pancuronium	nACh	0.08 mg/kg (2–4 mg) q30–90min
Rocuronium	nACH	0.6 mg/kg (60–100 mg)
Vecuronium	nACH	0.08 mg/kg (5–10 mg) over 1–3 mins, then 0.5–0.1 mg/kg/h (2–8 mg/h)
Cisatracurium	nACH	5–10 μg/kg/min
Miscellaneous		
Insulin		0.1 U/kg/h (Follow institutional protocols)
Glucagon		5–10 mg then 1–5 mg/h
Octreotide	Somatostatin analog	50 μg then 50 μg/h
Phenytoin	Antiepileptic	20 mg/kg (1–1.5 g) over 20–30 mins
Fosphenytoin	Antiepileptic	20 mg/kg (1–1.5 g) over 10 mins
Phenobarbital	Barbiturate	20 mg/kg (1–1.5 g) over 20 mins
Thiopental	Barbiturate	3–5 mg/kg (200–400 mg) over 2 mins
Mannitol	Osmotic	1.5–2 g/kg over 30–60 mins, repeat q6–12h to keep osm 310–320
Naloxone	Opioid antagonist	0.4–2 mg q2–3min to total 10 mg
Flumazenil	Benzo antagonist	0.2 mg over 30 s, then 0.3 mg over 30 s, may repeat 0.5 mg over 30 s to max 3 mg
Fentanyl	Opioid	50–100 μg then 50–unlimited μg/h

EQUATIONS

Metabolic

Anion Gap: Na – (Cl + Bicarb)

Delta/Delta = (actual anion gap – normal gap)/(normal HCO_3 – actual HCO_3)

Total body water (TBW) = weight (kg) × 0.6 (use 0.5 if female/elderly, 0.6 for infants)

Corrected Na = measured Na + (2.4 × [measured gluc –100])

Calculated osmoles = (2 × Na) + (gluc/18) + (BUN/2.8) + (EtOH/4.6)

Osmolal gap = measured osmoles – calculated osmoles (nl)

$$\textbf{Estimated Cr clearance} = \frac{[140 - \text{age (y)}] \times \text{wt (kg)}}{\text{Serum Cr (mg/dL)} \times 72} \times (0.85 \text{ in women})$$

Pediatric fluid maintenance (4-2-1 Rule):

$$(4 \text{ cc/kg for 1st 10 kg}) + (2 \text{ cc/kg for 2nd 10 kg}) + (1 \text{ cc/kg for remainder kg})$$

Hyponatremia:

$$\Delta[\textbf{Na}]/\textbf{liter infusate} = \frac{[\text{Na}]_{\text{infusate}} \times [\text{Na}]_{\text{serum}}}{\text{TBW} + 1}$$

$$\textbf{Rate of infusion (mL/h)} = \frac{1000 \times [\text{TBW} \times (\text{desired Na} - \text{serum Na})]}{[\text{Na (mmol/L)}]_{\text{infusate}} \times \text{time (h)}}$$

Hypernatremia:

Free water deficit = total body water × [(140/serum Na) – 1]

$$\Delta[\mathbf{Na}]/\textbf{liter infusate} = \frac{([Na]_{infusate} + [K]_{infusate}) - [Na]_{serum}}{TBW + 1}$$

$$\textbf{Total infusion (L)} = \frac{\text{Desired [Na (mEq/L)] – Serum [Na (mEq/L)]}}{\Delta\text{[Na]/liter infusate}}$$

Rate of infusion (mL/h) = total infusion (mL)/24 h

Cardiopulmonary

A-a gradient = $PAO_2 - PaO_2$ (nl ≈ 4 + [age/4])
Stroke volume = cardiac output/heart rate

$$\textbf{Mean arterial pressure} = \frac{[SBP + (DBP \times 2)]}{3} \text{(nl 70–100 mmHg)}$$

PROCEDURES

Common ED Procedures *(italicized procedures are discussed below)*	
Type	**Procedures**
Respiratory	Airway mgmt (Section XVII: Airway Management), mechanical ventilation (see above), *thoracentesis, tube thoracostomy*
Cardiac	Cardiac pacing, *pericardiocentesis,* resuscitative thoracotomy
Vascular	*Arterial puncture/catheterization,* peripheral IV, *central venous catheterization* & CVP monitoring, venous cutdown, *IO placement*
Anesthesia	Conscious sedation, nerve blocks
Skin & soft tissue	Wound closure, FB removal, *I&D*
GI	*Nasogastric intubation,* balloon tamponade of esophageal varices, *paracentesis,* anorectal procedures
Orthopedic	Fracture/dislocation reductions, splinting, arthrocentesis, compartment pressure measurement
GU	Bladder catheterization (urethral, suprapubic)
OB	Emergency delivery, resuscitative hysterotomy
Neuro	*Lumbar puncture,* Dix–Hallpike/Epley maneuver
Ophtho	Eye irrigation, FB removal, lateral canthotomy
ENT	Peritonsillar abscess drainage, ear canal & nasal FB removal, drainage of auricular hematoma
Dental	Dental nerve blocks, abscess drainage, mandibular reduction

---

Arterial Puncture and Catheterization

Purpose

- Puncture to obtain ABG; catheterization for continuous real-time BP monitoring, or need for repeat arterial blood sampling

Equipment

- Puncture: Local anesthetic, 3-mL syringe, 22-gauge needle (or insulin syringe)
- Catheterization: Arm board, tape, angiocath (size depends on artery cannulated), U/S for real-time guidance, guidewire, pressure tubing, pressure transducer, suture, needle driver, sterile dressing

Positioning

- Ideally placed in the radial or femoral artery; brachial & axillary are also useable, but they are terminal (no collateral supply), so worse prognosis if thrombosis occurs

Procedure

- Sterilize area, use sterile gloves, but generally drape & gown are not required
- Puncture: Use U/S to identify radial or femoral artery, aligning target artery w/ the centerline of the U/S. Insert needle and puncture under real-time sonographic guidance, confirming tip of needle in the center of vessel before advancing guidewire
- Catheterization: Immobilize wrist in slight dorsiflexion using tape/arm board, skin wheal w/ lidocaine in awake pt, insert needle as above until flash is observed and needle tip visualized in center of vessel on U/S, pass guidewire into artery, advance catheter to hub along the guidewire, remove wire, check flow, attach to pressure tubing, suture in place, apply sterile dressing

Complications

- Hematoma, AV fistula, pseudoaneurysm, bleeding, PAIN. *Rarely:* Catheter infxn, thrombosis or stenosis of artery, hand/limb ischemia

---

Central Venous Catheterization

Purpose

- Rapid volume resuscitation, emergency venous access, administration of spec medicines (ie, pressors, high-concentration electrolytes), CVP monitoring
- Sometimes used when peripheral access is not obtainable, but 1st consider external jugular, basilic, or cephalic vein catheterization, or IO access

Choice of Site

- Each site has advantages & disadvantages. Overall, no compelling evidence that one site is uniformly superior to others, or definite difference in infxn risk. CDC recommends weighing risk/benefits for each pt, but avoiding femoral when possible ("*Guidelines for the Prevention of Intravascular Catheter-related Infections*," 2024, CDC: www.cdc.gov).

Comparison of Types of Central Venous Catheterization

Site	Pros	Cons	Comments
Internal jugular	Bleeding easily controlled Low mechanical cx rate when used w/ U/S	Intermediate risk of infxn	U/S guidance is now the standard of care for IJ
Infraclavicular subclavian	Lowest infxn rate, least obtrusive to awake pt	↑ Risk of PTX (mitigated by U/S)	± U/S guided
Supraclavicular subclavian	Practical for cardiac arrest	↑ Risk of PTX ↓ Bleeding control	± U/S guided
Femoral	Fast, practical during arrest	Thought to have ↑ risk of infxn	± U/S guided

Equipment

- Chlorhexidine, cap, mask, sterile drape/gloves/gown, catheter device kit (includes 1% lidocaine w/ 10-mL syringe & 25-gauge needle, catheterization needle/syringe, guidewire, scalpel, dilator, catheter, needle driver, scissors, suture, sterile dressing)

Positioning

- Supine pt, Trendelenburg position for IJ; can do subclavians upright (eg, in CHF)
- Internal jugular: Bedside U/S guidance recommended if available
  - Locate the IJ vein (compressible) & carotid artery (pulsatile, noncompressible) using a sterile U/S probe w/i the triangle created by the clavicle & the sternal & clavicular heads of the sternocleidomastoid muscle
  - Advance the needle toward the IJ vein & away from the carotid artery w/ needle at 30° angle to skin while observing the needle penetrate the vein on U/S toward ipsilateral nipple
  - Confirm venous cannulation via U/S once the wire is in place
- Infraclavicular: Use of U/S increases success rate and decreases cx rate vs landmark technique. Insert needle 2 cm inferior & 2 cm lateral to the angle of the clavicle (located along the middle third), point toward spot just superior to the suprasternal notch & advance just posterior to the clavicle
- Supraclavicular: Insert needle at the junction of the middle & medial thirds of the clavicle, just posterior to the clavicle, point toward the contralateral nipple
- Femoral: Palpate femoral artery, then advance needle at 45° angle to skin toward the head just medial to the palpable artery

Procedure
- Rate of CVL-associated infxn ↓ w/ use of observer & checklist (*NEJM* 2006;355:2725)
- Sterile technique. Attach catheterization needle to syringe, advance while aspirating
- Remove syringe once vein is entered & check for free return of nonpulsatile blood
- Place the curved end of the guidewire into the needle & advance, check that the wire passes easily, & advance to estimated location of SVC
- Remove the needle while keeping the wire in position
- Make a 1-cm incision through the dermis where the wire meets the skin
- Advance the dilator over the wire several centimeters, then remove the dilator
- Advance catheter over wire, advance to the estimated location of the SVC, remove wire
- Suture in place, cover w/ sterile dressing, obtain CXR to r/o PTX (for all but femoral lines)

Complications
- Arterial puncture (if needle/wire puncture & compressible, apply prolonged pressure). If a major artery was *dilated*, leave in place & consult IR & vascular surgery
- PTX: Always r/o w/ XR. Always stat XR if SOB during line placement
- Bloodstream infxn, air embolus, nerve injury (phrenic, brachial plexus, femoral)

Pearls
- A triple-lumen CVC has a slower infusion rate than most PIVs; consider percutaneous introducer if large-volume resuscitation needed

---

Incision and Drainage

Purpose
- Definitive tx of a soft tissue abscess

Equipment
- Consider bedside U/S prior to procedure to confirm fluid collection. Hemostat, scissors, forceps, scalpel, packing gauze or vessel loop, 1–2% lidocaine w/ 10-mL syringe & 25-gauge needle

Procedure
- Anesthetize skin over the most fluctuant area. Make a single, linear incision w/ scalpel over the abscess cavity. Make a second incision if planning loop drain placement
- Dissect wound using a hemostat & probe into all corners of the cavity to break up loculations & evaluate for an FB
- If performing vessel loop drainage: Pass hemostat into 1 incision, through abscess cavity, out the other incision, and pull vessel loop through, tying loosely above to secure

---

Intraosseous Catheterization

Purpose
- Rapid temporary vascular access in critically ill adults and children

Equipment
- IO needle w/ stylet & syringe, powered IO driver if available, gauze

Positioning
- Proximal humerus in adults; 1–2 cm above the surgical neck on the greater tubercle
- 2° in adults, 1° peds: Anteromedial aspect of the proximal tibia, 1–3 cm distal to the tibial tuberosity
- Secondary options include distal femur, distal tibia

Procedure
- Sterile technique. Advance IO needle/stylet perpendicular to the bone w/ firm pressure & a twisting motion until the cortex is penetrated, remove stylet, attach syringe & aspirate to correct positioning of the needle. Secure in place w/ gauze pads. Flush w/ small amount lidocaine (20–60 mg) in awake pts

Complications
- Infxn, bleeding, fracture, retained FB, pain

Lumbar Puncture

Purpose
- Dx of meningitis (in the absence of elevated ICP), SAH, idiopathic intracranial HTN, other infectious, inflammatory, neoplastic processes

Equipment

- Careful neurologic exam beforehand (avoid in any pt w/ focal neurologic findings w/o imaging), sterile technique, 20–22-gauge spinal or Whitacre needle, LP tray (w/ collecting tubes, lidocaine 1%, manometer/stopcock, 25-gauge needle, 10-cc syringe, sterile drapes)
- Consider U/S in obese pts to identify nonpalpable landmarks
- Consider CTH prior to procedure if concern for mass effect/elevated ICP

Positioning

- Lateral decubitus w/ shoulders/hips perpendicular to the bed (preferable & necessary to measure opening pressure) or sitting up on the edge of the bed
- Have the pt maximally flex neck, hips, & knees, & arch back, into a fetal position
- L4 spinous process is found at the intersection of a line b/w the spine & the iliac crests; enter through the interspace above or below this location

Procedure

- Anesthetize locally w/ lidocaine 1% using 25-gauge needle, then advance needle while aspirating → inject lidocaine into the interspinous ligament
- Advance spinal needle toward the umbilicus w/ bevel pointed toward the pt's side (left or right) until a "pop" or sudden decrease in resistance is felt → remove the stylet
- Once clear fluid is obtained, attach the manometer & record opening pressure
- If fluid is not found, replace the stylet, pull back the needle to the level of SQ tissue, confirm that you are in midline, & reangle your needle slightly
- Obtain at least 1 cc in each collecting tube (more if extensive studies are necessary)
- Replace stylet, remove needle, place sterile dressing over wound
- Tests: cell count (tubes #1, #4), protein/gluc (#2 or #3), Gram stain & culture (#2 or #3)

Complications

- HA (5–40%), localized infxn, epidural hematoma (rare), herniation (in cases of elevated ICP)
- Blood patch can be used to treat post-LP headache if refractory to analgesics and caffeine

---

Nasogastric Intubation

Purpose

- Aspiration of stomach contents in pts at risk for recurrent vomiting (eg, GI obstruction), stomach decompression during trauma or after intubation

Equipment

- 16- or 18-gauge NG tube, lubricant, 60-cc syringe, cup of water w/ straw, towel, tape, stethoscope, topical anesthetic jelly, nasal vasoconstrictor

Positioning

- Sitting up, chin down

Procedure

- Place towel over chest, estimate distance to stomach (from nose to earlobe to xiphoid)
- Lubricate tube, spray patent nare w/ vasoconstrictor, apply anesthetic jelly, wait a few minutes
- Advance tube posteriorly along the floor of the nose until it enters the oropharynx, then have pt continuously sip water through straw while the tube is advanced into esophagus; once in the esophagus, quickly advance the tube to the desired distance
- Confirm placement by insufflating the NG tube w/ air using 60-cc syringe & listening over stomach for gush of air, & aspiration of GI contents. Obtain upright CXR
- Secure tube using tape attached to the nose & wrapped around the tube from each side; tape should also be used to attach a 2nd segment of the NG tube to the gown

Complications

- Vomiting during placement, tracheal intubation, small risk of intracranial penetration (contraindicated in facial fractures), bleeding, esophageal rupture (hx of esophageal stricture/alkali injury), pain

---

Paracentesis

Purpose

- Diagnostic: Removal of peritoneal fluid in a pt w/ ascites to (a) diagnose the cause of new ascites; (b) assess for spontaneous bacterial peritonitis
- Therapeutic: Relieve sxs in pts w/ tense ascites (eg, hypoxia from mass effect)

Equipment
- Use bedside U/S prior to procedure to confirm ascites & identify large pocket
- Sterile technique
- 25-gauge needle, 1% lidocaine. For diagnostic tap, only need 20–22-gauge needle & large syringe to aspirate fluid. For therapeutic tap, use paracentesis kit w/ 18-gauge needle, catheter sheath, & vacuum-sealed collection bottles

Positioning
- Supine; identify entry site: Usually 4–5-cm cephalad & medial to anterior superior iliac spine, lateral to the rectus muscle sheath, being careful to avoid any visible veins

Procedure
- Check for severe coagulopathy prior to procedure
- Perform w/ real-time bedside U/S if possible. Use abd probe to assess depth of fluid pocket. Use vascular probe to ensure no superficial vessels (eg, epigastric arteries) near site of insertion
- Anesthetize locally w/ lidocaine 1% using 25-gauge needle
- Z-tract: Pull the skin 2-cm caudad before advancing the larger-bore needle, then place the needle perpendicular to the skin, advance needle slowly while occasionally aspirating, until ascitic fluid is aspirated, then release skin
- After aspirating fluid, advance catheter 1–2 cm & remove needle → connect catheter to stopcock, & collect fluid into sterile containers
- Fluid: Send for cell count, albumin, culture. Consider total protein, gluc, LDH, amylase, Gram stain.
- Administer albumin following large volume para. (if >5 L removed) in pts w/ cirrhosis

Complications
- Hypotension (can have severe fluid shifts in large-volume tap), ascitic fluid leakage, abd wall hematoma, infxn, hemoperitoneum, viscera perforation

---

Pericardiocentesis

Purpose
- Emergent tx of pericardial effusion/tamponade in a pt w/ cardiac arrest (often PEA) or periarrest; hemorrhagic tamponade is best treated w/ thoracotomy

Equipment
- 16- or 18-gauge spinal needle attached to a 30- or 60-cc syringe or pericardiocentesis kit

Positioning
- Supine pt, angle needle 30°–45° to the skin, insert b/w xiphoid process & left costal margin, aim needle toward left shoulder (parasternal technique: 90° angle above 5th/6th rib L sternal border)

Procedure
- Sterile technique. Bedside U/S guidance recommended if available. Advance needle slowly while aspirating until fluid is removed (presence of blood suggests ventricular puncture)

Complications
- "Dry tap," PTX, myocardial laceration, coronary vessel laceration, hemopericardium, ventricular penetration, visceral injury

---

Thoracentesis

Purpose
- Diagnostic eval (new/unclear etiology) or therapeutic tx of pl effusion

Equipment
- 20- or 22-gauge needle w/ catheter or thoracentesis kit

Positioning
- Pt sitting upright, needle angled 90° to skin, insert in intercostal space above rib (no lower than 8th intercostal space) in midscapular line

Procedure
- Sterile technique. Bedside U/S guidance is recommended for locating height of effusion & distance of lung from the parietal pleura

- Anesthetize locally w/ lidocaine 1% using 25-gauge needle, then advance needle while aspirating → inject lidocaine → advance while aspirating further, until pl fluid is aspirated
- Remove needle, make a small 0.5-cm incision at the insertion site, then insert 20- or 22-gauge needle w/ catheter → advance while aspirating
- After aspirating fluid, advance catheter & remove needle
- Connect catheter to stopcock, & collect fluid into sterile containers
- Goal: Diagnostic (50–100 mL), therapeutic (relief of dyspnea, up to 1,500 mL)
- Fluid: Send for LDH, protein, gluc, cell count, amylase, cytology, gram stain, culture
- Remove catheter during exhalation
- Obtain postprocedure CXR

Complications

- PTX, bleeding (caution if PLT <50,000 or >1.5 × nl PT/PTT), cough, infxn, hemothorax, diaphragmatic penetration

---

TUBE THORACOSTOMY

Purpose

- Drainage of air (PTX), blood (hemothorax), or fluid (pl effusion, empyema) in the pl space that threatens cardiac or pulmonary function

Equipment

- #10 scalpel, Kelly clamp, #0 or #1 suture, scissors, chest tube (24F minimum; should place 14F pigtail catheter via Seldinger technique for PTX or HTX in stable pts)

Positioning

- Supine pt, shoulder abducted (raised overhead), enter at midaxillary line @ 4th intercostal space (nipple line), lateral to pectoralis major. Perform procedural sedation if possible

Procedure

- Sterile technique
- Create wheal using lidocaine 1% w/ epinephrine (1:100,000) & a 25- or 27-gauge needle, then advance needle while aspirating, & infiltrate broadly through muscle, periosteum & parietal pleura, staying above the rib; ±intercostal nerve block (at level, above, & below)
- Make 3–4-cm incision parallel & just over rib, through skin & fat overlying the rib
- Perform blunt dissection w/ a Kelly down to the rib & just above it
- Apply firm pressure w/ the Kelly closed to pop through the parietal pleura
- Look/listen for rush of fluid or air. Leave Kelly in place & spread to open the pleura further
- Insert finger into the chest wall (Kelly still in place) to verify that it is the pl space (feel lung, ensure no abd organs)
- Keep finger in place, remove Kelly, pass the tube over finger while gently spinning the tube
- Typically, direct tube superiorly & posteriorly
- Rotate the tube 360° to ↓ kinking & ensure all the tube holes are in the pl space
- Attach to water seal or suction. Never clamp a chest tube
- Confirm placement: Condensation w/ respiration, bubbles in water seal w/ coughing, CXR
- Suture in place, place petroleum gauze over wound, cover w/ dry gauze & tape in place

Complications

- Infxn, intercostal vessel/nerve laceration, lung laceration, intra-abd entry, solid organ tube placement, subcutaneous placement

ABBREVIATIONS

1°	Primary
2°	Secondary
AAST	American Association for the Surgery of Trauma
A/C	Anticoagulation
A/P	Assessment and plan
a/w	Associated with
AAA	Abdominal aortic aneurysm
ABC	Airway, breathing, circulation
abd	Abdominal
ABG	Arterial blood gas
ABI	Ankle-brachial index
abnl	Abnormal
abnlty	Abnormality
Abs	Antibodies
abx	Antibiotics
AC	Acromioclavicular, Activated charcoal
ACE-I/ ACEI	Angiotensin-converting enzyme inhibitor
ACh	Acetylcholine
Ach	Acetylcholinergic
AChE	Acetylcholinesterase
AChE-inh	Acetylcholinesterase inhibitor
AChR	Acetylcholine receptor
ACS	Acute coronary syndrome
ACT	Artemisinin-based combination therapies
ADD-RS	Aortic dissection detection risk score
addx	Additional
ADH	Antidiuretic hormone
ADHD	Attention-deficit hyperactivity disorder
Admx	Admission
AED	Antiepileptic drug
AF	Atrial fibrillation
AFL	Atrial flutter
AG	Aminoglycoside
AGE	Arterial gas embolism
AI	Aortic insufficiency
AICD	Automatic implantable cardioverter defibrillator
AIDS	Acquired immunodeficiency syndrome
AIR	Appendicitis inflammatory response
AKA	Alcoholic ketoacidosis
AKI	Acute kidney injury
ALI	Acute lung injury
alk phos	Alkaline phosphatase
ALL	Acute lymphocytic leukemia
ALS	Amyotrophic lateral sclerosis
ALT	Alanine transaminase
ALTE	Apparent life-threatening event
AMI	Acute myocardial infarction
a-MI	Anterior myocardial infarction
AML	Acute myeloid leukemia
amox	Amoxicillin
amoxicillin clav	Amoxicillin/clavulanate
AMS	Acute mountain sickness, Altered mental status
ANC	Absolute neutrophil count
Ant.	Anterior
antichol	Anticholinergics
ANUG	Acute necrotizing ulcerative gingivitis
AoD	Aortic dissection
AOM	Acute otitis media
AP	Anterior posterior
APAP	Acetaminophen
APLAS	Antiphospholipid antibody syndrome
APS	Antiphospholipid syndrome
ARB	Angiotensin receptor blocker
ARDS	Acute respiratory distress syndrome
ARF	Acute renal failure
Art.	Artery
ARVD	Arrhythmogenic right ventricular dysplasia
AS	Aortic stenosis
ASA	Acetylsalicylic acid (aspirin)
ASD	Atrial septal defect
AST	Aspartate aminotransferase
asx	Asymptomatic
AT	Atrial tachycardia
ATN	Acute tubular necrosis
ATS	American Thoracic Society
AV	Aortic valve
AVA	Aortic valve area
AVB	AV block
AVM	Arteriovenous malformation
AVN	Atrioventricular node
AVNRT	AV nodal reentrant tachycardia
AVR	Aortic valve replacement
AVRT	AV reciprocating tachycardia
AZ	Arizona
b/c	Because
b/l	Bilateral
b/w	Between
BA	Balloon angioplasty
BAL	Blood alcohol level
B-ALL	B-cell acute lymphoblastic leukemia
Barb	Barbiturate
BB	Beta blocker
βB	Beta blocker
βBs	Beta blockers
BBB	Bundle branch block
BCVI	Blunt cerebrovascular injury
BCx	Blood cultures
bili	Bilirubin
Benzo	Benzodiazepine
BiPAP	Bilevel positive airway pressure
BiVAD	Biventricular assist device
BM	Bowel movement
BMP	Basic metabolic panel

BMS	Bare metal stent
BNP	Brain natriuretic peptide
BP	Blood pressure
BPH	Benign prostatic hyperplasia
BPPV	Benign paroxysmal positional vertigo
BRAT	Bananas, rice, applesauce, toast
BRBPR	Bright red blood per rectum
BRUE	Brief resolved unexplained event
BSUS	Bedside ultrasound
BVM	Bag-valve mask
BW	Body weight
bx	Biopsy
BZD	Benzodiazepines
c/b	Complicated by
c/f	Concerning for
c/o	Complaint of
c/s	Consult
c/w	Compared with
CA	Cancer
CA-ASB	Catheter-associated asymptomatic bacteriuria
CABG	Coronary artery bypass graft
CAD	Coronary artery disease
CAP	Community-acquired pneumonia
CAUTI	Catheter-associated urinary tract infection
CAUTI	Catheter-associated UTI
CBC	Complete blood count
CBD	Common bile duct
CCB	Calcium channel blocker
CCS	Canadian Cardiovascular Society
CCU	Coronary care unit
CD	Crohn dz, Contact dermatitis
CF	Cystic fibrosis
CHB	Complete heart block
CHD	Congenital heart disease
CHF	Congestive heart failure
Chg	Change
chgs	Changes
c/i	Contraindicated
CIs	Confidence intervals
CKD	Chronic kidney disease
CI	Contraindication
c/f	Concern for
C/L	Contralateral
CIWA	Clinical Institute Withdrawal Assessment of Alcohol
CMP	Cardiomyopathy
CMV	Cytomegalovirus
CN	Cranial nerve, Cyanide
CNS	Central nervous system
CO	Carbon monoxide, Cardiac output
CO_2	Carbon dioxide
Coags	Coagulation studies
COPD	Chronic obstructive pulmonary disease
CP	Chest pain
CPAP	Continuous positive airway pressure
CPK/CK	Creatine phosphokinase
CPP	Cerebral perfusion pressure
CPR	Cardiopulmonary resuscitation
Cr	Creatinine
CRAO	Central retinal artery occlusion
CRP	C-reactive protein
CRVO	Central retinal vein occlusion
CSF	Cerebrospinal fluid
CT	Computed tomography
CTA	Computed tomography angiography
CTD	Connective tissue disease
CTH	Chronic tension headache
CTV	Computed tomography venography
CTX	Ceftriaxone
CVA	Cerebral vascular accident
CVP	Central venous pressure
CVVH	Continuous venovenous hemofiltration
Cx	Culture
cx	Complications
CXR	Chest x-ray
d	Day(s)
D/C	Discharge
d/o	Disorder
DAI	Diffuse axonal injury
DBP	Diastolic blood pressure
DCCV	DC cardioversion
DCS	Decompression sickness
DDAVP	Desmopressin
DDD	Dual-chamber pacing
DDx/DX	Differential diagnosis
Dec	Decrease
DES	Drug-eluting stent
derm	Dermatology
Dex	Dexamethasone
DEET	Diethyltoluamide
DHE	Dihydroergotamine
DHF	Dengue hemorrhagic fever
DI	Diabetes insipidus
Diam	Diameter
DIC	Disseminated intravascular coagulation
diff	Differential
DIP	Distal interphalangeal joint
dispo	Disposition
DKA	Diabetic ketoacidosis
DL	Direct laryngoscopy
DLBCL	Diffuse large B-cell lymphoma
DM	Diabetes mellitus
DOAC	Direct oral anticoagulant
DOE	Dyspnea on exertion
DP	Dorsalis pedis
DPA	Diagnostic peritoneal aspiration
DPL	Diagnostic peritoneal lavage
DRE	Digital rectal exam
DRESS	Drug reaction with eosinophilia and systemic symptoms
Ds	Deaths

DTs	Delirium tremens
DTaP	Diphtheria, tetanus, pertussis; inactivated
DVT	Deep vein thrombosis
Dx	Diagnosis
Dysfxn	Dysfunction
dz	Disease
e/o	Evidence of
EA	Elder abuse
EBV	Epstein–Barr virus
ECG/EKG	Electrocardiogram
ECMO	Extracorporeal membrane oxygenation
ED	Emergency department
EDH	Epidural hemorrhage
EDOU	Emergency department observation unit
EDV	End-diastolic volume
EEG	Electroencephalogram
EF	Ejection fraction
EGD	Extraglottic device, Esophagogastroduodenoscopy
EHEC	Enterohemorrhagic *E. coli*
EIA	Enzyme immunoassay
EIEC	Enteroinvasive *E. coli*
EM	Emergency medicine
EMS	Emergency medical services
ENT	Otolaryngology
env	Environmental
EOM	Extraocular muscles
EP	Electrophysiologist
Epi	Epinephrine
EPSS	End-point septal separation
equiv	Equivalent
ERCP	Endoscopic retrograde cholangiopancreatography
ESBL	Extended-spectrum beta-lactamase
esp	Especially
ESR	Erythrocyte sedimentation rate
ESRD	End-stage renal disease
ETEC	Enterotoxic *E. coli*
Etiol	Etiology
EtOH	Ethanol
ETT	Endotracheal tube
eval	Evaluation
Ex	Exam
ext, extr	extremity
f/b	Followed by
f/u	Follow-up
FAST	Focused assessment with sonography for trauma
FB	Foreign body
FEna%	Fractional excretion of sodium
FEV$_1$	Forced expiratory volume in 1 second
FFP	Fresh frozen plasma
FH	Family history
FHH	Familial hypocalciuric hypercalcemia
FHx	Family history
FMC	First medical contact
FSG	Fingerstick glucose
FT-ABS	Fluorescent treponemal antibody absorption
FTT	Failure to thrive
Fx	Fracture
fxnl	Functional
G6PD	Glucose-6-phosphate dehydrogenase
GABA	Gamma-aminobutyric acid
GBS	Guillain–Barré syndrome, Group B streptococcus
GC	Gonococcal
GCS	Glasgow Coma Scale
gen	Generation
GER	gastroesophageal reflux
GERD	Gastroesophageal reflux
GFR	Glomerular filtration rate
GI	Gastrointestinal
GIB	Gastrointestinal bleeding
Gluc	Glucose
GNR	Gram-negative rods
GP	Glycoprotein
GPC	Gram-positive cocci
GSW	Gunshot wound
Gtt	IV drip
GU	Genitourinary
GVHD	Graft-versus-host disease
h	Hour(s)
H&P	History and physical
H/H	Hemoglobin/hematocrit
H/o	History of
h/o	History of
HA	Headache
HACE	High-altitude cerebral edema
HACEK	Haemophilus, Aggregatibacter, Cardiobacterium hominis, Eikenella, & Kingella
HAP	Hospital-acquired pneumonia
HAPE	High-altitude pulmonary edema
HBIG	Hepatitis B immunoglobulin
HCAP	Health care–associated pneumonia
HCC	Hepatocellular carcinoma
hCG	Human chorionic gonadotropin
hCG	Pregnancy test
Hct	Hematocrit
HCTZ	Hydrochlorothiazide
HD	Hemodialysis, Hemodynamically
HDCV	Human diploid cell vaccine
HEENT	Head, eyes, ears, nose, and throat
HELLP	Hemolysis, Elevated liver enzymes, and Low platelets
HFNC	High-flow nasal cannula
HFpEF	Heart failure with preserved ejection fracture
HFrEF	Heart failure with reduced ejection fracture
HGA	Human granulocytic anaplasmosis
HHS	Hyperosmolar hyperglycemic state

HI	Homicidal ideation
Hib	Haemophilus influenzae B
HIDA	Hydroxy iminodiacetic acid
HIT	Heparin-induced thrombocytopenia
HIV	Human immunodeficiency virus
HK	Hypokinesis
HLD	Hyperlipidemia
HME	Human monocytic ehrlichiosis
HOB	Head of bed
HOCM	Hypertrophic obstructive cardiomyopathy
hosp	Hospital
HPI	History of present illness
HPV	Human papillomavirus
HR	Heart rate
HRIG	Human rabies immune globulin
HS TnI	High-sensitivity troponin I
HSCT	Hematopoietic stem cell transplantation
HSM	Hepatosplenomegaly
HSP	Henoch–Schönlein purpura
HSV	Herpes simplex virus
HTN	Hypertension
HUS	Hemolytic–uremic syndrome
hypoK	Hypokalemia
HypoTN	Hypotension
hyperK	hyperkalemia
hx	History
I&D	Incision and drainage
IABP	Intra-aortic balloon pump
IBD	Inflammatory bowel disease
IBS	Irritable bowel syndrome
IBW	Ideal body weight
IC	Inhaled corticosteroids, Intracranial
ICH	Intracranial hemorrhage
ICP	Intracranial pressure
ICS	Inhaled corticosteroids
ICU	Intensive care unit
IDSA	Infectious Diseases Society of America
IFA	Immunofluorescence antibody
IIH	Idiopathic intracranial hypertension
IJ	Internal jugular
I/L	Ipsilateral
ILD	Interstitial lung disease
IM	Intramuscular
IMI	Inferior MI
Immuno-supp	Immunosuppression
inc	Including
Inf.	Inferior
infxn	Infection
INH	Isoniazid
inh	Inhibitor
inj	Injury
inflamma	Inflammatory
inpt	Inpatient
INR	International normalized ratio
IO	Intraosseous
IOP	Intraocular pressure
IPF	Idiopathic pulmonary fibrosis
IPH	Intraparenchymal hemorrhage
IR	Interventional radiology
iCal	Ionized calcium
irreg	Irregular
Irrig	Irrigation
ITP	Immune thrombocytopenic purpura
IUP	Intrauterine pregnancy
IV	Intravenous
IVC	Inferior vena cava
IVDU	Intravenous drug use
IVF	Intravenous fluids
IVIG	Intravenous immunoglobulin
IVP	Intravenous pyelogram
JVD	Jugular venous distension
JVP	Jugular venous pressure
Jxn	Junction
KUB	Kidney ureter bladder
L	Left
Lac	Laceration
LAD	Left-axis deviation
LAE	Left atrial enlargement
LAFB	Left anterior fascicular block
LAN	Lymphadenopathy
Lat	Lateral
LBBB	Left bundle branch block
LBP	Lower back pain
LCx	Left circumflex artery
LDH	Lactate dehydrogenase
LE	Lower extremity
LENIs	Lower extremity noninvasive study
LES	Lower esophageal sphincter
LFT	Liver function test
LGIB	Lower gastrointestinal bleeding
LH	Lightheadedness
LIJ	Left internal jugular
LLL	Left lower lobe
LLQ	Left lower quadrant
LMN	Lower motor neuron
LMP	Last menstrual period
LMWH	Low–molecular-weight heparin
LOC	Loss of consciousness
LP	Lumbar puncture
LPFB	Left posterior fascicular block
LR	Lactated Ringer's solution
LSD	Lysergic acid diethylamide
LUTS	Lower urinary tract symptoms
LV	Left ventricle
LVAD	Left ventricular assist device
LVEF	Left ventricular ejection fraction
lvl	Level
Lytic	Fibrinolytic
LVH	Left ventricular hypertrophy
LVO	Large-vessel occlusion
MAC	Mycobacterium avium complex

MAHA	Microangiopathic hemolytic anemia
malfxn	Malfunction
MAOI	Monoamine oxidase inhibitors
MAP	Mean arterial pressure
MAT	Multifocal atrial tachycardia
MCP	Metacarpophalangeal
MDI	Metered-dose inhaler
MDMA	Methylenedioxymethamphetamine
MDRO	Multidrug-resistant organism
MDS	Myelodysplastic syndrome
Meds	Medications
med d/c-ed	Medication discontinued
memb	Membrane
MEN	Multiple endocrine neoplasia
Mets	Metastases
mgmt	Management
MH	Malignant hyperthermia
MI	Myocardial infarction
Mid.	Middle
MINDS	Minnesota Detoxification Scale
mins	Minutes
MIS-C	Multisystem inflammatory syndrome in children
MM	Mucous membrane
mos	Months
mod	Moderate
MR	Mitral regurgitation
MRA	Magnetic resonance angiography
MRCP	Mental retardation and cerebral palsy, Magnetic resonance cholangiopancreatography
MRI	Magnetic resonance imaging
MRSA	Methicillin-resistant *Staphylococcus aureus*
MRV	Magnetic resonance venography
MS	Mitral stenosis, Multiple sclerosis
MSK	Musculoskeletal
MSM	Men who have sex with men
MSOF	Multisystem organ failure
MSSA	Methicillin-susceptible *Staphylococcus aureus*
MTX	Methotrexate
MV	Mitral valve
MVC	Motor vehicle collision
MVP	Mitral valve prolapsed
mx	Multiple
mx RCTs	Multiple RCTs
N/V	Neurovascular
n/v	Nausea/vomiting
NAAT	Nucleic acid amplification test
NAC	*N*-Acetylcysteine
NAPQI	*N*-acetyl-*p*-benzoquinone imine
NAT	Nonaccidental trauma
NC	Nasal cannula
NCHCT	Noncontrast head computed tomography
NEC	Necrotizing enterocolitis
neg	Negative
neur	Neuroma
neuro	Neurologic or neurology
neuro-psych	Neuropsychiatric
neurotox	Neurotoxicity
NGT	Nasogastric tube
NHL	Non-Hodgkin lymphoma
NIF	Negative inspiratory force
NIHSS	National Institutes of Health Stroke Scale
NIPPV	Noninvasive positive-pressure ventilation
NIV	Noninvasive ventilation
nl	Normal
NM	Neuromuscular
NMO	Neuromyelitis optica
NMS	Neuroleptic malignant syndrome
NNT	Number needed to treat
NPA	Nasopharyngeal airway
NPH	Normal pressure hydrocephalus
NPJT	Nonparoxysmal junctional tachycardia
NPO	Nil per OS
NPV	Negative predictive value
NRB	Nonrebreather
NS	Normal saline
NSAID	Nonsteroidal anti-inflammatory drug
NSGY	Neurosurgery
NSSTW	Nonspecific ST-wave changes
NSTEMI	Non–ST-elevation MI
NSTI	Necrotizing soft tissue infection
NSVT	Nonsustained ventricular tachycardia
NTG	Nitroglycerin
O&P	Ova & parasites
O/d	Overdose
o/p	Outpatient
o/w	Otherwise
O_2	Oxygen
OA	Osteoarthritis
Ob/Gyn	Obstetrics and Gynecology
OCP	Oral contraceptive pill
OD	Overdose
OE	Otitis externa
OHS	Obesity hypoventilation syndrome
OM	Otitis media/Osteomyelitis
OME	Otitis media with effusion
OMFS	Oral and maxillofacial surgery
ophtho	Ophthalmology
OR	Operating room
ORIF	Open reduction and internal fixation
OSA	Obstructive sleep apnea
OTC	Over-the-counter
otw	Otherwise
outpt(s)	Outpatient(s)
p/w	Presents with
PAD	Peripheral arterial disease

PAI Primary adrenal insufficiency
PAIR Puncture, Aspiration, Injection, Re-aspiration
PAT Paroxysmal atrial tachycardia
PCC Poison control center/ prothrombin complex concentrate
PCI Percutaneous coronary intervention
PCKD Polycystic kidney disease
PCN Penicillin
PCOM Posterior communicating artery
PCOS Polycystic ovary syndrome
PCP Primary care physician
PCR Polymerase chain reaction
PCWP Pulmonary capillary wedge pressure
PDA Patent ductus arteriosus
PE Physical exam
PE Pulmonary embolism
PEA Pulseless electrical activity
PEEP Positive end-expiratory pressure
PEFR Peak expiratory flow rate
PEG Percutaneous endoscopic gastrostomy
pen VK Penicillin V potassium
PEP Postexposure prophylaxis
PERC Pulmonary embolism rule-out criteria
periph peripheral
PFO Patent foramen ovale
PGE_1 Prostaglandin E_1
PID Pelvic inflammatory disease
PIP Proximal interphalangeal joint
PJP *Pneumocystis jirovecii* pneumonia
PKD Polycystic kidney disease
pl Pleural
PLT Platelet
PM Pacemaker
PMH Past medical history
PMR Polymyalgia rheumatica
PNA Pneumonia
PND Paroxysmal nocturnal dyspnea
PNES Psychogenic nonepileptic seizures
PO Per Os (By Mouth)
POC Point of care
POC Products of conception
POCUS Point-of-care ultrasound
PORT Pneumonia Patient Outcomes Research Team
pos Positive
poss DC Possible DC
pPCI Primary percutaneous coronary intervention
PPE Personal protective equipment
PPI Proton pump inhibitor
ppl People
pPlat Plateau pressure
PPM Permanent pacemaker
PPV Positive predictive value, positive pressure ventilation
ppx Prophylactic
PQRST Palliation, quality, radiation, severity, timing
PRBC Packed red blood cell
pred Prednisone
PrEP Pre-exposure prophylaxis
PRES Posterior reversible encephalopathy syndrome
prev Previous
Pre-TP Pretest probability
PRN As needed
PRWP Poor R-wave progression
PS Pulmonary stenosis
psa/PsA Pseudomonas
PSI Pneumonia Severity Index
PT Prothrombin time, Posterior tibialis
PTHrP Parathyroid hormone–related protein
pt(s) Patient(s)
PT/PTT Prothrombin time/Partial thromboplastin time
PTX Pneumothorax
PUD Peptic ulcer disease
Pulm Pulmonary
pulm Pulmonary disease
PV Pulmonary valve
PVD Peripheral vascular disease
QTc Corrected QT interval
Qw Q wave
R Right
r/o Rule out
RABV Rabies virus
RAD Right axis deviation
RAE Right atrial enlargement
RBBB Right bundle branch block
RCA Right coronary artery
res Respiratory
req Requiring
RF Risk factor
RH Right heart
RIJ Right internal jugular
RLQ Right lower quadrant
RMSF Rocky Mountain spotted fever
ROM Range of motion
ROS Review of systems
ROSC Return of spontaneous circulation
RPR Rapid plasma reagin
RR Respiratory rate
RSI Rapid sequence intubation
RSV Respiratory syncytial virus
RT-PCR Reverse transcriptase polymerase chain reaction
RTA Renal tubular acidosis
RUG Retrograde urethrogram
RUQ Right upper quadrant
RUSH Rapid ultrasound for shock and hypotension
RV Right ventricle
RVH Right ventricular hypertrophy

Rx	Prescription
rxn	Reaction
s	Second(s)
s/p	Status post
s/s	Signs and symptoms
SAH	Subarachnoid hemorrhage
SBO	Small bowel obstruction
SBP	Systolic blood pressure
SCA	Subclavian artery
SCD	Sickle cell disease
SCFE	Slipped capital femoral epiphysis
SCI	Spinal cord injury
SCLC	Small cell lung cancer
SCM	Sternocleidomastoid
SDH	Subdural hemorrhage
SHx	Social history
SEA	Spinal epidural abscess
sens	Sensitive, Sensitivity
SES	Socioeconomic status
SEWS	Severity of alcohol withdrawal scale
SI	Suicidal ideation
SIADH	Syndrome of inappropriate antidiuretic hormone
SIDS	Sudden infant death syndrome
SIRS	Systemic inflammatory response syndrome
SJS	Stevens–Johnson syndrome
SLE	Systemic lupus erythematosus
SLR	Straight leg raise
SMA	Superior mesenteric artery
SOB	Shortness of breath
SOL	Signs of life
spec	Specific, Specificity
SS	Serotonin syndrome
SSRI	Selective serotonin reuptake inhibitor
SSSS	Staphylococcal scalded skin syndrome
ST	Sinus tachycardia
ST-T	ST-segment T-wave
STD	Sexually transmitted disease
STEMI	ST-segment elevation MI
SUBQ	Subcutaneous
SVC	Superior vena cava
SVR	Systemic vascular resistance
SVT	Supraventricular tachycardia
sxs	Symptoms
Synd	Syndrome
sz	Seizure
T+S	Type and screen
TAA	Thoracic aortic aneurysm
TACO	Transfusion-associated circulatory overload
tachy	Tachycardia
TAH	Total abdominal hysterectomy
TAH	Total artificial heart
TB	Tuberculosis
TBI	Traumatic brain injury
Tbili	Total bilirubin
TBSA	Total body surface area
tbsp	Tablespoon

TBW	Total body weight
T&C	Type and cross
TCA	Tricyclic antidepressants
TCP	Thrombocytopenia
Td	Tetanus-diphtheria
TdP	Torsade de pointes
TEE	Transesophageal echocardiogram
Tele	Telemetry
TEN	Toxic epidermal necrolysis
tfx	Transfusion
TIA	Transient ischemic attack
TID	Three times daily
TLICS	Thoracolumbar injury classification and severity scale
TM	Tympanic membrane
TMJ	Temporomandibular joint
TMP/SMX	Trimethoprim-Sulfamethoxazole
TOA	Tubo-ovarian abscess
TOF	Tetralogy of Fallot
tox	Toxicity
tPA	Alteplase
TP-PA	Treponema pallidum particle agglutination
Tpx	Transplant
TRALI	Transfusion-associated lung injury
TSH	Thyroid-stimulating hormone
tsp	Teaspoon
TSS	Toxic shock syndrome
TTE	Transthoracic echocardiogram
TTP	Thrombotic thrombocytopenic purpura
TTP	Tenderness to palpation
TURP	Transurethral resection of prostate
TV	Tidal volume
TV	Tricuspid valve
TVUS	Transvaginal ultrasound
TWI	T-wave inversion
tx	Treatment
TXA	Tranexamic acid
U/S	Ultrasound
UA	Urine analysis, Unstable angina
UAG	Urinary anion gap
UC	Ulcerative colitis
Ucx	Urine culture
UE	upper extremity
UFH/UH	Unfractionated heparin
UGIB	Upper gastrointestinal bleeding
UMN	Upper motor neuron
undx'ed	Undiagnosed
UOP	Urinary output
UPJ	Urinary pelvic junction
URI	Upper respiratory infection
US	Ultrasound
UTI	Urinary tract infection
V/D	Vomiting/diarrhea
V/Q	Ventilation/perfusion scan

VAD	Ventricular assist device
VA-ECMO	Veno-arterial extracorporeal membrane oxygenation
VAP	Ventilator-associated pneumonia
VBG	Venous blood gas
VCUG	Voiding cystourethrogram
VDRL	Venereal Disease Research Laboratory
VL	Video laryngoscopy
VNA	Visiting Nurse Association
VOC	Vaso-occlusive crisis
VRE	Vancomycin-resistant enterococcus
VS	Vital signs
VSD	Ventricular septal defect
VT	Ventricular tachycardia
VVI	Single-chamber ventricular pacing
vWD	Von Willebrand disease
vWF	Von Willebrand factor
VZV	Varicella zoster virus
w/	With
w/d	Withdrawal
w/i	Within
w/o	Without
w/u	Workup
WBC	White blood cell
WCT	Wide-complex tachycardia
wks	Weeks
WMAs	Wall motion abnormalities
WPW	Wolff–Parkinson–White syndrome
XRT	Radiation therapy
y/o	Year old
Y	Year(s)
Δ	Change

A

B

C

D

E

F

G

J

K

L

M

N

O

P

T

U

V

W

X

Y

Z